Register Now fo[...]
to Your [...]

SPRINGER PUBLISHING COMPANY
CONNECT

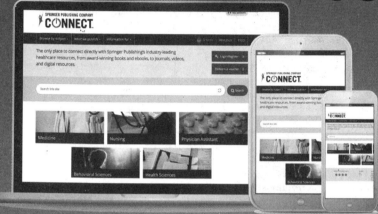

Your print purchase of *Intervention Research and Evidence-Based Quality Improvement, Second Edition* **includes online access to the contents of your book**—increasing accessibility, portability, and searchability!

Access today at:
http://connect.springerpub.com/content/book/978-0-8261-5571-9
or scan the QR code at the right with your smartphone
and enter the access code below.

MMHU66AR

Scan here for quick access.

SPRINGER PUBLISHING COMPANY
View all our products at springerpub.com

SPC

Bernadette Mazurek Melnyk, PhD, RN, APRN-CNP, FAANP, FNAP, FAAN, is the vice president for health promotion, university chief wellness officer, professor and dean of the College of Nursing at The Ohio State University (OSU), and professor of pediatrics and psychiatry at OSU's College of Medicine. She is a nationally/internationally recognized expert and researcher in intervention studies, evidence-based practice (EBP), child and adolescent mental health, and health and wellness, and is a frequent keynote speaker at national/international conferences on these topics. Dr. Melnyk has led the EBP movement in nursing and healthcare across the United States for the past two decades, and has consulted with hundreds of healthcare systems and academic institutions throughout the nation and globe on how to improve healthcare quality and population health outcomes through EBP. Her record as principal investigator includes more than $36 million of sponsored funding from federal agencies and foundations. She is editor of five books and has more than 345 publications, including two *American Journal of Nursing* Book of the Year awards. She is an elected fellow of the National Academy of Medicine, the American Academy of Nursing, the National Academies of Practice, and the American Association of Nurse Practitioners. She served a 4-year term on the United States Preventive Services Task Force and the National Institutes of Health (NIH) National Advisory Council for Nursing Research. Dr. Melnyk is currently a member of the National Quality Forum's Behavioral Health Steering Committee and the National Academy of Medicine's Action Collaborative on Clinician Wellbeing. She also serves as editor of the journal *Worldviews on Evidence-based Nursing.* Dr. Melnyk has received numerous national and international awards, including the inaugural National Institutes of Health/National Institute of Nursing Research Director's Distinguished Lectureship Award, the Lifetime Achievement Award by the National Organization of Nurse Practitioner Faculty, the Loretta Ford Award from the National Association of Pediatric Nurse Practitioners, and the Nancy Sharpe Cutting-Edge Award by the American Association of Nurse Practitioners. She also has been twice named an Edge Runner by the American Academy of Nursing and was inducted into Sigma Theta Tau International's Research Hall of Fame. Dr. Melnyk is the founder and executive director of the Helene Fuld Health Trust National Institute for Evidence-based Practice in Nursing & Healthcare, which is housed at the OSU College of Nursing. Dr. Melnyk founded the National Interprofessional Education and Practice Collaborative to advance the Department of Health and Human Services' Million Hearts® initiative to prevent 1 million heart attacks and strokes by 2017, which now has more than 150 participating academic institutions and organizations throughout the United States. She also created and chaired the first three National Summits on Building Healthy Academic Communities and founded the National Consortium for Building Healthy Academic Communities, a collaborative organization to improve population health in the nation's institutions of higher learning, for which she served as its first president.

Dianne Morrison-Beedy, PhD, RN, WHNP, FNAP, FAANP, FAAN, currently serves as chief Talent and Global Strategy officer and the Centennial Endowed Professor of Nursing at The Ohio State University. Prior to that, she was the dean of the University of South Florida (USF) College of Nursing, senior associate vice president of USF Health, and a professor of nursing, global health, and public health at USF. Dr. Morrison-Beedy has focused her research on HIV/AIDS risk reduction, especially for vulnerable adolescent girls. She has received more than $11 million in HIV prevention research funding and was inducted into the Sigma Theta Tau International Nursing Research Hall of Fame for developing an evidence-based sexual risk reduction intervention, the Health Improvement Project for Teens (HIPTeens), recognized by the Centers for Disease Control and the U.S. Department of Health and Human Services for its strong evidence for HIV/STI and pregnancy prevention. Internationally recognized as a scholar, administrator, and educator, she recently received two Fulbright awards—an administrator award (France) and a research scholar award (Scotland)—as well as an International Council of Nurses Global Leadership fellowship (Switzerland). Dr. Morrison-Beedy's interdisciplinary contributions also encompass serving as scientific reviewer for multiple HIV-related study sections and special emphasis panels at the NIH. In recognition of her contributions, she has been awarded the Florida Nursing Association Award for Research and the Association of Women's Health, Obstetric and Neonatal Nurses Award for Excellence in Research, the Association of Nurses in AIDS Care (ANAC) Research Recognition Award, Excellence in HIV Prevention Award, and the New York State Distinguished Nurse Researcher Award. She is an elected fellow in the American Academy of Nursing, the American Academy of Nurse Practitioners, and the National Academies of Practice. Dr. Morrison-Beedy served as faculty for Sigma Theta Tau International Chiron Nursing Leadership Program and Johnson & Johnson Maternal and Child Health Leadership Institute. She is a reviewer for numerous scientific journals and has more than 250 published articles and abstracts. Dr. Morrison-Beedy received her bacherlor's degree from Niagara University, her master's degree with a specialization in maternal and women's health nurse practitioner from the State University of New York at Buffalo, and her doctoral degree at the University of Rochester.

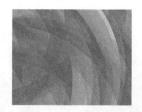

Intervention Research and Evidence-Based Quality Improvement

Designing, Conducting, Analyzing, and Funding

Second Edition

Bernadette Mazurek Melnyk, PhD, RN, APRN-CNP, FAANP, FNAP, FAAN

Dianne Morrison-Beedy, PhD, RN, WHNP, FNAP, FAANP, FAAN

EDITORS

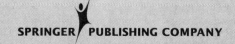

SPRINGER PUBLISHING COMPANY

Springer Publishing Company, LLC
11 West 42nd Street
New York, NY 10036
www.springerpub.com

Acquisitions Editor: Joseph Morita
Associate Managing Editor: Kris Parrish
Compositor: Graphic World

ISBN: 978-0-8261-5553-5
ebook ISBN: 978-0-8261-5571-9
Instructor's Manual ISBN: 978-0-8261-5549-8
Instructor's PowerPoints ISBN: 978-0-8261-5562-7

Instructor's Materials: Qualified instructors may request supplements by emailing textbook@springerpub.com

19 20 21 22 / 5 4 3 2

The author and the publisher of this Work have made every effort to use sources believed to be reliable to provide information that is accurate and compatible with the standards generally accepted at the time of publication. The author and publisher shall not be liable for any special, consequential, or exemplary damages resulting, in whole or in part, from the readers' use of, or reliance on, the information contained in this book. The publisher has no responsibility for the persistence or accuracy of URLs for external or third-party Internet websites referred to in this publication and does not guarantee that any content on such websites is, or will remain, accurate or appropriate.

Library of Congress Cataloging-in-Publication Data

Names: Melnyk, Bernadette Mazurek, editor. | Morrison-Beedy, Dianne, editor.
Title: Intervention research and evidence-based quality improvement :
   designing, conducting, analyzing, and funding / [edited by] Bernadette
   Mazurek Melnyk, Dianne Morrison-Beedy.
Other titles: Intervention research.
Description: Second edition. | New York, NY : Springer Publishing Company,
   LLC, [2019] | Preceded by Intervention research / Bernadette Mazurek
   Melnyk, Dianne Morrison-Beedy, editors. c2012. | Includes bibliographical
   references and index.
Identifiers: LCCN 2018010619 (print) | LCCN 2018011534 (ebook) |
   ISBN 9780826155719 | ISBN 9780826155535 (pbk.) | ISBN 9780826155719
   (ebook) | ISBN 9780826155498 (Instructor's Manual) | ISBN 9780826155627
   (Instructor's PowerPoints)
Subjects: | MESH: Clinical Trials as Topic | Research Design | Biomedical
   Research—methods | Ethics, Research | Financing, Organized | Research
   Report
Classification: LCC RA440.85 (ebook) | LCC RA440.85 (print) | NLM W 20.55.C5 |
   DDC 610.72/4—dc23
LC record available at https://lccn.loc.gov/2018010619

Printed in the United States of America.

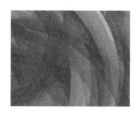

Contents

PART III: IMPLEMENTING INTERVENTION STUDIES

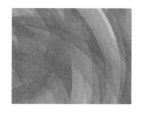

Contributors

Barbara E. Ainsworth, PhD, MPH, FACSM, FNAK Regents' Professor, School of Nutrition and Health Promotion, Arizona State University, Queen Creek, Arizona

Kimberly Arcoleo, PhD, MPH Associate Dean for Research, University of Rochester School of Nursing, Rochester, New York

Carol M. Baldwin, PhD, RN, CHTP, CT, NCC-BC, AHN-BC, FAAN Professor Emeritus; Southwest Borderlands Scholar, Deputy Director, PAHO/WHO Collaborating Centre to Advance the Policy on Research for Health, College of Nursing & Health Innovation, Arizona State University, Phoenix, Arizona

Barry B. Bercu, MD, FAAP Professor of Pediatrics, Molecular Medicine, and Molecular Pharmacology and Physiology, College of Medicine, University of South Florida, Tampa, Florida

Marion E. Broome, PhD, RN, FAAN Ruby Wilson Professor of Nursing, Dean of the School of Nursing, Duke University Health System, Durham, North Carolina

Cheryl L. Byers, MHA, CIP, CHRC Director, Protocol Review and Monitoring Systems and Regulatory Affairs, H. Lee Moffitt Cancer Center and Research Institute, Tampa, Florida

Luis Gabriel Cuervo, MD, MSc in Clinical Epidemiology Specialist in Family Medicine, Chevy Chase, Maryland

Jacqueline Dunbar-Jacob, PhD, RN, FAAN Dean and Distinguished Service Professor of Nursing, University of Pittsburgh School of Nursing, Pittsburgh, Pennsylvania

Julie Fleury , PhD, FAAN, FAHA Hanner Memorial Endowed Professor, Guy Hanner Professor of Nursing, College of Nursing and Health Innovation, Arizona State University, Phoenix, Arizona

Kevin D. Frick, PhD Professor Johns Hopkins Carey Business School, Baltimore, Maryland

Bonnie Gance-Cleveland, PhD, PNP, RNC, FAAN Loretta C. Ford Professor, University of Colorado, Morrison, Colorado

Sandra Glover Gagnon, PhD   Associate Professor, Department of Psychology, Appalachian State University, Boone, North Carolina

Linsey Grove, MPH, CPH, CHES   Chief Creative Officer and Owner, Eunoia Media Lab, LLC, St. Petersburg, Florida

Christine Hancock, BSc (Econ), RN   Founder and Director, C3 Collaborating for Health, London, United Kingdom, Past President, International Council of Nurses

Mary Beth Happ, PhD, RN, FAAN   Associate Dean of Research and Innovation, Distinguished Professor of Critical Care Research, The Ohio State University College of Nursing, Columbus, Ohio

Amanda A. Hastings, MSHL   Senior IT Data Analyst, Data Science and Clinical Data Management, WellCare Health Plans, Tampa, Florida

Colleen Keller, PhD, RN, FNP, FAAN   Regents' Professor and Foundation Professor in Women's Health, Arizona State University College of Nursing and Health Innovation, Phoenix, Arizona

Kevin E. Kip, PhD   Interim Chair, Distinguished USF Health Professor, University of South Florida, Tampa College of Public Health, Florida

Sharon M. Lawlor, MBA   Clinical Trials Program Specialist, NIH National Institute of Diabetes and Digestive and Kidney Diseases, Bethesda, Maryland

Kathryn B. Lindstrom, PhD, FNP-BC, ACHPN   Palliative Care Coordinator, Assistant Professor, School of Nursing, Vanderbilt University, Nashville, Tennessee

Catherine G. Ling, PhD, FNP-BC, FAANP   Associate Professor, Associate Dean for Graduate Clinical Programs, USF Health College of Nursing, Tampa, Florida

Ann Marie McCarthy, PhD, RN, FNASN, FAAN   Professor, Associate Dean for Research and Scholarship, College of Nursing, University of Iowa, Iowa City, Iowa

Sandee G. McClowry, PhD, RN, FAAN   Professor, New York University, New York

Usha Menon, PhD, RN, FAAN   Professor and Associate Dean of Research & Global Advances, University of Arizona College of Nursing, Tucson, Arizona

Shirley M. Moore, PhD, RN, FAAN   The Edward J. and Louise Mellen Professor of Nursing, Distinguished University Professor, Associate Dean for Research, Frances Payne Bolton School of Nursing Case Western Reserve University, Cleveland, Ohio

Cindy L. Munro, PhD, APRN-BC   Associate Dean of Research, University of South Florida College of Nursing, Apollo Beach, Florida

LaRon E. Nelson, PhD, RN, FNP, FNAP, FAAN   Scientist & OHTN Applied HIV Research Chair, St. Michael's Hospital, Li Ka Shing Knowledge Institute, Centre for Urban Health Solutions, Toronto, Ontario, Canada

Wanda K. Nicholson, MD, MPH, MBA   Professor, General Obstetrics and Gynecology, Director, Diabetes and Obesity Core, Center for Women's Health Research, UNC Health Care, Chapel Hill, North Carolina

Debra Parker Oliver, PhD, MSW   Paul Revare, MD, Family Professor of Family Medicine, School of Medicine, University of Missouri Health, Columbia, Missouri

Dónal P. O'Mathúna, PhD, MA, BSc (Pharm)   Associate Professor, School of Nursing & Human Sciences, Dublin City University, Ireland, and College of Nursing, The Ohio State University, Columbus, Ohio

Steven E. Pease, BS, MAS   Assistant Dean, Research and Finance Administration, University of Maryland School of Nursing, Baltimore, Maryland

Marlys R. Peck, PhD, MSW   Associate Professor, Central Missouri State University, Sedalia, Missouri

Rita H. Pickler, PhD, RN, FAAN   The FloAnn Sours Easton Professor of Child and Adolescent Health, Director, PhD and MS in Nursing Science Programs, The Ohio State University College of Nursing, Columbus, Ohio

Alicia G. Rossiter, DNP, FNP, PCPNP-BC, FAANP   Assistant Professor Director, Veteran to BSN Program, College of Nursing Military Liaison, University of South Florida College of Nursing, Tampa, Florida

Margaret Roudebush, MNO   Assistant Dean for Research Administration, Center for Research and Scholarship, Frances Payne Bolton School of Nursing, Case Western Reserve University, Cleveland, Ohio

Souraya Sidani, PhD   Professor, Daphne Cockwell School of Nursing, Ryerson University, Toronto, Ontario, Canada

Barbara A. Smith, PhD, RN, FAAN   Professor and Interim Vice Dean of Academic Affairs, University of South Florida, Tampa, Florida, and Professor, Florida State University, Tallahassee, Florida

Laura A. Szalacha, EdD   Director of Research Methods and Statistics, Professor, University of Arizona College of Nursing, Tucson, Arizona

Mindy B. Tinkle, PhD, RN, WHNP-BC, FAAN   Associate Professor, University of New Mexico College of Nursing, Albuquerque, New Mexico

Sharon Tucker, PhD, RN, FAAN   Grayce Sills Endowed Professor in Psychiatric-Mental Health Nursing and Director of the Implementation Science and Systematic Review Core, The Helene Fuld Health Trust National Institute for Evidence-Based Practice in Nursing and Healthcare College of Nursing, The Ohio State University, Columbus, Ohio

Peter A. Vanable, PhD   Associate Provost for Graduate Studies, Dean of the Graduate School, Professor of Psychology, Syracuse, New York

Constance Visovsky, PhD, RN, ACNP, FAAN   Associate Dean and Associate Professor, College of Nursing, University of South Florida, Tampa, Florida

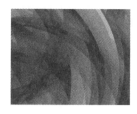

Foreword

As we near the end of the second decade of the millennium, a focus on rigorous and relevant intervention research and evidence-based practice continues to be an essential component of our nation's efforts to achieve a high-performing learning health system. Despite progress in reducing the number of uninsured and significant public and private sectors investments in improvement activities, we are still failing to provide consistent, high-quality, safe care to everyone. In fact, the latest National Healthcare Quality and Disparities Report from the Agency for Healthcare Research and Quality underscores the need: Progress is seen for only 52% of quality measures for which trend data are available and disparities in care are only improving for 16% of outcome measures.

We must do better, and this comprehensive updated volume from Melnyk and Morrison-Beedy will be a tremendous resource for researchers and clinicians alike. Its detailed, step-by-step approach to designing, implementing, analyzing, and scaling interventions into real-world settings will assist novice and skilled researchers alike. The inclusion of comparative effectiveness research is notable as health systems, clinicians, and patients want and need to make choices between available alternatives—understanding which intervention "works" for which patients in which settings. Of particular value is the attention to interventions that are sensitive to culture, race/ethnicity, and gender as well as the inclusion of considerations of diverse care settings. At the same time, as healthcare costs continue to rise and challenge payers, providers, and patients, we must heed the call from Melnyk and colleagues to focus on the "so what" questions. We should target our interventions to achieve the most impact. Evidence-based quality improvement requires dedicated resources from health systems and understanding the costs and cost-effectiveness—a critical aspect too often ignored by experts—is addressed in this volume.

The next decade of intervention studies and evidence-based quality improvement must not build just on what we know, but capitalize on the many opportunities for disruptive innovation and leveraging the increasing volume, variety, and velocity of data types. These forces, together with the trend toward multiside studies and team science, present significant opportunities for intervention research and evidence-based quality improvement. There also is a growing community of researchers and health system leaders impatient with the status quo and eager to partner to achieve better care for their patients. This growth is evident each year at the Conference on the Science of Dissemination and Implementation in Health as well as in the increasing number of healthcare delivery science centers being established in health systems and academic health centers. Every one of them should have a copy of this volume!

Lisa Simpson, MB, BCh, MPH, FAAP
President and CEO
AcademyHealth

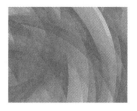

Preface

Imagine you hear about a wonderful product that has just been developed that could enhance your quality of life; it is far better than what is available to you currently. The word on the street is that people really need this product—it could change their lives for the better. You, your friends, and your family are really interested in getting access to this product. There is only one issue: it will not be available to you or others for 10, 15, or maybe 20 years. Disappointed? Upset? Frustrated? Unfortunately, this is often the typical scenario with evidence-based interventions that have been rigorously tested and found to be effective through research. It typically takes years, even decades, to translate research-based interventions into real-world clinical settings to improve healthcare quality and people's health outcomes. This long research–practice time gap does not sit well with either of us as we are truly passionate about making a positive difference in the health and well-being of people, families, and communities through intervention, development, testing, and translation. As friends and colleagues for almost three decades, we had the opportunity to have multiple discussions about how best to conduct meaningful and rigorous research that would target these unmet needs. After our doctoral programs, both of us pursued our dreams of making a difference through rigorous programs of intervention research. We went through the typical "character builders" of every step involved in intervention work, beginning with pilot studies that were eventually funded by the National Institutes of Health (NIH) as full-scale randomized controlled trials.

The first edition of our book, *Intervention Research: Designing, Conducting, Analyzing, and Funding,* included many of the lessons that we learned and tricks of the trade that we compiled into one user-friendly reference where others could learn from those who have successfully traveled down the intervention pathway. We were grateful that the first edition met your expectations and was also recognized by the *American Journal of Nursing* as the Research Book of the Year in 2012. In this second edition, we knew we had to extend the reach and impact of the book by addressing the ongoing dilemma of the "prolonged time to translation" of intervention research to clinical practice. Therefore, additional content on how to move research-based interventions more quickly into real-world settings has been added. **Qualified instructors may obtain access to an ancillary instructor's manual and instructor's PowerPoints by emailing textbook@springerpub.com.**

With the current confusion that exists in academia and healthcare regarding the preparation and role of individuals with clinical doctorates (e.g., the Doctor of Nursing Practice [DNP]), we begin this new edition with tackling the difference between "generating evidence" through intervention research versus "using evidence" through evidence-based quality improvement. Therefore, whether your passion lies in generating versus using evidence to improve real-world outcomes, we hope that this book will assist you in realizing your dreams through intervention work and evidence-based quality improvement.

Abraham Lincoln said that the best way to predict the future is to create it; so keep on dreaming, discovering, and delivering to transform healthcare and improve lives!

Warm regards,

Bernadette "Bern" Mazurek Melnyk and
Dianne Morrison-Beedy

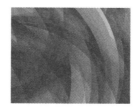

Acknowledgments

It usually takes an awesome team to accomplish a major initiative, such as the production of a book. Thanks and recognition go to my wonderful friend, colleague, and coeditor, Dr. Dianne Morrison-Beedy, who embarked on this dream and journey with me, weathering the "character-builders" along the course of the way. I also want to thank and acknowledge each of our terrific contributors, without whom this book would not have been possible. In addition, I want to recognize my supportive husband, John, and my three wonderful daughters, Kaylin, Angela, and Megan, who sacrificed time with me over the years so that I could pursue my dreams. Kathy York also deserves special recognition because she has been the "wind beneath my wings" for more than a decade, as well as my colleagues, study teams, students, and research participants from whom I have learned a lot. Finally, I credit two incredibly special people for my success—my dad Joe Mazurek, who gave me a spirit of never-ending determination, and my sister Chris, who was my "lifeline" during many of my life's challenges and who always encouraged me to "just get out there and do it!"

Bernadette Mazurek Melnyk

For this edition of our book, I am thinking a bit broader and deeper about acknowledgements. To my friend, colleague, idea partner, and coeditor Bernadette—30 years later and we are still such a good team. It is always a pleasure to bring our many dreams to reality. Also, at the top of the list are my dear husband Michael, son Mason, and daughter Megan. They are my life and my inspiration for trying to be part of the "change in the world" I am hoping to see in nursing and healthcare. I also thank my parents who always told me that I could do great things in this world that may require much effort (witness this book), but my dreams were possible. Now to you, our readers—my acknowledgement is to each of you. You are reading this book to gain a better understanding of how your creative ideas combine with rigorous science to produce an impact on real people. I applaud you on your efforts. Keep going in the face of adversity, grant rejections, manuscript revisions, or idea bashing. You will come out successful on the other end! What I have learned over the past year, however, is this: take care of yourself as you pursue your dreams; no one can really do that for you. All the essentials of health we try to convey and encourage our patients and families to undertake are just as important for us as individuals. So if you have not made an appointment for a checkup in a long time, make it. If you are thinking about having a snack, take the time to make yourself a delicious and healthy meal. If you need a break from reading this book, get up and take a walk. If you need to catch up on sleep, it is okay to put work away and go to bed early. Take care of yourself. This way you will still be around to contribute to research that transforms health and healthcare (and read our next edition!). Stay healthy and happy—you need to do that for you.

Dianne Morrison-Beedy

Intervention Research
and Evidence-Based
Quality Improvement

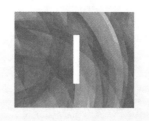

Setting the Stage

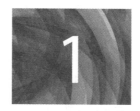

1

Generating Evidence Through Intervention Research Versus Using Evidence in Evidence-Based Practice/ Quality Improvement

Bernadette Mazurek Melnyk & Dianne Morrison-Beedy

> How wonderful that no one needs to wait a single
> moment to improve the world. —*Anne Frank*

GENERATING VERSUS USING EVIDENCE

Although billions of dollars are invested in funding research projects annually worldwide, few findings from research are actually used in real-world settings to improve quality of healthcare or population health outcomes. It takes years, even decades, for published research findings to be translated to and used in clinical settings in the form of evidence-based care. Individuals who have attained their PhD are educated and skilled in conducting rigorous research, whereas individuals with clinical doctorates in fields such as nursing, pharmacy, psychology, physical therapy, and audiology (e.g., doctor of nursing practice [DNP], doctor of pharmacy [PharmD], doctor of psychology [PsyD], doctor of physical therapy [DPT], and doctor of audiology [AuD]) are well prepared to use evidence generated from rigorous research in clinical practice to ultimately improve healthcare quality and outcomes (Melnyk, 2013). Unlike the PhD degree that is heavily focused on generating new knowledge/evidence through rigorous research, the clinical doctorate is a professional degree that focuses on knowledge, skills, and competencies required for the highest level of clinical practice. Healthcare professionals with clinical doctorates and point-of-care clinicians should bring questions or areas of care that need more evidence to PhD-prepared scientists so that they can design and lead rigorous research studies to inform best practice. Individuals with clinical doctorates and point-of-care clinicians can be integral members of research teams that conduct intervention research and, therefore, should understand its critical components. However, their emphasis should be on the rapid translation of evidence generated from research into practice to improve clinical care and patient outcomes.

Research is a systematic process used to generate new knowledge or evidence. **Clinical research** studies people, or data or samples of tissue from people, to understand health and disease. This type of research discovers how best to detect, diagnose, treat, and prevent disease (https://www.cancer.gov/publications/dictionairies/cancer-terms/def/clinical-research).

GENERATING EVIDENCE THROUGH INTERVENTION RESEARCH

Intervention research works best to improve outcomes in order to make a difference in what matters most to you. Although developing and testing interventions can be a challenging and lengthy process, establishing the efficacy of a new intervention or treatment that improves the health of a population for whom you care deeply and desire to improve outcomes is rewarding both personally and professionally. Although there are numerous areas in health, social sciences, and education that could benefit from intervention research, the majority of studies conducted are **nonexperimental** in design. As a result, the strongest **level of evidence** that is needed to change practice, influence policy, and positively impact population health outcomes is often lacking.

Intervention studies, also known as **experimental research**, are the only type of research that allows us to draw conclusions about cause and effect relationships between an intervention or treatment and an **outcome**. A **true experiment** or **randomized controlled trial** (RCT) is the strongest type of intervention study for testing **cause and effect relationships**. There are three components required in a true experiment (see Exhibit 1.1). First, there is an experimental intervention in which the investigator actually "does something" to some but not all of the participants in the study (the intervention group). Second, a comparison intervention or control group is needed to compare the effects of the experimental intervention on outcomes between those who received it and those who did not. Third, **random assignment** (randomly assigning subjects to the experimental or attention groups by probability, such as flipping a coin) is used to place participants in either the experimental group or the comparison/control group. The National Institutes of Health defines a **clinical trial** as a research study in which one or more human subjects are prospectively assigned to one or more interventions (which may include placebo or other control) to evaluate the effects of those interventions on health-related biomedical or behavioral outcomes (see https://grants.nih.gov/policy/clinical-trials/definition.htm).

EXHIBIT 1.1 Components of True Experiments

An intervention or treatment
A comparison or control group
Random assignment of participants to experimental or comparison/control groups

Examples of research questions that would be best answered by intervention studies or clinical trials include the following:

- In adolescents with anxiety (the designated population), what is the effect of cognitive behavioral skills building (the experimental intervention) versus an education-only intervention (the comparison condition) on substance use (the outcome)?
- In patients with hypertension (the designated population), what is the effect of providing on-site counseling by a pharmacist (the experimental intervention) versus written information in a pamphlet (the comparison intervention) on medication adherence (the outcome)?
- In critically ill patients (the designated population), what is the effect of early ambulation (the experimental intervention) versus continuous bed rest (comparison condition) on episodes of ventilator-associated pneumonia (the outcome)?
- In elementary school children (the designated population), what is the effect of an after-school mentoring program (the experimental intervention) versus individual tutoring (the comparison intervention) on academic performance (the outcome)?

THE TYPICAL PROGRESSION OF RESEARCH

Nonexperimental designs (e.g., qualitative, descriptive, and predictive research) are best suited when constructs need to be described (e.g., the grief process for parents whose child has died) or there is a desire to determine relationships among variables (e.g., whether there is a relationship between exercise and hypertension in older adult men or whether depression predicts substance use in adolescents). Experimental designs are used when an investigator would like to establish causality (i.e., whether certain treatments or intervention strategies cause changes in selected outcomes).

The following diagram represents the typical progression of research.

Qualitative Research → Descriptive Research → Predictive Research → Experimental Research

There are three criteria that are necessary to establish causality: (a) the independent variable (i.e., the treatment) must precede the dependent variable (i.e., the outcome); (b) there must be a strong relationship between the intervention and the outcome; and (c) the relationships between the treatment and the outcome cannot be explained as being due to the influence of other variables. For example, an investigator is testing the effects of a 6-week cognitive behavioral therapy program versus a 6-week yoga program in reducing fear of flying in adults. The week before the subjects are scheduled to complete the follow-up questionnaire to measure their fear of flying, the study participants learn about a major airline crash that kills 179 people. If the final results of the study reveal no differences between the two intervention groups on their fear of flying, the investigator could not conclude that cognitive behavioral therapy or yoga is ineffective in reducing fear of flying because a major confounding variable occurred—that of the airline crash.

Programs of research are frequently halted at the descriptive or predictive stage and investigators never move to developing and testing interventions that could positively impact outcomes in individuals, families, and communities. This scenario is common because researchers are often limited in the knowledge and skills needed to design, conduct, analyze, and fund intervention studies. This book provides useful information to prepare you for an exciting journey as an interventionist with a focus on "real-world" advice and wisdom from investigators who have successfully traveled down that road.

USING RESEARCH EVIDENCE IN EVIDENCE-BASED PRACTICE

Evidence-based practice (EBP) is a lifelong problem-solving approach to the delivery of care that integrates (a) the best evidence from well-designed research studies, (b) a clinician's expertise, including assessment from the patient's history and condition as well as availability of healthcare resources, and (c) a patient's preferences and values (see Figure 1.1; Melnyk & Fineout-Overholt, 2015). As seen in Figure 1.1, when clinicians integrate these three elements in a context of caring, it results in evidence-based clinical decision making and the best patient outcomes. A culture and environment that support and empower clinicians to implement evidence-based care are necessary to sustain EBP. Findings from multiple studies indicate that the consistent implementation of EBP results in high-quality, safe, and cost-effective care with improved population health outcomes and enhanced clinician satisfaction, known as the quadruple aim in healthcare (Bodenheimer & Sinsky, 2014; Melnyk, Fineout-Overholt, Giggleman, & Choy, 2017; Tucker, 2014).

The seven steps of EBP are as follows:

0. Develop a spirit of inquiry.
1. Ask the question in PICO(T)—Patient population; Intervention or area of interest; Comparison intervention or group; Outcomes; and Time, if indicated—format.
2. Search for the evidence (using key words from the PICO[T] question).
3. Critically appraise the evidence.
4. Integrate the evidence with clinician expertise and patient preferences to make an evidence-based clinical decision.
5. Evaluate the outcome.
6. Disseminate the outcome. (Melnyk & Fineout-Overholt, 2019)

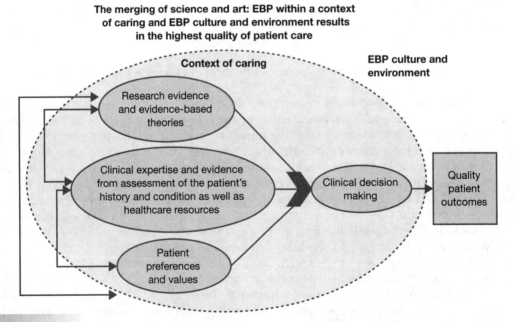

FIGURE 1.1 Evidence-based practice (EBP) within a culture and environment that supports it results in the highest quality, safe, and cost-effective care.

Melnyk, B. M., & Fineout-Overholt, E. (2019). *Evidence-based practice in nursing & healthcare: A guide to best practice* (4th ed.). Philadelphia, PA: Wolters Kluwer/Lippincott Williams & Wilkins.

Clinicians from all disciplines should have the knowledge and skills to implement the seven steps of EBP, including the process of how to search for evidence to answer their clinical questions and to critically appraise research studies and clinical practice guidelines, to facilitate the highest level of care. However, even with all of the positive outcomes that result from the delivery of evidence-based care, multiple barriers persist in healthcare systems throughout the United States and world that prevent clinicians from consistently implementing EBP.

These barriers include: (a) inadequate knowledge and skills in EBP, especially in the critical appraisal and synthesis of evidence as well as outcomes evaluation; (b) lack of leader/ manager support; (c) misperceptions that EBP takes too much time; (d) organizational politics and a culture of "that is the way it is done here"; (e) a lack of EBP mentors to work with point-of-care clinicians; (f) negative attitudes toward research; and (g) continued teaching of rigorous research in academic programs instead of teaching the steps of EBP in a way that clinicians become skilled to implement it efficiently in real-world practice settings (Melnyk, Gallagher-Ford, & Fineout-Overholt, 2016; Melnyk, Fineout-Overholt, Gallagher-Ford, & Kaplan, 2012; Wilson et al., 2015). Thus, facilitators need to be put into place in healthcare systems to ensure the consistent and sustained implementation of EBP by all healthcare providers. These should include culture, structure, and resources that support EBP; evidence-based policies and procedures; continuing education offerings that build clinicians' EBP knowledge and skills to meet the EBP competencies; and a critical mass of EBP mentors who can work with point-of-care clinicians on the implementation of evidence-based care (Melnyk & Fineout-Overholt, 2015; Melnyk, Gallagher-Ford, & Fineout-Overholt, 2016; Melnyk, Gallagher-Ford, Thomas, et al., 2016; Stetler, Ritchie, Rycroft-Malone, & Charns, 2014; ten Ham, Minnie, & van der Walt, 2016).

EVIDENCE-BASED QUALITY IMPROVEMENT

EBP and evidence-based quality improvement (QI) have become drivers of enhancements in clinical practice and improvements in patient outcomes. However, there is often confusion and a lack of clarity between QI and EBP (Hockenberry, 2014; Mick, 2015; Shirey et al., 2011). Unlike intervention research that is conducted to generate new knowledge, QI uses a systematic process to analyze existing data and improve its processes and/or outcomes for a specific patient population (Kring, 2008; Shirey et al., 2011).

Healthcare institutions use various QI models to improve care and outcomes. A commonly used model is the Plan, Do, Study, Act (PDSA) model. In the PDSA model, a change is planned once a problem that needs improvement is identified (Plan; e.g., a healthcare system has a high rate of rehospitalizations in adult patients with congestive heart failure). Second, the plan is formed and carried out (Do; e.g., leaders provide their opinion on the problem and develop a plan on what should be done to decrease rehospitalization rates, followed by implementation of the plan). Third, the results are analyzed (Study; e.g., did rehospitalization rates improve with the change in practice?). Fourth, action strategies are decided upon to continue to improve and sustain the outcome (Act; e.g., a permanent change in practice). In many QI models, a comprehensive review and critical appraisal of the body of research evidence available is usually not conducted. Unfortunately, QI strategies are frequently implemented based on what people think may improve the problem instead of using the best evidence to drive an improvement in outcomes (Melnyk, Buck, & Gallagher-Ford, 2015). This frequently used brainstorming tactic is popular because it can be conducted quickly and ideas can be generated and implemented rapidly. However, major problems in this approach are that the solutions are usually ideas, and the process used is usually trial and error. If the goal of the QI process is to find the best solution with the most likely chance of successful resolution of the problem, then the current fast fix approach needs to be replaced with a thoughtful evidence-based approach (Melnyk, Buck, & Gallagher-Ford, 2015). Incorporating the first steps in the EBP process into QI models can strengthen their effectiveness and no doubt improve the outcomes achieved. For example, in the planning phase of the PDSA model, if a PICO(T) question was asked followed by a search for and critical appraisal and synthesis of evidence conducted, implementation would be based on the best evidence and likely yield positive impact.

In summary, high-quality intervention research is necessary to generate needed evidence to guide clinical practice. Once generated, the evidence from rigorous research needs to be rapidly translated into real-world clinical settings. The consistent use of EBP and evidence-based QI by healthcare systems along with the generation of rigorous research when there is no high-quality evidence to guide practice leads to the highest quality of healthcare and best population health outcomes.

Key Points From This Chapter

- It takes years, even decades, for published research findings to be translated to and used in clinical settings in the form of evidence-based care.
- Individuals with research doctorates (i.e., PhDs) have the education and skills to lead and conduct rigorous intervention research studies that generate evidence for practice, whereas those with clinical doctorates should be experts in translating the evidence generated from research into clinical practice to improve healthcare quality and patient outcomes.
- Individuals with clinical doctorates should bring important clinical questions that need evidence to PhD-prepared researchers and participate as members of intervention research teams with an understanding of key research concepts.
- Research is a systematic process used to generate new knowledge or discover new evidence.
- Intervention research is all about learning what treatments or strategies work best to improve outcomes.
- EBP is a lifelong problem-solving approach to the delivery of care that integrates the best evidence from well-designed research studies with a clinician's expertise and a patient's preferences and values.
- Evidence-based QI uses a systematic process to analyze existing data and improve processes and/or outcomes for a specific patient population based on a thorough search and critical appraisal of a body of evidence.
- The consistent use of EBP and evidence-based QI by healthcare systems, along with the generation of rigorous intervention research when there is no high-quality evidence to guide practice, leads to the highest quality of cost-effective healthcare and best population health outcomes.

REFERENCES

Bodenheimer, T., & Sinsky, C. (2014). From triple to quadruple aim: Care of the patient requires care of the provider. *Annals of Family Medicine, 12*(6), 573–576. doi:10.1370/afm.1713
Hockenberry, M. (2014). Quality improvement and evidence-based practice change projects and the institutional review board: Is approval necessary? *Worldviews on Evidence-Based Nursing, 11*(4), 217–218. doi:10.1111/wvn.12049

Kring, D. L. (2008). Research and quality improvement: Different processes, different evidence. *MEDSURG Nursing, 17*(3), 162–169.

Melnyk, B. M. (2013). Distinguishing the preparation and roles of Doctor of Philosophy and Doctor of Nursing Practice graduates: National implications for academic curricula and health care systems. *Journal of Nursing Education, 52*(8), 442–448. doi:10.3928/01484834-20130719-01

Melnyk, B. M., Buck, J., & Gallagher-Ford, L. (2015). Transforming quality improvement into evidence-based quality improvement: A key solution to improve healthcare outcomes. *Worldviews on Evidence-Based Nursing, 12*(5), 251–252. doi:10.1111/wvn.12112

Melnyk, B. M., & Fineout-Overholt, E. (2019). *Evidence-based practice in nursing & healthcare: A guide to best practice* (4th ed.). Philadelphia, PA: Wolters Kluwer/Lippincott Williams & Wilkins.

Melnyk, B. M., Fineout-Overholt, E., Gallagher-Ford, L., & Kaplan, L. (2012). The state of evidence-based practice in US nurses: Critical implications for nurse leaders and educators. *Journal of Nursing Administration, 42*(9), 410–417. doi:10.1097/NNA.0b013e3182664e0a

Melnyk, B. M., Fineout-Overholt, E., Giggleman, M., & Choy, K. (2017). A test of the ARCC© model improves implementation of evidence-based practice, healthcare culture, and patient outcomes. *Worldviews on Evidence-Based Nursing, 14*(1), 5–9. doi:10.1111/wvn.12188

Melnyk, B. M., Gallagher-Ford, L., & Fineout-Overholt, L. E. (2016). *Implementing the evidence-based practice (EBP) competencies in healthcare: A practical guide for improving quality, safety, and outcomes.* Indianapolis, IN: Sigma Theta Tau International.

Melnyk, B. M., Gallagher-Ford, L., Thomas, B. K., Troseth, M., Wyngarden, K., & Szalacha, L. (2016). A study of chief nurse executives indicates low prioritization of evidence-based practice and shortcomings in hospital performance metrics across the United States. *Worldviews on Evidence-Based Nursing, 13*(1), 6–14. doi:10.1111/wvn.12133

Mick, J. (2015). Addition of a decision point in evidence-based practice process steps to distinguish EBP, research and quality improvement methodologies. *Worldviews on Evidence-Based Nursing, 12*(3), 179–181. doi:10.1111/wvn.12084

Shirey, M. R., Hauck, S. L., Embree, J. L., Kinner, T. J., Schaar, G. L., Phillips, L. A., … McCool, I. A. (2011). Showcasing differences between quality improvement, evidence-based practice, and research. *Journal of Continuing Education in Nursing, 42*(2), 57–68. doi:10.3928/00220124-20100701-01

Stetler, C. B., Ritchie, J. A., Rycroft-Malone, J., & Charns, M. P. (2014). Leadership for evidence-based practice: Strategic and functional behaviors for institutionalizing EBP. *Worldviews on Evidence-Based Nursing, 11*(4), 219–226. doi:10.1111/wvn.12044

ten Ham, W., Minnie, K., & van der Walt, C. (2016). Integrative review of benefit levers' characteristics for system-wide spread of best healthcare practices. *Journal of Advanced Nursing, 72*(1), 33–49. doi:10.1111/jan.12814

Tucker, S. (2014). Determining the return on investment for evidence-based practice: An essential skill for all clinicians. *Worldviews on Evidence-Based Nursing, 11*(5), 271–273. doi:10.1111/wvn.12055

Wilson, M., Sleutel, M., Newcomb, P., Behan, D., Walsh, J., Wells, J. N., & Baldwin, K. M. (2015). Empowering nurses with evidence-based practice environments: Surveying Magnet®, Pathway to Excellence®, and non-Magnet facilities in one healthcare system. *Worldviews on Evidence-Based Nursing, 12*(1), 12–21. doi:10.1111/wvn.12077

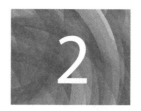

Setting the Stage for Intervention Research and Evidence-Based Quality Improvement: The "So What," "What Exists," and "What's Next" Factors

Bernadette Mazurek Melnyk & Dianne Morrison-Beedy

> The important thing is not to stop questioning. —*Albert Einstein*

THE "SO WHAT" FACTORS IN INTERVENTION RESEARCH AND EVIDENCE-BASED QUALITY IMPROVEMENT

One of the fundamental building blocks that lays the foundation for intervention work and evidence-based quality improvement (EBQI) is the "so what" factor. The "so what" factor is a term we are using to describe the development and conduct of research and EBQIs with high impact potential to improve important outcomes. The following questions are ones upon which all investigators need to reflect as they begin to design new intervention studies, and all clinicians and healthcare leaders need to ask themselves before embarking on EBQI projects:

- **"So what"** is the prevalence of the problem and is it modifiable through an intervention or evidence-based practice change?
- **"So what"** will be the end outcome of the study or project once it is completed?
- **"So what"** difference will the study or EBQI project make in improving health, educational or healthcare quality, costs, and, most importantly, patient, family or community outcomes?

- **"So what"** will others do with the study or project's outcomes (e.g., clinicians, health-care systems, schools, public health departments)?
- **"So what"** actions will you take to translate your study's findings into real-world settings or sustain the improvements from the EBQI project?
- **"So what"** is the chance that others will adopt and implement your intervention or EBQI practice change, based on its feasibility, reproducibility, and cost?

We must focus more on the "so what" factors as investigators and clinicians craft new studies and build programs of research and EBQI initiatives focusing on problems that are amenable to change. Planting the "so what" seeds is the first step in designing a successful intervention study or EBQI project. Without this approach, we risk continuing to generate a large number of research findings that are disseminated through publications and presentations but, to a large extent, do not make it into the real world to positively impact outcomes.

IMPACT, SIGNIFICANCE, AND INNOVATION: CRITICAL ELEMENTS FOR INTERVENTION STUDIES AND EBQI PROJECTS

Studies and EBQI projects that address the "so what" factors often have high overall impact, significance, and innovation. **Impact** is the probability of whether the study or project will exert a sustained powerful influence on the field or on important outcomes. The topic of **significance** questions whether the study or EBQI project addresses an important problem or a critical barrier to progress in the field or clinical area along with the question of "If the aims of the study or EBQI project are achieved, how will scientific knowledge, technical capability, and/or clinical practice and health outcomes be advanced?"

Specifically for research studies, questions to consider when determining **innovation** include: (a) Does the study employ novel concepts, approaches, or methods? (b) Are the aims original and innovative? (c) Does the project challenge existing paradigms or develop new methodologies or technologies? Other ways of looking at innovation include: (a) the problem is one that has not been previously studied; (b) the solution has not been previously suggested; (c) the population has not been included in prior studies; (d) the outcomes have not been previously measured; and (e) the research methods have not been previously used (Sechrest & Babcock-Parziale, 2007). These three criteria (i.e., impact, significance, and innovation) are frequently used by federal funders, including the National Institutes of Health, when reviewing grant applications (see https://grants.nih.gov/grants/how-to-apply-application-guide/format-and-write/write-your-application.htm).

FIVE ESSENTIAL INGREDIENTS FOR CONDUCTING INTERVENTION STUDIES AND EVIDENCE-BASED QUALITY IMPROVEMENT PROJECTS

There are five Ps that need to be considered as essential when launching an intervention study or EBQI project:

- **P**revalence of the problem and the "So What" factor
- **P**assion, which is critical for engagement and sustainability
- **P**lanning, which includes the details necessary to conduct a scientifically rigorous study or impactful EBQI project
- **P**ersistence, which is key to getting through all of the "character builders" that accompany intervention research or EBQI

■   **P**atience, a virtue developed through building an intervention study or EBQI project that makes a difference in outcomes

After considering the "so what" factors, the second and probably the most important element in embarking on intervention research or EBQI is passion. An important quote to remember when embarking on this type of research or project is that "Nothing happens unless first a dream" (Carl Sandburg). A dream of what it is that you want to accomplish, specifically the impact or difference that you want to make in outcomes (e.g., decreasing depression rates in adolescents, reducing preterm birth, decreasing length of hospital stay for critically ill patients, or improving graduation rates of at-risk students), is critical to ensure success. Keeping that dream in front of you every day and keeping it bigger than your fears will assist you in overcoming the obstacles that you are sure to face along your journey. Many times researchers and clinicians are convinced by others to embark on a topic about which they are not passionate in order to respond to a funding opportunity. Although funding is essential to conduct many projects, the work will be laborious if you do not have passion for the research or EBQI project upon which you are embarking. It is often possible to refine your work to an area of funding opportunity and still keep the passion alive for what is most important to you.

The third important element for conducting intervention studies or EBQI projects is planning. Meticulous planning of every element of the study or project is necessary in order to have successful implementation and completion. As part of the planning, it is critical to comprise a team that is also passionate about the topic, dedicated to the project, and willing to "go the extra mile" to successfully complete it. If you are a novice at intervention research or EBQI, your team may consist of "me, myself, and I." However, remember that you can also establish a team of colleagues and mentors to assist you with your early work.

> Setting a goal is not the main thing. It is deciding how you will go about achieving it and staying with that plan. —*Tom Landry*

The fourth essential ingredient for conducting intervention research or EBQI projects is persistence. Whether planning and implementing a study or EBQI project or writing a grant application to fund the project, there will no doubt be several "character builders" along the course of the way. These might include: having to rewrite several institutional review board applications; grant application rejections; and unexpected participant attrition to name just a few. Thinking through potential barriers and generating strategies to overcome them before they occur and staying steadfast through the "character builders" is important for a project's successful completion.

> Character consists of what you do on the third and fourth tries. —*John Albert Michener*

Finally, patience is a virtue that is necessary for designing, conducting, and funding intervention work or EBQI initiatives. Every aspect of intervention or EBQI work provides plenty of opportunity to develop your staying power.

> Patience, persistence and perspiration make an unbeatable combination for success. —*Napoleon Hill*

OTHER MAJOR FACTORS TO CONSIDER FOR INTERVENTION RESEARCH

Feasibility of the study is another important consideration for intervention work. Questions pertaining to feasibility should include the following: (a) Do you have the time to be lead or principal investigator on the project? (b) Can the study be conducted in a reasonable amount of time? (c) Are the sites in which you are proposing to conduct the study amenable to the project? (d) Will a sufficient number of subjects be attainable to reach your study's goal for sample size? (e) Is the intervention practical to administer and not overly burdensome to subjects? (f) Are study materials, such as instruments to measure outcomes, readily available or will they need to be designed? (g) Is there sufficient funding for the study? (h) Are you able to comprise a team with the skills and dedication needed to conduct the study?

Ethical issues are always an important aspect to consider when conducting intervention research. Specifically, you need to determine whether what you will be asking of participants is ethical and does not lead to undue subject burden. The amount of subject burden, as well as benefits of study participation, is scrutinized heavily by members of an institutional review board along with grant reviewers. In particular, conducting intervention studies with vulnerable populations (e.g., prison populations, pregnant women, and children) presents its own challenges in assuring protection of human subjects. Specific issues regarding human subjects and ethical considerations are covered in detail in later chapters.

Level of ambitiousness of the project is another important consideration for intervention research. Many investigators propose to conduct intervention studies that are complex with large sample sizes in a short period or they try to achieve multiple study aims with a very limited budget. Being overly ambitious with a study can result in limited success of the project, which is why thoughtful planning up front is essential for intervention work. When planning an intervention study, think realistically rather than grandiose. As a general rule of thumb, it often takes twice as long to conduct each phase of the study than you think that it will. Obtaining the perspective of other investigators who have conducted similar work can provide you with "guesstimates" of appropriate timelines for various study activities. However, remember that these perspectives will be greatly influenced by whether the investigator already had an established team and ongoing relationships with study sites and the target population.

OTHER MAJOR FACTORS TO CONSIDER FOR EVIDENCE-BASED QUALITY IMPROVEMENT PROJECTS

Assembling a terrific team that is skilled and dedicated also is important for planning EBQI projects. These projects can be conducted at the unit (e.g., in an emergency room or on a surgical unit) or system-wide level. If conducting the project throughout an entire hospital or healthcare system (e.g., planning to implement an evidence-based intervention to reduce falls in hospitalized adults), careful planning with the entire team that will be responsible for implementation of the evidence-based practice change is essential. A close collaboration with the individuals who conduct data analytics for the system also will be important in order for you to evaluate the impact of the EBQI change on the outcome (i.e., in this example, whether a decrease in fall rates was achieved). Buy-in from leadership for the evidence-based change also will be important for the success of the project. Use evidence to present a compelling case of why the EBQI project is needed, including the return on investment (ROI) that is expected (e.g., a decrease of 10% in falls of hospitalized patients would save the hospital $500,000 annually).

THE "WHAT EXISTS" FACTOR IN INTERVENTION RESEARCH AND EBQI PROJECTS

After addressing the "so what" factors and the associated questions, it is critical to conduct a thorough review, critical appraisal, and synthesis of the literature. For planning intervention studies, this literature search will help you to determine the state of the science and how the study that you are proposing extends what is known in the field. Most intervention research tests a new intervention or compares two interventions that have already been supported as efficacious through prior research (i.e., comparative effectiveness trials). Intentionally replicating a prior intervention study is totally acceptable; in fact, replication studies are needed to generate **systematic reviews,** the strongest level of evidence (i.e., **Level 1 evidence**) needed to change clinical practice (Melnyk & Fineout-Overholt, 2015). However, "unknowing replication" (i.e., repeating a prior study without knowledge that it has already been conducted because a thorough literature search was not performed) will place your project's viability at risk and lead to character-building experiences. One such critical experience could be when grant reviewers point out that the study being proposed has already been completed and funding is denied due to lack of due diligence or minimal impact on the field.

For EBQI projects, a thorough search for and critical appraisal of the body of evidence is absolutely necessary. Determining the best evidence-based intervention or protocol that could be implemented in a practice change to result in improved outcomes for your population of interest is a key component of EBQI.

When conducting a thorough literature search, it is important to first formulate a **PICO(T)** (P = **P**atient/**p**articipant population; I = **I**ntervention of interest; C = **C**omparison intervention; O = **O**utcome; T = **T**ime) **question** (Melnyk & Fineout-Overholt, 2015). For example: In premature infants (P), how does massage (I) versus music (C) affect oxygen saturation (O) in the neonatal intensive care unit; or: In overweight women (P), how do group walking classes (I) versus daily use of a pedometer (C) affect body mass index (0) after 3 months? The PICO(T) format helps you to identify key words or phrases that, when entered successively and combined, expedite the locating of relevant articles in massive research databases, such as MEDLINE, CINAHL, ERIC, or Psycinfo. For the second PICO(T) question posed on overweight women, the first key phrase to be entered into the database would be "overweight women," a subject so common that tens of thousands of citations and abstracts will be generated. The second term to be searched would be "group walking classes," followed next by "pedometer" and the remaining key words in the PICO(T) question. The final step of the search is to combine the results of the searches for each of the terms entered earlier. Using this strategy narrows the results to studies pertinent to the PICO(T) question. Use of a PICO(T) question to conduct a thorough literature search will result in a more expedited search and lead to the elimination of nontargeted studies and those that are irrelevant to the question. Setting limits on the search, such as "English" or "human language," also is helpful in eliminating animal studies or those published in foreign languages.

Once the literature search is conducted and studies pertinent to your area of interest are retrieved, it is useful to then place each study within a table that assists you in looking across the studies to identify similarities as well as differences (see Table 2.1). Following completion of the tabling of these published studies, it is important to synthesize the literature so that strengths and limitations of the body of prior work in the field can be identified. When this process is completed, you will more readily be able to describe how your proposed study will extend the science in the area or drive an evidence-based practice change that will improve outcomes for your population of interest.

AUTHOR(S), TITLE OF STUDY, AND YEAR	PURPOSE OF STUDY AND CONCEPTUAL FRAMEWORK	SAMPLE AND SETTING	STUDY DESIGN AND INTERVENTIONS	OUTCOME VARIABLES WITH MEASURES, INCLUDING VALIDITY AND RELIABILITY	FINDINGS	MAJOR STRENGTHS AND LIMITATIONS

TABLE 2.1 Recommended Format for Tabling Studies From the Literature Review

THE WHAT'S NEXT FACTOR: FORMULATING RESEARCH QUESTIONS AND STUDY HYPOTHESES FOR INTERVENTION STUDIES

For intervention studies, the next step after conducting the literature review is to formulate your research questions and hypotheses. If there is very little or no prior work in the area, or if you will be testing a novel intervention for the first time in a pilot study, you might pose only research questions for your study without hypotheses that provide predictive direction.

Characteristics of a well-formulated research question include one that:

■ Addresses a significant problem that is amenable to change
■ Is feasible
■ Is innovative
■ Focuses on a topic for which you have much passion
■ Is formatted in a way that will extend the science or knowingly replicate prior work
■ Is ethical
■ Clearly delineates the independent (intervention) and dependent (outcome) variables
■ Is focused on a single question

Examples of poorly and well-formed research questions are included in Table 2.2. Hulley, Cummings, Browner, Grady, and Newman (2013) use the pneumonic FINER as a way to formulate research questions, which represents Feasible, Interesting, Novel, Ethical, and Relevant to clinical practice.

Some studies will pose primary and secondary research questions. In intervention studies, secondary research questions typically focus on explaining the process through which the intervention works (e.g., Do cognitive beliefs mediate the effects of the experimental intervention on healthy lifestyle behaviors?) or identifying factors that might moderate the effects of the experimental intervention (e.g., How does gender impact the effects of the experimental intervention on healthy lifestyle behaviors?).

Hypotheses. A **hypothesis** is a predictive statement about the relationship between variables. In intervention studies, the hypothesis delineates how you expect the experimental intervention to impact the study's outcome (s). Hypotheses are used to establish the basis for tests of statistical significance. Examples of hypotheses that flow from the research questions

TABLE 2.2 Examples of Poorly and Well-Formed Research Questions

POORLY FORMED RESEARCH QUESTIONS	WELL-FORMED RESEARCH QUESTIONS
How does counseling of parents by a primary care provider affect children?	In preschool children with behavioral problems, what is the effect of one-on-one counseling of parents by a primary care provider versus group counseling on the children's behavioral problems?
How would exercise affect women's self-worth and body fat?	In overweight women, what is the effect of exercise three times weekly versus exercise one time per week on weight loss?
	In overweight women, what is the effect of exercise three times weekly versus exercise one time per week on their self worth?
Is it effective to provide SSRIs to adults with depression?	In depressed adults, what is the effect of Prozac versus a placebo on depressive symptoms?

SSRIs, selective serotonin reuptake inhibitors.

TABLE 2.3 Examples of Well-Formulated Hypotheses

Preschool children (the designated population) whose parents receive one-on-one counseling from a primary care provider (the experimental intervention/independent variable) versus group counseling (the comparison intervention/independent variable) have fewer behavioral problems 3 months after the intervention (the outcome/dependent variable).

Overweight women (the designated population) who exercise three times per week (the experimental intervention/independent variable) versus those who exercise one time per week (the comparison intervention/independent variable) will have more weight loss at 6 months follow-up (the outcome/dependent variable).

Overweight women (the designated population) who exercise three times per week (the experimental intervention/independent variable) versus those who exercise one time per week (the comparison intervention/independent variable) will have better self-concept (the outcome/dependent variable).

Depressed adults who receive Prozac (the experimental intervention/independent variable) versus those who receive a placebo (the control condition) will have fewer depressive symptoms at 4 months follow-up (the outcome/dependent variable).

in Table 2.2 are outlined in Table 2.3. In each of the examples, the population of interest is clearly defined, and the expected change in the outcome variable as a result of the treatment is delineated.

Whenever possible, hypotheses should be simple (i.e., containing one independent variable and one dependent variable) instead of complex, which means they contain more than one independent or dependent variable. For example, following is a complex hypothesis with two dependent variables: High school students who receive two interactive classes on anger management versus those who watch a video on anger management will report less anger and have fewer disruptive behaviors in the classroom. Complex hypotheses are not readily testable with one statistical test, which is why it is more favorable to compose single hypotheses.

THE "WHAT'S NEXT" FACTOR IN EVIDENCE-BASED QUALITY IMPROVEMENT PROJECTS

After a thorough search for and critical appraisal of the evidence is accomplished to answer your PICO(T) question, a decision can now be made about whether or not a practice change will be implemented to improve an important "so what" outcome or multiple outcomes in your population of interest. Specific steps in conducting an EBQI project are covered in Chapter 3.

In summary, intervention research and EBQI projects provide you with the opportunity to have a profound impact on outcomes and the things that matter most to you. Along with the excitement of developing and conducting intervention studies or EBQI projects come the "character building" experiences faced by everyone. Carefully incorporating the "So What," "What Exists," and "What Next" factors as you are beginning your work allows you to remain relevant, focused, and impactful; these characteristics are critical for designing, conducting, and analyzing intervention work or EBQI projects. Including these critical components will enhance your chances of successful funding as well. The five Ps (prevalence, passion, planning, persistence, and patience) should be the first items you place in your suitcase of knowledge and skills. Now let us get going—we have many stops along the journey we will take in this book. Your suitcase will be filled with ideas and advice at the end of your trip so that you can be highly successful in accomplishing your dreams and making a real-world positive impact!

FORMING INTERPROFESSIONAL TEAMS FOR SUCCESS

"It is all about the team." You may have heard this saying before, and it is never more relevant than when we consider successful intervention research and EBQI projects. The team that you establish and bring together will be composed of people with diverse unique skills and perspectives, which you will need to successfully navigate the gentle flow and raging rivers that are the waters of a research study or EBQI project. You also may have heard the saying, "There is no I in Team." Although technically true, the principal investigator (PI) and EBQI project leader is in a very critical role as the captain of the ship.

As research and EBQI projects become more rigorous in their approaches, assembling a transdisciplinary team with members who possess distinct skill sets but who also can cross-cover for each other in their roles is a critical task that the PI or EBQI project leader must undertake at the onset. One of the true joys in conducting research and EBQI projects is the opportunity to hear the experiences of and problem solving used by others outside of your own perspective. Actively partnering with professionals across disciplines to create a robust team that is nimble in both function and thought can help ensure successful intervention research and EBQI projects.

Personnel usually represent the largest component of a project's budget. Therefore, it is imperative that enough "hands on deck" are available to get the work done without wasteful redundancy. However, the team will be at risk as will the project if team members cannot cover each other's roles in emergency situations; thus, cross-training of team members is an important step in the initial phases of the project. The PI or EBQI leader must determine who will be cross-trained and for what roles as the entire team cannot be expected to be functional in every aspect of the project. Creating an effective focused project team is a key responsibility of the PI or EBQI leader. In doing so, the PI or EBQI leader should define and communicate the goals of the project and empower team members to take ownership over their areas of responsibility. It is the PI or EBQI leader's responsibility to provide the support, resources, and strategies to ensure successful completion of the project, but this is done within the parameters of the grant or project as well as with feedback and input from team members.

Having the perspectives of those from other disciplines or experiences not only is helpful but also can actually provide the PI or EBQI project leader a lifeline when faced with challenges and dilemmas not personally encountered during previous studies or projects.

Establishing a work environment where team members hold each other accountable for meeting project timelines, prioritizing tasks, and providing ongoing feedback on project successes and challenges in "real time" is a critical responsibility of the PI or EBQI project leader. Creating a culture of open communication and providing ongoing education and training of team members with regular evaluations are important human resources (HR) functions of the PI/EBQI leader, which can often be neglected because of the focus on the "science" or "substance" of the project, oftentimes to the extreme detriment to the study. The PI/EBQI leader should capitalize on the value of having a transdisciplinary team, encouraging team members to share information and delegating problem-solving tasks to the team. Regular standing meetings are critical as is the flexibility for impromptu face-to-face or video meetings or calls to address unpredictable situations or "character builders" that will surely arise during the course of the study. Incorporating brainstorming of ideas and building consensus help to secure team members' commitment to changes in initial approaches and protocols.

It is still not unusual to hear that PI or EBQI project leaders think they have formed a transdisciplinary team because they have a biostatistician as a member of the group. However, having team members with a broad array of backgrounds is conducive to successful research and EBQI projects. Team members within the same discipline but with different training and skills sets are also imperative for true translational endeavors. For instance, although a nurse with a PhD can serve as PI on a research study, including those with clinical doctorates will provide additional views on clinical and pragmatic integration of the project. The same philosophy holds true for EBQI projects led by those with clinical doctorates. Ultimately, the research or project being conducted successfully is only as good as the team conducting it, so giving sufficient time and attention to this critical component of intervention work will help lay the scaffolding for a strong study or EBQI project.

Key Points From This Chapter

- There exists a major gap between available evidence-based interventions and the health, social, and educational needs of society.
- Experimental studies are the only type of research that supports intervention cause and effect relationships.
- The "So What" factors address problem prevalence, significance, impact, and translatability.
- The "What Exists" factors addresses the need to assess the state of evidence by conducting a thorough review and critical appraisal of the literature using the PICO(T) method of forming the question to guide the search.
- The "What's Next" factor in intervention research targets the need for focused, clearly delineated research questions and hypotheses.
- The "What's Next" factor in EBQI projects outlines the specific steps in making an evidence-based practice change to improve outcomes.
- Prevalence, passion, planning, persistence, and patience are essential ingredients for successful intervention work and EBQI projects.
- Transdisciplinary teams that respect one another's roles, work well together, and communicate effectively are important for the success of intervention research and EBQI projects.

REFERENCES

Hulley, S. B., Cummings, S. R., Browner, W. S., Grady, D. G., & Newman, T. B. (2013). *Designing clinical research* (4th ed.). Philadelphia, PA: Lippincott Williams & Wilkins.

Melnyk, B. M., & Fineout-Overholt, E. (2015). *Evidence-based practice in nursing & healthcare: A guide to best practice* (3rd ed.). Philadelphia, PA: Wolters Kluwer/Lippincott Williams & Wilkins.

Sechrest, L., & Babcock-Parziale, J. B. (2007). *Writing effective research proposals.* Fairfax, VA: Public Interest Research Services.

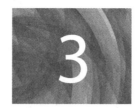

Designing, Conducting, and Evaluating Outcomes of Evidence-Based Quality Improvement Projects

Bernadette Mazurek Melnyk

> Quality is never an accident; it is always the result of high intention, sincere effort, intelligent direction and skillful execution; it represents the wise choice of many alternatives. —*William A. Foster*

BACKGROUND

Although the United States spends more money on healthcare than any western world country, it is ranked 37th in health outcomes (Murray & Frenk, 2010). Further, medical errors are the third leading cause of death in America affecting 400,000 people annually (Makary & Daniel, 2016). There is no doubt that continuous quality improvement (QI) in healthcare systems is desperately needed. In an attempt to improve outcomes, many hospitals and healthcare systems have created **QI** or **outcome management (OM)** programs or committees that are responsible for monitoring quality of care and patient outcomes and making practice changes to improve them.

QI has been defined as a systematic process used by healthcare systems to analyze existing data and improve its processes and/or outcomes for a specific patient population (Kring, 2008; Shirey et al., 2011). It consists of using patient data/outcomes (i.e., internal evidence compared with external evidence that is generated from rigorous research) to improve clinical care and outcomes. In many models, QI does not involve a search for and critical appraisal and synthesis of evidence to determine the best interventions or process improvement strategies but, instead, uses ideas for solutions generated by healthcare leaders. When improvements are based on a thorough search for and critical appraisal and synthesis of the literature and the best evidence is implemented along with the monitoring of outcomes, it is known as **evidence-based quality improvement (EBQI**; Melnyk, Buck, & Gallagher-Ford, 2015). Ideally, EBQI projects should follow the seven steps of the evidence-based practice (EBP) process:

Step #0. Cultivate a spirit of inquiry within an EBP culture and environment (background/ significance of the clinical problem).

Step #1. Ask the burning clinical question in PICO(T) format, (i.e., Population, Intervention, Comparison intervention, Outcome, [Time, if relevant]).

Step #2. Search for and collect the most relevant best evidence.

Step #3. Critically appraise the evidence (i.e., rapid critical appraisal [RCA], evaluation, and synthesis).

Step #4. Integrate the best evidence with one's clinical expertise and patient/family preferences and values in making a practice decision or change.

Step #5. Evaluate outcomes of the practice decision or change, based on evidence.

Step #6. Disseminate the outcomes of the EBP decision or change. (Melnyk & Fineout-Overholt, 2019)

DESIGNING AND CONDUCTING AN EVIDENCE-BASED QUALITY IMPROVEMENT PROJECT

Most EBQI or EBP implementation projects are undertaken because a healthcare leader or clinician identifies a clinical problem (e.g., the number of cases of ventilator-associated pneumonia [VAP] in the ICU has escalated, infection rates on postoperative patients have skyrocketed, length of stay following mental health hospitalization in adolescents has increased, or the prevalence of depression in college students has increased). Once a clinical problem is identified (Step #0 in the seven steps of EBP), a PICO(T) question should be formed (e.g.: In ICU-ventilated patients [Population of interest], how does early ambulation [Intervention of interest] versus turning side to side every 4 hours [Comparison intervention] affect the prevalence of VAP [Outcome] 6 months after implementation [T; Step #1 in EBP]?). Then, the keywords from the PICO(T) question, separately and combined, are entered into the databases being used to search for the evidence to answer the question (Step #2 in EBP). Once the search is conducted and relevant studies found, critical appraisal and synthesis of the evidence are conducted to determine the best intervention to decrease the prevalence of VAP (Step #3 in EBP). If the conclusion from the systematic search and critical appraisal of a body of studies indicates that early ambulation in the ICU improves the prevalence of VAP, a change in practice is then planned and implemented (Step #4 in EBP). After a period (e.g., 6 months), the rate of VAP is determined to assess whether early ambulation resulted in a decreased prevalence of VAP (Step #5 in EBP). The last step (#6) in the EBP process is disseminating the outcomes of the EBQI or EBP change project and determining how best to sustain them. In this case, the project, including the outcome, would be shared with colleagues in the organization, presented at professional conferences, or published in a professional journal.

DATA GATHERING FOR EVIDENCE-BASED QUALITY IMPROVEMENT PROJECTS

Accessing data that is housed within healthcare settings for EBQI projects typically comes from sources such as electronic health records, QI or human resource departments, administration, or clinical systems. Being clear and specific about the data that is needed is very important. Asking for data in a format that can be easily used is important, such as in an electronic format. Collecting data that is already available in electronic format can prevent errors and numerous hours needed for data entry when measures are collected in a paper format. Once data have been acquired for analysis, statistical tests may be conducted using spreadsheet software or the data file can be easily transferred to statistics software for further analysis (Brewer & Alexandrov, 2015).

Unlike data generated from research, the data gathered for EBQI projects is not meant to be generalized to other practice settings across the country but rather to be used for decisions about patient care in the setting in which it is generated. When data sources that exist are not available to assess important outcomes of interest, it is important to decide what measures and processes will be used to collect the needed data (Brewer & Alexandrov, 2015).

ASSESSING PROCESSES AND OUTCOMES IN EVIDENCE-BASED QUALITY IMPROVEMENT PROJECTS

Outcomes happen as a result of a healthcare intervention, practice, or treatment that can be quantified (e.g., number of rehospitalizations, infection rates, number of complications, and length of stay in days). They can be assessed by objective measures or self-report (Hockenberry, Brown, & Rodgers, 2014). For example, if you implemented a new evidence-based cognitive behavioral therapy–based depression program for adolescents in primary care (the intervention), it would be important to assess the prevalence of depression (the outcome) before implementing the new program and 6 months after implementing the program. If the number of depressed adolescents in your practice average 16 per month before implementing the program and four per month after implementation of the program, you could conclude that the evidence-based cognitive behavioral therapy–based program was effective in decreasing depression rates. It is important to differentiate **process measures** from outcomes. Process measures are those factors or variables that influence outcomes. For example, an action that is a process measure that may impact the rate of VAP (the outcome of care) might include how many times a patient is turned in 24 hours.

In today's healthcare system where emphasis is placed on delivering high-quality care at reduced costs, it is important to measure **"so what" outcomes** (e.g., those that are important to the healthcare system). Examples of "so what" outcomes include core performance metrics (e.g., infection rates, falls, catheter-associated urinary tract infections), length of stay, complication rates, rehospitalizations, and costs. Because these types of metrics are currently tied to reimbursement rates for hospitals and healthcare systems, including them in EBQI or EBP implementation projects is of utmost importance. Cost outcomes also are important to include as the current healthcare system is cost driven and places high importance on return on investment. If the focus of EBQI projects is on "soft outcomes," such as patient uncertainty or caring, it is highly unlikely that hospitals and healthcare systems will be interested in investing resources into making a practice change. Table 3.1 outlines important steps in assessing process and outcome data for an EBQI project.

EXAMPLES OF EVIDENCE-BASED QUALITY IMPROVEMENT PROJECTS

The following are five excellent examples of EBQI projects, three conducted as part of doctor of nursing practice (DNP) degree projects. The DNP is a clinical doctorate that, like other clinical doctorates (e.g., doctor of pharmacy [PharmD], doctor of psychology [PsyD], doctor of physical therapy [DPT], doctor of audiology [Au.D.]), should prepare individuals for

TABLE 3.1 Steps in Assessing Process and Outcome Data for an EBQI Project
1. Identify the "so what" outcomes and processes that are important to measure when an EBP change is planned.
2. Determine where the outcome data is located in your organization and who owns the data (e.g., director of QI) so that it can be collected and analyzed.
3. Be clear and specific about the data that you are requesting.
4. Decide on the time frames when the outcome data will be collected.
5. Collect and record the baseline data.
6. Collect and record the outcome data after the EBP change is made for a specified period.
7. Use the data to determine whether the EBP change should be sustained or further refined for the continued improvement of outcomes.

EBP, evidence-based practice; EBQI, evidence-based quality improvement; QI, quality improvement.

Source: Adapted from Melnyk, B. M. (2016). The evidence-based practice competencies related to outcomes evaluation. In B. M. Melnyk, L. Gallagher-Ford, & E. Fineout-Overholt (Eds.), *Implementing the evidence-based practice (EBP) competencies in healthcare. A practical guide for improving quality, safety, & outcomes* (pp. 129–142). Indianapolis, IN: Sigma Theta Tau International.

the highest level of clinical practice, including expertise in EBP and EBQI, versus the PhD, which prepares individuals to conduct rigorous research. Individuals with clinical and research doctorates should work closely together to rapidly translate the best evidence-based interventions into real-world settings to improve healthcare quality and population-based outcomes.

USING THE EVIDENCE TO REDUCE VENTILATOR-ASSOCIATED PNEUMONIA IN AN ADULT ICU

Joyce Zurmehly, PhD, DNP, RN, NEA-BC, ANEF

Background/Significance of the Problem (Step #0 in EBP)

Pneumonia accounts for 47% of all hospital-acquired infections, second only to urinary tract infections (Augustyn, 2007). VAP occurs as a result of pulmonary inflammation after intubation. Critically ill patients have been identified as those affected primarily by VAP, with an incidence rate as high as 90% (O'Keefe-McCarthy, Santiago, & Lau, 2008). For patients receiving mechanical ventilation, the risk of pneumonia increases by 6 to 21 times because they are admitted to an ICU with harmful bacteria already in their system. With VAP so prevalent, the Institute of Healthcare Improvement (IHI) launched a 5-million lives campaign identifying prevention as a top priority, thereby reducing deaths (American Association of Critical Care Nurses [AACN], 2010; Institute for Healthcare Improvement [IHI], 2010). For a year, the IHI reviewed studies performed in hospitals throughout Scotland. These studies included a daily oral care regimen of 0.12% chlorhexidine solution for ventilator patients. In May 2010, after reviewing the Scotland studies that showed improved outcomes, the IHI added the same daily oral care regimen to the ventilator care bundles given to ICUs in hospitals throughout the United States. These care bundles have been promoted as a means of improving patient outcomes by grouping evidence-based interventions together with quality care (Tolentino-Delosreyes, Ruppert, & Shiao, 2007; Westwell, 2008).

At the project hospital, the rates of VAP were tracked through hospital infection control surveillance. The VAP rate was defined by the National Healthcare Safety Network (NHSN) as the number of infections per 1,000 ventilator days. In 2009, surveillance showed that the VAP rate for the study hospital was 10.75 cases. The state and national rates were 6.49 cases and 5.50 cases, respectively. Therefore, this rate was approximately 50% above the state and national averages.

The PICO(T) Question (Step #1 in EBP)

In the adult ICU mechanically ventilated patient (P), how does the use of an antiseptic agent (chlorhexidine swab; I) versus the use of toothettes (C) affect the incidence rate of VAP (O) over a 3-month period (T)?

Search for the Evidence (Step #2 in EBP)

A systematic review of the literature was conducted on the basis of the PICO(T) question. The literature search consisted of the following databases: Cochrane Database of Systematic Reviews, Cumulative Index to Nursing and Allied Health Literature (CINAHL), MEDLINE, the Joanna Briggs Institute of EBP Database, as well as governmental sources such as the Centers for Disease Control and Prevention (CDC) and Centers for Medicare & Medicaid Services (CMS) websites. The search was focused on the keywords specific to VAP: "ventilator bundle," "VAP," "and evidence-based guidelines." After abstracts were reviewed, articles were excluded if they did not specifically indicate bundled practices for VAP. Fifteen studies were identified and reviewed. Six additional studies were identified from the bibliographies of key references. Twelve studies were accepted on the basis of inclusion criteria.

Critical Appraisal of the Evidence (Step #3 in EBP)

When the literature was searched, a total of 435 references were obtained. During review of the initial list, 71 duplicates were extracted and another 203 were excluded because they were published before the 1995 CDC VAP clinical practice guideline was available. The remaining 161 references were submitted to three VAP inclusion criteria: (a) adult mechanically ventilated, (b) ICU setting, and (c) nurse-driven prevention techniques. On the basis of the inclusion criteria, another 120 failed, leaving 41 potentially relevant studies. A total of 32 studies and findings were included with recommendations for standard-of-care practices to prevent VAP. The evidence summary reflecting the state of the science for preventing VAP strongly supported the inclusion of 0.12% chlorhexidine gluconate (CHG) swabbing solution as a nursing intervention.

Integration of the Evidence With a Clinician's Expertise and a Patient's Preferences and Values in Making a Decision/Implementation (Step #4 in EBP)

After a review of EBP material and guidelines, the project leader and hospital's policy review committee implemented a new oral care protocol for mechanically ventilated patients. With ICU nurses as the target, a VAP program was developed using evidence-based clinical guidelines.

Research from the AACN (2010) and the IHI (2010) was analyzed. The recommendations included nursing interventions, specifically, brushing the teeth of patients undergoing mechanical ventilation at least three times a day and oral swabbing every 12 hours with 0.12% CHG swabbing solution. The recommendation for oral care was integrated into the prevention program for the nurses in ICU.

Evaluation of Outcomes (Step #5 in EBP)

The measurement and monitoring components included evaluation of patient VAP rates during a period extending from 3 months before to 3 months after the intervention. During the 6-month period, a total of 180 mechanically ventilated patients were enrolled in the project. Overall ventilator days were significantly decreased in the postintervention group ($p < 0.01$). Subsequently, during the postintervention period, only one episode of VAP occurred during a total of 421 ventilator days among 854 total patient days. This is equivalent to an infection rate of 4.8 patients per 1,000 ventilator patient days, 2.7% of the total sample of 180 patients. Of the 180 patients in the ICU, five had VAP; four of 95 cases (2.2%) occurred before intervention and one of 85 cases (0.5%) occurred after intervention. During the postintervention period, the infection rate was 1.8 per 1,000 ventilator days, a decrease of 62.5% compared with the preintervention period. The results of this project suggested that oral care with tooth brushing at least three times per day and oral swabbing every 12 hours with 0.12% CHG solution and sustained by nursing care and actions successfully decreased the incidence of VAP.

Dissemination (Step #6 in EBP)

The project leader disseminated the results of the project to internal and external audiences. Internally, reports were provided to the Hospital Quality Council and Executive Leadership. Externally, an article was published in 2013 in the *Journal of Continuing Education in Nursing* (Zurmehly, 2013).

EVIDENCE-BASED PRACTICE IN ACTION: CLUSTERED ASSIGNMENTS DECREASE PATIENT FALLS AND IMPROVE STAFF ENGAGEMENT

Barbara Potts, MS, RN, APRN-CNS, ACCNS-AG, Laura Droll, MS, RN, NE-BC, Stephanie Ferry, BSN, RN-BC, Caitlin Wears, BSN, RN-BC, January Belcher, RN-BC, Matthew Shirzadian, BSN, RN-BC, and Amy M. Knupp, PhD, RN, APRN-CNS, CPPS

Background/Significance of the Problem (Step #0 in EBP)

Healthcare organizations are expected to provide patient safety and deliver high-quality patient care. Process breakdowns within organizations often lead to patient dissatisfaction, disenchanted clinicians, and missed opportunities for optimal patient outcomes (Minnier et al., 2012). One medical unit within a tertiary academic medical center in the Midwest was provided an opportunity to improve its staffing model and ultimately impact the areas of quality, patient experience, and staff engagement. The following statement of opportunity was developed by the unit staff:"There is a perception of lack of time to appropriately address patient needs, which may be impacting patient safety, patient experience, and staff engagement."

Retrospective quality metrics related to patient falls, patient experience scores, and staff nurse engagement scores for the specific nursing unit were reviewed to understand the unit's baseline metrics from the previous 2 years. Fall data showed a total of 26 patient falls: zero with major injury for the fiscal year 2015 (FY15); 26 patient falls, one with major injury (fracture) for fiscal year 2016 (FY16); and 16 patient falls, one with major injury (fractures) for the first 5 months of fiscal year 2017 (FY17; see Table 3.2). Data indicated no improvement in patient fall outcomes across this 2.5-year time period. In addition, a major injury resulting from a patient fall was reported in each of the last two fiscal years.

TABLE 3.2 Quality: Patient Falls

METRIC	FY15	FY15 TARGET[a]	FY16	FY16 TARGET	FY17 (YTD[b])	FY17 TARGET
Falls	26	21.6	26	23.4	16	19.5
Falls with injury	0	0	1	0	1	0

[a]Target was based on a goal reduction compared with the previous fiscal year.
[b]YTD, year to date (first half of fiscal year).
FY15, fiscal year 2015; FY16, fiscal year 2016; FY17, fiscal year 2017.

TABLE 3.3 Patient Experience

METRIC	FY15	FY15 TARGET[a]	FY16	FY16 TARGET	FY17 (YTD[b])	FY17 TARGET
HCAHPS Overall	66.7%	79%	62.8%	79.4%	64.1%	79.5%

[a]Target was determined by internal benchmarking.
[b]YTD, year to date (first quarter).
FY15, fiscal year 2015; FY16, fiscal year 2016; FY17, fiscal year 2017; HCAHPS, Hospital Consumer Assessment of Healthcare Providers and Systems.

TABLE 3.4 Staff Engagement

	2013 RESULTS	2013 TIER GROUP	2015 RESULTS	2015 TIER GROUP
Medical unit	4.33	Tier 1	4.12	Tier 2

Patient experience metrics were reviewed using the data provided by Hospital Consumer Assessment of Healthcare Providers and Systems (HCAHPS; CMS, 2014). The unit patient experience scores for this 2.5-year time period are shown in Table 3.3. This "overall" metric measures the percentage of patients who respond with a 9 or 10 (0 being the lowest and 10 the highest) to this question: Using a number from 0 to 10, what number would you use to rate this hospital? Data indicated no improvement in overall patient experience across the reporting periods.

The terms "satisfaction" and "engagement" when referring to staff experience are often used interchangeably. The organization measures staff engagement every other year. Staff engagement metrics were reviewed using the biannual unit data provided by Press Ganey, from both 2013 and 2015 staff engagement surveys. Press Ganey is an outside consulting group with expertise in organizational development and caregiver engagement, assisting in the building of resilient patient-centered cultures (Press Ganey, 2017). The unit scores are reflected in Table 3.4. Staff engagement is based on employees' (a) willingness to recommend the organization to their family, friends, and colleagues; (b) pride in affiliation with the organization; and (c) overall satisfaction in employment. On the basis of the results, units are categorized into Tier 1 (≥4.15), Tier 2 (≥3.80 and <4.15), and Tier 3 (<3.8), with Tier 1 representing the highest employee engagement.

Nursing Unit Description
This 27-bed medical nursing unit cares primarily for patients with hepatology disease but also serves patients admitted to the hospital with other general medical conditions. The unit is located in an aging building within the academic health system and consists of a long

250-foot corridor with both private and semiprivate patient rooms. The unit uses an existing nursing care delivery model that includes registered nurses (RNs), patient care associates (PCAs), and unit clerical associates (UCAs). The average RN-to-patient ratio is 1:5, the average PCA-to-patient ratio is 1:10, and there is typically one UCA on duty for the entire unit for each shift. One charge nurse is staffed per shift and also is assigned an average of one to three patients. The charge nurse assigns patients to RNs based on perceived nursing workload and patient acuity and assigns patients to PCAs based on geographical zones, attempting to decrease the size of their work area and keep them closer to their assigned patients. Although unit geography was typically considered when making PCA assignments, the practice was not often considered when building RN assignments. This meant that an RN could be assigned five patients in any part of the long 250-foot straight corridor.

Workgroup

The nursing unit leadership team, in conjunction with the director of nursing quality, assembled an EBP workgroup of unit staff members to develop an updated staffing model, using the allocated resources to optimize patient safety, patient experience, and staff engagement. The EBP workgroup, representing both night shift and day shift, was composed of four RNs (both staff nurses and charge nurses), three PCAs, one UCA, the nursing unit leadership team (i.e., nurse manager, assistant nurse manager, and clinical nurse specialist), and the director of nursing quality. The EBP workgroup timeline included a total of five 2-hour meetings, spanning over a 2-month period.

Retrospective unit data from the previous 2 years and specific to patient quality, experience, and staff engagement were reviewed with the EBP workgroup. In addition, unit quality metrics for the current fiscal year were reviewed. Then the EBP workgroup developed the following primary purpose statement: To develop an updated staffing model that uses the allocated resources in the most ideal manner to optimize patient safety (specifically patient falls), patient experience, and staff engagement. A secondary purpose was also developed: To define and standardize the roles involved with the ideal process.

The PICO(T) question (Step #1 in EBP)

Because the topic for review was related to improving patient safety and experience as well as staff engagement, use of the intervention PICO template was warranted (Melnyk & Fineout-Overholt, 2015). In the adult-hospitalized patient (P), how does a new nursing care delivery model (I), compared with the existing nursing care delivery model (C), optimize patient safety, patient experience, and staff engagement (O)? The EBP workgroup defined patient safety specifically as reducing patient falls, which also factored into searching the literature.

Search for the Evidence (Step #2 in EBP)

A comprehensive literature review was initiated, using the CINAHL database. CINAHL was chosen because this project focused on nursing quality, specifically patient falls, and patient experience. Terms from the PICO question were used to generate search results as well as other key words, such as "primary nursing," "team nursing," "pod nursing," and "fall prevention." The search yielded over 2,400 articles that were filtered to "literature from the past 10 years" and then filtered using the key words just listed.

Critical Appraisal of the Evidence (Step #3 in EBP)

Concentrating on the purpose statement developed by the EBP workgroup, the themes of patient safety and experience, "pod" nursing, and nursing satisfaction were the foci when applying the RCA to the literature (Fineout-Overholt, Melnyk, Stillwell, & Williamson,

2010c). The RCA yielded a total of 10 applicable articles, which are summarized in the literature summary table (Appendix A). As illustrated in Table 3.5, of the 10 articles, two articles were Level V evidence (Fineout-Overholt, Melnyk, Stillwell, & Williamson, 2010a; i.e., one article was a systematic review of qualitative studies and one article was a descriptive study). The majority of the articles were Level VI evidence (evidence implementation projects). The final article was Level VII evidence (consensus opinion). As seen in Table 3.6, the body of literature revealed that patient experience can be positively impacted with a pod nursing design. Improved response times when answering call lights and the perception of more nursing time spent at the patient bedside were demonstrated with the pod nursing

TABLE 3.5 Levels of Evidence Table

	1	2	3	4	5	6	7	8	9	10
Level I: Systematic review or meta-analysis										
Level II: Randomized controlled trial										
Level III: Controlled trial without randomization										
Level IV: Case–control or cohort study										
Level V: Systematic review of qualitative or descriptive studies	X						X			
Level VI: Qualitative or descriptive study (includes evidence implementation projects)		X	X	X	X	X		X	X	
Level VII: Expert opinion or consensus										X

TABLE 3.6 Synthesis Table

	1	2	3	4	5	6	7	8	9	10
Outcome										
Pod design improves patient satisfaction	↑	↑					—		↑	
Pod design improves patient safety	↑	↑	↑						↑	
Improve teamwork; improve nursing satisfaction	↑	↑	↑	↑				↑	↑	
More nursing time at bedside	↑						↑			
Improved response time answering call lights			↑		↑					
RN non–value-added time tasks						↑				
Nurse aide not being used to full potential						↑				↑
Inadequate staffing leads to higher costs/poorer outcomes							↑	↑		
Decrease length of stay									↑	

↑, positive correlation; ↓, negative correlation; —, neutral correlation.

design. From a nursing perspective, the pod nursing design also was associated with improved teamwork and nursing satisfaction. Most importantly, patient safety was improved with the pod nursing design, specifically a reduction in patient falls. The EBP workgroup concluded that the pod nursing design supported each aspect of the group's defined purpose statement related to reducing patient falls, improving patient experience, and increasing staff engagement.

Integration of the Evidence With a Clinician's Expertise and a Patient's Preferences and Values in Making a Decision/Implementation (Step #4 in EBP)

The EBP workgroup was assembled and educated on QI processes, after which the project purpose statements were developed. Members were assigned to review different articles and were responsible for reporting their summaries to the workgroup during the meetings. The EBP workgroup detailed the unit's current workflow related to staffing and patient care assignments and then discussed the article findings to develop an ideal workflow process. The workgroup considered various factors when creating the ideal workflow, such as patient population, unit geography, and staffing resources. The articles inspired the workgroup members to question the existing practice for making patient care assignments. The literature challenged the workgroup to consider including patient location and unit geography when assigning patients.

The nurses in the EBP workgroup used their clinical expertise in discussing the physiological characteristics of a typical patient on the unit. As a medical unit with a high volume of patients with hepatology disease, most patients are considered a high risk for falls and falls with injury related to their physiological deconditioning. Many of the patients have encephalopathy resulting in confusion, impulsiveness, and poor decision making. Because of these patient characteristics, frequent monitoring is necessary for maintaining patient safety; however, frequent monitoring can be difficult when assignments are spread out across a 250-foot corridor. Patient preferences were considered in creating the ideal workflow based on the supporting literature. The patient perception of more nursing time at the bedside along with an improved response time to call lights impacted the ideal workflow design.

The EBP workgroup then created an ideal workflow, which was coined "clustered assignments." The group considered the unit geography and defined the clusters so that patient assignments would be in groupings, encompassing smaller areas. The borders of the clusters were considered fluid, to allow consideration for varying patient acuity and throughput. The charge nurse is responsible for making both RN and PCA assignments using the clustering care model. The goal in making assignments is to allow caregivers to stay geographically located. Implementation of clustered assignments included an educational plan, a rollout date, and a process for feedback and evaluation. The EBP workgroup members facilitated education and implementation of the project. The targeted rollout date was chosen to allow a 6-month comparison of the existing workflow to the clustered assignment workflow and the impact on previously discussed metrics for the unit.

Evaluation of Outcomes (Step #5 in EBP)

Informal, anecdotal feedback was gathered from the workgroup members throughout project implementation. A feedback board was available in the staff break room where staff members were encouraged to share comments and concerns. Themes generated from staff feedback included quicker response time to call lights, improved efficiency because of a reduction in steps, and more help available when needed. One nurse posted, "I feel like I can provide better quality care!"

The quality metric of patient falls and falls with injury was established as an outcome measure at the initiation of the EBP project. In review, the first half of FY17 fall data included 16 total falls with one fall as a major injury. At the completion of the EBP project, the last half of FY17 fall data reflected six falls, zero with major injury (Figure 3.1). Patient falls were decreased by 62.5% from the first half of FY17 to the last half of FY17. The percent of change was calculated by taking the difference between the number of falls in the first half of FY17 and the number of falls in the last half of FY17 (16 − 6 = 10). Then the decrease (10) was divided by the original number (16) and multiplied by 100 (10/16 = 0.625 × 100 = 62.5%).

In addition to patient falls and patient falls with injury, the HCAHPS patient experience metrics was established as an outcome measure at the initiation of the EBP project. A question level comparison of the unit's HCAHPS patient experience scores for 6 months pre-and postclustering assignments is illustrated in Figure 3.2. Demonstrated improvement is noted in two specific domains: (a) nurse communication and (b) responsiveness. The following statements showed improvement: (a) Nurses explain in ways you understand (6.7% increase), (b) Nurses treat you with courtesy/respect (7.8% increase), (c) Call button help comes as soon as you wanted it (13.2% increase). Although it is difficult to isolate the impact of a single intervention on patient experience data, it is certainly favorable that the most improved question over this time period is "call button help comes as soon as you wanted it."

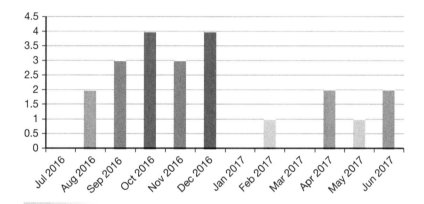

FIGURE 3.1 Patient falls: fiscal year 2017 (July 2016–June 2017).

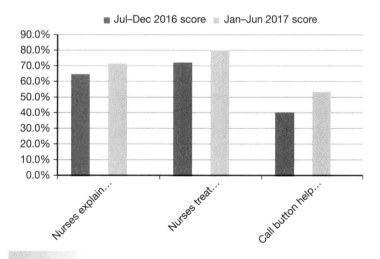

FIGURE 3.2 Patient experience: question level–cluster impact.

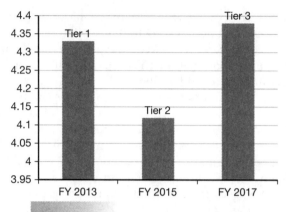

FIGURE 3.3 Staff engagement scores.

Along with patient falls and patient experience, staff engagement was selected as an outcome measure for the clustered assignment EBP project. As previously suggested, the nursing unit had decreased from Tier 1 to Tier 2 on the employee engagement spectrum between FY13 and FY15. In conjunction with the EBP project implementation, the workgroup requested an off-cycle staff engagement survey to evaluate this outcome measure. A pulse survey was administered 4 months into the implementation of the EBP project. As noted in Figure 3.3, the unit's staff engagement scores improved from Tier 2 (4.12) to Tier 1 (4.38).

Dissemination (Step #6 in EBP)

Outcomes of this EBP project continue to be shared at many venues. Success with this project is being viewed as an exemplar within our medical center, and other nursing units have been implementing the process of geographically clustering patient care assignments. Several other units have sent staff representatives to shadow on this unit to seek information about the clustered assignment nursing care delivery model. EBP workgroup members have presented the outcomes at the system level shared governance council, as well as to individual units desiring to replicate and implement this care delivery model. Internal dissemination within the organization has also included poster presentations on clustered assignments for the 2017 annual safety fair and the 2017 nursing excellence fair. In addition, this project was accepted and presented by members of the EBP workgroup at the 2017 annual convention of the Academy of Medical-Surgical Nurses. The EBP workgroup members will continue to explore and welcome further means of disseminating the process and outcomes.

HOSPITAL-ACQUIRED PRESSURE INJURY PREVENTION IN INTENSIVE CARE

Shannon Appelfeller, BSN, RN, CCRN, SN III and
Colleen O'Leary MSN, RN, AOCNS®

Background/Significance of the Problem (Step #0 in EBP)

Pressure ulcers occur on any area of skin or underlying tissue that has been damaged by unrelieved pressure or pressure in combination with friction and shear. These typically occur over bony prominences in immobilized patients (Swafford, Culpepper, & Dunn, 2016).

The National Database of Nursing Quality Indicators (NDNQI) has made hospital-acquired pressure injuries (HAPIs) one of the quality indicators that facilities must track and report. In addition to NDNQI results, at our comprehensive cancer center, selected staff nurses participate in quarterly skin rounds on patients on their units as part of their quality initiatives pertaining to HAPI detection and prevention. The results of both are then reviewed for any possible trends. In February 2016, the ICUs, including the Neurosciences Critical Care Unit (NCCU), the medical ICU (MICU), and the surgical ICU (SICU) experienced almost double the number of pressure injuries typically seen in these ICUs (see Figure 3.4). As a result, a group consisting of nurse managers, PCAs, RNs, and nurse educators and clinical nurse specialists gathered to determine next steps.

The PICO(T) question (Step #1 in EBP)

The group identified that there was inconsistent practice among nurses and PCAs in the prevention of HAPIs. In addition, there was not an identified group to lead efforts to reduce HAPIs. Because of this, their PICO question was: "In patients in the ICUs, how does the use of a skin rounding team with specific interventions compared to individual nurse interventions affect the incidence of HAPIs?"

Search for the Evidence (Step #2 in EBP)

A review of the literature included the keywords: "Pressure ulcers," "prevention," "ICU," "management," "evidence-based practice pressure ulcers," and "skin injury." The search engines used were CINAHL, EbscoHost, and PubMed. In addition, internal audit results were reviewed.

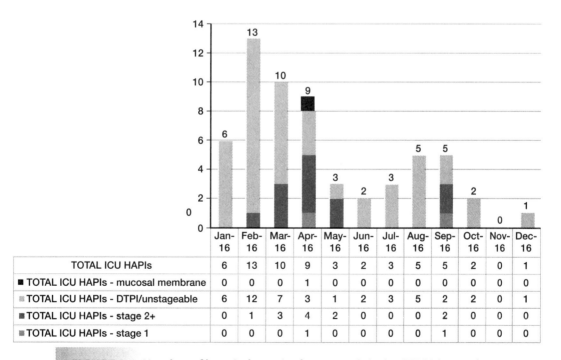

	Jan-16	Feb-16	Mar-16	Apr-16	May-16	Jun-16	Jul-16	Aug-16	Sep-16	Oct-16	Nov-16	Dec-16
TOTAL ICU HAPIs	6	13	10	9	3	2	3	5	5	2	0	1
■ TOTAL ICU HAPIs - mucosal membrane	0	0	0	1	0	0	0	0	0	0	0	0
▨ TOTAL ICU HAPIs - DTPI/unstageable	6	12	7	3	1	2	3	5	2	2	0	1
■ TOTAL ICU HAPIs - stage 2+	0	1	3	4	2	0	0	0	2	0	0	0
■ TOTAL ICU HAPIs - stage 1	0	0	0	1	0	0	0	0	1	0	0	0

FIGURE 3.4 Number of hospital acquired pressure injuries (HAPIs) over time.

Critical Appraisal and Synthesis of the Evidence (Step #3 in EBP)

Eight articles were found on the prevention of skin injuries and after critically appraising all of the articles, five were found to be of use to the group (see Table 3.7). The interventions that appeared in these articles that were chosen included turning the patient every 2 hours, assessing the Braden Scale every 8 hours, using a low air loss mattress, assessing and providing adequate nutrition, positioning of any tubes, bathing with chlorhexidine gluconate (CHG) wipes, and using a barrier protective cream (Cooper, 2013; Gage, 2015).

Integration of the Evidence With a Clinician's Expertise and a Patient's Preferences and Values in Making a Decision/Implementation (Step #4 in EBP)

In addition to the interventions mentioned in the articles, we chose to use foam wedges when turning patients to assist in keeping them on the appropriate side and began to use protective bandages. Weekly skin assessments also were increased by a skin rounding team that included the RN, nurse manager, nurse educator, and wound nurse. Finally, a skin champion was identified on each unit that is responsible for ensuring that these interventions were occurring on each unit.

Evaluation of Outcomes (Step #5 in EBP)

NCCU had a decrease in HAPIs by 67% after implementing the program. After the second month, the NCCU had a 100% decrease in HAPIs and stayed at that rate for 3 months Figure 3.5. MICU and SICU did not have results as significant but had an overall decrease in the HAPI trend. The MICU rates started decreasing after 2 months of the implemented interventions, and they consistently had less than two HAPIs per month. The SICU HAPI rates started trending downward as the interventions were implemented (Figures 3.6 and 3.7).

TABLE 3.7					
	1	2	3	4	5
Level I: Systematic review or meta-analysis			x		
Level II: Randomized controlled trial					
Level III: Controlled trial without randomization					
Level IV: Case–control or cohort study					
Level V: Systematic review of qualitative or descriptive studies					
Level VI: Qualitative or descriptive study (includes evidence implementation projects)	x	x			x
Level VII: Expert opinion or consensus				x	

Source: Cooper, K. L. (2013). Evidence--based prevention of pressure ulcers in the intensive care unit. *Critical Care Nurse, 33*(6), 57–66. doi:10.4037/ccn2013985; Gage, W. (2015). Preventing pressure ulcers in patients in intensive care. *Nursing Standard, 29*(26), 53–61. doi:10.7748/ns.29.26.53.e9657; Swafford, K., Culpepper, R., & Dunn, C. (2016). Use of a comprehensive program to reduce the incidence of hospital--acquired pressure ulcers in an intensive care unit. *American Journal of Critical Care, 25*(2), 152–155. doi:10.4037/ajcc2016963

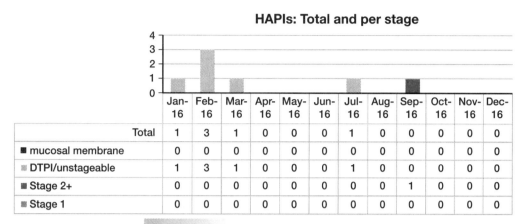

HAPIs: Total and per stage

	Jan-16	Feb-16	Mar-16	Apr-16	May-16	Jun-16	Jul-16	Aug-16	Sep-16	Oct-16	Nov-16	Dec-16
Total	1	3	1	0	0	0	1	0	0	0	0	0
■ mucosal membrane	0	0	0	0	0	0	0	0	0	0	0	0
▨ DTPI/unstageable	1	3	1	0	0	0	1	0	0	0	0	0
■ Stage 2+	0	0	0	0	0	0	0	0	1	0	0	0
▨ Stage 1	0	0	0	0	0	0	0	0	0	0	0	0

FIGURE 3.5 NCCU HAPI rates over time.

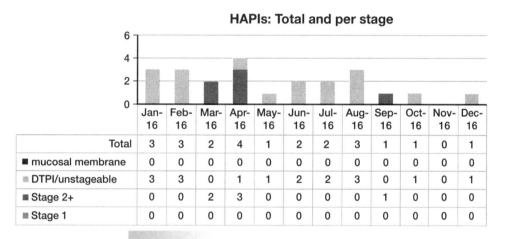

HAPIs: Total and per stage

	Jan-16	Feb-16	Mar-16	Apr-16	May-16	Jun-16	Jul-16	Aug-16	Sep-16	Oct-16	Nov-16	Dec-16
Total	3	3	2	4	1	2	2	3	1	1	0	1
■ mucosal membrane	0	0	0	0	0	0	0	0	0	0	0	0
▨ DTPI/unstageable	3	3	0	1	1	2	2	3	0	1	0	1
■ Stage 2+	0	0	2	3	0	0	0	0	1	0	0	0
▨ Stage 1	0	0	0	0	0	0	0	0	0	0	0	0

FIGURE 3.6 MICU HAPI rates across time.

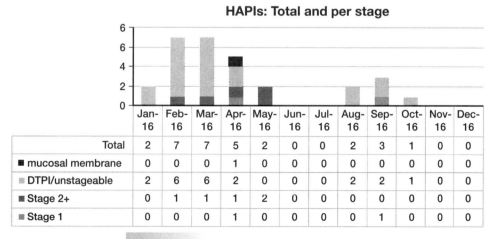

HAPIs: Total and per stage

	Jan-16	Feb-16	Mar-16	Apr-16	May-16	Jun-16	Jul-16	Aug-16	Sep-16	Oct-16	Nov-16	Dec-16
Total	2	7	7	5	2	0	0	2	3	1	0	0
■ mucosal membrane	0	0	0	1	0	0	0	0	0	0	0	0
▨ DTPI/unstageable	2	6	6	2	0	0	0	2	2	1	0	0
■ Stage 2+	0	1	1	1	2	0	0	0	0	0	0	0
▨ Stage 1	0	0	0	1	0	0	0	0	1	0	0	0

FIGURE 3.7 SICU HAPI rates across time.

Dissemination (Step #6 in EBP)

The team shared its interventions and outcome data with all of our health system critical care areas and presented a poster at a Patient Safety Fair. The poster was acknowledged as one of the top posters and winner at the fair out of more than 70 posters. Improvement in HAPI rates is continuously monitored in the ICUs with audits conducted by the nurses. This will ensure adherence to the new interventions and, when it is found that the interventions are not being followed, "in the moment" education will be completed. Minimizing the number of pressure injuries acquired in the hospital will promote positive patient outcomes, ensure quicker healing, minimize incurred costs from HAPIs, and increase quality of life for our patients.

IMPLEMENTATION OF AN EVIDENCE-BASED PRACTICE PROTOCOL TO REDUCE CATHETER-ASSOCIATED URINARY TRACT INFECTIONS IN A LONG-TERM ACUTE CARE HOSPITAL

Joyce Zurmehly, PhD, DNP, RN NEA-BC, ANEF

Background/Significance of the Problem (Step #0 in EBP)

In the United States, advances in technology, aging population, and chronicity of diseases have resulted in a patient population classified as "chronic critically ill" (CCI; Kahn et al., 2015). The CCI patient survives an initial critical illness only to suffer prolonged dependency and the need for longer term therapeutic interventions. Also, improvements in critical care have resulted in shorter stays and shifts to long-term acute care hospitals (LTACHs) for CCI patients.

LTACH patients are frequently admitted with urinary catheters. Many are critically ill with multiple risk factors resulting in immune exhaustion, leaving them vulnerable to healthcare-associated infections (HAIs), including catheter-associated urinary tract infections (CAUTIs). Indwelling urinary catheters are primary sources of bacteremia in healthcare settings; CAUTIs are the second most frequently diagnosed HAI and the most common cause for hospitalization with a bacterial infection (Genao & Buhr, 2012). Annually, an estimated 720,000 CAUTIs occur, accounting for more than 13,000 deaths (CDC, 2018) and estimated costs of $340–$450 million (Strouse, 2015).

In addition to urinary catheter presence, duration (catheter days) also contributes to CAUTI risk. Likelihood increases 3% to 7% daily; by 1 month, the risk is nearly 100% (IHI, 2011). In LTACHs, there is a potential for a higher incidence of inappropriately retained indwelling urinary catheters because of a misunderstanding of their necessity or lack of clear removal orders. LTACHs have a higher rate than almost all other healthcare sites for CAUTI-pooled mean rates and urinary catheter device use ratios (CDC, n.d.; NHSN, 2014). Patients in LTACHs depend on nurses to provide optimal care, including controlling nosocomial-type infections.

Several evidence-based CAUTI prevention guidelines exist that support a decrease of catheter days through nurse-led initiatives. This EBQI project was implemented within a large LTACH where CAUTI incidence was tracked through infection control surveillance. The CAUTI Standardized Infection Ratio (SIR) goal rate was defined by CMS in 2015 as 1.03 per 1,000 catheter days (CDC, 2015). In 2015, surveillance showed the CAUTI rate for the study LTACH was above the national rate (CDC, 2018). Thus, CAUTIs became a target for rate reduction. This project's purpose was to develop and implement a nurse-led, EBP urinary catheter protocol (UCP) and measure the impact on catheter days and CAUTI rates among CCI patients in a large LTACH. Goals included meeting national quality metric benchmarks for CAUTIs and implementing education, based on current best practice evidence.

PICO(T) (Step #1 in EBP)

The goal of this project was to implement a nurse-led, EBP UCP to reduce CAUTI. Literature to support this project was collected based on the following PICO(T) question: In the adult long-term acute care patient (P), how does the implementation of a nursing UCP on admission (I) compared with no protocol (C) affect CAUTI rates (O) over a 3-month period?

Search for the Evidence (Step #2 in EBP)

A systematic review of the literature was conducted focused on the PICO(T). The search strategy included an electronic database search of published and unpublished articles extracted from PubMed, MEDLINE, CINAHL, and the Cochrane database for systematic and peer reviews to identify keywords within the title used to describe relevant interventions. A systematic search of the literature was done using the keywords: "EBP," "catheter urinary tract infection," "urinary tract infection," "LTACH CAUTI rates," "nursing intervention," "effects on nursing education," "decreasing CAUTIs," "indwelling urinary catheter," "education," and "clinical practice guidelines." Boolean searches using keywords such as "CAUTI," "CAUTI rates," and "indwelling urinary catheter" found 375 total articles and 75 direct articles that matched nursing interventions used to decrease CAUTIs. When LTACH was added, the search narrowed to 37 individual articles, two systematic reviews, and six major guidelines that addressed the PICO(T) question.

Critical Appraisal of the Evidence (Step #3 in EBP)

To determine whether the literature identified in the search was "relevant, valid, and reliable, and applicable to the clinical question" (Fineout-Overholt, Melnyk, Stillwell, & Williamson, 2010b, p. 52), a RCA was undertaken. In appraising the level of the evidence based on the 16 individual studies and one systematic review were incorporated in the body of evidence to be synthesized. An evaluation table was developed to organize studies, and synthesis tables were used to distinguish similarities, differences, and common themes among the findings in the pertinent studies (Fineout-Overholt et al., 2010c, Part II). On the basis of the appraisal and synthesis of the evidence, discrepancies were noted between the research evidence, best practice, and the current practice in the LTACH. It was evident that a practice change was needed to provide the best care possible to the patients.

Integration of the Evidence With a Clinician's Expertise and a Patient's Preferences and Values in Making a Decision/Implementation (Step #4 in EBP)

Highlights from the literature review were summarized and used to plan an intervention. Current nursing practices were evaluated against CDC recommendations. On the basis of the findings, practice changes were identified, with the goal of improving CAUTI rates among LTACH patients. Next, stakeholders were identified to act as CAUTI champions to support change, remove barriers, and act as champions for evidence-based care. The CAUTI champions revised the existing admissions protocol to include current best practice, with an emphasis on first assessment upon admission into the LTACH.

The new CAUTI protocol was developed and reviewed by content experts and the CAUTI champions. The CAUTI program was developed integrating the best practice evidence-based aspects of previous studies of intervention programs into a multidimensional protocol algorithm. The project was first introduced to the nurses via the secure email server as well as in monthly staff meetings.

Before implementing the new protocol, systemwide educational sessions were provided via synchronous elearning sessions to all nurses. Toolkits were available and included a copy of the new policy and protocol, the electronic medical record (EMR) flow chart outlining processes, and a urinary catheter kit with supplies for any RN to use. Moreover, each nurse received a quick reference pocket guide to use as a resource with CDC indications of catheter device usage. The toolkit information included best practices, with information on topics related to CAUTI, epidemiology and scope of the problem, risk factors, definitions, prevention, strategies to reduce CAUTI, and the new UCP.

Evaluation of Outcomes (Step #5 in EBP)

Evaluation of outcomes included patient CAUTI rates. There were 115 qualifying patient admissions during this evaluation period. Primary outcomes measured were number of catheter days and hospital-acquired CAUTI rates. Overall urinary catheter days decreased from 2,697 to 2,423, a reduction of 274 catheter days (10.1%). CAUTI rates were calculated using the number of hospital-acquired urinary tract infections/number of catheter days × 1,000. After the education sessions, CAUTI incidence decreased from 13 to 3 (77%). This number represented a statistically significant ($z = 1.0, p < .03$, two tailed) reduction of CAUTIs following the educational intervention. Subsequently, the hospital-acquired CAUTI rate per 1,000 catheter days decreased from 4.82 to 1.24 (74%) although the total number of patient days increased by 1.3%. The absolute risk reduction (ARR) to determine event rates was 3.58 infections per 1,000 catheter days.

Dissemination (Step #6 in EBP)

The team disseminated the results of the project at internal and external meetings. Internally, reports were provided to the quality council and committees across the organization including a final report being sent to the leadership group. Externally, the project has been submitted for publication and is currently under review.

AN EVIDENCE-BASED PROTOCOL TO IMPROVE TREATMENT COMPLIANCE AND DECREASE TIME TO TREAT FOR EMPLOYEES EXPOSED TO INFECTIOUS DISEASES

Reginald R. Pryear Jr., DNP, MBA, RN, NEA-BC and
David P. Hrabe, PhD, RN, NC-BC

Background/Significance of the Problem (Step #0 in EBP)

Healthcare professionals, particularly nurses, are often exposed to microorganisms that can cause serious or even lethal infections (Efstathiou, Papastavrou, Raftopoulos, & Merkouris, 2011). As one example in the United States, invasive meningococcal disease has a high morbidity rate with 75,000 cases occurring annually resulting in 26,000 to 42,000 hospitalizations (Harrell & Hammes, 2012). Because exposure to meningitis can lead to serious complications for the healthcare provider and/or lead to secondary exposures, it is vital for hospital staff members to be seen as soon as an exposure is identified (Stuart et al., 2001).

Because healthcare is now considered to be a high-hazard and high-risk industry for both patients and workers (The Joint Commission, 2012), employee health departments of healthcare organizations are reshaping their screening and treatment protocols to protect their employees from contracting virulent infectious diseases. As manager of a large, midwestern medical center's Employee Health Department, Dr. Pryear noted that during a 2-year time frame, 679 employees had significant exposures to three infectious diseases: tuberculosis, Neisseria meningitis, and varicella. A closer examination of 1-year events showed that out of the 13 exposure events, only 44% of hospital staff members were seen in the optimal time frame and that the majority (56%) of staff members were screened outside of the optimal time frame or were never screened at all.

The purpose of this DNP project was to create an evidence-based protocol to improve treatment compliance as well as "time to treat" among employees exposed to select infectious diseases by moving the point of care from central Employee Health to on-site screening and expanding service hours to better accommodate physicians, advanced practice providers, residents, medical students, nurses, PCAs, respiratory therapists, and housekeepers from all three shifts.

The PICO(T) Question (Step #1 in EBP)

The PICO(T) question for this project was: "In hospital staff members (Population) who have been exposed to select infectious diseases, does on-site screening and treatment (Intervention) versus centralized screening and treatment (Comparison) impact time to treat and compliance within the appropriate time frame (Time)?" Key words from the PICO(T) question were used to search CINAHL, PubMed, and Cochrane databases.

Search for the Evidence (Step #2 in EBP)

The search terms that were used in the databases were "meningitis" and "protocol" (425 articles), "meningitis" and "hospital worker" (9 articles), and "meningitis" and "hospital-acquired infections" (51 articles). In addition, "varicella and protocol" (17) and "varicella and hospital worker" were used (35). "Tuberculosis" and "protocol" (199) were also used. Furthermore, "occupational health services" and "health screenings" (555) were used. Finally, occupational "health screenings" and "point-of-care testing" were used (6). After the initial search, another search was conducted and key search words were used to obtain additional information. Search terms were broadened to include "infectious diseases" and "on-site screening and treatment" (16). There were no time limits placed on the search. Information that was found ranged from 1978 to 2014. On further review, six articles related to "barrier removal" and "reducing time to treat" were chosen for critical appraisal.

Critical Appraisal and Synthesis of the Evidence (Step #3)

After critically evaluating the evidence, two themes that could apply to this project emerged. The first theme was to remove or address barriers that make it more difficult for staff to be screened and treated. van Dulmen et al. (2007; Level VII Evidence) and Bender, Milgrom, and Apter (2003; Level VII Evidence) posited that removing technical barriers such as location and time limitations improved patient adherence.

The second theme, point-of-care screening to improve time to treat and patient engagement, was identified in several different settings. Renaud et al. (2008; Level II Evidence) conducted a randomized trial in the emergency department (ED) using point-of-care testing to successfully reduce time to treat. Singer, Ardise, Gulla, and Cangro (2005; Level IV Evidence) trialed point-of-care testing in the emergency room for patients with chest pain to improve turnaround time and facilitate treatment. Laurence et al. (2009; Level II Evidence) found that patient satisfaction with point-of-care testing improved and that patients thought having immediate feedback was important to being more engaged in their treatment. Gialamas et al. (2009; Level II Evidence) found similar positive responses by patients and also noted that point-of-care testing was very useful to providers because they could make immediate decisions based on the results and discuss the results/plan of care with the patient in a more timely manner. Although the settings where these studies occurred were in the ED and general practice, it was reasoned that point-of-care screening with expanded hours would remove existing barriers to decrease time to treat, improve compliance, and would be beneficial in the employee health context.

Integration of the Evidence With a Clinician's Expertise and a Patient's Preferences and Values in Making a Decision/Implementation (Step #4 in EBP)

Feedback from hospital staff members during past exposures indicated that employees found it difficult to be screened in the Employee Health office because of the distance from their work unit and the time it took to do so. In addition, employees reported that Employee Health's typical business-day hours of operation were another significant barrier. Clearly, the employees' experience was inconsistent with the medical center's mission to provide excellent clinical service. The evidence reviewed for the project provided easy-to-implement and low-cost practices to address employee concerns. As a result of the feedback and a review of evidence, a protocol was developed to provide on-site screenings at hours convenient to employees and was approved as a QI project through standardized institutional review board (IRB) protocols. The project was reviewed for relevancy and feasibility through the medical center's Feasibility Review Committee.

An opportunity to implement on-site screening occurred within the specified time frame (details have been redacted to maintain confidentiality). A male patient was admitted to the medical center ED for a gunshot wound to the chest. Over the next 3 days, he was taken to the operating room (OR) and eventually transferred to the SICU. On the fourth day of admission, specimens were collected from a Broncho Alveolar Lavage (BAL) and antibiotics were started for a suspected infection. On the evening of the 7th day of admission, laboratory tests confirmed *Neisseria meningitidis*[1]. On the 8th day of admission, the Clinical Epidemiology Department issued an exposure notification memo to the ED, OR, SICU, Anesthesia Department, and Respiratory Therapy Department. Because *Neisseria meningitidis* requires droplet isolation, all employees who had contact with the patient's respiratory secretions for 4 admission days during the time the patient was not being treated for meningitis needed to be identified by the appropriate manager and consequently screened by the Employee Health Department. Once identified, employees were personally evaluated to determine whether they provided care during the unprotected period. The Employee Health staff was quickly assembled to develop screening days and times for this exposure, as well as securing a location within proximity of the majority of exposed staff. Six on-site screening clinics were scheduled over 4 days and at various times to serve different shifts.

Evaluation of Outcomes (Step #5 in EBP)

The following measures were used to evaluate the effect of the project on key project outcome indicators:

- Percentage of employees seen within the optimal time frame
- Percentage of employees seen beyond the optimal time frame
- Percentage of employees never seen
- Overall satisfaction score with point-of-care screening/treatment
- Cost and time savings

Implementing on-site screening improved the overall compliance of healthcare workers seen within the optimal time frame. The percentage of healthcare workers who were never screened decreased dramatically from 53% (in previous exposures of the same type) to 2%. A delay in initially identifying the presence of the disease resulted in most employees not being seen within the optimum 3-day time frame, but 94% of healthcare workers on the exposure list were seen within 3 days of identification. Excluding the

---

[1]*Neisseria meningitidis* is a Gram-negative bacterium that leads to meningitis. *Neisseria meningitidis* will be referenced as meningitis moving forward throughout this document.

delayed diagnosis time period, this pilot project improved the number of healthcare workers seen in the first 3 days of notification. The percentage of employees who were treated with Cipro (the antibiotic of choice) in this incident was higher than in past, similar exposures: 32 of 89 employees (35.9%) compared with 30 of 110 (27.3%).

There were several healthcare workers who were not on the exposure list but who presented for screening representing 18 employees who would not have otherwise been screened. Because of point-of-care screening, they were made aware of a potential exposure through word of mouth from colleagues and chose to self-identify as being at risk. Postexposure prophylaxis was recommended for 32 of the 89 (35.9%) workers on the exposure list and 10 of 18 (55.6%) of those who self-identified. After the screening process was complete, screened employees were asked to complete a survey. The survey consisted of five questions related to (a) satisfaction with location, (b) screening times, (c) service, (d) provided information, and (e) an open-ended question. Seventy-eight employees out of 105 employees who were screened completed the survey (74% response rate).

There was a high level of satisfaction from this pilot project related to questions 1 to 4 (93.2%–99.1% indicated "very satisfied"). Employees indicated in the open-ended question that they were very satisfied with this new process, and they felt it was very convenient for them to be screened. The Employee Health staff received written feedback such as "everything was perfect and convenient," "very easy to stop for screening," and "everything seemed very forward and helpful." Two ED staff members indicated that the location was not ideal for them.

Historically, the majority of employees who have been exposed to infectious diseases were either not screened in a timely manner or were not seen at all. The main focus of this pilot project was to implement a point-of-service screening approach to improve two key outcomes: the proportion of employees seen within 10 days of the event and the proportion of employees who were seen.

Travel time and wait time were decreased when Employee Health staff screened and treated employees on the unit. Owing to the range of employees who were screened during an exposure, the Medical Center's average employee rate of $30/hour was used to calculate the projected savings. Employee Health accrued minimal overtime to implement the project. On analysis, the project to improve treatment compliance, time to treat, and employee satisfaction was found to be budget neutral.

Overall, this intervention was successful because it was received positively by staff and it accomplished the goals that were established. The Employee Health staff screened physicians, residents, anesthesiologists, nurses, respiratory therapists, nurses' aides, sitters, and housekeeping staff. For each staff member, the process took less than 4 minutes, including the time it took for employees to complete the satisfaction survey. The vast majority of staff were appreciative that the Employee Health staff came to their department. One of the anesthesiologists shared relief for not having to leave his assigned area, noting that time constraints would have made it difficult otherwise. As a result of on-site screening, time to treat and compliance were greatly improved. This success lends support to use this project's approach in future exposures to provide better support for the employees.

Dissemination (Step #6 in EBP)
Project results were disseminated internally to both hospital Infection Prevention Committees for this medical center. They track all exposure events and assist with advocating for additional resources in the future. The project results were also shared at the Nurse Executive Council, which is a gathering of chief nursing officers and various nursing leaders throughout the medical center. This is to inform them about the screening and treatment of their staff. External dissemination activities included presenting this project at Ohio State University's College of Nursing during a public oral defense. Following that, a poster was presented at the Midwest

Nursing Research Society in April of 2017. This conference provides opportunities for students to learn about innovative research projects and new scientific methods and enables them to have thoughtful discussions with other nursing faculty and students throughout the country.

Historically, the majority of employees who were exposed to infectious diseases were either not screened in a timely manner or were not seen at all. The main focus of this pilot project was to implement a point-of-service screening approach to improve two key outcomes: the proportion of employees seen within 10 days of the event and the proportion of employees who were never seen. Overall, this intervention was successful because it accomplished the established goals and was positively received by staff. For each staff member, the process took less than 4 minutes, including the time it took for employees to complete the satisfaction survey.

Although the project successfully reduced the time to treat and overall compliance with screening, some systems issues were not addressed by this project. One limitation that was not addressed in this project is the manual identification of exposed employees. Creating this list is labor intensive and takes a great deal of time to complete. The Employee Health staff must rely on managers to generate an accurate list in a timely manner. Another area of concern is about those employees who were never notified of the exposure but who self-identified for screening. Without implementation of on-site screening, the active word-of-mouth activity would not have occurred and these employees would not have been screened and treated. Automated identification would address this issue.

Prior to the project, finding space that was proximal to exposed employees' work areas was a concern. Fortunately for this project, finding space was not an issue. For future exposures, however, not having proximal space is an important barrier to overcome.

Key Points From This Chapter

- QI has been defined as a systematic process used by healthcare systems to analyze existing data and improve its processes and/or outcomes for a specific patient population.
- Not all QI models or projects are evidence based.
- Incorporation of the search for and critical appraisal of a body of evidence to guide best practice decisions should be incorporated into QI, which then transforms it to EBQI.
- It is important to incorporate "so what" outcomes (i.e., those that are currently important to the healthcare system, such as core performance metrics and cost) into EBQI projects.
- EBQI should follow the seven-step EBP process.

REFERENCES

American Association of Critical Care Nurses. (2010). American Association of Critical Care Nurses practice alert: Ventilator-associated pneumonia. Retrieved from https://www.aacn.org/clinical-resources/practice-alerts/ventilator-associated-pneumonia-vap

Augustyn, B. (2007). Ventilator-associated pneumonia: Risk factors and prevention. Critical Care Nurse, 27(4), 32–36, 38–39; quiz 40.

Bender, B., Milgrom, H., & Apter, A. (2003). Adherence intervention research: What have we learned and what do we do next? *Journal of Allergy and Clinical Immunology, 112*(3), 489–494.

Brewer, B. B., & Alexandrov, A. W. (2015). The role of outcomes and quality improvement in enhancing and evaluating practice changes. In B. M. Melnyk & E. Fineout-Overholt (Eds.), *Evidence-based practice in nursing & healthcare: A guide to best practice* (3rd ed., pp. 224–234). Philadelphia, PA: Wolters Kluwer.

Centers for Disease Control and Prevention. (n.d.). Operational guidance for long term care hospitals to report catheter-associated urinary tract infection (CAUTI) data to CDC's NHSN for the purpose of fulfilling CMS's quality reporting requirements. Retrieved from http://www.cdc.gov/nhsn/PDFs/LTACH/8-6-2012-LTCH-CAUTI-Guidance.pdf

Centers for Disease Control and Prevention. (2015). National Healthcare Safety Network. Retrieved from http://www.cdc.gov/nhsn

Centers for Disease Control and Prevention. (2018). Urinary tract infection (catheter-associated urinary tract infection [CAUTI] and non-catheter-associated urinary tract infection [UTI]) and other urinary system infection [USI]) events. Retrieved from http://www.cdc.gov/nhsn/pdfs/pscmanual/7psccauticurrent.pdf

Centers for Medicare & Medicaid Services. (2014). HCAHPS: Patients' perspectives of care survey. Retrieved from https://www.cms.gov/Medicare/Quality-Initiatives-Patient-Assessment-Instruments/HospitalQualityInits/HospitalHCAHPS.html

Cooper, K. L. (2013). Evidence-based prevention of pressure ulcers in the intensive care unit. *Critical Care Nurse, 33*(6), 57–66. doi:10.4037/ccn2013985

Efstathiou, G., Papastavrou, E., Raftopoulos, V., & Merkouris, A. (2011). Factors influencing nurses' compliance with standard precautions in order to avoid occupational exposure to microorganisms: A focus group study. *BMC Nursing, 10*(1), 1. doi:10.1186/1472-6955-10-1

Fineout-Overholt, E., Melnyk, B. M., Stillwell, S. B., & Williamson, K. M. (2010a). Critical appraisal of the evidence: Part III: The process of synthesis: Seeing similarities and differences across the body of evidence. American Journal of Nursing, 110(11), 43–51.

Fineout-Overholt, E., Melnyk, B. M., Stillwell, S. B., & Williamson, K. M. (2010b). Evidence-based practice step by step: Critical appraisal of the evidence: Part I. *American Journal of Nursing, 110*(7), 47–52. doi:10.1097/01.NAJ.0000383935.22721.9c

Fineout-Overholt, E., Melnyk, B. M., Stillwell, S. B., & Williamson, K. M. (2010c). Evidence-based practice, step by step: Critical appraisal of the evidence: Part II: Digging deeper—examining the 'keeper' studies. *American Journal of Nursing, 110*(9), 41–48. doi:10.1097/01.NAJ.0000388264.49427.f9

Friese, C. R., Grunawalt, J. C., Bhullar, S., Bihlmeyer, K., Chang, R., & Wood, W. (2014). Pod nursing on a medical/surgical unit: Implementation and outcomes evaluation. *Journal of Nursing Administration, 44*(4), 207–211. doi:10.1097/NNA.0000000000000051

Gage, W. (2015). Preventing pressure ulcers in patients in intensive care. *Nursing Standard, 29*(26), 53–61. doi:10.7748/ns.29.26.53.e9657

Genao, L., & Buhr, G. (2012). Urinary tract infections in older adults residing in long term care facilities. *Annals of Long-Term Care: Clinical Care and Aging, 20*(4), 33–38.

Gialamas, A., Yelland, L. N., Ryan, P., Willson, K., Laurence, C. O., Bubner, T. K., … Beilby, J. J. (2009). Does point-of-care testing lead to the same or better adherence to medication? A randomized controlled trial: The POCT in general practice trial. *Medical Journal of Australia, 191*(9), 487–491.

Hall, C., McCutcheon, H., Deuter, K., & Matricciani, L. (2012). Evaluating and improving a model of nursing care delivery: A process of partnership. *Collegian, 19*(4), 203–210.

Harrell, T., & Hammes, J. S. (2012). Meningitis admitted to a military hospital: A retrospective case series. *Military Medicine, 177*(10), 1223–1226.

Hockenberry, M. J., Brown, T. L., & Rodgers, C. C. (2014). Implementing evidence in clinical settings. In B. M. Melnyk & E. Fineout-Overholt (Eds.), *Evidence-based practice in nursing & healthcare: A guide to best practice* (3rd ed., pp. 202–223). Philadelphia, PA: Wolters Kluwer.

Institute for Healthcare Improvement. (2010). Implement the ventilator bundle: Daily oral care with chlorhexidine. Retrieved from http://www.ihi.org/IHI/Topics/CriticalCare/IntensiveCare/Changes/IndividualChages/DailyOralCarewithChlorhexidine.htm

Institute for Healthcare Improvement. (2011). How-to guide: Prevent catheter-associated urinary tract infections. Retrieved from http://www.ihi.org/resources/Pages/Tools/HowtoGuidePreventCatheterAssociatedUrinaryTractInfection.aspx

The Joint Commission. (2012). *Improving patient and worker safety opportunities for synergy, collaboration and innovation.* Oakbrook Terrace, IL: Author. http://www.jointcommission.org

Kahn, J. M., Le, T., Angus, D. C., Cox, C. E., Hough, C. L., White, D. B., & … Carson, S. S. (2015). The epidemiology of chronic critical illness in the United States. *Critical Care Medicine, 43*(2), 282–287. doi:10.1097/CCM.0000000000000710

Kring, D. L. (2008). Research and quality improvement: Different processes, different evidence. MEDSURG Nursing, 17(3), 162–169.

Laurence, C. O., Gialamas, A., Bubner, T., Yelland, L., Willson, K., Ryan, P., & Beilby, J. (2009). Patient satisfaction with point-of-care testing in general practice. *British Journal of General Practice*, 60(572), e98–e104. doi:10.3399/bjgp10X483508

Makary, M. A., & Daniel, M. (2016). Medical error: The third leading cause of death in the U.S. *BMJ, 353*, i2139. doi:10.1136/bmj.i2139

Melnyk, B. M. (2016). The evidence-based practice competencies related to outcomes evaluation. In B. M. Melnyk, L. Gallagher-Ford., & E. Fineout-Overholt, (Eds.), *Implementing the evidence-based practice competencies in healthcare: A practical guide for improving quality, safety & outcomes* (pp. 129–142). Indianapolis, IN: Sigma Theta Tau International.

Melnyk, B. M., Buck, J., & Gallagher-Ford, L. (2015). Transforming quality improvement into evidence-based quality improvement: A key solution to improve healthcare outcomes. *Worldviews on Evidence Based Nursing, 12*(5), 251–252. doi:10.1111/wvn.12112

Melnyk, B. M., & Fineout-Overholt, E. (2015). *Evidence-based practice in nursing & healthcare: A guide to best practice* (3rd ed.). Philadelphia, PA: Wolters Kluwer.

Melnyk, B. M., & Fineout-Overholt, E. (2019). *Evidence-based practice in nursing and healthcare. A guide to best practice* (4th ed.). Philadelphia, PA: Wolters Kluwer.

Minnier, T. E., Brownlee, K., Kosko, R., Kowinsky, A., Martin, S. C., McLaughlin, M., & ... Young, J. (2012). Reliable and variable rounder care delivery model for nursing assistants and patient care technicians. *Nurse Leader, 10*(5), 28–35. doi:10.1016/j.mnl.2012.07.005

Murray, C. J., & Frenk, J. (2010). Ranking 37th: Measuring the performance of the U.S. health care system. *New England Journal of Medicine, 362*, 98–99. doi:10.1056/NEJMp0910064

National Healthcare Safety Network. (2014). Catheter-associated urinary tract infection outcome measure. Retrieved from http://www.hospitalsafetyscore.org/media/file/CAUTI.pdf

O'Keefe-McCarthy, S., Santiago, C., & Lau, G. (2008). Ventilator-associated pneumonia bundled strategies: An evidence-based practice. Worldviews on Evidence-Based Nursing, 5(4), 193–204. doi:10.1111/j.1741-6787.2008.00140.x

Press Ganey. (2017). Caregiver experience: Achieve cultural transformation across the organization. Retrieved from http://www.pressganey.com/consulting/caregiver-experience

Renaud, B., Maison, P., Ngako, A., Cunin, P., Santin, A., Hervé, J., ... Roupie, E. (2008). Impact of point of-care testing in the emergency department evaluation and treatment of patients with suspected acute coronary syndromes. Academic Emergency Medicine, 15(3). 216–224. doi:10.1111/j.1553-2712.2008.00069.x

Rudisill, P. T., Callis, C., Hardin, S. R., Dienemann, J., & Samuelson, M. (2014). Care redesign: A higher-quality, lower-cost model for acute care. Journal of Nursing Administration, 44(7/8), 388–394. doi:10.1097/NNA.0000000000000088

Shirey, M. R., Hauck, S. L., Embree, J. L., Kinner, T. J., Schaar, G. L., Phillips, L. A., ... McCool, I. A. (2011). Showcasing differences between quality improvement, evidence-based practice, and research. Journal of Continuing Education in Nursing, 42(2), 57–68. doi:10.3928/00220124-20100701-01

Singer, A. J., Ardise, J., Gulla, J., & Cangro, J. (2005). Point-of-care testing reduces length of stay in emergency department chest pain patients. *Annals of Emergency Medicine, 45*(6), 587–591. doi:10.1016/j.annemergmed.2004.11.020

Stefancyk, A. L. (2009). Improving processes of care: Making changes that hit and miss. American Journal of Nursing, 109(6), 36–37. doi:10.1097/01.NAJ.0000352470.81295.ee

Strouse, A. C. (2015). Appraising the literature on bathing practices and catheter-associated urinary tract infection prevention. Urologic Nursing, 35(1), 11–17.

Stuart, J. M., Gilmore, A. B., Ross, A., Patterson, W., Kroll, J. S., Kaczmarski, E. B., ... Monk, P. (2001) Preventing secondary meningococcal disease in health care workers: Recommendations of a working group of the PHLS meningococcus forum. *Communicable Disease and Public Health, 4*(2), 102–105.

Swafford, K., Culpepper, R., & Dunn, C. (2016). Use of a comprehensive program to reduce the incidence of hospital-acquired pressure ulcers in an intensive care unit. *American Journal of Critical Care. 25*(2), 152–155. doi:10.4037/ajcc2016963

Tolentino-DelosReyes, A. F., Ruppert, S. D., & Shiao, S. Y. (2007). Evidence-based practice: Use of the ventilator bundle to prevent ventilator-associated pneumonia. *American Journal of Critical Care, 16*(1), 20–27.

van Dulmen, S., Sluijs, E., van Dijk, L., de Ridder, D., Heerdink, R., & Bensing, J. (2007). Patient adherence to medical treatment: A review of reviews. *BMC Health Services Research, 7,* 55. doi:10.1186/1472-6963-7-55

Westwell, S. (2008). Implementing a ventilator care bundle in an adult are unit. *Nursing in Critical Care, 13*(4), 203–207. doi: 10.1111/j.1478-5153.2008.00279.x

Zurmehly, J. (2013). Oral care education in the prevention of ventilator-associated pneumonia: Quality patient outcomes in the intensive care unit. *Journal of Continuing Education in Nursing, 44*(2), 67–75. doi:10.3928/00220124-20121203-16

APPENDIX A

1. Brackett, T., Comer, L., & Whichello, R. (2013). Do lean practices lead to more time at the bedside? *Journal For Healthcare Quality: Official Publication of the National Association for Healthcare Quality, 35* (2), 7 –14. doi:10.1111/j.1945-1474.2011.00169.x

FIRST AUTHOR (YEAR)	CONCEPTUAL FRAMEWORK	DESIGN/ METHOD	SAMPLE/ SETTING	MAJOR VARIABLES STUDIED (AND THEIR DEFINITIONS)	MEASUREMENT	DATA ANALYSIS	FINDINGS	APPRAISAL: WORTH TO PRACTICE
Brackett, (2013) Do lean practices lead to more time at the bedside?		Systematic review				1. Articles that discuss application of lean or TCAB 2. Articles based on actual case studies of lean principles or TCAB 3. Literature reviews related to lean processed or TCAB	TCAB goal to improve care, improve experience of care, improve teamwork, improve nursing satisfaction, nurse retention and added value Decrease in harm from falls, a decrease in code events, and decreased admissions Six of 10 decreased falls Increase in nursing spending more time at bedside	Keywords: nursing quality, six sigma/lean, transforming care at the bedside TCAB used PDSA cycles "It is evident that our success is a result of the nurses being at the bedside, caring and interacting with patients and using the principles of lean"

2. Donahue, L. (2009). A pod design for nursing assignments: Eliminating unnecessary steps and increasing patient satisfaction by reconfiguring care assignments. *American Journal of Nursing, 109* (11), 38–40. doi:10.1097/01.NAJ.0000362019.47504.9d

FIRST AUTHOR (YEAR)	CONCEPTUAL FRAMEWORK	DESIGN/ METHOD	SAMPLE/ SETTING	MAJOR VARIABLES STUDIED (AND THEIR DEFINITIONS)	MEASUREMENT	DATA ANALYSIS	FINDINGS	APPRAISAL: WORTH TO PRACTICE
Donahue, (2009) A pod design for nursing assignments: Eliminating unnecessary steps and increasing patient satisfaction by reconfiguring care assignments		TCAB	Thirty-eight-bed cardio-thoracic and vascular surgery unit, academic medical center. Pods covered 100 feet each	Divided unit into four pods composed of 10, 10, nine, and nine patients each. Two RNs per pod	1. Spaghetti diagram of nurse without pod, then same nurse in pod 2. Patient satisfaction scores 3. Time devoted to value-added patient care		1. Erratic spaghetti diagram prior to pod implementation, after implementation spaghetti diagram less erratic but improved workflow 2. Consistent and sustained improvement in patient satisfaction scores after implementation 3. Time value-added care increased	The pod design for care assignments has improved patient satisfaction by increasing the visibility and accessibility of nurses and enhanced nurses' ability to provide safe and reliable care

(continued)

3. Friese, C. R., Grunawalt, J. C., Bhullar, S., Bihlmeyer, K., Chang, R., & Wood, W. (2014). Pod nursing on a medical/surgical unit: Implementation and outcomes evaluation. *Journal Of Nursing Administration, 44* (4), 207–211. doi:10.1097/NNA.0000000000000051

4. Hall, C., McCutcheon, H., Deuter, K., & Matricciani, L. (2012). Evaluating and improving a model of nursing care delivery: A process of partnership. *Collegian, 19* (4), 203–210. doi:10.1016/j.colegn.2012.07.003

FIRST AUTHOR (YEAR)	CONCEPTUAL FRAMEWORK	DESIGN/METHOD	SAMPLE/SETTING	MAJOR VARIABLES STUDIED (AND THEIR DEFINITIONS)	MEASUREMENT	DATA ANALYSIS	FINDINGS	APPRAISAL: WORTH TO PRACTICE
Friese, (2014) Pod nursing on a medical/ surgical unit: Implementation and outcomes evaluation	Physical and process redesign	Quality improvement project	Thirty-two-bed MS unit University of Michigan Health System	Divided unit into four pods composed of eight patients each Two RNs per pod	1. Patient outcomes satisfaction 2. Call lights—total # of calls recorded by system 3. Falls with/without injury per 1,000 patient-days 4. Nurse outcomes satisfaction—5-item questionnaire 5. Overtime—incremental overtime reported to HR on monthly basis	1. Patient satisfaction—Press Ganey satisfaction survey 2. Total # of calls registered in nurse call system 3. Falls—falls data from event reporting system 4. 5-item paper questionnaire 5. Overtime report as submitted to HR	Overall nursing satisfaction increased from 84.8 to 86.9; # of call lights decreased over study period, showing a linear decline over study period. Total falls demonstrated similar linear decline over study period	Improved workflow, improved teamwork, staff reported increased efficiency; will need to use nurse servers to have supplies readily available in all areas of unit
Hall, (2012) Evaluating and improving a model of nursing care delivery: A process of partnership	PAR Cyclic participatory process of gaining evidence used to bring change to the workplace	General surgical ward in private hospital	Evaluating and improving the model of nursing care delivery to patients	Qualitative theme identification	Descriptive and interpretive approach	Lack of shared understanding of the "Team Nursing" approach	Patient-centered care was linked to increased job satisfaction for nursing staff	

FIRST AUTHOR (YEAR)	CONCEPTUAL FRAMEWORK	DESIGN/ METHOD	SAMPLE/ SETTING	MAJOR VARIABLES STUDIED (AND THEIR DEFINITIONS)	MEASUREMENT	DATA ANALYSIS	FINDINGS	APPRAISAL: WORTH TO PRACTICE
Minnier, (2012) Reliable and variable rounder care delivery model for nursing assistants and patient care technicians	Redesign model of care	Quality project	Thirty-six-bed MS unit in academic women's hospital	Predictable or unpredictable tasks for PCAs Two PCAs assigned to 18 patients each to complete predictable tasks One PCA serves as VR covering all 36 patients for unpredictable tasks	1. Response time to call lights 2. Blood work turnaround time 3. Patient return to unit and seen by staff 4. Managing interruptions		Response to call lights (time) decreased from 1 to 14 minutes to 0 to 2 minutes Blood test turnaround time decreased from 10 to 150 minutes to 8 to 28 minutes Patients returning to unit time decreased from 9 minutes to 2 minutes	Helping staff at all levels to understand the design flaws in traditional work distribution; engaging the staff to understand the concepts of predictable and unpredictable work

5. Minnier, T. E., Brownlee, K., Kosko, R., Kowinsky, A., Martin, S. C., McLaughlin, M., & . . . Young, J. (2012). Reliable and variable rounder care delivery model for nursing assistants and patient care technicians. *Nurse Leader, 10* (5), 28 –35. doi:10.1016/j.mnl.2012.07.005

FIRST AUTHOR (YEAR)	CONCEPTUAL FRAMEWORK	DESIGN/ METHOD	SAMPLE/ SETTING	MAJOR VARIABLES STUDIED (AND THEIR DEFINITIONS)	MEASUREMENT	DATA ANALYSIS	FINDINGS	APPRAISAL: WORTH TO PRACTICE
Musanti, (2012) Partners in caring: An innovative nursing model of care delivery	Promoting action of research		600-bed Magnet® facility		1. RN work time 2. Documentation 3. NA work	Standard quality improvement time study	1. RN spend 20% in non-value-added time (delegatable tasks) 2. Documentation taking 18% of time, redundant at time 3. NA work load too high, not being used to full potential	Implemented a clinical coordinator type position Recommen-dation for only certified NA Use of rapid cycle change process

6. Musanti, R., O'Keefe, T., & Silverstein, W. (2012). Partners in caring: An innovative nursing model of care delivery. *Nursing Administration Quarterly, 36* (3), 217–224. doi:10.1097/ NAQ.0b013e318258c256

(continued)

FIRST AUTHOR (YEAR)	CONCEPTUAL FRAMEWORK	DESIGN/ METHOD	SAMPLE/ SETTING	MAJOR VARIABLES STUDIED (AND THEIR DEFINITIONS)	MEASUREMENT	DATA ANALYSIS	FINDINGS	APPRAISAL: WORTH TO PRACTICE
7. O'Brien-Pallas, L., Meyer, R. M., Hayes, L. J., & Wang, S. (2011). The Patient Care Delivery Model–an open system framework: Conceptualisation, literature review and analytical strategy. *Journal of Clinical Nursing, 20* (11-12), 1640–1650. doi:10.1111/j.1365-2702.2010.03391.x								
O'Brien-Pallas, (2011) The patient care delivery model–an open system framework: Conceptualisation, literature review and analytical strategy		Systematic review					PCDM input, throughput and output are all factors of PCDM	PCDM is supported in the literature; PCDM needs a supportive work environment to enable good quality care When nursing units are inadequately staffed, it results in higher costs and poorer outcomes for patients and nurses
8. O'Connell, B., Duke, M., Bennett, P., Crawford, S., & Korfiatis, V. (2006). The trials and tribulations of team-nursing. *Collegian, 13* (3), 11–17. doi:10.1016/S1322-7696(08)60527-2								
O'Connell, (2006) The trials and tribulations of team-nursing	To review the team nursing approach to care	Descriptive evaluative design Quantitative/ qualitative	Two medical wards private hospital	1. Delivery of patient care 2. Teamwork 3. Role clarity and allocation of tasks 4. Team communication		Focus groups transcribed verbatim SPSS for quantitative data	Expected LOS needs to be communicated to patients and families	Team approach reinforces the RNs role as delegator and coordinator of care Minimizing barriers and enhancing the favorable factors of nursing practice to optimize delivery of patient care

FIRST AUTHOR (YEAR)	CONCEPTUAL FRAMEWORK	DESIGN/ METHOD	SAMPLE/ SETTING	MAJOR VARIABLES STUDIED (AND THEIR DEFINITIONS)	MEASUREMENT	DATA ANALYSIS	FINDINGS	APPRAISAL: WORTH TO PRACTICE
9. Rudisill, P. T., Callis, C., Hardin, S. R., Dienemann, J., & Samuelson, M. (2014). Care Redesign: A higher-quality, lower-cost model for acute care. *Journal Of Nursing Administration, 44* (7/8), 388–394. doi :10.1097/NNA.0000000000000088								
Rudisill, (2014) Care Redesign: A higher-quality, lower-cost model for acute care		Novel nursing care redesign	One MS unit at each of three hospital sites in Alabama, Tennessee, Mississippi	Balance caregiver workload; improve quality of care and nursing satisfaction	1. Clinical outcome data for falls, HCAHPS, LOS 2. Nurse satisfaction 3. Patient satisfaction 4. LOS	Paired-samples test for nursing satisfaction	Statistically significant improvement in nurse satisfaction. Patient satisfaction improved in three of eight domains. Most clinical quality indicators improved. LOS decreased by 0.39 days on average	Plan to assess patient care needs and review in huddles every 4 hours to maintain equity; e ach person working to their scope of practice. Mixed model of care: RN-UAP
10. Stefancyk, A. L. (2009). Improving processes of care: Making changes that hit and miss. *American Journal of Nursing, 109* (6), 36–37. doi:10.1097/01.NAJ.0000352470.81295.ee								
Stefancyk, (2009) Improving processes of care: Making changes that hit and miss	Pilot project			Value-added processes Documentation			Decentralizing supplies decreased the amount of distance for supply to task, which added value (time)	Decentralizing linen a big hit; moving frequently used clinical supplies to the patient's bedside. This project was implemented prior to EMR; however, the concept of double documen-tation applies with the EMR

EMR, electronic medical record; HCAHPS, Hospital Consumer Assessment of Healthcare Providers ans Systems; HR, human resources; LOS, Length of stay; MS, medical-surgical; NA, nurse assistant; PAR, Participatory Action Research; PCA, patient care associate; PCDM, Patient care delivery model; PDSA, Plan-Do-Study-Act; SPSS, Statistical Package for the Social Sciences; TCAB, Transforming Care at the Bedside; UAP, unlicensed assistive personnel; VR, Variable Rounder.

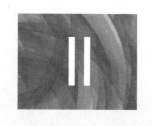

Designing Intervention Studies

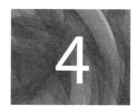

4

Using Theory to Guide Intervention Research

Julie Fleury & Souraya Sidani

The important thing is to never stop questioning. —*Albert Einstein*

Theory has an integral role in the design of interventions and studies aimed at evaluating the effects of interventions consisting of single or multiple components. Theory provides an understanding of the problem that the intervention targets, the nature of the intervention and/or its components, and the mechanisms underlying the anticipated improvement in outcomes. It also guides sample selection, operationalization of the intervention, and the specification of outcomes. Results of theory-based intervention evaluation indicate who benefits from the intervention, delivered in what context, and how the intervention and/or its components produce(s) changes in the outcomes. This knowledge is useful for translating research findings to practice and in making relevant decisions regarding the application of the intervention and/or its components in the practice setting. In this chapter, the role of theory in intervention studies is reviewed. Strategies for developing interventions are briefly described. The contribution of theory to the design of interventions and pertinent evaluation studies is clarified and illustrated with examples. Finally, sources for generating theory are identified and illustrated with examples from the literature.

ROLE OF THEORY IN INTERVENTION STUDIES

Leaders in social, behavioral, and health sciences have emphasized the importance of theory as a guide for intervention design and evaluation. At the simplest level, a theory is an explanation of why a phenomenon occurs the way it does. Theory reflects a body of knowledge that organizes, describes, predicts, and explains a phenomenon. In intervention research, theory or theoretical frameworks allow us to better represent the complexity of the situation under study. Frameworks clarify the problem targeted by the intervention, providing information on the determinants or factors causing the problem, the population experiencing the problem, the specific intervention strategies likely to address the determinants and/or to alleviate or improve management of the problem, the important steps or links of the transformation process the intervention brings about, and the specific outcomes indicating the effectiveness of intervention. Thus, theoretical frameworks guide the development of interventions that are more likely to permit strong causal inference and interpretable results (Sidani, 2015). This information is essential for developing and expanding the knowledge base for clinical practice and assisting clinicians in selecting and prescribing the most appropriate interventions.

Theoretical frameworks foster a systematic approach to intervention development and implementation that allow us to move beyond a simplistic, outcomes-focused approach to examining the central processes underlying intervention effects (Prestwich et al., 2014). In many instances, intervention effects are observed, but conclusions underlying the mechanisms for change remain isolated, without comprehensive understanding of the theory underlying intervention development, implementation, and evaluation. Theory-based interventions are central to addressing, in a sound and responsive manner, needs in the promotion of health, prevention, and management of illness as well as eliminating disparities in health and healthcare among vulnerable and underserved populations.

The use of theory as a basis for intervention design stems from an internally consistent group of relational statements specifying how the problem of interest comes about, and how that problem may be prevented, managed, or resolved. Theoretical frameworks guiding interventions are directly testable, including an integrated set of concepts, existence statements, and relational statements that link the problem to be addressed with relevant intervention strategies and the expected series of changes leading to the achievement of intended outcomes. This approach enhances sensitivity in intervention design by decreasing trial and error in design and implementation. In addition, theoretical frameworks direct the specification of various aspects of an intervention evaluation study, which contributes to enhanced validity of conclusions. Use of theoretical frameworks enables the investigator to identify what constitutes the intervention and what does not, what components or elements of the intervention are crucial, and where variation is possible, reducing the possibility of alternative rival hypotheses and strengthening internal validity (Sidani, 2015). A theory-based approach enhances construct validity through clear operationalization of the intervention, which enhances fidelity of implementation, and through specification of the intervention goals from which the outcomes are derived. Accordingly, the selected outcomes are sensitive to the intervention and the likelihood of detecting significant hypothesized effects is improved.

Theoretical frameworks are effective guides for research, practice, and the development of interventions that improve the health of the public. As a guide to intervention research, theoretical specificity allows for (a) accurate conceptualization of the problem targeted by the intervention, as well as specification of the population responsive to the intervention, (b) specification of the critical inputs that operationalize the intervention, (c) delineation of contextual factors that influence the implementation and outcomes of the intervention, including characteristics of the target population, interventionists, and setting or environment that **moderate** the effects of the intervention on outcomes, and (d) understanding of the mechanisms or processes of change yielding the expected or desired outcomes, including identification of specific **mediators** of change that can determine why an intervention was or was not successful.

Despite the acknowledged strengths of theory-based intervention research, the explication of theory in intervention development and evaluation and, in particular, the theoretically predicted mechanisms of change have been limited. Conn, Cooper, Ruppar, and Russell (2008) reviewed the published reports of 141 studies that evaluated nursing interventions. They found that, in general, the interventions under evaluation were incompletely described; 27% reported enough detailed information to replicate the intervention in another study or translate the intervention into practice. These authors indicate that although about half (52%) of the studies referenced a theoretical framework on which the intervention under evaluation was based, there was minimal explanation of the linkages between the concepts in the framework and the content of the intervention. In response to these concerns, Michie and Prestwich (2010) developed an objective approach for assessing the extent to which behavioral interventions are theory-based, as well as the degree to which intervention development and evaluation are informed by theory. Similarly, there are a very limited number of studies that clearly articulate the mechanism explaining the effects of the intervention on the selected outcomes. Hoffmann et al. (2014) introduced the Template for Intervention Description and Replication (TIDieR), an approach for specifying dimensions of interventions including characterizing the delivery and the content domain of activities that comprise the intervention.

Understanding the problem requiring management, the specific aspects of the problem addressed by the intervention, the components or elements characterizing the intervention, and the mechanism or processes underlying its effects are critical for implementing the intervention and attaining the beneficial outcomes in the context of practice. Such an understanding is generated through the application of a careful and systematic process for developing interventions.

STRATEGIES FOR INTERVENTION DEVELOPMENT

There is limited consensus on the processes central to the development of theory-based interventions. Recent frameworks have been proposed, including the Medical Research Council (MRC) framework (Craig et al., 2013), intervention mapping (IM; Kok et al., 2016), behavioral change techniques (BCT; Michie et al., 2016), and the realist approach to evaluation (Pawson & Manzano-Santaella, 2012). In addition, the multiphase optimization strategy trial (MOST) has been suggested as a strategy to build multicomponent interventions and optimize their effectiveness (Collins, Dziak, Kugler, & Trail, 2014). Although useful in providing investigators with a structured process to map intervention mechanisms to relevant aspects of the problem requiring management and to identify active intervention components that best contribute to positive outcomes, these frameworks and strategies do not explicitly explain the role of theory in intervention design. The problem-solving approach represents a useful alternative that emphasizes the clear delineation of the links between the problem and the elements or components of the intervention carefully selected to address the problem; these links also inform the specification of the mechanisms underlying the intervention effects on outcomes.

Medical Research Council Framework
The MRC framework (Craig et al., 2013) addresses approaches for developing and evaluating complex interventions using a stepwise approach starting with identifying existing evidence in support of the intervention, identifying and developing theory, and progressing to modeling, feasibility, evaluation, and implementation phases. In the MRC framework, context is central to intervention design and evaluation, including socioeconomic background, the health service systems, the characteristics of the population, the prevalence or severity of the condition studied, and how these factors change over time. Identifying existing evidence in support of the intervention clarifies what is known about similar interventions and evaluation methods. Identifying and developing theory reflects an understanding of the processes of change, drawing on empirical data and supported by preliminary research. Modeling

involves hypothesizing and **testing** both what to target (e.g., behavioral determinants of the problem) and how to do this (e.g., techniques to change these determinants). Modeling of the intervention both depends on, and informs, understanding of the underlying problem. Feasibility approaches are recommended to explore key uncertainties regarding intervention acceptability, compliance, delivery of the intervention, participant recruitment and retention, and proposed effect size. Evaluation includes selection of methodological choices, including primary and secondary outcome variables. Process evaluation is used to address fidelity of intervention implementation, clarify causal mechanisms, and identify contextual factors associated with variation in outcomes. Additional key tasks include identifying barriers to application of the intervention and considering the best achievable combination of intervention components and intensity. Implementation includes dissemination of results as widely as possible, with further research to assist and monitor the process of implementation.

Intervention Mapping

Kok et al. (2016) describe a process for intervention development, implementation, and evaluation of behavioral change interventions. This process integrates theory and evidence in (a) assessment of needs or problem analysis identifying what needs to be changed and for whom; (b) development of matrices of program objectives reflecting behaviors and behavioral determinates; (c) selection of theory-based intervention methods and practical strategies to change behavioral risk factors for health problems; (d) production of program components; (e) anticipation of program adoption, implementation, and sustainability; and (f) anticipation of process and effect evaluation. IM outlines a process from the recognition of a need or problem to the identification of a solution. Products such as program matrices, planning documents, and program materials are developed throughout each step of the process. The role of theory is most relevant during the phase of selecting program strategies relevant to each program objective where theory may guide the choice or the development of strategies to accomplish program objectives. Accordingly, interventions based on the IM approach do not have an exclusive focus on one theory, but rather they reflect a combination of the most promising theoretically derived intervention strategies for a given problem.

Behavioral Change Techniques

This approach is designed to clarify the link between intervention BCT and mechanisms of action (Michie et al., 2016). The BCT framework is designed to characterize interventions as well as provide a system for matching intervention strategies to a behavioral target, a target population, and the context in which the intervention will be delivered. The BCT approach has included a causal analysis of behavior and conditions specific to individuals in their social and physical environment, and the changes needed for a specified behavioral target to be achieved. Interventions are designed and selected according to an analysis of the nature of the behavior, the mechanisms that need to be changed to bring about behavioral change, and the interventions needed to change these mechanisms. Michie and Prestwich (2010) present a theory-coding scheme for assessing the extent to which theory has been applied to developing and evaluating interventions targeting behavioral change. The coding scheme includes six categories related to (a) reference to theory in intervention design, (b) targeting relevant theoretical constructs in intervention strategies, (c) using theory to select participants or tailor interventions, (d) measurement of relevant theoretical constructs, (e) testing mediation effects, and (f) refining theory. Understanding how theory has been applied and tested in a given body of literature provides empirical support for theory selection. Michie et al. (2015) introduced the BCT Taxonomy, a formalized approach to characterizing BCT. BCT are operationally defined to facilitate a common dialogue and description. Current research is focused on developing matrices of hypothesized links between behavioral change techniques, specific mechanisms of action, and behavioral theory (Michie et al., 2016).

Realist Evaluation Approach

The realist approach is a theory-driven strategy for evaluating single- or multiple-component interventions. It is concerned with determining not only the net effects of an intervention on outcomes, but also with generating an understanding of what intervention or components work, for whom, in what circumstances, in what respects, over which duration, and how or why (Pawson & Manzano-Santaella, 2012; Salter & Kothari, 2014).

The realist approach to evaluation assumes there is an underlying theory behind the working of an intervention. The middle-range theory explains variations in outcomes observed following the interventions relative to mechanisms and contexts; it is configured as Context–Mechanism–Outcome (CMO). Mechanisms represent how the intervention and its components are received, interpreted, and acted upon by patients to produce the outcomes (Dalkin, Greenhalgh, Jones, Cunningham, & Lhussier, 2015). Contexts are the environmental (physical and sociopolitical) and personal (physical, psychological, and sociocultural) factors that affect the implementation of the intervention, the patients' reactions and responses to the intervention, and hence, the changes in intended outcomes (Bonell, Fletcher, Morton, Lorenc, & Moore, 2012). The outcomes reflect improvement in patients' health problems or behaviors.

The application of the realist evaluation approach requires the development of the just mentioned middle-range theories before or as part of the evaluation study. This can be accomplished by reviewing and synthesizing relevant theoretical and empirical literature that informs a priori generation of the theory to guide the design and conduct of the study, and/or by incorporating qualitative methods (e.g., interviews with the persons who developed, implemented, and received the intervention) to explore the contextual factors and the mechanisms underlying the effectiveness of the intervention (Pawson & Manzano-Santaella, 2012).

Multiphase Optimization Strategy

The multiphase optimization strategy trial (MOST) is used to optimize the effectiveness of the intervention. This is done by first dismantling the intervention into its components; these include the specific and nonspecific elements that contribute to the outcomes. Second, factorial or fractional factorial designs are carried out to identify (a) the components that are active and lead to best outcomes, (b) the components that are inactive and have minimal or detrimental effects on outcomes, and (c) the extent to which one component impacts the effects of others. The results will help to revise the intervention to optimize its effects, by omitting ineffective components (Collins et al., 2014).

These frameworks and evaluation strategies provide an important guide for specifying intervention strategies and intended outcomes and offer general templates for mapping behavioral change intervention strategies to behavioral determinants. Building on these frameworks, efforts are needed to clearly articulate the nature of the links that are created when mapping intervention strategies to behavioral determinants, clarifying the mechanisms through which intervention strategies achieve effects. Without understanding these links, it will be difficult to derive the testable hypotheses, derived from the intervention middle-range theories, needed to further intervention science. Detail on the nature of the problem of interest, the context of the problem, how to use theory to conceptualize the problem of interest, and how to design an intervention responsive to the problem of interest allows greater specificity in intervention development and testing. Understanding the causal links between the problem of interest, intervention strategies, mediating variables, and intended outcomes permits an intervention to be delivered in a responsive manner, rather than in a mechanical or stereotypic format. Rothman et al. (2016) and Pawson and Manzano-Santaella (2012) have called for theory testing and refinement using a programmatic approach to clarify the underlying causal processes of behavioral change and the conditions under which these processes occur. To achieve this goal, an approach to intervention design is needed which furthers knowledge about the mechanisms underlying a theory-based intervention and the problem it is designed to address. The problem-solving approach to intervention development, which has guided our work with colleagues and students for over a decade, represents such an approach.

Problem-Solving Approach

The problem-solving approach fosters understanding the problem requiring remediation; specifying populations experiencing the problem; clarifying the intervention in terms of critical inputs needed to address the problem, including components, implementation issues and exogenous factors; and identifying the expected outcomes of the intervention. These elements are integrated to form a theory that is used to explain for whom, why, and how the intervention works in producing the outcomes, under what circumstances, and to guide the design of an intervention evaluation study. The next sections discuss what each element is about and how it contributes to the study design. Exhibit 4.1 is a list of questions to be addressed when clarifying each element of the theory.

EXHIBIT 4.1 The Problem-Solving Approach to Intervention Design

---

UNDERSTANDING THE PROBLEM OF INTEREST

- What are the manifestations and characteristics of the problem?
- What intensity, severity, and duration cause it to be labeled as a problem?
- What are the relevant antecedents to consider?
- When does the problem exist?
- What are the causative, associative, and contributing factors?
- At what level is the problem amenable to change?
- How do you want the problem to change—what are the desired outcomes?
- What would the change look like?
- Which theory best fits with the identified problem?
- How does the selected theory help to explain the problem?
- How does the theory identify how the problem comes about?
- How does the theory identify how the problem worsens or improves?
- How does the theory address antecedents and/or consequences of the problem?
- How does clinical knowledge support use of the theory?
- Does the theory reflect the experiences of the population?

SPECIFYING THE POPULATION

- Who has the problem of interest?
- Who is susceptible?
- Under what conditions is that population susceptible?
- How will you measure the existence of the problem?
- How does the problem change over time, place, events, or people?

MEDIATING PROCESSES

- Are the mediators proposed consistent with the problem of interest?
- Do the mediators explain how change will occur?
- Do the mediators clarify underlying mechanisms for change?
- Are the mediators composed of variables that are changeable?
- Is there a logical link between intervention critical inputs and mediators?
- Can the critical inputs be expected to have a direct effect on mediators?
- In what ways will critical inputs lead to change in mediators?

(continued)

EXHIBIT 4.1 The Problem-Solving Approach to Intervention Design *(continued)*

INTERVENTION THEORY—PROGRAM

- What theory addresses the change desired?
- What is the empirical support for the theory in designing intervention?
- In what ways are the focus and assumptions of the intervention theory consistent with the problem theory?
- Are there clear mechanisms for the change outlined consistent with the problem?
- Are the nature and content of the intervention critical inputs clearly specified?
- How do the specification of intervention critical inputs characterize what is necessary, what is sufficient, and what is optimal to produce the expected effects?
- In what ways do the intervention critical inputs reflect theoretical foundations?
- Is there a logical link between critical inputs and mediators?
- Can the critical inputs be expected to have a direct effect on mediators?
- In what ways will critical inputs lead to change in mediators?
- Is the context for use of the theory clearly specified?
- Is the theory relevant to the population of interest?
- Is the theory gender and culturally relevant?
- Is the theory developmentally appropriate?

STRENGTH AND DOSE

- How are the strength and dosage of the intervention characterized?
- What is the range within which the planned intervention is likely to show treatment effects?
- What is the minimal level necessary to deliver the intervention at effective strength?

EXOGENOUS FACTORS

- What are the individual factors that may affect treatment processes?
- What are the contextual or environmental factors that may affect treatment processes?

IMPLEMENTATION ISSUES

- What aspects of the treatment delivery system are relevant to consider?

TREATMENT FIDELITY STRATEGIES DESIGN

- Is the treatment dose, including number, frequency, and length of contacts specified?
- What strategies are in place to ensure a fixed dose in treatment delivery across participants and study conditions?
- What strategies are in place to record deviations from protocol?
- What mechanisms are in place to track the number, frequency, and duration of contacts?
- Is there a comprehensive, scripted treatment manual developed with objectives and content for each session of treatment delivery?
- What strategies are in place for externally monitoring sessions and providing feedback to interventionists?
- What strategies are in place for interventionist self-monitoring of sessions?

INTERVENTIONIST TRAINING

- How will training be standardized across interventionists?
- How will skill acquisition in interventionists be measured?
- How will change in interventionist skills be minimized?

(continued)

EXHIBIT 4.1 The Problem-Solving Approach to Intervention Design *(continued)*

INTERVENTION DELIVERY

- What mechanisms are in place to evaluate the extent to which interventions were delivered as intended regarding content and dose?
- How will contamination across interventions be minimized when delivered by the same interventionist?
- What mechanisms are in place to standardize intervention delivery?

INTERVENTION RECEIPT

- How will you verify that participants understand the information provided?
- How will you verify that participants can use the behavioral skills or evoke the subjective state they are trained to use?
- How will issues that interfere with receipt of the intervention be addressed?

ENACTMENT OF TREATMENT SKILLS

- What strategy can be applied to verify that participants use the cognitive, behavioral, and motivational skills and strategies provided in the intervention in the appropriate life situations?
- How will issues that interfere with enactment be addressed?

IDENTIFYING THE PRODUCT OF THE INTERVENTION

- What is the nature and form of the selected outcomes?
- What is the timing of treatment effects expected?
- What are the minimal magnitudes of effects thought to be clinically relevant?
- What is the maximal magnitude of effects thought to be likely?

CONTRIBUTION OF THE ELEMENTS OF INTERVENTION THEORY

Understanding the Problem

An important function of theory in intervention design is to guide the researcher in understanding the nature and characteristics of the problem targeted by the intervention. In general, there has been limited discussion in the literature around analyzing the nature of the problem of interest as the starting point for design of theory-based interventions. Therefore, one of the first steps in developing relevant theory-based interventions is the in-depth exploration of the problem in need of treatment.

Conceptualization of the problem specifies those "natural or social causes of the problem" and provides a comprehensive understanding of the nature of the problem, its manifestations, determinants, or factors that cause the problem, the conditions under which the problem comes about and may change over time, and the relevant consequences of the problem. Understanding these characteristics of the problem is critical for generating intervention strategies that are consistent with and responsive to them. For instance, interventions targeting the initiation of behavioral change differ from those targeting behavioral maintenance. Variations in the characteristics of the problem require interventions of different nature and with different goals and structure. Thus, before we develop the intervention, we need to specify the characteristics of the problem that the intervention is designed to address. Failure to clearly outline the nature of the problem beyond its behavioral manifestation limits our ability to tie the problem clearly to an intervention. In a review of physical activity interventions, Keller, Fleury, Sidani, and Ainsworth (2009) note that few of the studies reviewed specified the problem under investigation from a theoretical, rather than behavioral, perspective. Many intervention studies outline intervention components, but do not clearly specify the problem to which the intervention is directed. Instead, the focus of the research is on specific behaviors, disease states, or health-related outcomes, inferring that outcomes of the intervention reflect the problem addressed by the intervention.

This may not always be the case; the problem to be targeted may be related to a determinant of a behavior or health state (e.g., lack of motivation to engage in physical activity) or the conditions under which the problem comes about (e.g., unsafe neighborhood). Although specifying the nature of the problem is helpful as a beginning step in problem specification, additional exploration of the problem characteristics is required to identify which is amenable to change and, therefore, can be meaningfully addressed by the intervention. Problem definition goes beyond the recognition of disease processes, such as obesity, diabetes, or cardiovascular disease, to detail its essential attributes or experiences such as failure to maintain dietary changes consistent with limited self-monitoring skills or lack of self-efficacy to engage in physical activity and its determinants or causative factors. Slippage between the specification of the problem and the intervention increases error in the design of the intervention, which results in limited, if any, effectiveness of the intervention in addressing the problem, and reduces our ability to make valid causal inferences. Even when interventions are effective, if the problem is not clearly specified, the ability to replicate intervention findings is limited.

Our emphasis on understanding the problem in intervention research is to call attention to the need to carefully design interventions that are responsive to an identified problem. Understanding the problem requires clarification of the nature of the problem, its manifestations, causative factors, and level of severity, and using this information to identify a theory that explains these characteristics of the problem (see Exhibit 4.1). Specificity in understanding the problem may come from qualitative and descriptive data that identify the relevant dimensions of the problem, when the problem occurs, as well as how the problem may look or come about differently given different social conditions and populations. Descriptive data may provide important information about problem manifestations, particularly given differing social conditions and different populations, the level of problem severity, and the most significant determinants of the problem such as perceptions, beliefs, personal enabling skills, and social enabling factors that should be taken into account when developing an intervention (Thornton et al., 2017).

Qualitative methods have been considered necessary for developing valid and valued interventions that acknowledge (a) cultural and contextual factors that facilitate the effectiveness of intervention, (b) social and ecological validity of intervention, and (c) attention to the specific needs and resources of the target population (Duggleby & Williams, 2016). Similarly, epidemiological and community-based data can provide direction for identifying concrete problems in communities. Descriptive and qualitative data may be helpful in identifying individual and community experiences in problems of living or taking people's problems as a starting point to determine if intervention makes a difference to those problems in practice. Our understanding of the problem allows us to address the manifestations of the problem through questions such as "How would you know the problem if you saw it?" Manifestations of the problem typically include patterns of signs and symptoms experienced in association with the problem. Specificity in understanding manifestations of the problem may come from descriptive or clinical data that specify the relevant dimensions, when the problem occurs as well as how the problem may present differently given different social conditions and populations. It is important to frame understanding of the manifestations of the problem as it relates to a specific condition, population, or behavior rather than assuming generalizability across conditions. In a critique of the transtheoretical model (TTM), Hutchison, Breckon, and Johnston (2009) note that although the TTM has been widely applied in interventions designed to promote physical activity, no attempts have been made to ascertain whether different change processes occur in initiating physical activity behavioral change beyond those specified by the TTM. Thus, different processes of change, or manifestations of the problem of limited motivation to engage in behavioral change, may exist for sedentary individuals compared to smokers or those with a poor diet.

There are typically multiple determinants or causative factors for a problem. These are likely to differ in scope, with some focused on individual function, resources, or cognitions as the source of the problem, whereas others focus on community, organizational, or policy factors. For example, possible determinants of physical inactivity may include diminished functional status, lack of social support, perception of an unsafe environment for activity, or public policy, which limits the construction of walking trails or neighborhood parks (Thornton et al., 2017). By carefully considering the determinants or causative factors associated with a problem beyond its behavioral manifestation, we are better able to target our intervention strategies to address the specific factor and subsequently the problem in a responsive and systematic way.

The problem also is characterized by its intensity, severity, and duration. Understanding these characteristics involves the identification of patterns such as the presence and perceived burden of symptoms that accompany a particular problem; changes in psychosocial and functional status across the trajectory of chronic illness; or perceived capability, opportunity, and motivation related to problem maintenance. Our understanding of the level of problem severity may be addressed through questions such as, Where and when can change be expected and which outcomes are central? Attention to these characteristics helps to ensure that the problem is addressed in ways that will produce the desired effects with interventions of appropriate nature and/or dose. For instance, recommendations for diet and physical activity will differ for people with varying levels of weight excess.

Considering when the problem exists or when the risk of the problem is greatest may help to understand variations in problem intensity and frequency that take place naturally over time or that are associated with particular conditions. For example, descriptive data on the maintenance of physical activity following cardiac rehabilitation shows that the risk of relapse is greatest within 2 weeks following completion of a monitored program. Specification of the trajectory of the problem allows us to localize the most effective time for intervention delivery through questions such as, How does the problem change over time, place, events, or people? Determining the appropriate time for intervention allows us to target the intervention delivery to when the problem achieves a level of sufficient intensity to require intervention. When timing is not considered, interventions may be given without considering when the intervention is most likely to produce the greatest effect, potentially leading to incorrect conclusions about its effectiveness. Clinical and descriptive data, particularly those derived from longitudinal observations, may guide determination of the most appropriate time for intervention delivery.

Desired outcomes reflect both achievable and clinically meaningful changes in the problem. However, our understanding of the problem guides the specification of outcomes. Expected outcomes will differ in nature, timing of when the changes are expected to occur, and the expected pattern of change after implementation of an intervention.

The nature and characteristics of the problem can be integrated in a **theory of the problem**. It models the processes that produce the problem needing attention. Problem theory may be judged according to how clearly it addresses the phenomenon of concern or explains the problem requiring intervention. It provides a framework for deciding what characteristic of the problem is treatable, when and at what level it is treatable, for what populations, under what conditions, and for what desired outcomes. The problem theory gives directions for delineating intervention strategies or ways that will successfully address the problem and produce the desired outcomes. Knowledge of the conditions under which the intervention is expected to work is necessary for generalization of its effects, for improvement or refinements of the intervention, and for clinical applicability.

The problem theory offers an appropriate grounding for stating the research topic to be investigated in an intervention evaluation study, for identifying the study target population and setting, for delineating the participants' eligibility criteria, and for justifying the timing for the delivery of the intervention. Specifically, adequate definitions of the problem rely on a specification of the nature of the problem and its characteristics as experienced by the target population. Particular attention to the degree to which the conceptualization of the problem reflects the experience of the target population is critical. Such descriptions, tied to clear conceptualization of the problem, are needed for selecting appropriate samples and assessing the applicability of findings to other populations. Often, it is assumed that there is a shared meaning for constructs. However, culture determines perceptual, explanatory, and behavioral responses to health, health problems, and treatment. In order for a theory to adequately represent the problem in a specific population, the main concepts in the theory must be recognizable to the population and reflect identifiable events in their lives.

The adequacy of problem theory may be judged according to how clearly it explains the problem under investigation. In selecting a problem theory, it might be helpful to explore available theories that have been generated to explain the problem. Typically, theories are chosen that have been used successfully in previous pertinent research. However, evaluation of the degree to which these theories reflect the experience of the population of interest is needed, particularly among vulnerable groups that have traditionally been absent from clinical studies. A challenge for researchers and clinicians is to identify, develop, or refine the multiple theories, or derive the problem theory through (a) conceptual analysis of available theoretical, empirical, and clinical literature resulting in the generation of a meaningful and coherent combination of various factors within a broad framework that comprehensively explain the problem; (b) integrating empirical, quantitative, and/or qualitative evidence as is done in literature review or meta-analysis to clarify the problem; and (c) carefully designing and carrying out descriptive correlational studies that serve as early exploratory efforts to establish the characteristics of the problem, encompassing its nature, severity of its presentation, manifestations, and determinants or causative factors, in different populations and under different conditions.

Specifying the Population Experiencing the Problem

Conceptualization of the problem targeted by the intervention provides relevant information for specifying participants' characteristics or attributes that might determine response to the intervention, including the nature, course, and manifestation of the problem. Effective intervention planning is based on how the problem is experienced by the target population and how the proposed intervention will address the problem in that population. Knowledge of "for whom, and under what circumstances" the intervention works is necessary to maximize treatment **effectiveness**. A systematic evaluation of intervention effectiveness requires that the intervention be given to individuals who are experiencing the problem or its determinants that are treatable by the intervention. Participants who do not have the problem of interest cannot be helped by treatment, no matter how well the intervention is designed. In this case, results of evaluation indicate the interventions are not effective in addressing the problem, a potentially incorrect conclusion. Participant homogeneity in response to treatment is necessary to detect significant treatment effects in an experimental study or randomized clinical trial. In contrast, heterogeneity will produce variability in response to treatment reflected in increased variance in outcomes. Careful sample selection is needed to enhance homogeneity. Sample selection proceeds from our understanding of who has the problem or relevant determinants that are targeted by the intervention. Inclusion criteria reflect characteristics of the problem that are addressed by the intervention, meaning that we select those individuals who experience the problem as delineated in the problem theory because they are likely to respond to the intervention. In some instances, the conceptualization of the problem indicates the condition under which the problem occurs; that is, it will tell us that the problem is inherent in a given situation. For example, lack of resources for physical activity or an unsafe environment might be inherent to residents of a given neighborhood; in other situations we may not know when the problem will occur exactly. For example, social cognitive theory does not guide us in knowing when a lack of self-efficacy might occur, so it is necessary to assess these perceptions as part of inclusion criteria. Characteristics of the problem must be measureable in some way to ensure that the sample is homogenous on what matters. A lack of specificity in problem identification creates the risk of delivering a theoretically relevant intervention to those who may not need the treatment. For example, Allison and Keller (2004) tested an intervention based on social cognitive theory and designed to promote maintenance of physical activity among older persons following graduation from cardiac rehabilitation. It was proposed that risk for relapse was due to low levels of efficacy expectations; levels of efficacy were not measured as part of study inclusion criteria. Failure to show significant changes in self-efficacy following the intervention was because of participants having high scores on measures of self-efficacy at baseline, creating a ceiling effect. Thus, in this case, the problem was poorly conceptualized, the sample selection was not well specified, and the intervention was delivered to those who did not need it.

To build intervention science and to facilitate knowledge translation, we need to improve our understanding about how interventions function as participant characteristics vary. The major chronic illnesses—heart disease, diabetes, stroke, and cancers—are disproportionately common among vulnerable populations defined as those who live in poverty, have limited education, live in rural areas with limited access to healthcare, and the very old. Such populations may respond differently to interventions that were successful in the majority populations. Thus, there is a need to know whether interventions have differential effects upon participants with varying characteristics of vulnerability. This, in turn, will increase our understanding of the processes through which the intervention operates with certain participants and not with others. Identifying the responsiveness of different groups to different or same interventions can yield important information about the benefits of the intervention for at-risk individuals. It is likely that different people change their behavior for different reasons. A key will be to determine what interventions work with what groups of people and understand when to select the optimal time frame for intervention.

Attention in intervention research has recently shifted to the development and evaluation of tailored and stage-matched interventions, which require a specific focus on sample selection and intervention delivery. In tailored interventions, specific levels or types of treatment are matched to specific participants' characteristics assessed at pretreatment, using validated algorithms. This design may improve the efficiency and cost-effectiveness of interventions by delivering treatment in a way that is consistent with and responsive to individuals' profiles. Depending on the focus of the intervention, tailoring variables may include individual, family, or context characteristics. Collins, Murphy, and Bierman (2004) introduced the use of **adaptive interventions** as a perspective on research-based prevention and treatment. An adaptive intervention assigns different doses of certain intervention components across individuals and/or within individuals across time. More recent applications include Just-in-Time Adaptive Interventions (JITAIs) designed to address the changing needs of individuals by providing the type and amount of intervention support needed, when it is needed. Advances in mobile technology have fostered real-time, individualized approaches responsive to the intervention needs of participants, with doses assigned on the basis of decision rules linking characteristics of the individual with specific levels and types of intervention components. Articulating the links between doses and types of treatment and participant or problem characteristics optimizes intervention effects. Prior research may be helpful in specifying these relationships, as will relevant theory and clinical experience.

Identifying Mediating Processes

Mediating processes specify the mechanism underlying the intervention effects as a cause–effect sequence between an intervention and an ultimate outcome (Teixeira et al., 2015). The sequence states how an intervention leads to desired changes in the ultimate outcome, clarifying the essential process of change beyond a simple input–output model. Few interventions can be viewed as working directly on the ultimate outcome; nearly all have their effects through some **mediating variables** such as reactions to the intervention, knowledge, self-efficacy, or perception of social norms. These mediator variables are critical cognitions, behaviors, or attitudes that must be changed by the intervention in order for the desired outcomes to occur (see Exhibit 4.1). The change process is contingent upon accurate specification and manipulation of mediating variables; interventions are more likely to be effective if the mediating variables are strongly related to the desired ultimate outcome and if the intervention clearly targets change in the mediating variables at acceptable levels. The potential effect of an intervention is characterized by the relationship between mediators and specified ultimate outcome, so specifying the mediating variables helps to clarify the change process.

Theory should clearly specify relevant mediators. The mediators chosen need to be consistent with and reflect the mechanisms for change connecting the intervention or its components with the intended ultimate outcome. Further, mediators must be amenable to change by the intervention, and the degree of change in the mediators following treatment delivery must be measured in a standardized way. Accordingly, theory guides the selection of instruments for measuring the proposed mediators, the delineation of the time at which and the pattern of changes in mediators are expected, and the plan for data analysis. The analysis is concerned with examining the extent to which the intervention has direct effects on the mediating variables and indirect effects on the desired ultimate outcome. The links will clarify the mechanisms for change and allow a greater understanding of how intervention strategies are expected to lead to desired outcomes. Knowledge of why and how the intervention works is necessary for its careful application in practice.

Developing the Intervention to Address the Problem

Theory offers explanations of the problem amenable to treatment, indicates the nature of relevant intervention strategies that could successfully address the problem, as well as the processes mediating the intervention effects on the ultimate outcome. The design of theory-based intervention involves feedback or movement between the conceptualization of the problem and the specification of key elements of the intervention designed to treat or prevent the problem. Thus, the intervention is developed in the context of the problem and is specifically developed to address the deficits identified in or to promote the strengths inherent to the problem. Determining what makes the problem better or worse helps to clarify the specific components of the intervention, or identify the related antecedent or associative factors. Together, they specify the structure and content of the intervention, including critical inputs, components, treatment strength, and intervention dose and timing. As such, they provide a basis for explaining how an intervention exerts its influence on outcomes and further understanding of what interventions work, for whom, and under what conditions. When these elements are considered, the possibility of alternative rival hypotheses about the intervention's contribution to the outcomes is minimized, thereby strengthening **internal validity** (i.e., the degree to which we can say that the change in the outcome is due to the intervention, not extraneous/confounding variables).

The theory guides the operationalization of the intervention; it specifies the nature and dose of the intervention necessary to produce the expected effects. The intervention is operationally defined according to the central concepts of the theory as the critical inputs that define the intervention. Intervention science cannot be advanced without clear identification of the specific actions and the conditions under which an intervention is delivered. The intervention is operationally defined in terms of its "active ingredients" or specific elements that are responsible for creating change in mediating variables and/or outcomes. The active ingredients are activities or strategies that constitute the intervention; they represent what is to be done and what is necessary, sufficient, and optimal to produce the desired outcomes. In addition, the theory specifies the mode for intervention delivery and the strength and dose required to bring about desired change in the outcome in the target population. This level of specificity enables identification of what comprises treatment and what does not, thus clarifying the critical aspects of the intervention and the possibility for variation in treatment delivery, minimizing the possibility of alternative or rival hypotheses, and strengthening internal validity. To achieve specificity, the essential elements or features of the intervention are identified and separated from the less important ones. This is important to (a) distinguish the intervention from others (this will guide the selection of an appropriate comparison treatment, which should not incorporate the theoretically active ingredients of the intervention under evaluation), and (b) develop instruments to assess and monitor fidelity of intervention implementation by interventionists and adherence to treatment by participants. Keller et al. (2009) found that despite differing theoretical perspectives guiding interventions to promote physical activity, studies reviewed incorporated similar intervention approaches, designed to enhance cognitive and behavioral processes of change, decisional balance, self-efficacy, social support, self-regulation, and outcome expectancy. The similarity of intervention approaches across studies reviewed blurs the theoretical specificity of treatments and limits our ability to clearly evaluate the efficacy of one perspective over another. A greater level of specificity in operationalization of interventions that are consistent with relevant theory is needed to maintain construct validity of the intervention implementation. The current state of intervention research has provided little guidance on how to best manipulate mediating variables to obtain behavioral change. Greater theoretical specificity in developing critical inputs that target theoretical mediators may address this concern (Teixeira et al., 2015). Similarly, specificity in how constructs are operationalized will foster the effective blending of different behavioral theories as a guide for intervention, recognizing how each contributes uniquely to the intervention and specified outcomes.

Treatment strength refers to the likelihood that an intervention can achieve the desired ultimate outcome. Investigators use information from theory, descriptive research, and prior intervention to propose the amount or format for intervention delivery needed to produce a measurable effect. Strong treatments contain large amounts of the "active ingredients," which lead to change in the outcomes. If treatment strength is low relative to the problem of interest, it is unlikely that significant change will be achieved. Although evaluation of intervention strength is viewed as essential in pharmaceutical treatments, where the dose continuum is largely a matter of quantity and frequency, few theory-based interventions in the behavioral and social sciences have evaluated treatment strength.

Treatment strength may be characterized as including several factors central to intervention design and testing, including clarity in intervention conceptualization and operationalization, treatment dose, and fidelity in treatment implementation. Treatment strength is enhanced by a clear theoretical rationale for intervention design, with specified links that tie the intervention's critical inputs to mediating processes and outcomes. A key consideration is the conceptual relevance of the treatment or specification of what treatments will address which problems; if a treatment does not address the problem of interest, strength is irrelevant. To evaluate treatment strength, we must be able to identify what treatment addresses which problem of interest, as well as what constitutes treatment and what is not consistent with theory, and where treatment delivery might vary without jeopardizing its integrity and effectiveness. This level of conceptual specificity will foster the development and use of detailed treatment manuals and protocol to guide interventionist training, determine intervention dose and delivery, and evaluate treatment fidelity. A standardized protocol adds clarity and facilitates intervention delivery as designed, which keeps it from becoming contaminated or weakened over time. Standardization may include developing a protocol that describes the nature of the intervention activities, specifies the sequence of activities to be performed, and provides details for the procedures to be carried out (Sidani & Braden, 2011). Procedures for quantifying the strength of intervention may include a quantitative synthesis of past research to summarize components of "strong" interventions, expert review and evaluation of intervention strength, and programmatic research to systematically test intervention of different strengths. Methods to ensure treatment strength include the use of a scripted protocol, training of the interventionist, a structured review of information shared with participants, and intervention delivery audit and monitoring.

The dose of an intervention represents the amount, frequency, and duration with which the treatment is given to produce changes in mediating and/or outcome variables. Response to treatment is often characterized as a dose–response relationship. Amount refers to the quantity of the treatment that should be given. Frequency refers to the number of times the treatment is to be given over a specified time. Duration refers to the total length of time the treatment is to be implemented for the expected changes in outcomes to be achieved. Intervention dose may be characterized in different ways, depending on the focus and mechanisms for intervention delivery. A "dose" of an intervention might be a telephone call, session attendance, the number of contacts or minutes engaged with a lay health advisor, completion of an online educational module, or number of postings or minutes engaged in an online support group. Dose might be carried out weekly, biweekly, or monthly and continue over 6 weeks, 8 weeks, or 6 months. The optimal dose of the intervention needed to achieve effects may be determined through clinical experience, programmatic research on the intervention, or an integrative review of intervention studies. One approach to determining dose may be to test interventions in which different dose levels are implemented and compared. The process of quantifying intervention dose includes developing a measure assessing intervention amount, frequency, and duration that reflects the dose received by participants. Intervention dose may be quantified by sessions attended or telephone calls received; a log in which participants document what they did, when, how frequently, and for what length of time. Quantifying intervention dose allows for a dose–response analysis in evaluation of intervention effects, which assists in identifying or confirming the optimal dose for producing relevant outcomes (Conn & Chan, 2016).

Treatment fidelity refers to the methodological strategies used to monitor and enhance the reliability and validity of intervention conceptualization and implementation. When there is a high degree of monitoring and control over factors associated with the delivery of intervention, it is possible to evaluate the efficacy of a theory-based intervention, or compare the impact of two or more treatments on an outcome with validity. Unless treatment is implemented with fidelity, the extent to which the intervention under evaluation is the primary mechanism for the observed changes in the outcomes will remain unclear. Further, intervention strength is dependent on treatment fidelity, with low fidelity decreasing the strength of the intervention. Bellg et al. (2004) outline five areas to conceptualize and maintain treatment fidelity: (a) study design, (b) training providers, (c) delivery of treatment, (d) receipt of treatment, and (e) enactment of treatment skills.

Treatment fidelity related to study design includes a strong and identifiable integration of theory within the conceptualization of the problem targeted by the intervention, operationalization of the intervention, specification of mediating processes, and specification of the ultimate outcome (Ibrahim & Sidani, 2015). Approaches to maintain treatment fidelity specific to study design are intended to ensure that the intervention is consistent with the underlying theory, allowing an accurate test of theory-based interventions. The effect of an intervention can be accurately evaluated when the research design does not confound treatment effects with extraneous differences between treatment groups or treatment and comparison groups. Treatment fidelity is strengthened with the development and use of a standardized manual and protocol for implementing the intervention as conceptualized. Careful delivery of the intervention as specified in the manual or protocol decreases the potential for contamination across treatment groups. To date, intervention research targeting behavioral change has shown variable fidelity to theory in study design, limiting judgments about the contribution and explanatory power of health behavioral theories, informed comparison among theories, and systematic intervention replication (Keller et al., 2009).

Training of the interventionists is an important area to consider in maintaining fidelity. Variability in intervention delivery will make it less likely that significant effects will be achieved and will introduce alternative explanations for intervention effects. Treatment fidelity is enhanced with standardized interventionist training in the theory underlying the problem and the intervention, the protocol for intervention delivery, and any procedures specific to participant contact or follow-up. Standardized training of interventionists to performance criteria is continuous throughout the study period. Methods of training may include standardized training materials, conducting role-playing, and observing intervention delivery for consistency with the manualized protocol. The risk for slippage in the implementation of the intervention over time may be addressed by interventionist-training booster sessions, regular review of session audio or videotapes for consistency with the manualized protocol, and review of interventionist documentation of intervention delivery. The adequacy of training in both theory and intervention implementation is evaluated and monitored for each interventionist both during and at regular intervals after the training process.

Treatment fidelity processes monitor and improve implementation of the intervention so that it is delivered as intended (Moore et al., 2015). In testing theory-based interventions, significant treatment effects are observed in the form of differences between the outcomes for the intervention group and those for the comparison group. Thus, the clear specification of the content and activities constituting the intervention and the comparison treatment conditions and strategies to support their consistent delivery is essential to enhance internal validity. A primary challenge to treatment fidelity is variability in treatment implementation either across interventionists and participants and/or over time. If the delivery of intervention changes over time, or if it is inconsistent because of different interventionists, across participants in different sites or at different time points over the study period, then variability in participant response to treatment ensues; this, in turn, decreases the likelihood of finding significant intervention effects. Indeed, process evaluation of a randomized trial to promote self-management in primary care patients showing no significant effects (Kennedy et al., 2013) revealed that the intervention as designed was not delivered to most patients (Kennedy et al., 2014). Another challenge is limited contrast or difference in treatment delivered to the intervention and comparison groups. The difference between groups, specific to the theoretically active ingredients of the intervention, represents the strength of the intervention effects on the desired outcomes. Treatment conditions without clearly specified content and clear differentiation will reduce any differences found in outcomes between the intervention and comparison groups. In addition, monitoring intervention delivery requires strategies for quantifying the dose proposed to produce the desired change in outcomes. Abildgaard, Saksvik, and Nielsen (2016) outline qualitative and quantitative approaches to evaluating the intervention process. Quantitative approaches include the use of process evaluation scales measuring key aspects of the intervention and degree of implementation (Havermans et al., 2016). Process evaluation scales document the extent to which the intervention content was relayed, activities were performed, and dose was offered in accordance with those specified in the treatment manual and protocol. The use of validated process evaluation scales during intervention delivery may allow investigators to better understand factors that limit or promote implementation of the intervention, such as a lack of time or group dynamics, and better inform future research. Process evaluation scales completed by the interventionist following each session may highlight areas of weakness or alterations in treatment delivery and reinforce the need to address these issues with the interventionists. Randomly audio- or videotaping treatment sessions may be helpful as a post hoc evaluation of treatment delivery. Comparison of what was delivered to what was specified in the treatment manual and protocol identifies discrepancies that should be accounted for at the data analysis stage. Regular review of process evaluation data and feedback to interventionists may strengthen the skills for providing the treatment and support the standardization of intervention delivery across interventionists, participants, and sites. A qualitative approach to process evaluation includes collecting and analyzing data through interviews, focus groups, field notes, or observation. Qualitative approaches to process evaluation may help to explain unexpected results of an intervention as well as clarify intervention mechanisms (Greasley & Edwards, 2015).

According to Bellg et al. (2004), receipt of treatment involves processes that monitor and improve the ability of participants to understand and perform the necessary behavioral skills and cognitive strategies central to treatment delivery. Treatment receipt evaluates participant use of behavioral skills (physical activity monitoring) or cognitive strategies (self-regulation) that have been developed as part of the intervention. Methods for evaluation include review of homework assignments, documenting strategies used to achieve personal goals, or review of physical activity calendars.

Enactment of treatment consists of processes to monitor and improve the ability of participants to perform the necessary behavioral skills and cognitive strategies in relevant real-life settings (Bellg et al., 2004). Enactment evaluates the extent to which participants use specific behavioral skills or cognitive strategies at the appropriate time and setting in daily life. Enactment evaluation may include self-report of behavior over time, use of monitoring devices such as accelerometers to evaluate physical activity patterns at home, or telephone calls to monitor the use of coping strategies.

Careful consideration of the timing and conditions for implementing the intervention contributes to consistency in treatment delivery and to internal validity. Timing refers to providing the intervention when it will be most responsive to the problem and most effective in creating change. Similar to biological treatments designed to prevent or treat illness, behavioral interventions require sensitivity to a timing factor. When timing is not considered, interventions are given without considering when the intervention is most likely to produce the greatest effect.

The conditions for delivery of an intervention should be consistent with those specified in the intervention theory. To rule out alternative explanations for intervention effects, it is important to distinguish the "active ingredients" of the intervention from the elements associated with its delivery methods and context. Issues in treatment implementation are aspects of the delivery system relevant to providing the specific intervention. These issues refer to the resources needed to carry out the intervention, including material supplies and human skills that facilitate the delivery of the intervention as planned. Intervention delivery targeting individuals or groups, at one or multiple sessions, may differ by population and setting and will reflect how the intervention is packaged for a given study (format of information, color, language, pictures used), the delivery plan developed (information through audiotape delivery, Internet delivery, mail delivery), and the identification of settings that facilitate the implementation of the intervention as designed. Understanding of conditions may come from analysis of the context under which successful interventions have been delivered, acknowledgement of conditions guiding descriptive or pilot work, clinical knowledge of the importance of settings, the timing of intervention delivery, and the role of supportive or unsupportive situations in resolving the problem. For example, an understanding of community ecology can lead to a better match with community-based health promotion interventions, including developing new and existing leadership, strengthening community organizations, and furthering organizational collaboration (Fleury & Lee, 2006). Thus, a thorough understanding of the multiple conditions under which interventions might best be delivered, including attention to intervention feasibility and cost, has the potential to facilitate the identification of interventions that are effective.

Context includes characteristics of participants and interventionists, and environmental factors that may influence intervention implementation. Relevant participants' characteristics may include demographic profile (age, gender, education level), personality traits (locus of control), or personal beliefs (cultural values). Characteristics of the interventionist may include personal and professional attributes necessary for treatment delivery such as communication skill, educational background, beliefs about the treatment, or competence in treatment delivery. Environmental factors encompass physical and psychosocial features of the environment; they relate to the convenience of the setting in which treatment is given to participants; a setting that is clean, safe, private, and quiet; availability of resources necessary for treatment delivery; and the organizational culture of the setting reflecting prevailing norms and policies.

Clarifying the Outcomes of the Intervention

In contrast to a black box approach to intervention design and evaluation, the application of theory allows a more comprehensive modeling and **measurement** of the processes accounting for the ultimate outcome expected as a result of the interventions. The outcomes reflect the resolution or successful management of the problem targeted by the intervention. They are the reason for which the intervention is given and form the criteria for evaluating intervention effectiveness. Thus, outcomes selected are consistent with the target problem and responsive to the intervention. Theory determines (a) the nature of the anticipated outcomes, including clinical end points, functional status, or changes in knowledge, attitudes, and motivation; (b) the points in time at which changes in outcomes are expected to occur; and (c) the expected pattern of change in outcomes after delivery of the intervention. The nature of the outcomes refers to aspects of the problem that the intervention is designed to address and the ultimate goals of the intervention. By specifying the logic that connects intervention critical inputs to mediating and outcome variables, theory identifies the outcomes that can reasonably be expected. Without this specification, there is not a clear basis for selection of meaningful outcomes that are responsive to the intervention and of instruments to validly measure outcomes. The timing refers to the point at which the changes in the outcomes are expected to take place following intervention delivery. Some changes occur during or immediately after intervention delivery, whereas others appear over time. The pattern of change refers to the trajectory, or the direction and rate of change in the outcomes over time. The theoretical perspective, clinical experience, and descriptive data can provide direction for when to best measure change; change may be targeted on the basis of theoretically important times, at multiple time points to investigate trends over time, or at clinically important times. Many studies measure outcomes immediately following the treatment, or posttest, with limited justification for the timing of measurement. This approach to outcome measurement implies that effects have an immediate onset and peak following intervention delivery, but other patterns of change are possible. Different outcomes might have different patterns of change, with some most pronounced immediately following the intervention and others at some later time. Choosing appropriate times for outcome measurement is required to detect important intervention effects; otherwise, we may be looking in the wrong place at the wrong time.

SOURCES FOR GENERATING THEORY

There are several sources of theory available to guide the design interventions. Donaldson and Lipsey (2006) note that the choice of theory requires clarifying assumptions about the etiology of the problem the intervention attempts to address and the mechanisms by which change can be achieved. Three approaches may be helpful in providing an explanation of the problem and the mechanisms by which change may be achieved.

Middle-range theories, which may be derived from relevant grand theory, can guide intervention development and testing focused on a limited aspect of experience in a particular situation of interest. A middle-range theory has a focus on specific health experiences, health and illness problems, or certain patient populations; it provides clearly articulated concepts and relationships, which can be tested empirically through systematic research. Theory may be developed through qualitative research and practice observations or through logical analysis and synthesis of existing theory (Liehr & Smith, 2017). Middle-range predictive theory allows the prediction of relationships between concepts, or how changes in a phenomenon occur. Shearer (2011) describes the iterative process guiding the development and testing of her middle-range theory of health empowerment, leading to a theory-based health empowerment intervention. Beginning with qualitative methods, Shearer identified aspects of the lived experience of health empowerment, including contextual factors and interpersonal factors positively associated with health empowerment. In quantitative testing of this emerging theory, Shearer and Reed (2004) examined the relationships among contextual factors, interpersonal factors, and purposeful participation in health behaviors. Although the study findings partially supported the theoretical propositions, the limited variance in behaviors explained by contextual and interpersonal factors warranted further study. A second qualitative study with older women clarified the social support needs and resources and contextual factors used to facilitate health empowerment (Shearer & Fleury, 2006). Social-contextual resources in the revised theory reflected perceived supportive relationships and opportunities for nurturance and the exchange of information and materials to foster health empowerment. A third qualitative study with homebound older women (Shearer, 2009) clarified the role of personal resources as the unique characteristics of each woman, including inherent strength as self-capacity that promoted change and growth. Health empowerment was defined as a relational process emerging from a woman's recognition of personal resources and social-contextual resources, which results in a transformation in awareness of and belief in ability to knowingly participate in the changes inherent in health and health outcomes. The health empowerment intervention was developed to enhance awareness of personal resources and social-contextual resources, to foster purposeful participation in the attainment of personally valued health goals, resulting in well-being. Elements of the intervention are self-capacity building, social network building, and building social service utilization. The interventionist works in concert with an older woman and engages in a participatory process in which the interventionist listens and encourages the older adult to talk, share, and enact her health goals (Shearer, 2009).

Meleis (2010) presents a middle-range theory of transition and outlines an empirically supported framework to articulate and characterize the relationships between theory concepts. The use of inductive and deductive reasoning guided evaluation of the utility of different concepts of the framework and identified additional emerging concepts. Through a series of five studies, the framework was able to specify (a) types and patterns of transitions; (b) properties of transition experiences; (c) transition conditions, including facilitators and inhibitors; (d) process indicators; (e) outcome indicators; and (f) intervention critical inputs. Understanding the properties and conditions inherent in the transition process guides understanding of the complexities of the problem, the development of intervention critical inputs consistent with the problem, mediating processes, and outcome variables, as well as the conditions under which theory-based interventions might be most effective.

Qualitative and mixed-methods research may provide opportunities to gather information required to understand the etiology of certain problems and the mechanisms by which change can be achieved as a basis for intervention design. The primary purpose of qualitative inquiry is to capture the meaning of phenomena and relationships among concepts as they occur naturally, and as reflected in thoughts, language, and behavior, from the perspective of the participants. Morse (2017) describes qualitative outcome analysis (QOA), a procedure designed to qualitatively identify intervention strategies and examine outcomes. QOA builds on a completed qualitative study, moving from an understanding of individual experiences to identifying and applying interventions. Using qualitative methods, the processes, stages, and phases that occur during the course of a given phenomenon are described to the extent that a theory is developed, and the factors that alter the course of the phenomenon are recorded. Through QOA, a series of steps are outlined, which begin with identification of the behavioral manifestations of the phenomenon, clarifying and documenting the dynamics of the problem, identifying strategies to modify the problem, evaluating the efficacy of the strategies developed, and modifying and reevaluating the intervention strategies used.

Sullivan-Bolyai, Bova, and Harper (2005) present qualitative description as a relevant method for assessing, developing, and refining interventions to serve vulnerable populations and reduce health disparities. The goal of qualitative description is descriptive and interpretive validity to provide interventions that (a) focus on factors that promote access and use of services, (b) are acceptable and understandable to those experiencing the problem of interest, and (c) are sensitive to the cultural context of those experiencing the problem. The inclusion of formative qualitative research before intervention development may establish the need for intervention, define key constructs in a culturally valid manner, foster understanding of the factors that influence the outcomes, and identify key resources related to the intervention.

Natasi et al. (2007) present a heuristic for research and intervention development that uses an iterative research-intervention process. The research process begins with formative data to test a proposed conceptual model developed on the basis of existing theory and research. Qualitative research methods are used to identify and define the concepts specific to a particular culture or context. Findings from the qualitative research are used to construct a modified model and develop assessment and intervention tools to test the model. Evaluation research involves the triangulation of qualitative and quantitative methods to examine acceptability, social validity, cultural specificity, integrity, and effectiveness of interventions. The repeated application of mixed methods across cultures, contexts, and populations can be used to develop a theory that reflects both universal and culturally specific concepts, as well as address local cultural and contextual needs.

Intervention design may proceed from an integration of concepts either proposed by related theories or consistently found to be related. Although integration of theories may result in stronger interventions, a clear rationale is needed for the added value of this approach in furthering understanding of the problem, or providing an innovative explanation of the mechanisms by which change can be achieved. The blending of theories in intervention design requires an understanding of the strengths and limitations of different theoretical perspectives, as well as the underlying assumptions of each theory and the congruence of assumptions across theories. Treatment fidelity in intervention design requires clear specification of the contributions of each theoretical perspective as critical elements of the intervention. Specificity in construct definition as well as clear links between intervention theory and the critical elements chosen for the intervention are needed to evaluate specific predictors from theory and provide meaningful guidelines for intervention development targeting these constructs. Specification of the unique contribution of each theoretical perspective to intervention design will further empirical support for the contribution of combined theory to conceptual understanding of theory-based interventions.

Published reports of individual studies that evaluate the effectiveness of interventions or of meta-analytic studies that synthesize the empirical evidence of intervention effects may provide a guide for selecting the most relevant theory with empirical support. However, these reviews may offer a limited perspective on complex issues and often produce conflicting findings.

Given these approaches to theory identification and development, investigators are encouraged to consider what constitutes a relevant theory and how a theory might address a problem experienced by a given population (Exhibit 4.2). However, the literature on theory evaluation and application as a basis for intervention design and testing is very limited. Prochaska, Wright, and Velicer (2008) outline criteria for evaluating theory based on perspectives from the philosophy of science (Dubin, 1977; Kuhn, 1977). Theory is evaluated according to which concepts are considered as explaining the phenomenon of interest, including (a) conceptual clarity, or that concepts are well defined and can be measured reliably and validly; (b) consistency, or the articulation of a logical and unified set of relationships between concepts; and (c) parsimony, the statement of concepts and relationships in the simplest manner possible because complexity makes operationalization for intervention development and testing of the full theory difficult. When evaluating theory as a basis for intervention, the clarity and relevance of underlying assumptions, concept definitions, and construct validity are essential.

Theory is further evaluated according to support for how concepts in the theory are related, including (a) testability, or the extent to which concepts can be operationalized and measured, and propositions can be examined; (b) predictability, or empirical support for the theory in predicting future change, or patterns of expected correlations either at one point in time or longitudinally; and (c) explanatory, or evidence of causality, such as that found in randomized controlled trials testing theory-based interventions. When evaluating theory as a basis for intervention, the empirical support for theoretical propositions, explanatory power, and predictive ability related to the problem of interest will guide theory selection. Evaluation moves beyond the review of individual studies to include integrative review or meta-analysis; attention to testing of the complete theory is important in determining the contribution to theory-based interventions.

EXHIBIT 4.2 Evaluating Theory Relevance

- What theories have been used in prior research?
- Which contains well-defined concepts that are operationalized, explicit, and internally consistent?
- Is there evidence for shared meaning for concepts?
- Which has conceptual definitions consistent with underlying assumptions?
- Which explains the problem of interest in the least complex manner possible?
- What descriptive work has been done?
- What is the strength of empirical work?
- To what extent are the relevant theoretical concepts measured?
- To what extent has prior research targeted relevant theoretical concepts in intervention design?
- To what extent has prior research clarified the theoretical basis for intervention critical inputs?
- To what extent does the intervention change targeted theoretical concepts?
- Are theoretical claims congruent with evidence in explaining why change occurred and why it did not?
- How has prior research characterized participant inclusion criteria or tailored intervention to measureable relevant concepts?
- To what extent does the theory generate new questions and ideas and add to the knowledge base?
- To what extent does the theory generalize to other situations, places, and times?
- To what extent have concepts been demonstrated to mediate the effect of the intervention?

Theory also is evaluated according to its relevance across populations, settings, and behaviors, including (a) productivity, or the amount of knowledge and research that a theory has produced; (b) generalizability, or the number of problems and populations to which a theory can validly be applied, including replicability of hypothesized patterns of relationships among concepts; and (c) utility, or the usefulness and efficacy of the theory in designing and evaluating theory-based interventions. When evaluating theory as a basis for intervention, the extent to which theory is relevant to different populations as well as changing problems and experiences will guide selection. Evaluation includes recognition of the extent to which theory can facilitate processes of health and well-being within and among human systems across a diversity of environments.

Key Points From This Chapter

- Theory provides an understanding of the problem that the intervention targets, the nature of the intervention, and the mechanisms underlying the anticipated improvement in outcomes.
- Theory fosters a systematic approach to intervention development and implementation that allow us to move beyond a simplistic, outcomes-focused approach to examining the central processes underlying program effects.
- Theory helps investigators to identify both outcomes and mediating processes that specify a cause and effect sequence between an intervention and outcome.

REFERENCES

Abildgaard, J. S., Saksvik, P. Ø., & Nielsen, K. (2016). How to measure the intervention process? An assessment of qualitative and quantitative approaches to data collection in the process evaluation of organizational interventions. *Frontiers in Psychology, 7,* 1380. doi:10.3389/fpsyg.2016.01380

Allison, M. J., & Keller, C. (2004). Self-efficacy intervention effect on physical activity in older adults. *Western Journal of Nursing Research, 26*(1), 31–46. doi:10.1177/0193945903259350

Bellg, A. J., Borrelli, B., Resnick, B., Hecht, J., Minicucci, D. S., Ory, M., … Czajkowski, S. (2004). Enhancing treatment fidelity in health behavior change studies: Best practices and recommendations from the NIH behavior change consortium. *Health Psychology, 23*(5), 443–451. doi:10.1037/0278-6133.23.5.443

Bonell, C., Fletcher, A., Morton, M., Lorenc, T., & Moore, L. (2012). Realist randomised controlled trials: A new approach to evaluating complex public health interventions. *Social Science & Medicine, 75,* 2299–2306. doi:10.1016/j.socsimed.2012.08.032

Collins, L. M., Murphy, S. A., & Bierman, K. L. (2004). A conceptual framework for adaptive preventive interventions. *Prevention Science, 5*(3), 185–196. doi:10.1023/B:PREV.0000037641.26017.00

Conn, V. S., & Chan, K. C. (2016). How much, how often, how long? Addressing dosage in intervention studies. *Western Journal of Nursing Research, 38*(1), 3–4. doi:10.1177/0193945915605067

Conn, V. S., Cooper, P. S., Ruppar, T. M., & Russell, C. L. (2008). Searching for the intervention in intervention research reports. *Journal of Nursing Scholarship, 40*(1), 52–59. doi:10.1111/j.1547-5069.2007.00206.x

Craig, P., Dieppe, P., Macintyre, S., Michie, S., Nazareth, I., & Petticrew, M. (2013). Developing and evaluating complex interventions: The new Medical Research Council guidance. *International Journal of Nursing Studies, 50,* 587–592. doi:10.1016/j.ijnurstu.2012.09.010

Dalkin, S. M., Greenhalgh, J., Jones, D., Cunningham, B., & Lhussier, M. (2015). What's in a mechanism? Development of a key concept in realist evaluation. *Implementation Science, 10,* 49–55. doi:10.1186/s13012-015-0237-x

Donaldson, S. I., & Lipsey, M. W. (2006). Roles for theory in contemporary evaluation practice: Developing practical knowledge. In I. Shaw, J. C. Greene., & M. M. Mark (Eds.), *The handbook of evaluation: Policies, programs, and practices* (pp. 56–75). Thousand Oaks, CA: Sage.

Dubin, R. (1977). *Theory building*. New York, NY: Free Press.

Duggleby, W., & Williams, A. (2016). Methodological and epistemological considerations in utilizing qualitative inquiry to develop interventions. *Qualitative Health Research, 26*(2), 147–153. doi:10.1177/1049732315590403

Fleury, J., & Lee, S. M. (2006). The social ecological model and physical activity in African American women. *American Journal of Community Psychology, 37*(1–2), 129–140. doi:10.1007/s10464-005-9002-7

Greasley, K., & Edwards, P. (2015). When do health and well-being interventions work? Managerial commitment and context. *Economic and Industrial Democracy, 36*(2), 355–377. doi: 10.1177/0143831X13508590

Havermans, B.M., Schelvis, R.M.C, Boot, C.R.L., Brouwers, E.P.M, Anema, J.R., & van der Beek, A.J. (2016). Process variables in organizational stress management intervention evaluation research: A systematic review. *Scandinavian Journal of Work, Environment & Health, 42*(5):371–381.

Hoffmann, T. C., Glasziou, P. P., Boutron, I., Milne, R., Perera, R., Moher, D., … Michie, S. (2014). Better reporting of interventions: Template for Intervention Description and Replication (TIDieR) checklist and guide. *BMJ, 348*, g1687. doi:10.1136/bmj.g1687

Hutchison, A. J., Breckon, J. D., & Johnston, L. H. (2009). Physical activity behavior change interventions based on the transtheoretical model: A systematic review. *Health Education & Behavior, 36*(5), 829–845. doi:10.1177/1090198108318491

Ibrahim, S., & Sidani, S. (2015). Fidelity of intervention implementation: A review of instruments. *Health, 7*, 1687–1695. doi:/10.4236/health.2015.712183

Keller, C., Fleury, J., Sidani, S., & Ainsworth, B. (2009). Fidelity to theory in PA intervention research. *Western Journal of Nursing Research, 31*(3), 289–311. doi:10.1177/0193945908326067

Kennedy, A., Bower, P., Reeves, D., Blakeman, T., Bowen, R., Chew-Graham, C., … Rogers, A. (2013). Implementation of self-management support for long term conditions in routine primary care settings: Cluster randomized controlled trial. BMJ, *346*, f2882. doi:10.1136/bmj.f2882

Kennedy, A., Rogers, A., Bown, R., Lee, V., Blakeman, T., Gardner, C., … Chew-Graham, C. (2014). Implementing, embedding and integrating self-management support tools for people with long-term conditions in primary care nursing: A qualitative study. *International Journal of Nursing Studies, 51*, 1103–1113. doi:10.1016/j.ijnurstu.2013.11.008

Kok, G., Gottlieb, N. H., Peters, G. J., Mullen, P. D., Parcel, G. S., Ruiter, R. A., … Bartholomew, L. K. (2016). A taxonomy of behavior change methods: An intervention mapping approach. *Health Psychology Review, 10*(3), 297–312. doi:/10.1080/17437199.2015.1077155

Kuhn, T. S. (1977). Second thoughts on paradigms. In F. Suppe (Ed.), *The structure of scientific theories* (2nd ed.). Urbana: University of Illinois Press.

Liehr, P., & Smith, M. J. (2017). Middle range theory. A perspective on development and use. *Advances in Nursing Science, 40*(1), 51–63. doi:10.1097/ANS.0000000000000162

Meleis, A. I. (2010). Theoretical development of transitions. In A. I. Meleis (Ed.), *Transitions theory: Middle-range and situation-specific theories in nursing research and practice* (pp. 13–51). New York, NY: Springer Publishing.

Michie, S., Carey, R. N., Johnston, M., Rothman, A. J., de Bruin, M., Kelly, M. P., & Connell L. E. (2016). From theory-inspired to theory-based interventions: A protocol for developing and testing a methodology for linking behavior change techniques to theoretical mechanisms of action. *Annals of Behavioral Medicine, 52*(6), 501–512. doi:10.1007/s12160-016-9816-6

Michie, S., & Prestwich, A. (2010). Are interventions theory-based? Development of a theory coding scheme. *Health Psychology, 29*(1), 1–8. doi: 10.1037/a0016939

Michie, S., Wood, C. E., Johnston, M., Abraham, C., Francis, J. J., & Hardeman, W. (2015). Behaviour change techniques: The development and evaluation of a taxonomic method for reporting and describing behavior change interventions. *Health Technology Assessment, 19*(99), 1–188. doi:10.3310/hta19990

Moore, G. F., Audrey, S., Barker, M., Bond, L., Bonell, C., Hardeman, W., … Baird, J. (2015). Process evaluation of complex interventions: Medical Research Council guidance. *BMJ, 350*, h1258. doi:10.1136/bmj.h1258

Morse, J. M. (2017). *Analyzing and conceptualizing the theoretical foundations of nursing*. New York, NY: Springer Publishing.

Nahum-Shani, I., Hekler, E. B., & Spruijt-Metz, D. (2015). Building health behavior models to guide the development of just-in-time adaptive interventions: A pragmatic framework. *Health Psychology, 34*(Suppl.), 1209–1219. doi:10.1037/hea0000306

Natasi, B.K., Hitchcock, J., Sarkar, S., Burkholder, G., Varjas, K., & Jayasena, A. (2007). Mixed methods in intervention research. *Journal of Mixed Methods, 1*(2), 164–182.

Pawson, R., & Manzano-Santaella, A. (2012). A realist diagnostic workshop. *Evaluation, 18*(2), 176–191. doi:10.1177/1356389012440912

Prestwich, A., Sniehotta, F. F., Whittington, C., Dombrowski, S. U., Rogers, L., & Michie, S. (2014). Does theory influence the effectiveness of health behavior interventions? Meta-analysis. *Health Psychology, 33*(5), 465–474. doi:10.1037/a0032853

Prochaska, J. O., Wright, J. A., & Velicer, W. F. (2008). Evaluating theories of health behavior change: A hierarchy of criteria applied to the transtheoretical model. *Applied Psychology, 57*(4), 561–588. doi:10.1111/j.1464-0597.2008.00345.x

Rothman, A. J., Baldwin, A. S., Burns, R. J., & Fuglestad, P. T. (2016). Strategies to promote the maintenance of behavior change: Moving from theoretical principles to practice. In M. Diefenbach, S. Miller-Halegoua., & D. Bowen (Eds.), *Handbook of health decision science* (pp. 121–132). New York, NY: Springer.

Salter, K. L., & Kothari, A. (2014). Using realist evaluation to open the black box of knowledge translation: A state-of-the-art review. *Implementation Science, 9*, 115. doi:10.1186/s13012-014-0115-y

Shearer, N. B. C. (2009). Health empowerment theory as a guide for practice. *Geriatric Nursing, 30*(Suppl. 2), 4–10. doi:10.1016/j.gerinurse.2009.02.003

Shearer, N. B. C. (2011). Creating a nursing intervention out of a passion for theory and practice. In P. G. Reed & N. B. C. Shearer (Eds.), *Nursing knowledge and theory innovation: Advancing the science of practice* (pp. 85–94). New York, NY: Springer Publishing.

Shearer, N. B. C., & Fleury, J. (2006). Social support promoting health in older women. *Journal of Women & Aging, 18*(4), 3–17. doi:10.1300/J074v18n04_02

Shearer, N. B. C., & Reed, P. G. (2004). Empowerment: Reformulation of a non-Rogerian concept. *Nursing Science Quarterly, 17*, 253–259. doi:10.1177/0894318404266325

Sidani, S. (2015). *Health intervention research: Understanding research design and methods*. London, UK: Sage

Sidani, S., & Braden, C. J. (2011). *Design, evaluation, and translation of nursing interventions*. New York, NY: Wiley-Blackwell.

Sullivan-Bolyai, S., Bova, C., & Harper, D. (2005). Developing and refining interventions in persons with health disparities: The use of qualitative description. *Nursing Outlook, 53*(3), 127–133. doi:10.1016/j.outlook.2005.03.005

Teixeira, P. J., Carraça, E. V., Marques, M. M., Rutter, H., Oppert, J. M., De Bourdeaudhuij, I., ... Brug, J. (2015). Successful behavior change in obesity interventions in adults: A systematic review of self-regulation mediators. *BMC Medicine, 13*, 84. doi:10.1186/s12916-015-0323-6

Thornton, C. M., Kerr, J., Conway, T. L., Saelens, B. E., Sallis, J. F., Ahn, D. K., ... King, A. C. (2017). Physical activity in older adults: An ecological approach. *Annals of Behavioral Medicine, 51*, 159–169. doi:10.1007/s12160-016-9837-1

Nuts and Bolts of Designing Intervention Studies

Bernadette Mazurek Melnyk, Dianne Morrison-Beedy, & Shirley M. Moore

> To accomplish great things, we must not only act, but also dream;
> not only plan, but also believe. —*Anatole France*

Now that you have determined the "so what" factors for your research, conducted the literature review to assess the state of the science, delineated how your work will be innovative and extend the science in the area, formulated your research questions/hypotheses, and crafted the theoretical/conceptual framework that will guide your intervention and selection of study variables, it is time to determine the type of **research design** that you will need to best answer your research question(s) and test your hypothesis/hypotheses.

The research design is the foundation or backbone of a study (Hulley, Cummings, Browner, Grady, & Newman, 2013). It is the overall plan for answering the study question(s) or testing the hypotheses, which includes:

- The strategies that will be used to control for **confounding variables**
- The exact times that the intervention(s) will be implemented
- The number of times that data will be collected

A good design is one that (a) appropriately answers the **research question**, (b) lacks **bias**, (c) controls for **extraneous/confounding variables**, and (d) has sufficient **power**, which is the ability to detect **statistically significant findings** (Melnyk, Morrison-Beedy, & Cole, 2015).

When beginning to design your study, it is helpful to conduct a "research design workout" with your team and develop an outline of the various components of the research you are planning (see Table 5.1). Research design workouts are meetings held with members of your team to complete the study outline and discuss issues regarding the study's methods

TABLE 5.1 Example of a Completed Outline for an Intervention Study

The study's purpose	What is the main purpose of the study?
	The purpose of this study is to determine the efficacy of the COPE program versus an attention control program on the process and outcomes of parental coping with a preterm infant and premature infants' length of stay in the NICU.
Research questions(s)	What question(s) will the study answer?
	What is the effect of the COPE program on the process and outcomes of parental coping with a preterm infant?
	What is the effect of the COPE program on premature infants' length of stay in the NICU?
Significance/background/ the "so what" factor	Why is this study important to conduct? How will it extend the science in the area or improve clinical practice?
	More than 500,000 premature infants are born in the United States every year, and the healthcare costs associated with preterm birth are exorbitant.
	There is a high incidence of depression and other negative outcomes in parents of premature infants.
	Prematurely born children have a high incidence of adverse developmental, emotional, and academic outcomes through the adolescent years.
Innovation	What is innovative about the study?
	Unlike prior studies with parents of preterm infants, this is the first study to test a theory-based reproducible intervention program with parents of preterm infants that commences within 2 to 4 days after admission to the NICU. Early intervention may be key to future successful programs because evidence has supported that once a negative parent–infant interaction trajectory is started, changes are difficult to initiate and sustain.
Theoretical/conceptual framework	What theory or theories will guide the intervention and selection of study variables?
	Self-regulation and control theories will guide the intervention and selection of study variables.
	One component of the COPE intervention is driven by self-regulation theory (Johnson & Leventhal), which contends that the provision of concrete objective information before/during an upcoming stressful experience creates a cognitive schema of what to expect and increases understanding, predictability, and confidence that in turn enhances both emotional and functional coping outcomes. Therefore, providing parents with concrete objective information about how their infants differ from full-term infants should enhance their understanding, predictability, and confidence (i.e., their beliefs about their infant), which should in turn lead to less negative emotion (i.e., depression and anxiety) and more involvement in their infant's care (i.e., the functional outcome of coping).

(continued)

TABLE 5.1 Example of a Completed Outline for an Intervention Study *(continued)*	
	The second component of the COPE intervention is driven by control theory (Carver & Scheier), which contends that a discrepancy between a current state and a preexisting standard or goal motivates behaviors that serve to decrease the discrepancy. However, certain conditions or barriers (e.g., anxiety, lack of confidence or knowledge, the environment) may block the initiation of behaviors once the discrepancy is recognized. Parents of premature infants experience a discrepancy between the role they expected (their parenting standard) and their role as experienced (in the NICU). Providing parents with education and practice in parenting behaviors specific to their situation as well as the permission to do so will remove the typical barriers and allow them to participate more in their infants' care.
Subjects	What are the sampling criteria and the sampling design?
	The sampling criteria will include the following: (a) mothers and fathers should be aged 18 years and older; (b) they should be able to read and speak English; (c) they should have no history of another infant in the NICU; and (d) infant gestational age should be between 26 and 34 weeks.
	The sampling design will be one of convenience at two NICUs in the northeast region of the United States.
Variables Independent variable	What is the independent variable (the intervention) and will it be reproducible and cost efficient for others to implement if the study supports its efficacy? Can the varying needs of individuals be met using a single uniform intervention and dose?
	Random assignment to the COPE intervention, a four-phase educational–behavioral intervention program or a four-phase attention control program.
Dependent variables	What is the dependent variable(s)?
	Parental anxiety and depression during the NICU stay and up to the infants' 2 years of age.
	Parental interaction in the NICU with their infant.
	Infant cognitive development.
Mediating variable	What is the mediating variable (the variable through which the intervention is expected to produce its effects)?
	Parental beliefs about their infant and their role.
Moderating variable(s)	What are potential moderating variables (variables that could influence the intervention's effect on the outcome[s])?
	Educational level; SES.
Cost variable	Infant length of stay in the NICU.
Potential confounding variables with solutions	What are the potential confounding variables and how will you control for them?
	Acuity of infant illness: Exclude infants with Grade III or IV hemorrhage; record illness severity so if different between the study groups, it can be controlled statistically.

(continued)

TABLE 5.1 Example of a Completed Outline for an Intervention Study *(continued)*	
Statistical issues	What are the hypotheses?
	Parents who receive the COPE program will report less depression than parents who receive the attention control program.
	Infants whose parents receive the COPE program will have a shorter length of stay in the NICU than infants of parents who receive the attention control program.
Sample size and power	What is the needed sample size to find statistically significant differences between or among the study groups?
	The number of subjects to obtain a power of .8 at the .05 level of significance and medium effect size is 144 mothers and 144 fathers using multivariate analysis of variance tests with repeated measures. Twenty percent of additional subjects will be added for potential attrition from the study.
	What are the best analyses to answer the study question(s) or test the hypotheses?
	Multivariate analysis of variance tests with repeated measures will be used for statistical analyses. Analysis of covariance will be used if study groups are found to be unequal on baseline demographic and/or clinical variables and those variables are correlated with the dependent variables.

COPE, Creating Opportunities for Parent Empowerment; NICU, neonatal intensive care unit; SES, socioeconomic status.

and protocol. These meetings also are a good time to discuss and agree on roles that each person will have in the study as well as in the writing of grant applications to fund the work. It is important that a statistician be part of your team and that he or she is involved in the study from its earliest planning stage. There is nothing more frustrating to statisticians than to be asked to join a research team after a study has already been planned.

> Coming together is a beginning. Keeping together is progress.
> Working together is success. *—Henry Ford*

EXPERIMENTAL OR INTERVENTION STUDY DESIGNS

Experimental designs are used to test the effects of an intervention or treatment on an outcome. They are the designs that need to be used when an investigator is interested in generating evidence to support causality (i.e., being able to say that the intervention causes a change in the dependent variable or outcome, such as giving a baby a pacifier causes a reduction in crying 1 hour later).

An experimental or intervention program of research usually follows a five-phase development sequence, beginning with a feasibility study in which the intervention is developed and tested with a small number of subjects to assess acceptability of the intervention and their responses to it (e.g., whether they thought it was helpful and why; see Table 5.2). Next, a pilot study is conducted before embarking on a full-scale **randomized controlled trial (RCT)**. A pilot study allows you to assess the preliminary effects of a new intervention as well as provides an opportunity to assess study burden and the best times for collecting measures. Essentially, a pilot study is helpful in working out potential "glitches" in the intervention or study protocol before embarking on a full-scale trial. After efficacy of an intervention is established through a full-scale RCT, the next study that should be conducted in a program of intervention research is an **effectiveness trial**. Effectiveness trials are conducted in real-world practice settings to determine whether the outcomes that were achieved in an efficacy RCT can be reproduced in real-world settings. The National Institutes of Health has a similar trajectory for phases of clinical trials (see Table 5.3).

TABLE 5.2 The Five-Phase Development Sequence of Experimental or Intervention Research	
Phase I	Basic research that is exploratory and descriptive in nature and that establishes the variables that may be amenable to intervention or in which the content, strength, and timing of the intervention are developed, along with the outcome measures for the study.
Phase II	Pilot research (i.e., a small-scale study in which the intervention is tested with a small number of subjects so that the feasibility of a large-scale study is determined and alternative strategies are developed for potential problems).
Phase III	Efficacy trials in which evaluation of the intervention takes place in an ideal setting and clinical efficacy is determined (in this stage, much emphasis is placed on internal validity of the study and preliminary cost-effectiveness of the intervention).
Phase IV	Effectiveness of clinical trials in which analysis of intervention effect is conducted in clinical practice and clinical effectiveness is determined, as is cost-effectiveness (in this stage, much emphasis is placed on external validity or generalizability of the study).
Phase V	Effects on public health in which wide-scale implementation of the intervention is conducted to determine its effects on public health.

Source: From Whittemore, R., & Grey, M. (2002). The systematic development of nursing interventions. *Journal of Nursing Scholarship, 34*(2), 115–120. doi:10.1111/j.1547-5069.2002.00115.x

TABLE 5.3 The National Institutes of Health Phases of Clinical Trials	
PHASE	**PURPOSE**
I	To test a new biomedical or behavioral intervention in a small group for the first time to establish safety (e.g., a pilot study with 20–80 subjects)
II	To study the biomedical or behavioral intervention in a larger group of people to determine efficacy and to further evaluate safety (e.g., a trial with 100–300 subjects)
III	To study the efficacy of the biomedical or behavioral intervention in large groups (e.g., 1,000–3,000 subjects) by comparing the intervention to other standard or experimental interventions as well as to monitor adverse effects
IV	To monitor the effectiveness of the approved intervention in the population and to collect information about any adverse effects associated with widespread usage

THE RANDOMIZED CONTROLLED TRIAL OR TRUE EXPERIMENT

The gold standard for experimental studies is the RCT or a true experiment because it is the strongest design for testing cause and effect relationships. Three characteristics must exist to meet the criteria for a RCT; the study must have

- An experimental group that receives the treatment or intervention;
- A comparison or **attention control group** that receives a different intervention than the experimental group;
- **Random assignment** or **randomization**, which is a strategy used to assign subjects to experimental or comparison/attention control groups by probability (e.g., using a random numbers table or tossing a coin).

RCTs are the strongest designs for controlling extraneous or confounding variables, which strengthens **internal validity** of a study. Internal validity is the ability to say that it was the intervention or treatment that caused a change in the **dependent variable** or **outcome**, not other confounding variables. Random assignment helps to ensure that the study groups are similar at the start of the study before the treatments are delivered. If subjects are not equivalent on baseline demographic and clinical characteristics at the start of the study, it would be impossible to conclude that it was the intervention itself that was responsible for the difference in outcomes between the groups. As a hypothetical example to illustrate this point, an experimental study was conducted to determine the effects of a 6-week cognitive behavioral therapy intervention (the experimental intervention) versus yoga (the comparison intervention) on state anxiety in college students with high stress levels. At the start of the study, before the interventions were delivered, state anxiety of the two groups of students was measured with a well-known valid and reliable state anxiety measure. Following the 6-week interventions, state anxiety was again measured. Findings indicated that students in the cognitive behavioral therapy group had a state anxiety mean score of 45 and the yoga students had a mean score of 50 at baseline, before their interventions. At the end of the trial, the cognitive behavioral therapy group had a mean score of 40 and the yoga students had a mean score of 45. However, because the students did not begin the trial with similar levels of state anxiety (assessed by statistical analysis), it could not be concluded that cognitive behavioral therapy is more effective than yoga.

Types of True Experimental Designs

Exhibits 5.1 to 5.10 depict the various types of true experimental designs. In the exhibits, R indicates random assignment, X represents an intervention or treatment (X_1 indicates the experimental intervention, and X_2 and X_3 indicate that the subjects received comparison or attention control interventions different from the experimental intervention), and O indicates when the outcome assessment or observation was performed (O_1 indicates the first time that the outcome assessment was collected, and O_2 and O_3 indicate that the outcome assessment was collected for the second and third time).

These exhibits were first used to depict experimental designs in a classic landmark book by Campbell and Stanley in 1963 and are still widely used today. In the exhibits, time moves from left to right, and subscripts are used to designate different groups or various measurement points.

The Two-Group Randomized Controlled Trial With Pretest/Posttest Design and Structurally Equivalent Comparison Group

The two-group RCT with pretest/posttest and a structurally equivalent comparison group is the strongest design for testing cause and effect (Exhibit 5.1). In this type of experiment, subjects are randomly assigned to receive either the experimental intervention or a comparison

EXHIBIT 5.1 Two-Group Randomized Controlled Trial With Pretest/Posttest Design and Structurally Equivalent Comparison Group

R O_1 X_1 O_2

R O_1 X_2 O_2

Note: R, random assignment; X, intervention/treatment with X_1 being the experimental intervention and X_2 being the comparison/attention control intervention; O, observation/outcome measurement with O_1 being the first time that the variable is measured at baseline and O_2 being the second time that it is measured after the intervention.

EXHIBIT 5.2 Two-Group Randomized Controlled Trial With Posttest-Only Design

R X_1 O_1

R X_2

Note: R, random assignment; X, intervention/treatment with X_1 being the experimental intervention and X_2 being the comparison/attention control intervention; O, observation/outcome measurement with O_1 being the first time that the variable is measured after the intervention.

or attention control intervention. Controlling for time and attention with an attention control group is important in experimental studies because if differences are found between the study groups at the end of the project, the inference can be made that the differences are truly because of the effects of the intervention and not just because the experimental group received "something." Although **pretesting** (gathering assessments from the subjects on the study's measures prior to the start of the interventions) can sensitize the subjects to measures that will be used in the study, pretesting allows the investigator to assess equivalence between the study groups on baseline demographic and clinical variables.

Two-Group Randomized Controlled Trial With Posttest-Only Design
In a two-group RCT with posttest-only design, subjects are not pretested on any measures before they receive their interventions (see Exhibit 5.2). The advantage to this design is that there is no pretest effect or sensitization to the measure(s) that will be used at the follow-up assessments. However, the major disadvantage to this design is that baseline data is unknown, so the investigator cannot be certain that the subjects are equal on baseline demographic and clinical variables. Although the major reason for using random assignment is that, by probability, there is a good chance that subjects will be equal on demographic and baseline variables at the start of the study, one cannot be absolutely certain that this will be the case because there is always the chance that probability may deal a "dirty hand," with the result being unequal study groups at baseline.

Two-Group Randomized Controlled Trial With Long-Term Repeated Measures Follow-Up
The two-group RCT with long-term repeated measures follow-up allows you to determine both the short- and long-term effects of an intervention, which is important in assessing sustainability of the intervention's effects on outcomes over time (see Exhibit 5.3). Disadvantages of this design are that it is more costly because of the longer term follow-up of subjects and that attrition of subjects may be a problem, which threatens the internal validity of the study.

EXHIBIT 5.3 Two-Group Randomized Controlled Trial With Long-Term Repeated Measures Follow-Up

R	X_1	O_1	O_2	O_3
R	X_2	O_1	O_2	O_3

Note: R, random assignment; X, intervention/treatment with X_1 being the experimental intervention and X_2 being the comparison/ attention control intervention; O, observation/outcome measurement with O_1 being the first time that the variable is measured, O_2 being the second time the variable is measured, and O_3 being the third time the variable is measured.

EXHIBIT 5.4 Two-Group Randomized Controlled Trial Without an Attention Control Group

R	X_1	O_1
R		O_1

Note: R, random assignment; X, intervention/treatment with X_1 being the experimental intervention; O, observation/outcome measurement with O_1 being the first time that the variable is measured after the intervention.

Two-Group Randomized Controlled Trial Without an Attention Control Group

The major disadvantage to the two-group RCT without an attention control group is that intervention effects may solely be related to giving the intervention group "something" (see Exhibit 5.4). The control group in this design does not receive a structurally equivalent intervention that is of equal time and attention to the experimental group. The absence of a structurally equivalent attention control group is a major flaw in many intervention studies. For example, a study is designed with the purpose of determining the efficacy of a 1-hour stress reduction intervention for surgical patients on their postoperative stress levels. The experimental intervention consists of a social worker teaching patients in the treatment group about deep breathing and imagery in a 1-hour preoperative session. However, the control group receives only the typical preoperative "standard of care" that is given to all surgical patients prior to their operation, which includes a pamphlet with tips on how to reduce stress but no time with a social worker. If the findings from the study reveal that the experimental group subjects report significantly less stress after their operations than the control group subjects, it may be due only to the fact that a social worker spent an hour of time with them and not be the result of the actual content of the intervention (i.e., deep breathing and imagery exercises).

Three-Group Randomized Controlled Trial

A three-group RCT allows an investigator to compare the efficacy of providing subjects with a comparison or structurally equivalent attention control intervention and a pure control condition (no type of intervention; see Exhibit 5.5). Disadvantages of this design are that additional subjects are needed, which will incur additional costs.

Solomon Four-Group Design

The advantage of a Solomon four-group experimental design is that it allows the investigator to separate the effects of pretesting, before the intervention is delivered, on the outcome(s) (see Exhibit 5.6). Disadvantages include the need for more subjects and additional study costs.

EXHIBIT 5.5 Three-Group Randomized Controlled Trial

R	X_1	O_1
R	X_2	O_1
R		O_1

Note: R, random assignment; X, intervention/treatment with X_1 being the experimental intervention and X_2 being the comparison/attention control intervention; O, observation/outcome measurement with O_1 being the first time that the variable is measured after the intervention.

EXHIBIT 5.6 The Solomon Four-Group Design

R	O_1	X_1	O_2
R		X_1	O_2
R	O_1	X_2	O_2
R		X_2	O_2

Note: R, random assignment; X, intervention/treatment with X_1 being the experimental intervention and X_2 being the comparison/attention control intervention; O, observation/outcome measurement with O_1 being the first time that the variable is measured before the intervention, and O_2 being the second time the variable is measured after the intervention.

EXHIBIT 5.7 A 2 × 2 Factorial Experiment

		EDUCATION	
		YES	**NO**
EXERCISE	**YES**	Education and exercise	Exercise only
	NO	Education only	Neither education nor exercise

Note: A 2 × 2 factorial experiment results in four study groups: (a) a group of subjects who receive both education and exercise, (b) a group of subjects who receive education only, (c) a group of subjects who receive exercise only, and (d) a group of subjects who receive neither education nor exercise.

2 × 2 Factorial Experiment

A **2 × 2 factorial experiment** is a true experiment that allows an investigator to study the separate and combined effects of interventions (i.e., two or more interventions or treatments; see Exhibit 5.7). For example, if a clinician was interested in the separate and combined effects of two different interventions, education and exercise, on weight loss in overweight adults, this type of design would result in four study groups:

1. A group of subjects who receive education only
2. A group of subjects who receive exercise only

3.   A group of subjects who receive both education and exercise
4.   A group of subjects who receive neither education nor exercise

A major strength of this study is that it can be determined if the combination of education and exercise results in more weight loss than either education or exercise alone. Disadvantages to this design include additional subjects and costs.

QUASI-EXPERIMENTAL INTERVENTION STUDIES

Quasi-experiments are studies in which the independent variable is manipulated (an intervention or treatment is delivered), but there is a lack of at least one of the other two properties of true experiments (i.e., random assignment or a comparison/control group; see Exhibit 5.8).

Although quasi-experimental designs are sometimes conducted for practical, ethical, or feasibility reasons, they are not as strong as true experiments in their ability to support causality. In addition, there are threats to internal validity in quasi-experiments that weaken the ability to say that it was the intervention or treatment that caused a change in outcomes, not other extraneous/confounding variables. Therefore, whenever possible, it is best to use a true experimental design with random assignment and a comparison/control group. However, there are times when quasi-experiments are necessary because real-life circumstances may exist that prohibit your ability to randomly assign subjects to treatment groups. For example, if you are conducting an intervention study in a high school setting, you may be prohibited from randomly assigning students to different intervention groups if the principal is not in favor of this strategy. As another example, if you are conducting an intervention study in a hospital that accommodates four patients to a room, you would not want to randomly assign individual patients to the treatment or control conditions as **cross-contamination** (some part of the experimental intervention diffuses to subjects in the control group) could be a major problem that confounds your study's results. If individual randomization by subject is not feasible, it is often possible to introduce some level of random assignment into a study (e.g., randomly assigning schools or patient rooms to treatment or comparison/control conditions). In quasi-experiments in which random assignment is not used, pretesting is especially important to assess whether the study groups are equal on demographic and clinical variables at the start of the study (Melnyk et al., 2015). Even if the study groups are fairly similar at the start of a quasi-experimental study, you cannot be absolutely sure that there are no other unexplored differences that exist between the groups that might affect the findings in the study. If only posttests are conducted in a quasi-experiment, it will be very difficult to have confidence in the study's findings because it will not be known if the groups were similar at commencement of the study. Conversely, when random assignment is used in true experimental studies, it is very likely that the study groups will be similar on pretest measures.

EXHIBIT 5.8   A Quasi-Experimental Study That Lacks Random Assignment

O_1 X_1 O_2

O_1 X_2 O_2

Note: X, intervention/treatment with X_1 being the experimental intervention and X_2 being the comparison/attention control intervention; O, observation/outcome measurement with O_1 being the first time that the variable is measured at baseline and O_2 being the second time that it is measured after the intervention.

EXHIBIT 5.9 A Quasi-Experimental Time Series Design

| O_1 | O_2 | O_3 | O_4 | X | O_5 | O_6 | O_7 | O_8 |

Note: X, intervention/treatment; O, observation/outcome measurement with $O_1, O_2, O_3,$ and O_4 being collected before the intervention, and $O_5, O_6, O_7,$ and O_8 being collected after the intervention.

EXHIBIT 5.10 A Preexperiment

| X | O_1 |

Note: There is no random assignment or no comparison/control group. X is the intervention, and O_1 is the outcome measure/observation.

Another type of quasi-experimental study is the interrupted time series design (see Exhibit 5.9). In this intervention study, there is neither random assignment nor a comparison/attention control group. Instead, there is first a series of pretest measures followed by an intervention, which is subsequently followed by a series of posttest measures. This type of design is used most commonly in community intervention studies. For example, adolescent pregnancy rates might be tracked over a number of years and then followed by an intervention. After delivery of the intervention for some length of time, pregnancy rates are tracked for several more years. Major threats to internal validity with the time series design are **history**, which is when some event unrelated to the intervention accounts for the change in outcome(s), and **maturation** (i.e., when subjects change merely with the passage of time and the change in their outcome[s] has nothing to do with the experimental intervention).

PREEXPERIMENTAL INTERVENTION STUDIES

Preexperiments lack both random assignment and a comparison/attention control group (see Exhibit 5.10). They are extremely weak in internal validity because there are too many competing explanations for the study's findings. These designs are used most often when an intervention is first being developed to test its feasibility and acceptability.

COMPARATIVE EFFECTIVENESS RESEARCH

A great deal of recent attention and funding by federal agencies has been devoted to **comparative effectiveness research** (CER), which is the comparison of effective interventions among patients in typical patient care settings, with decisions that are tailored to meet individual patient needs (i.e., which interventions are most effective for which patients; Sox & Greenfield, 2009). A major objective of CER is to provide **evidence-based information** to assist consumers, clinicians, and payers in making better informed clinical and health policy decisions by providing evidence on the effectiveness, benefits, and harms of different treatment options (e.g., two different medications, surgery versus medication; Luce et al., 2009;

Agency for Healthcare Research and Quality [AHRQ], 2011). The evidence to inform these decisions is generated from clinical trials that compare drugs, treatment devices, tests, or ways to deliver healthcare (AHRQ, 2011). However, unfortunately, many clinical trials have excluded certain subgroups of patients based on age, sex, and race/ethnicity as well as failed to measure important health and long-term outcomes, which limits the ability of clinicians, administrators, insurers, and policy makers to make good informed decisions.

CER uses various methodologies, including RCTs and **systematic reviews**, which are typically used to develop **evidence-based clinical practice guidelines**. For example, because you are interested in determining the most effective treatment for depressed adults, you review the literature and discover that both cognitive behavioral therapy and interpersonal therapy have been empirically supported in RCTs to reduce episodes of depression. However, an RCT has never been conducted that compares cognitive behavioral therapy to interpersonal therapy with depressed adults to determine the more effective treatment. Therefore, you decide to conduct a two-group RCT in which you will compare the two treatments to determine which is more effective in the treatment of depression in culturally diverse adults. In your study, you also will monitor for adverse effects of the treatments.

The Institute of Medicine issued 100 topic priorities for CER that can be accessed at http://www.nationalacademies.org/hmd/~/media/Files/Report%20Files/2009/Comparative EffectivenessResearchPriorities/CER%20report%20brief%2008-13-09.pdf. A few of the priorities listed in the top quartile include

- Comparing the effectiveness of school-based interventions involving meal programs, vending machines, and physical education at different levels of intensity in preventing and treating overweight and obesity in children and adolescents;
- Comparing the effectiveness of treatment strategies for atrial fibrillation, including surgery, catheter ablation, and pharmacological treatment;
- Comparing the effectiveness of clinical interventions to reduce the incidence of infant mortality, preterm births, and low birth rates, especially among African American women.

DESIGNING THE EXPERIMENTAL AND CONTROL INTERVENTIONS

The investigator has many important decisions to make when it comes to designing an intervention. Guiding these decisions should be, first and foremost, the state of the science in the area and a clear understanding of what interventions currently exist, their strengths and limitations, and for which populations they have been developed and in which they have been tested. Having a clear understanding of the literature should help you to identify gaps and determine what direction seems logical and is needed. Identifying what current interventions are being used or having evidence obtained in scientifically rigorous trials will be the basis for your next step. If you are adapting an intervention, you may even ask yourself—could this intervention that has been empirically supported in the literature still be as effective if it were briefer or provided in a different format or to a different population?

Interventions that are theoretically driven may be more effective than those that are not and provide a framework for understanding the relationships between constructs identified as influential on the outcome of interest. Whether it be understanding how (a) patients cope with stress and illness, (b) teens change high-risk behaviors, (c) parents discipline their children, or (d) teachers motivate underperforming students, understanding how the conceptual pieces fit together is an essential component of intervention development. Without a theory serving as your guide, choosing which constructs to investigate and manipulate could be like going on a wild goose chase. When designing intervention components, it is important to address each of the key theoretical constructs. Interventions that measure changes in theoretically driven constructs yet have intervention strategies that target only some of the constructs face the risk that what really drives change in critical outcomes is not being manipulated.

An important consideration for developing your intervention is the "**dose**" needed to change the study's outcome. Dose refers to the amount of the intervention that the participants receive—whether it be hours, sessions, videos watched, phone calls made, pills taken, meals eaten, miles swam—to change the dependent variable/outcome. Balance is again a key—what dose will be sufficient to make a measureable impact on your outcome(s), yet not be excessive so that time, money, and effort are, in a sense, wasted? Early on in your intervention work, the choice is to err on the side of a sufficient (even if overly sufficient) dose so that an intervention effect is identifiable. Ultimately, when designing an intervention, there must be a balance between effectiveness of the treatment and its safety. In addition, the intervention must not be overly burdensome to the participants. Incentives for study participation may allay some of this burden, but remember that these incentives will not exist when your intervention is translated into practice or community settings. Will people still participate in your program or will others implement your intervention treatment when there is no incentive involved? A key question ultimately is whether your intervention will be adaptable and usable in the real world. These issues must be considered in designing your intervention study. With future work, your intervention can be refined to allow further tapering of the dose required to affect change in outcome(s).

For example, guided by the information, motivation, behavioral skills model (Fisher, Fisher, Bryan, & Misovich, 2002), an intervention was developed to reduce HIV risk in adolescent girls. This model posits three key constructs that predict HIV behavioral risk reduction: (a) information, (b) motivation, and (c) behavioral skills. To develop the Health Improvement Project for Teens (HIP Teens) intervention, the principal investigator (PI) and research team developed multiple intervention strategies (e.g., role-playing, games, team-building exercises) that addressed these three key constructs (Morrison-Beedy, Carey, Aronowitz, Mkandawire, & Dyne, 2002; Morrison-Beedy, Carey, Kowalski, & Tu, 2005; Morrison-Beedy, Carey, Seibold-Simpson, Xia, & Tu, 2009). Based on previous findings from effective interventions for other at-risk populations, 8 hours of intervention were determined to be an adequate dose of treatment. The decision was made to divide the dose into four 2-hour sessions to decrease burden on participants (versus a single 8-hour dose) and facilitate attendance. Predicting that all participants would not attend every session because of scheduling conflicts, illness, forgetfulness, and other factors, it was critically important that intervention strategies addressed *each* of the key constructs (IMB) at *every* session. This approach would ensure dosing on all constructs for participants. Had the intervention placed all activities addressing a construct on 1 day only (e.g., all information in session one), participants who did not attend that session would not be dosed on that construct. If, ultimately, the construct of information was identified as the predominant predictor of behavioral change, then those participants who did not receive information strategies would most likely not change their behavior. This "lack" of intervention dosing could, depending on the number who did not attend session one, dilute the true impact of the intervention and lead to results that would not reach statistical significance. Thus, the need to carefully map out your intervention with a focus on adequate dosing on all constructs is essential.

Among the many choices that you will face as you design your intervention is whether you should test one specific intervention or integrate two different interventions into one "new" treatment. In early HIV prevention interventions, the focus was on interventions that provided information to participants. As the epidemic continued, new interventions that provided behavioral skills–training were tested. Subsequently, combination interventions (providing both information and skills) were developed and tested with improved effects on risk behaviors. Although single-treatment approaches are easier to design and implement in research and real-world settings, it is the state of the science that drives the development and testing of single versus combination interventions and thus impacts your intervention decision making as an investigator.

Developing an effective experimental intervention requires directed attention to its tailoring for your specific population. Factors such as gender, race/ethnicity, educational level, and socioeconomic status must be considered—there is no skipping this important step. Conducting formative work (e.g., focus groups, interviews) with participants during intervention development is an appropriate first step in designing your intervention. It provides the opportunity to craft an intervention that truly "fits" your population and addresses cultural, developmental, and social realities that will impact its utility. Grant reviewers will expect this tailoring of the intervention as "one size does not fit all."

Devoting time to developing a credible control condition also is important. Whenever possible, it is best to design a **structurally equivalent attention control intervention** to control for the time and attention being spent with participants in the experimental group. As an example, in an intervention study to determine the efficacy of the COPE program for parents of preterms on parental depression and anxiety, the experimental group of parents received audiotaped and written information that prepared them for what behaviors to expect in their preterm infants and how best to parent them (Melnyk et al., 2006). The attention control intervention group also received audiotaped and written information of the same length as the COPE program, but the information in the control program focused on policies and procedures within the neonatal intensive care unit and did not contain any of the information contained in the COPE program. Intervention effects can be diluted if the control condition contains ingredients that may positively impact the outcome variable. For example, if the control condition in the COPE study contained information about stress reduction for parents, differences in anxiety between the two study groups would be diminished. It is important for the comparison intervention to be just as engaging as the experimental condition to prevent differential attrition from occurring in the comparison/control group.

Some studies have used "standard of care" in a setting as a control condition. Although using standard of care can function as a control condition, it does not typically control for time, attention, and intervention strategies as a comparison condition and may be identified by reviewers as a substantial limitation in a study's design. In drug studies, a placebo pill is typically provided as the comparison condition. Conversely, participants in a "no attention" control condition receive absolutely no type of intervention or attention and would just complete data collection measures. Designing a study with a "no attention" control condition is usually seen as a major flaw with far too many threats to internal validity. Ethical concerns also may be raised by reviewers about control conditions if those participants are not offered the experimental intervention at the completion of the study.

After you have developed or tailored your experimental and control interventions, a critical next step is to document them in a manner that will ensure that they are delivered to participants as you have "envisioned" them. Writing a manual that outlines, in as much detail as possible, "what" the intervention is, how it should be provided, and how much time should be allotted for each component is essential. It should be clear where flexibility exists in providing the treatment and where it does not. This manual is used to train the personnel providing the intervention and as a tool to assess for intervention "drift." Drift occurs when the intervention is initially provided in one manner (as you intended it to be) and, over time, inconsistency creeps in to how the intervention is being delivered. This drift can occur for many reasons, including inconsistent training of those persons providing the intervention, lack of enthusiasm, and attention to detail as the job becomes more routine or lacks expectations. Ultimately, it is impossible to determine the effects of an intervention if its delivery changes throughout the course of the study.

In developing the HIP Teens risk reduction program for adolescent girls, the intervention protocol manual contained a detailed outline of content, strategies for addressing difficulties encountered during each of the intervention sessions, and equipment or supplies needed for each of the sessions. The intervention was provided to over 700 girls in small groups (6–9 participants) led by two trained facilitators. The approximate time to be allotted for each intervention strategy was determined and documented in the manual. Attending to time allocation for each component in the intervention helped to ensure that some groups of girls did not receive extensive dosing on one construct (e.g., knowledge), whereas other groups received only brief exposure to the intervention strategy intended to affect that construct. Following construction of the study's protocol manual, measures were developed to assess the intervention's fidelity (i.e., providing the intervention in the exact manner in which it was designed to be delivered; see Chapter 15 for discussion on Maintaining Intervention Fidelity). Assuring that the intervention is carried out consistently in the manner it was intended is one of the greatest challenges you will face in intervention research.

Blinding of the investigator, the data collectors, or the participants occurs when details regarding which participants are receiving the experimental intervention versus those receiving the control or comparison condition are concealed. Reducing the risk of bias in an intervention study can be accomplished with blinding, which is fairly easy. When data collectors are not exposed to any intervention components and function independent of those who provide the intervention or when the investigator has access to only de-identified data, then blinding is possible. In some studies, it is difficult to blind participants. For example, those who experience side effects from the intervention are difficult to blind in a study.

Designing an intervention requires focused attention on multiple issues. These include deciding on a theoretical framework to guide your study, balancing safety versus effect, testing single versus combination interventions, and determining appropriate dosing of the treatment. In addition, tailoring the intervention to your population, manualizing the intervention to enhance reproducibility and consistent administration, constructing methods and measures to ensure intervention fidelity, and determining the appropriateness of blinding investigators, team personnel, and participants are required. Although this list is not comprehensive, investigators who tackle these issues will be better equipped to design and conduct scientifically rigorous intervention studies. Many of the strategies for intervention development discussed in this section can be implemented and refined during pilot work.

DESIGNING PILOT STUDIES

The Chinese philosopher Lao-tzu once said, "A journey of 1,000 miles begins with a single step." This also holds true for the wise investigator who, before implementing a full-scale intervention study, conducts pilot work as a preliminary step. Pilot studies can answer many questions and point out "glitches in the system" that need correction. You may be eager to begin testing your intervention and look forward with anticipation to the impact it may have on your outcome(s) of interest. Congratulations! That motivation and drive will lay the foundation for your successful program of research. Conducting this groundwork to assess the feasibility and acceptability of your project will be key to ensuring your ability to carry out your future work.

The preliminary steps taken in a pilot study can be invaluable. Pilot studies lay the foundation for future full-scale studies by providing reliability and validity data on measures, determining appropriate timing for their administration, and eliciting participants' responses to the intervention (e.g., whether they believe it was helpful, culturally sensitive, developmentally appropriate, and engaging). This pilot work is useful for refining your intervention timetable as well as data collection and coding plans. Pilot studies are the perfect opportunity to develop and document study procedures and work out the "kinks" in protocols. One key function of the pilot can be to estimate the preliminary **effect size** of the intervention itself, which indicates the strength of impact that the intervention had on the study's outcome(s). All these components are at the very heart of a successful intervention study. Unless other investigators have already laid this foundation, you will need to conduct pilot work before any full-scale intervention study. Certainly, agencies that fund research intervention studies (e.g., the National Institutes of Health, the Agency for Healthcare Research & Quality) will not provide monetary support for a full-scale clinical trial without promising pilot work.

Time devoted to a pilot study also allows you to establish working relationships with the agency or program in which recruitment will be conducted. Intervention details can be worked out and methods for enrolling and retaining participants refined. In addition, a pilot study will offer you a good look at the true "pool" of potential participants, including an opportunity to gain a clearer understanding of what facilitates or hinders enrollment and retention. This preliminary study can shed light on the recruitment and retention procedures that are most effective and provide you with data on participant characteristics and demographic distributions. The data collected from a pilot study then assist you in determining if you will meet planned recruitment numbers needed for the full-scale study as well as gender and minority enrollment.

Pilot studies are usually conducted in a brief time period. This differs from the intervention study and its targeted outcome. For example, a pilot of a tutoring intervention for failing high school students may have final passing grades as its outcome. This study would naturally require a longer follow-up period. However, another option might be to assess the change in grades by semester instead of annually, which would require a shorter follow-up period (exam grades being a proxy for final grades). Conversely, many pilot studies can be conducted in a brief time period. You may be able to recruit all of your participants in 1 day (depending on the setting) and have them complete baseline measures, followed shortly thereafter by the intervention. An important point is that your pilot study should reflect the protocol for your planned full-scale study as much as possible. It is up to you as the investigator to determine which aspects are most critical to pilot. You may feel very successful recruiting a sample of participants from a currently existing support group for women affected by interpersonal violence (IPV) and then providing your 8-hour intervention in one big weekend "blitz." However, if your full-scale intervention protocol is actually designed for women *newly* admitted to domestic violence shelters who will then receive eight hourly intervention sessions attached to their weekly counseling groups, your pilot may provide you with limited information. Recruiting a sample that was somewhat more "accessible" (although they experienced a history of IPV) and providing the intervention in a manner different from what you plan to do in the full-scale study (one 8-hour session versus eight 1-hour sessions) does not truly reflect your plans for the full-scale study. The time you invest in having your pilot study mirror your planned study protocols will reap many benefits.

The opportunity to do a "dress rehearsal" of study procedures is a tremendous benefit of the pilot study. It is helpful for you, the investigator, to go through the protocol as a study participant and assess from the subject's point of view how things are working (Morrison-Beedy et al., 2002). Community or clinical site relationships also can be built or strengthened during the pilot study; their commitment to the larger project may be secured once they see how the program will function within their setting.

Most often, the ultimate objective of intervention studies is to provide evidence of long-term positive impact on the target population; creating a treatment with "holding power" or sustainability is the aim of most investigators. The goal in the pilot study is to assess whether your intervention makes a difference in outcome(s) in the short run. Often, this difference is quantified as effect sizes versus statistical significance (which requires a larger sample size).

Determining the effect size (i.e., an estimate of the extent of impact that the intervention made on the outcome of interest) for the main outcome variable in a pilot study will provide you with data needed to determine the needed sample size for your full-scale study (Mays & Melnyk, 2009). Effect sizes are easy to calculate and typically are not influenced by sample size. They are computed with the Cohen's *d* statistic in a statistical analysis program or calculated by subtracting the mean score on the outcome variable of the control group from the mean score of the experimental group and dividing by the pooled or average standard deviation (Mays & Melnyk, 2009). A small effect size is .2; a medium effect size is .5; and a large effect size is .8 or greater (Cohen, 1988). A mistake that investigators often make is to conduct a pilot study and determine the effect size of their intervention on the major study outcome but not use this information in calculating the sample size for their full-scale study. For example, in a study of a peer group intervention to reduce substance use in teens, the findings revealed that the intervention produced a small positive effect on daily marijuana use (the main outcome). However, in the proposal for their full-scale study, the investigators reported that their power and sample size determinations are based on a medium effect size (which is the common size used by many investigators when calculating sample size). A reviewer would then determine that the sample size proposed in this study is too small—it is underpowered; it needed to be powered to detect a small, not a medium, effect. Similarly, if pilot findings indicate the pilot intervention has a large effect on the outcome, fewer subjects will be needed. Reviewers will be looking for an accurate sample size estimation based on effect size from the pilot study. Effect sizes also should be determined in full-scale trials so that the impact of the intervention on the study's outcome(s) can be assessed (Mays & Melnyk, 2009). Reporting of effect sizes in published studies also allows investigators to compare findings across intervention trials.

No pilot study looks exactly like another. Pilots can focus on gathering participants' responses to protocols, psychometric evaluation of instruments, trialing the intervention in a feasibility study with a small number of participants (e.g., 15–20), or conducting a randomized controlled pilot trial with short-term follow-up assessments with 40 to 50 participants. Pilot studies can ultimately help you reduce costs and effort in the full-scale study and, just as important (or maybe even more so), they can help to minimize the trials and tribulations faced by investigators during the course of an intervention study. They provide evidence to reviewers of your ability to carry out the work, to successfully recruit and retain participants, and to provide the intervention. The data obtained from your pilot work will help you craft the case in your proposal as to why the next step in this area of research should be *your* study.

DETERMINING SAMPLE SIZE FOR INTERVENTION STUDIES

One of the greatest mistakes investigators make is not planning to enroll enough subjects in an intervention study. This results in a lack of power, which is the ability to detect statistically significant differences between study groups. Conversely, some investigators enroll far too many subjects, which is unnecessary and costly. Enrolling a suitable number of subjects is an important goal and should be determined in the early phase of designing an intervention study.

Developing hypotheses is an important first step in determining sample size as they form the basis for tests of statistical significance and are needed to compare findings across intervention/treatment groups (Hulley et al., 2013). A **null hypothesis** contends that there is no association between the treatment and outcome variables (e.g., there is no difference in depression between adults who receive an antidepressant and those who receive cognitive behavioral therapy). A null hypothesis forms the basis for testing statistical significance because the goal of intervention studies is to reject the prediction that there is no difference between treatment groups. An **alternative hypothesis** contends that there is indeed an association between the intervention and outcome variables. **Research hypotheses** are usually one sided (i.e., the direction of the relationship between the intervention and outcome is specified, such as adults who receive cognitive behavioral therapy have less depression than those who receive an antidepressant), whereas an alternative hypothesis states only that an association exists but does not specify a direction (e.g., there is an association between cognitive behavioral therapy and depression).

Next, an appropriate statistical test should be determined (e.g., independent *t*-test, analysis of variance) along with the expected effect size, which is an estimation of how large an impact the intervention will have on the primary outcome variable. Effect size estimates are best determined from an intervention pilot study or by reviewing literature of similar interventions.

Following formulation of the most important hypothesis and selection of a statistical test and effect size, an **alpha (a)** and **beta (β)** should be set. If you have more than one important hypothesis, the sample size for the study should be calculated on which hypothesis needs the largest sample (Hulley et al., 2013). Alpha (i.e., the level of statistical significance, depicted as ∞) is the probability of making a Type I error (i.e., rejection of the null hypothesis when it is actually true). It is common practice to set the alpha at .05, meaning that 5 times out of 100, the results are likely to be due to chance and not due to true differences between the study groups. You may choose to set a lower alpha (i.e., more restrictive, such as .01) if a study has significant treatment risks to patients as with drug trials. On the contrary, if you know that you do not have enough subjects to fully power your study (e.g., in a pilot trial), you may choose to set the alpha at a higher level ($p = .10$) to avoid the probability of making a Type II error, which is called beta (β). A Type II error is when an investigator accepts a false null hypothesis (i.e., that there is no difference between treatment groups when one actually exists). Most studies set the β at .20. Thus, the power in this study would be .80, and the investigator would have an 80% chance of being able to detect a statistically significant intervention effect.

Once all of these criteria are determined, a sample size can be calculated. Options for calculating sample size include sample size tables (Cohen, 1988) or statistical software packages. Attrition rate should be taken into consideration in calculating the sample size. Sample size estimates are based on the final number of participants needed at the end data collection point in a study. For example, if you require a sample size of 100 participants for statistical testing (based on your sample size calculation), but you anticipate a 20% attrition rate across the duration of your study, then 120 participants should be enrolled at the outset of your study.

PLANNING STUDY MEASURES THAT TAP THE STUDY OUTCOMES

When designing an intervention study, it is best to choose valid and reliable measures that have been used with similar study populations. It is important that you measure variables that tap every key construct in your study. Detailed information about measurement is included in Chapter 10.

ASSESSING THE PROCESS THROUGH WHICH THE INTERVENTION WORKS WITH MEDIATING VARIABLES

The primary aim of intervention studies is to determine the impact of an intervention/treatment on outcomes. However, because it is important to explain the process through which interventions work to extend the science and create an understanding of intervention effects, investigators should consider exploring mediating variables when conducting an intervention study. A **mediating variable** is a variable through which the intervention

EXHIBIT 5.11 The Mediating Effects of the COPE Intervention on Anxiety and Depression in Parents of Premature Infants

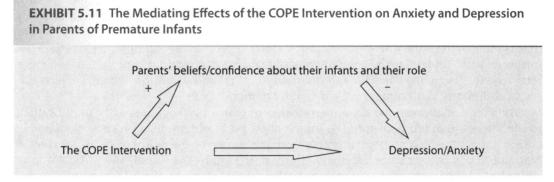

Parents' beliefs/confidence about their infants and their role

+ −

The COPE Intervention   Depression/Anxiety

COPE, Creating Opportunities for Parent Empowerment.

produces its effects on the outcome(s). For example, in an RCT with 260 low-birth-weight premature infants and their parents by Melnyk et al. (2006), findings indicated that parents who received an educational–behavioral intervention (i.e., COPE) had less parental anxiety and depression in the neonatal intensive care unit than parents who received an attention control program. The effects of COPE on parental anxiety and depression were mediated by the parents' cognitive beliefs/confidence about their infants and their role (see Exhibit 5.11). Specifically, COPE enhanced parents' beliefs/confidence, which, in turn, reduced their anxiety and depression. Therefore, the effects of COPE were mediated through parental beliefs (Melnyk, Crean, Feinstein, & Fairbanks, 2008). Mediating variables should be derived from the theoretical/conceptual framework and be an integral part of intervention work.

ASSESSING FACTORS THAT MAY INFLUENCE THE IMPACT OF THE INTERVENTION ON OUTCOMES WITH POTENTIAL MODERATORS

Moderating variables are those variables that may influence or change the relationship between the intervention/treatment and outcome(s). In the prior example using the COPE intervention with parents of premature infants, educational status of the parents or prior experience with a preterm infant could influence the intervention effects. Specifically, parents with higher levels of education or prior experience with a preterm infant could benefit more from the COPE intervention than parents with lower levels of education or no prior experience with a preterm infant. Testing of moderating variables allows investigators to determine for what populations the interventions work best. Common moderators explored by investigators when conducting experimental research include gender, race/ethnicity, and socioeconomic status. More specific information on moderating and mediating variables is covered in Chapter 22.

DESIGNING ADAPTIVE INTERVENTIONS

Speeding Up Knowledge About Effective Interventions: The Adaptive Intervention Approach

Tailoring behavioral interventions to the specific needs of any given participant in a randomized clinical trial presents challenges for an investigator in that the gold standard approach to test an intervention is to standardize or "fix" the composition and level of the intervention components during the trial. The goals of the fixed intervention approach are to enhance the validity of the study findings by maintaining precision in the specific cause (components and dose of the intervention) that produce the effects and to increase the replicability of the study. This approach assumes that all individuals in the study will respond to all components of an intervention in the same way. However, we know that people respond differently to the same intervention. In contrast to the fixed intervention approach is another approach to behavioral intervention design, the **adaptive intervention**, which does not assume that all subjects will respond similarly to all components of an intervention.

An adaptive intervention is an intervention in which participant-specific modifications to the intervention are built into the intervention protocol based on process, mediator, or outcome measures taken on participants over the course of the study (Collins, Murphy, & Bierman, 2004). To assure the internal validity of the study, the use of such variables must be limited to the intervention arm(s) and to the specific purpose of modifying an *individual* participant's intervention based on observed values (Collins et al., 2004). This approach is different from the use of clinical judgment for tailoring at the time of delivery of an intervention in that, in the adaptive intervention design, explicit decision rules are developed a priori that link characteristics of an individual or environment with specific levels and types of program components (Murphy, Collins, & Rush, 2007). The primary aim of an adaptive intervention is to maximize the strength of the intervention. Another aim is to maximize replicability of the intervention. In what follows, a description of the design principles for the development of an adaptive intervention is provided, including a sample adaptive intervention protocol. The advantages and challenges of using adaptive interventions are discussed.

Principles for the Design of Adaptive Interventions

There are four design principles for the creation of an adaptive intervention:

- Selecting the tailoring variables
- Measuring the tailoring variables
- Derivation of the decision rules
- Optimal implementation of the decision rules

Selecting the Tailoring Variables. The first step in the design of an adaptive intervention is to select the tailoring variables (Collins, Murphy, Nair, & Strecher, 2005). The tailoring variables are those variables that are expected to moderate the effect of the treatment component. It is expected that the level or type of intervention an individual needs varies according to the tailoring variables. For example, in a weight loss behavioral intervention program, initial weight on entrance to the program may be a tailoring variable because morbidly obese individuals in the program may benefit from additional counseling sessions than the planned group-delivered intervention. In interventions that are delivered over a long time, the tailoring variable can be used to adjust for an individual on an ongoing basis according to individual changes on the tailoring variable. Thus, a process variable, mediator, or intermediate outcome variable may be a candidate tailoring variable. For example, adherence to an exercise routine may be a mediating variable in a weight loss program that could be designated as a tailoring variable. In this situation, a value would be set for a minimum amount of exercise in a given period on which participants would be monitored on an ongoing basis and individual participants falling below the exercise threshold value would be provided with supplemental counseling/assistance using a specified protocol.

Pretreatment variables also can serve as tailoring variables. For example, in a study of weight loss in overweight adolescents, screening for binge eating at entrance to the study may identify a subset of participants who can benefit from treatment for binge eating in addition to the standard intervention provided to the majority of participants who are not binge eaters. In this case, the adaptive intervention allows resources to be expended more appropriately and reduces disenfranchisement of intervention participants who may not need a component in a weight loss program regarding binge eating. Several examples of tailoring variables are displayed in Table 5.4. It is important to remember that the goal of an adaptive intervention is to maximize the intervention for *each* participant in the study, thus achieving optimal impact overall.

Measuring the Tailoring Variables. The second step in the development of an adaptive intervention protocol is the measurement of the tailoring variables. The quality of the measurement of the tailoring variables is crucial. Invalid and unreliable measures of the tailoring variable may result in inappropriate dosage of the adaptive intervention. Also, unreliability in the measurement of the tailoring variables introduces random error into the dosage assignment decision, which results in random error in the intervention itself, thus reducing the strength of the adaptive intervention.

Derivation of the Decision Rules. Essential to the adaptive intervention design process is the development of a set of prespecified decision rules on key variables for adaptation. In the traditional tailored intervention approach, investigators usually adjust their intervention for any one individual on an ad hoc basis. This often results in uneven application of the intervention and in difficulty in replicating the intervention and interpreting study findings. In an adaptive intervention, good decision rules assure that components of the intervention are delivered in the intended intensity to the intended individuals. Table 5.4 provides examples

TABLE 5.4 Sample Items From the IMPACT Study Adaptive Intervention Protocol

TYPE OF VARIABLE	VARIABLE	VALUE	REVIEW INTERVAL	CHANGE IN INTERVENTION
Moderator	Obesity level	≥the 99th percentile	Baseline	Assignment of a personal "health coach" to the child throughout the study (1–2 hr/month maximum contact time)
Moderator	Parental involvement	If a parent does not consent for self to participate or comes to less than half of the sessions	Beginning of study and at monthly intervals thereafter	Assignment of a personal "health coach" to the child (1–2 hr/month maximum contact) unless parent is involved more than one-half of the sessions/month
Mediator	Dietary intake	<5 fruits/veggies eaten on >3 days/week	End of third session and at each session thereafter until back to ≥5 fruits/veggies days/week	Session with a coach following each lapse; choose from menu of options including having a registered dietician review family recipes
Process	Family-designed experiments	<2 in each quarter	Quarterly throughout study	One personal session with a health coach to reteach and problem-solve with family re: family experiments; coach then follows up with family every 2 weeks for 3 months

of a set of decision rules in a protocol format. There are three characteristics of good decision rules. First, they must accurately reflect the underlying model of the study. A pathway
analysis of the relations among the tailoring variables, treatment dosage, and outcome is necessary to derive valid decision rules and provide the scientific rationale for the adaptation.
Second, good decision rules are objective; they state the dosage to be given and the values on
the measure of the tailoring variables. Last, good decision rules comprehensively reflect all
of the anticipated incidences of the tailoring variable. The underlying principle in assigning
decision rules is that to achieve the desired treatment effect, different dosages or types of
treatment may be needed for different individuals. In designing the decision rules, investigators should ask themselves, "If we were to give this dosage to people with this characteristic
on the tailoring variables, what treatment effect would be expected?"

Optimal Implementation of the Decision Rules. Last, there must be optimal implementation of the
decision rules. Decision rules are established in advance and are applied uniformly across
participants in an intervention arm of the study. Every dosage decision should be made using
identical rules, and the decision rules are applied identically to any participant with the
same values on the tailoring variables. There should be no exceptions made on an ad hoc
basis. Infidelity in treatment implementation introduces random error into the intervention,
thus lessening its effectiveness. The same procedures to assure intervention fidelity in a fixed
intervention protocol should be applied to an adaptive intervention protocol.

Example of an Adaptive Intervention Protocol

Table 5.4 provides an example of an adaptive intervention protocol designed for a study of one
of the authors. The IMPACT study is a randomized trial to determine the efficacy of behavioral
interventions to decrease obesity in urban youth in Cleveland, Ohio. The study includes multiple
intervention arms to test interventions of differing conceptual approaches to promote weight
management in adolescents and their families. Table 5.4 is a modified version of a protocol developed by the study investigators as a way to display the elements of the adaptive intervention
for one arm of the IMPACT study. A similar adaptive protocol table was constructed for all intervention arms of the study, and each table differs in its set of tailoring variables consistent with
the underlying conceptualizations and components unique to the respective intervention. The
adaptive intervention protocol tables for all intervention arms include the following elements:
(a) the type or category of variable on which an adaptation is made, (b) the tailoring variables
selected, (c) the value of a tailoring variable that will trigger the implementation of the adaptive
intervention protocol, (d) the review intervals at which data on a tailoring variable will be monitored, and (e) the specific adaptation that will be made to the intervention.

   To construct the adaptive intervention protocol shown in this table, the study team first
gave careful consideration to the selection of the tailoring variables. This involved reviewing
the conceptual model underlying the intervention and how it was expected to achieve its
results, including the hypothesized mediating and moderating variables. The understanding of the pathways and relations of the study variables assisted the team in considering
how the intervention components might differently affect any given child in the study. For
example, child level of obesity at entrance to the study (morbidly obese, not morbidly obese)
and the level of parent/guardian involvement in the intervention program (parent attending
less than half of the intervention group education sessions) were thought by the study team
to be possible moderators of a child's response to the intervention.

   Similarly, dietary intake was thought to be a mediating variable in this weight management
intervention, and, thus, the study team decided that monitoring levels of dietary intake over
time in individual children would provide information about the need to adapt the intervention
dose for the children not responding to the diet-education component of the intervention. In
this responsive intervention protocol, dietary intake was operationalized as fruit and vegetable

intake because this was a fairly easily measured indicator of the dietary intake goals of the intervention. Finally, a process variable thought to be central to the successful use of the behavioral strategies taught in this intervention arm was selected as a tailoring variable. This process variable was the number of self-designed experiments completed by the families to change some aspect of their daily routine, which was the major behavioral change technique taught in this family systems intervention. A threshold value of less than two family experiments in a 3-month period (intervention period of 1 year) was set and will be monitored quarterly. The table indicates the threshold values for all of the tailoring variables and the review period for monitoring the values for implementation of the adapted intervention protocol.

In the IMPACT study, the interventions are delivered in groups of 12 to 15 families and, thus, adaptations for the tailoring variables consist of the addition of a set level of individual coaching sessions for a child whose values on the tailoring variable indicate that an improved response to the intervention might be achieved with a larger, more intense dose. For example, for the tailoring variable, level of parental involvement in the study and children who do not have at least one parent/guardian participating in at least half of the group intervention sessions in a given period will receive personal coaching sessions throughout the study in addition to the group-delivered components. Note that the exact dose to be provided is described to be an additional 1 to 2 hours of individualized coaching each month.

Of course, not all adaptations will consist of an increase in the dose of an intervention component. Adaptations can also consist of a reduction or omission of a particular intervention component as well. This delivery of a lower level of the intervention might be done when some of the participants are found at the beginning of the intervention program to already possess a particular knowledge or set of skills that is taught in the standard protocol. Of course, this adaptation (omitting a portion of the program for these individuals) would be accomplished by applying a set of predetermined decision rules. This adaptation, rather than the one-size-fits-all approach to intervention delivery, may reduce participant disenfranchisement with the study and more efficiently use their time. This approach also allows greater efficiency in the use of study resources.

Challenges in the Use of Adaptive Interventions

There are several challenges or cautions that should be considered in the design and use of adaptive interventions. First, investigators must consider just how many tailoring variables are practical in an adaptive intervention protocol. Considerable time and resources may be needed to identify the tailoring variables and to develop clear decision rules, as well as to conduct the ongoing measurement needed to determine the participants' values on the respective tailoring variables. In addition, study resources are needed to perform the fidelity monitoring needed to assure optimal implementation of the adaptive protocol.

Another caution is that most decision rules are incomplete. Developing rules that can be universally applied is not easy; addressing all possible situations that may arise in the application of the rules is difficult and can lead to interventionists reverting to clinical judgment in situations not covered in the protocol. Such deviations from protocol increase potential threats to the replicability and validity of the intervention.

Another important issue is the strength of the evidence to support the decision rules. When multiple-component behavioral interventions are "packaged," there are often varying degrees of evidence to support the hypothesized effect size of any one component or the composite of components included in the intervention. The effect size can be even more difficult to determine for an adaptation made in an intervention tailored on individual characteristics (moderating variables). The potency of adaptive interventions, however, can be improved by the use of newer intervention design studies, such as the Sequential Multiple Assignment Randomized Trial (SMART Trial; Collins, Murphy, & Strecher, 2007) or the Multiphase

Optimization Strategy (MOST; Collins et al., 2011; Collins et al., 2007). These new methods of intervention development use a series of small randomized trials and factorial designs to identify the most potent components to include in an intervention program (Chakraborty, Collins, Strecher, & Murphy, 2009; Collins, Dziak, & Li, 2009).

Remember, an adaptive intervention is a set of tailoring variables and decision rules whereby an intervention is changed in response to characteristics of the individual program participant or the environment to produce optical outcomes for each participant. This approach acknowledges that the varying intervention needs of individuals may not be met by using a single uniform composition and dose. Adaptive interventions can enhance the potency of an intervention, reduce waste, and potentially increase compliance because of the individualization of the treatment.

Pragmatic Trials. Sensible, Realistic, Useful—These are all terms that can be used to describe **pragmatic trials**. Assessing the benefits of an intervention or treatment under ideal scientific conditions evaluates the efficacy of an intervention. This type of study is oftentimes referred to as an "explanatory trial," which typically recruits a population that is relatively homogenous and aims to further our understanding of whether an intervention makes a difference in a specific outcome or it does not. This type of trial stresses internal validity or control. In contrast, pragmatic trials focus on testing an intervention in a population that is similar to where the intervention is meant to be used in real life. It is often heterogeneous or very diverse in regard to many of the so-called "inclusion criteria" of participants than would be considered in an efficacy trial. For example, if the intervention is meant to address care of the diabetic patient, the population using a pragmatic trial would be diverse in age, race, medical history, and other criteria. Pragmatic trials look at how to logistically and reasonably roll out the trial using a real-world approach and to assess the effectiveness of the intervention using measures that are easily understood and could be used by employees, clinicians, patients, and leaders who are not necessarily well versed in research methods. By addressing clinical questions that are important to every day practice, pragmatic trials test interventions in an environment that is as close to that in which it will be implemented in real life. Scientific criteria for approaching selection of participants, addressing retention and attrition and assessing outcomes are still adhered to in pragmatic trials. Important aspects that reduce bias in the scientific study, such as randomization, blinding, treating both groups equally and analyzing data from all participants originally randomized in the study must be adhered to in a pragmatic trial (Williams & Gilchrest, 2015). Efficacy or explanatory trials assess whether a treatment works under ideal scientific, rigorous conditions, though pragmatic trials ask how does the intervention work in the real world and is it still useful. Efficacy and effectiveness trials are like the Yin and Yang of intervention research—both are needed to develop interventions that are scientifically reproducible and translatable to communities.

In summary, designing an intervention study requires thoughtful planning and meticulous detail. Keeping your dream alive and your passion burning for intervention research will fuel your energy as you plan your study. Attention to small details in the planning stage while keeping "the big picture" in mind will help ensure your study's success.

Key Points From This Chapter

- Conduct a "research design workout" to convene members of your research team, including a statistician, to develop the study and its protocol.
- Whenever possible, design a true experiment with a comparison or structurally equivalent attention control condition instead of a quasi-experiment or preexperiment because it is the strongest study for supporting cause and effect relationships

(i.e., being able to say that it was the treatment that caused a change in outcome[s] and not other confounding/extraneous variables).

- If random assignment by individual subject is not possible, consider introducing some other type of randomization into the study (e.g., randomly assigning schools or patient rooms).
- Conduct a pilot study to work through important details of the study's methods and protocol before embarking on a full-scale trial.
- Use an intervention's effect size on a primary outcome variable from a pilot study or comparable intervention studies to determine sample size for your full-scale intervention trial.
- Explore mediating and moderating variables as part of the study's design.
- Conduct a pragmatic trial when you are interested in taking a real-world approach to assess the effectiveness of an intervention using measures that are easily understood and could be used by employees, clinicians, patients, and leaders who are not necessarily well versed in research methods.
- Consider an adaptive intervention when varying needs of individuals may not be met using a single uniform intervention and dose.

REFERENCES

Agency for Healthcare Research and Quality. (2011). Effective health care program. Retrieved from http://www.iom.edu/Reports/2009/ComparativeEffectivenessResearchPriorities.aspx

Campbell, D. T., & Stanley, J. C. (1963). *Experimental and quasi-experimental designs for research*. Chicago, IL: Rand McNally.

Chakraborty, B., Collins, L. M., Strecher, V. J., & Murphy, S. A. (2009). Developing multicomponent interventions using fractional factorial designs. *Statistics in Medicine, 28*(21), 2687–2708. doi:10.1002/sim.3643

Cohen, J. (1988). *Statistical power analysis for the behavioral sciences* (2nd ed.). London, UK: Routledge Academies.

Collins, L. M., Baker, T. B., Mermelstein, R. J., Piper, M. E., Jorenby, D. E., Smith, S. S., … Fiore, M. C. (2011). The multiphase optimization strategy for engineering effective tobacco use interventions. *Annals of Behavioral Medicine, 41*(2), 208–226. doi:10.1007/s12160-010-9253-x

Collins, L. M., Dziak, J. J., & Li, R. (2009). Design of experiments with multiple independent variables: A resource management perspective on complete and reduced factorial designs. *Psychological Methods, 14*(3), 202–224. doi:10.1037/a0015826

Collins, L. M., Murphy, S. A., & Bierman, K. L. (2004). A conceptual framework for adaptive preventive interventions. *Prevention Science, 5*(3), 185–196. doi:10.1023/B:PREV.0000037641.26017.00

Collins, L. M., Murphy, S. A., Nair, V. N., & Strecher, V. J. (2005). A strategy for optimizing and evaluating behavioral interventions. *Annals of Behavioral Medicine, 30*(1), 65–73. doi:10.1207/s15324796abm3001_8

Collins, L. M., Murphy, S. A., & Strecher, V. (2007). The multiphase optimization strategy (MOST) and the sequential multiple assignment randomized trial (SMART): New methods for more potent eHealth interventions. *American Journal of Preventive Medicine, 32*(Suppl. 5), S112–S118. doi:10.1016/j.amepre.2007.01.022

Fisher, J. D., Fisher, W. A., Bryan, A. D., & Misovich, S. J. (2002). Information-motivation-behavioral skills model-based HIV risk behavior change intervention for inner-city high school youth. *Health Psychology, 21*(2), 177–186. doi:10.1037/0278-6133.21.2.177

Hulley, S. B., Cummings, S. R., Browner, W. S., Grady, D. G., & Newman, T. B. (2013). *Designing clinical research* (4th ed.). Philadelphia, PA: Lippincott Williams & Wilkins.

Luce, B. R., Kramer, J. M., Goodman, S. N., Connor, J. T., Tunis, S., Whicher, D., & Schwartz, J. S. (2009). Rethinking randomized clinical trials for comparative effectiveness research: The need for transformational change. *Annals of Internal Medicine, 151*(3), 206–209. doi:10.7326/0003-4819-151-3-200908040-00126

Mays, M. Z., & Melnyk, B. M. (2009). A call for reporting of effect sizes in research reports to enhance critical appraisal and evidence-based practice. *Worldviews on Evidence-Based Nursing, 6*(3), 125–129. doi:10.1111/j.1741-6787.2009.00166.x

Melnyk, B. M., Crean, H. F., Feinstein, N. F., & Fairbanks, E. (2008). Maternal anxiety and depression after a premature infant's discharge from the neonatal intensive care unit: Explanatory effects of the creating opportunities for parent empowerment program. *Nursing Research, 57*(6), 383–394. doi:10.1097/NNR.0b013e3181906f59

Melnyk, B. M., Feinstein, N. F., Alpert-Gillis, L., Fairbanks, E., Crean, H. F., Sinkin, R. A., ... Gross, S. J. (2006). Reducing premature infants' length of stay and improving parents' mental health outcomes with the Creating Opportunities for Parent Empowerment (COPE) neonatal intensive care unit program: A randomized, controlled trial. *Pediatrics, 118*(5), e1414–e1427. doi:10.1542/peds.2005-2580

Melnyk, B. M., Morrison-Beedy, D., & Cole, R. (2015). Generating evidence through quantitative research. In B. Melnyk & E. Fineout-Overholt (Eds.), *Evidence-based practice in nursing & healthcare: A guide to best practice* (3rd ed., pp. 439–475). Philadelphia, PA: Wolters Kluwer/Lippincott Williams & Wilkins.

Morrison-Beedy, D., Carey, M. P., Aronowitz, T., Mkandawire, L., & Dyne, J. (2002). An HIV risk-reduction intervention in an adolescent correctional facility: Lessons learned. *Applied Nursing Research, 15*(2), 97–101. doi:10.1053/apnr.2002.29530

Morrison-Beedy, D., Carey, M. P., Kowalski, J., & Tu, X. (2005). Group-based HIV risk reduction intervention for adolescent girls: Evidence of feasibility and efficacy. *Research in Nursing & Health, 28*(1), 3–15. doi:10.1002/nur.20056

Morrison-Beedy, D., Carey, M. P., Seibold-Simpson, S. M., Xia, Y., & Tu, X. (2009). Preliminary efficacy of a comprehensive HIV prevention intervention for abstinent adolescent girls: Pilot study findings. *Research in Nursing & Health, 32*(6), 569–581. doi:10.1002/nur.20357

Murphy, S. A., Collins, L. M., & Rush, A. J. (2007). Customizing treatment to the patient: Adaptive treatment strategies. *Drug and Alcohol Dependence, 88*(Suppl. 2), S1–S3. doi:10.1016/j.drugalcdep.2007.02.001

Sox, H. C., & Greenfield, S. (2009). Comparative effectiveness research: A report from the Institute of Medicine. *Annals of Internal Medicine, 151*(3), 203–205. doi:10.7326/0003-4819-151-3-200908040-00125

Whittemore, R., & Grey, M. (2002). The systematic development of nursing interventions. *Journal of Nursing Scholarship, 34*(2), 115–120. doi:10.1111/j.1547-5069.2002.00115.x

Williams, H. C., & Gilchrest, B. A. (2015). Clinical trials submitted to the JID: Place your bet and show us your hand. *Journal of Investigative Dermatology, 135*, 325–327. doi:10.1038/jid.2014.478

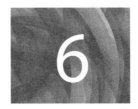

Designing Interventions That Are Sensitive to Culture, Race/ Ethnicity, and Gender

Usha Menon

> By doubting we are led to questions, by questioning
> we arrive at the truth —*Peter Abelard*

The old adage that "one size fits all" has been shown to be ineffective in healthcare, especially when related to issues of health promotion and preventive care. When individuals are asymptomatic and fail to see a need to change behavior in the short term, it is difficult to bring about behavioral change. Eliciting behavioral change becomes especially challenging when coupled with healthcare beliefs that are rooted in cultural and spiritual mores.

Intervention development must be preceded by the understanding that changes in health and behavior are affected by multiple factors, such as social determinants, access issues, and the healthcare system itself (Smedley, Stith, & Nelson, 2003). Warnecke et al. (2008) developed a broad ecological framework for addressing multifactorial influences on health. Three levels of health determinants in this model are identified as "proximal," "intermediate," and "distal," and they encompass a wide range of variables from individual beliefs to healthcare system issues. Culture, race/ethnicity, and gender are embedded at various levels in this framework, allowing a broad interpretation of each factor and its impact on health, as well as affording the opportunity to study interactions among factors as well as their mediating and moderating effects.

When designing interventions, it is critical to focus our attention on culture, race/ ethnicity, and gender because these factors will often moderate or directly impact the efficacy of interventions. Given the scarcity of resources and research funding, it would be ideal to develop a common intervention strategy that takes into consideration several factors, including race/ethnicity and gender. When considering the growing obesity epidemic in the United States, high mortality rates from preventable and curable cancers, incidence of heart disease, and diabetes that could be prevented by diet and physical activity, it is critical to understand the underlying mechanisms and factors that affect health behavior, including culture, race/ethnicity, and gender, so that effective interventions can be developed that will have a positive impact on health outcomes.

RACE/ETHNICITY

The changing demography of the United States with substantive increases in the populations of racial and ethnic minorities along with changing worldviews on gender and sexuality underscore the need to design interventions that are sensitive to culture, race/ethnicity, and gender. This chapter focuses on strategies in designing interventions that are relevant or appropriate to different population subgroups whose beliefs and/or customs may differ from the majority, while noting that, given the nuances of such differences both within and between groups, there is no magic formula to follow. It is beyond the scope of this chapter to undertake a debate on the definitions of race and culture. For the purpose of this chapter and in keeping with contemporary scholarship, race is viewed as a social construct (Fisher, Burnet, Huang, Chin, & Cagney, 2007).

Race/ethnicity is clearly a risk factor for health. In some cases, an individual's race can determine biological pathways and underlying physiological mechanisms of responses to diseases. In other cases, the impact of race/ethnicity is mediated by other factors such as poverty, discrimination, and the lived environment, which can affect an individual's capacity to respond to environmental challenges and healthcare needs (Warnecke et al., 2008). In this chapter, the focus is on cultural constructions of race/ethnicity and how considerations of culture can impact health behavior and, consequently, the design of health interventions.

CULTURE

There remains ongoing debate about the definition of culture with multiple perspectives delivered from different disciplinary paradigms. Culture has been defined as the customary beliefs, norms, and traits of a racial, religious, or social group; and also as the shared values, goals, and practices within an organization. This definition, although somewhat simplistic, allows a broad characterization of culture for the purposes of defining the thoughts, beliefs, and behavioral processes of a subgroup. Broadly speaking, race/ethnicity might be subsumed under culture if focusing on social norms, traditional beliefs, and spiritual values related to health.

An individual's culture often defines its beliefs about healthcare, including preventative care, treatment, and end-of-life care. Traditional concepts regarding the causes and treatment of disease, healthcare, and norms of behavior for men or women are carried over from the country of origin. Immigrant minority communities may live in or close to enclaves of similar people, and traditional beliefs may be further reinforced through close ties with family and social networks (Shin, Kim, Juon, Kim, & Kim, 2000).

There are many traditional beliefs about the origins of diseases and their incidence. Several examples shown subsequently illustrate this point. For example, Koreans commonly believe that mystical and supernatural powers are potent forces in daily life and that a person becomes ill from the fate of fortune, devil's mischief, temporary separation of soul and body, moving residences on a bad day, violation of rules for not eating foods in the ancestral rites, misfortune, or past sins (Kendall, 1988).

For a woman who believes that health is determined by actions in a previous lifetime (*karma*), eating of hot or cold foods, curses, or God's will, a basic educational message on the importance of early screening for breast cancer will likely have little to no impression. Similarly, for a group that believes being "big-boned" or overweight may be seen as a sign of prosperity and health, simply teaching about the benefits of exercise to lose weight will likely have low impact (Stevens, 2010). The key to developing a successful intervention that also is culturally appropriate is to understand how to leverage those beliefs in an intervention to increase the impact of the intervention on the outcome of interest.

Enhanced understanding of cultural values, beliefs, and mores is based on formative work such as in-depth interviews, focus groups, and descriptive surveys. It also is imperative to note that formulaic interpretations of norms in communities can lead to erroneous information and emphasis on issues not culturally salient for a subgroup. According to the National Cancer Institute (2004), the Asian Americans/Pacific Islanders race/ethnicity category represents more than 25 ethnic groups with origins in East Asia, Southeast Asia, the Indian subcontinent, Polynesia, Melanesia, Hawaii, Guam, Samoa, and other Pacific islands. Each ethnic group is unique in language, culture, and health beliefs. The common tendency to group all Asian Americans and Pacific Islanders into one population group has hindered efforts to discover effective community and culturally responsive intervention strategies (Lee-Lin & Menon, 2005).

To illustrate this point further, consider the example of Asian Indian immigrants to the United States. Asian Indians are among the fastest growing Asian immigrant group in the United States and are concentrated in certain geographical locations, namely California, New York, New Jersey, Texas, Florida, and Illinois (U.S. Bureau of Census, 2007). However, Asian Indians in the United States constitute a more heterogeneous group than other Asian subgroups. Differences in lay language (14 major languages), province or state of origin (28 states), religion (five major religions), and race (at least four distinct racial types) have led to the formation of distinct subgroups ("One state, many worlds," 2013; Varshney, 1983). As such, assuming that beliefs held by one subgroup apply to all Asian immigrants would lead to interventions that are not culturally sensitive and, depending on the issue being discussed, may even have a negative impact by being embarrassing or incorrect.

GENDER

Gender may influence health outcomes from several perspectives. Here, the focus is on gender as defined by biological sex—male or female. From the perspective of social and cultural constructions of gender, however, it is important to note that contemporary thinking does allow for broader constructions of gender, such as with transgendered individuals. Depending on the study sample, it is important to incorporate either traditional or broader definitions of culture.

There are the diseases that occur only in men or are more common among women, respectively. Such gender-specific diseases include prostate cancer (males) or breast cancer (mostly females). In addition, some diseases are perceived to be male diseases (e.g., colon cancer), and women may need increased awareness and knowledge before perceptions of risk change for the better.

Culture and ethnicity also can influence gender roles. Social and cultural constructions of masculinity can influence health behaviors among men of various ethnicities, but there also are unique aspects within ethnicities indicating that formative research with the ethnic group or subgroup of interest is imperative. For example, in traditional Korean culture, gender roles are distinct; men retain authority as head of the household, and the most admirable virtue in a woman is obedience and devotion to her husband or father and family (Choi, 1995). Talking about health problems is considered a weakness that damages male power among Korean men. Among Hispanics, *machismo* and *caballerismo* refer to manliness within the Latino culture but have disparate meaning (Rivera-Ramos & Buki, 2011). *Machismo* is a pejorative term connoting hypermasculine qualities, such as aggression and antisocial behavior, often attributed to working-class Latino men, whereas *caballerismo* represents positive attributes and chivalrous qualities such as emotional connectedness and social responsibility (Rivera-Ramos & Buki, 2011). Although one may prevent a man from seeking healthcare, such as screening for prostate cancer (Rivera-Ramos & Buki, 2011), another might enhance health behaviors by emphasizing the notion of being healthy to be good fathers, husbands, brothers, sons, workers, and community members (Sobralske, 2006).

Among immigrant women, long-term gender discrimination may lead to problems with self-image and self-esteem, which can then directly impact healthcare-seeking behavior (Niaz & Hassan, 2006). Other culturally based factors that can hinder health promotion efforts directed at minority women are social prohibitions from discussing bodily experiences such as menstrual health, gastrointestinal ailments, breast-related health or menopause, and placing their health and welfare after that of their husbands and children (Choi, 1995; Park, 1987).

Designing Health Interventions

Research studies focus on and often compare three levels of health interventions—standard, targeted, and tailored (Strecher, Greenwood, Wang, & Dumont, 1999). Standard (generic or general) health interventions provide information to the general population of interest and often represent the most common approach. For example, the population of interest may be overweight adults and a common approach would be to encourage an increase in physical activity.

Targeted health messages are created to reach a defined population group and take into account shared characteristics of group members (Kreuter & Skinner, 2000; Kreuter, Strecher, & Glassman, 1999). Targeted education for overweight adolescent Latinos would include language-appropriate materials that also incorporate elements of Latino culture known to be commonly accepted. Targeting can be achieved by incorporating all or some of the five distinct strategies described by Kreuter, Lukwago, Bucholtz, Clark, and Sanders-Thompson (2003) later on in this chapter.

Tailored interventions are personalized to individual beliefs, knowledge, or other characteristics. Tailored messages are a combination of information or change strategies intended to reach a specific person on the basis of characteristics that are unique to that person and related to the outcome of interest that is usually derived from an individual assessment (Kreuter & Skinner, 2000). The decision to choose an intervention strategy—standard, targeted, or tailored—depends on multiple factors including the following:

- *Cost*: A standard intervention will likely cost the least, followed by targeted and then tailored strategies.
- *Delivery*: A tailored intervention will need either extended personal contact (e.g., in person or telephone or web based) or a technology-based strategy that is delivered via interactive computer, web, or phone.
- *Outcome of interest*: Consideration of the nature of the outcome is an important factor. Ongoing, long-term lifestyle changes, such as diet and physical activity, will take intensive interventions, perhaps tailored to the individual. Behavioral change (e.g., obtaining a yearly mammogram) may need less intensive strategies such as yearly reminders or provider recommendation after the initial education.

■ *Expected or known variance in attributes to be manipulated*:
  ■ *High variance*: Certain attributes or variables have increased variance within a group, such as barriers to cancer screening, which may extend to varied reasons for not getting a screening test. In such instances, tailoring provides the ideal strategy to reach every individual in the study with a personalized message relevant to their specific barriers (see Figure 6.1).
  ■ *Low variance*: Variables with low variance within a group can be addressed for the group as a whole with a targeted message. For example, a culturally based spiritual belief such as fatalism has been established as a commonly held notion among older African Americans (Powe, Daniels, & Finnie, 2005; Powe, Hamilton, & Brooks, 2006). As such, educational messages intended to address fatalism may be targeted to the entire group rather than individually tailored.

Other factors may weigh in to the decision to choose an intervention strategy, such as time and respondent burden, setting (e.g., home, clinic), and demographics (e.g., older adults, adolescents). An intervention strategy must be based on intimate knowledge of the population of interest and study design rather than selected only because of past effectiveness.

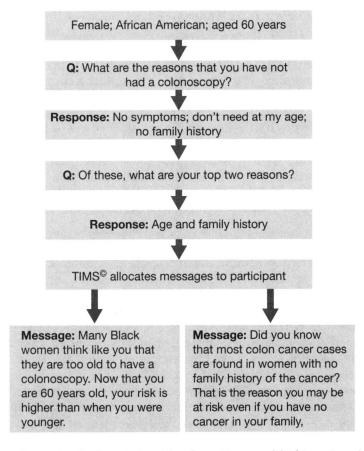

FIGURE 6.1 Example of tailored algorithm for a 60-year-old African American female.

TIMS ©, Tailored Intervention Messaging System.

Cultural Targeting

Kreuter et al. (2003) offer one of the most logical and intuitive frameworks published for cultural targeting. This framework is presented subsequently with illustrative examples of each strategy. They describe five strategies for cultural targeting. These are peripheral, evidential, linguistic, constituent-involving, and sociocultural strategies.

- *Peripheral strategies* use culturally sensitive packaging, including images and exemplars with individuals who look like the sample of interest. For example, in a study with Native Americans, brochures might contain images of Native Americans, colors favored by the community, and patterns or icons that are rooted in the culture. Such components are meant to capture the audience with immediate relevancy to them and/or their communities.
- *Evidential strategies* include drawing on evidence to support the magnitude of the problem in that community (e.g., enhancing perceived relevance by presenting evidence of the obesity epidemic among Hispanics). These messages increase perceptions of the significance of the problem being addressed.
- *Linguistic strategies* use the language of the target community (e.g., Spanish). This strategy goes beyond simply using the language but delves further into the construction of words with cultural meaning (i.e., the use of vernacular phrases and idioms that are common to the community). For example, when addressing teenagers, using contemporary vernacular may reach the audience better than text that is based on medical facts.
- *Constituent-involving strategies* include members of the target community in delivering the program, for example, lay health workers, facilitators, and peer support "buddies" from the target community. When using static media, such as print or DVDs, including quotations from popular opinion leaders in the target community can increase reach of the intervention.
- *Sociocultural strategies* discuss the health problem within the broader social and cultural values of the target community. A group's cultural values, beliefs, and behaviors are recognized, reinforced, and built upon to provide context and meaning to information and messages about a given health problem or behavior. These strategies may incorporate messages (e.g., wellness of the family or community begins with the individual; obesity is adversely affecting the Hispanic community's overall health).

Cultural Tailoring

The process of tailoring is described in detail elsewhere (Kreuter & Skinner, 2000; Menon & Wilkie, 2009). Briefly stated, tailoring involves the assessment of the variables of interest before intervention delivery and then personalizing messages based on the information gathered. Computer tailing is the most practical and long-term cost-effective method of tailoring (Menon & Wilkie, 2009). Although actual delivery of the intervention can occur through media, such as print or phone, or in person, the process of personalizing the intervention is usually accomplished by computer (Menon & Wilkie, 2009). Figure 6.1 illustrates the computer algorithms used in a tailored software program called Tailored Intervention Messaging System (TIMS; Menon et al., 2008). In TIMS, to tailor education to individual women on colon cancer screening, baseline information is entered into a database. Preprogrammed algorithms draw relevant messages for that individual (Figure 6.1). In this example, two messages address the woman's top two barriers for getting a colonoscopy. Gender, age, and race are woven into the messages, personalizing the text further to her. Although some of these interventions are delivered by computer, tailored scripts also can be used to guide phone-based or in-person counseling, mailed in printed materials, and delivered through interactive web or computer formats (Menon & Wilkie, 2009).

Additional Considerations in Developing an Intervention

In addition to race/ethnicity, culture, and gender as described earlier, other factors that need to be taken into consideration when developing an intervention are that it is important to (a) intervene on variables that are changeable; (b) examine demographics of the sample other than race/ethnicity and gender, such as language (translation methods, cultural language), health literacy, delivery medium (e.g., computer, mail), and take into consideration who is delivering the message (e.g., lay health workers, nurses, psychologists).

Variables that are mutable or changeable should be the focus of the intervention. Age and income may be nonchangeable factors within the context of a study. As such, they can only be measured, not altered, with an intervention, although targeted messaging can incorporate these factors. Some culturally based beliefs may not be changeable or it may be inappropriate to try to change them. For example, challenging a person's spiritual beliefs is offensive, but incorporating those beliefs in such a way as to leverage cultural aspects (see definitions of targeted and tailoring under the previous "Designing Health Interventions" section) will likely lead to a more effective intervention.

Interventions must fit into the lifestyle and environment of the individual, rather than be an external burden. Age, socioeconomic status, and education are additional factors to consider. Respondent burden can decrease intervention effectiveness. An older adult may not want to listen to a phone-based intervention for an hour. A single mother who works for hourly wages may not be able to take time off work to attend a group educational session on cancer screening.

Health literacy is another important consideration. For too many years, education was considered a proxy for literacy, but current data clearly underscore the need to understand the health literacy levels of our population groups and design interventions that take health literacy into consideration. According to results of the National Assessment of Adult Literacy, only 12% of adults have proficient health literacy. That is, almost 9 of 10 adults may lack necessary skills to manage their health and prevent disease (Kutner, Greenberg, Jin, & Paulsen, 2006). It is imperative to note that low health literacy rates exist not only among foreign-born individuals, but also among persons born in the United States and those who have been educated in the U.S. school systems.

Translation methods also can influence how intervention material is perceived. Many studies rely on back-translation to adapt materials to the target language from English. This commonly used method is fraught with limitations, and a committee or modified committee method will yield better translations that are appropriate to the community as a whole (Harkness, Van de Vijver, & Mohler, 2003). The medium of delivery of the intervention and the speaker related to the intervention also are important issues to factor into design. For example, an educational intervention delivered by a lay health worker implemented in a church setting would be written in language much different than an educational intervention on postchemotherapy symptom management delivered by a nurse in an oncology clinic.

In summary, although race and ethnicity are important contributors to health outcomes, they cannot be used as a proxy for culture. African Americans, for example, do not share a single monolithic culture; cultural subgroups may exist, and any African American may belong to one, none, or several of these (Kreuter et al., 2003). Traditional models and theories of behavioral change fail to take into account cultural nuances of health behavior. Existing frameworks place narrowly defined determinants of behavior (e.g., those from the health belief model; Champion & Skinner, 2008) in a specific relationship with one another, entirely isolated from social context (Burke, Joseph, Pasick, & Barker, 2009; Pasick & Burke, 2008). The effect of cognitive variables from the health belief model on breast cancer screening behavior was attenuated by variables of colonialism, discrimination and racism, healthcare experiences in the home country and the United States, religious and spiritual orientations, and perceptions of causes of illness and of the body (Joseph, Burke, Tuason, Barker, & Pasick, 2009). Researchers must reach outside the comfort of known models of behavioral change and use rigorous formative work to understand the cultural assumptions of their targeted communities.

A culturally based intervention that accounts for language or traditional beliefs by itself cannot alter the health behaviors of an individual. Key components proactively identify areas where a cultural intervention can improve behaviors and actively implement solutions using cultural practices, products, philosophies, or environments as vehicles that facilitate behavioral change of patients and practitioners (Fisher et al., 2007). This process is certainly time-intensive and requires rigorous formative research. In the long term, the payoff will be increased efficacy, effectiveness, and sustainability of health interventions.

Key Points From This Chapter

- Culture, race/ethnicity, and gender are important to consider when designing interventions.
- An individual's culture often defines his or her beliefs about healthcare.
- Standard (generic or general) health interventions provide information to the general population of interest and often represent the most common approach.
- Targeted health messages are created to reach a defined population group and take into account shared characteristics of group members.
- Tailored interventions are personalized to individual beliefs, knowledge, or other characteristics.
- It is important to use rigorous formative work to understand the cultural assumptions of targeted communities where interventions will be delivered.

REFERENCES

Burke, N. J., Joseph, G., Pasick, R. J., & Barker, J. C. (2009). Theorizing social context: Rethinking behavioral theory. *Health Education & Behavior, 36*(Suppl. 5), S55–S70. doi:10.1177/1090198109335338

Champion, V. L., & Skinner, C. S. (2008). The health belief model. In K. Glanz, B. K. Rimer, & K. Viswanath (Eds.), *Health behavior and health education: Theory, research, and practice* (4th ed., pp. 45–65). San Francisco, CA: Jossey-Bass.

Choi, S. H. (1995). The struggle for family succession and inheritance in a rural Korean village. *Journal of Anthropological Research, 51*, 329–346. doi:10.1086/jar.51.4.3630141

Fisher, T. L., Burnet, D. L., Huang, E. S., Chin, M. H., & Cagney, K. A. (2007). Cultural leverage: Interventions using culture to narrow racial disparities in health care. *Medical Care Research and Review, 64*(Suppl. 5), S243–S282. doi:10.1177/1077558707305414

Harkness, J. A., Van de Vijver, F. J. R., & Mohler, P. (2003). *Cross-cultural survey methods.* Hoboken, NJ: Wiley.

Joseph, G., Burke, N. J., Tuason, N., Barker, J. C., & Pasick, R. J. (2009). Perceived susceptibility to illness and perceived benefits of preventive care: An exploration of behavioral theory constructs in a transcultural context. *Health Education & Behavior, 36*(Suppl. 5), S71–S90. doi:10.1177/1090198109338915

Kendall, L. (1988). Healing thyself: A Korean shaman's afflictions. *Social Science & Medicine, 27*(5), 445–450. doi:10.1016/0277-9536(88)90367-x

Kreuter, M. W., Lukwago, S. N., Bucholtz, R. D., Clark, E. M., & Sanders-Thompson, V. (2003). Achieving cultural appropriateness in health promotion programs: Targeted and tailored approaches. *Health Education & Behavior, 30*(2), 133–146. doi:10.1177/1090198102251021

Kreuter, M. W., & Skinner, C. S. (2000). Tailoring: What's in a name? *Health Education Research, 15*(1), 1–4. doi:10.1093/her/15.1.1

Kreuter, M. W., Strecher, V. J., & Glassman, B. (1999). One size does not fit all: The case for tailoring print materials. *Annals of Behavioral Medicine, 21*(4), 276–283. doi:10.1007/BF02895958

Kutner, M., Greenberg, E., Jin, Y., & Paulsen, C. (2006). *The health literacy of America's adults: Results from the 2003 National Assessment of Adult Literacy* (NCES 2006–483). U.S. Department of Education. Washington, DC: National Center for Education Statistics.

Lee-Lin, F., & Menon, U. (2005). Breast and cervical cancer screening practices and interventions among Chinese, Japanese, and Vietnamese Americans. Oncology Nursing Forum, 32(5), 995–1003. doi:10.1188/04. ONF.995-1003

Menon, U., Szalacha, L. A., Belue, R., Rugen, K., Martin, K. R., & Kinney, A. Y. (2008). Interactive, culturally sensitive education on colorectal cancer screening. Medical Care, 46(9 Suppl. 1), S44–S50. doi:10.1097/MLR.0b013e31818105a0

Menon, U., & Wilkie, D. (2009). New approaches to conducting oncology nursing research using technology. In J. Phillips & J. Holmes (Eds.), *Advancing oncology nursing science*. Pittsburgh, PA: Oncology Nursing Society Press.

National Cancer Institute. (2004). Cancer clinical trials: A resource guide for outreach, education, and advocacy. Retrieved from https://pubs.cancer.gov/ncipl/detail.aspx?prodid=P921

Niaz, U., & Hassan, S. (2006). Culture and mental health of women in South-East Asia. *World Psychiatry, 5*(2), 118–120.

One state, many worlds, now what? (2013, June 25). Retrieved from https://www.economist.com/blogs/johnson/2013/06/language-identity-india

Park, S. I. (1987). Rural Korean housewives' attitudes toward illness. *Yonsei Medical Journal, 28*(2), 105–111. doi:10.3349/ymj.1987.28.2.105

Pasick, R. J., & Burke, N. J. (2008). A critical review of theory in breast cancer screening promotion across cultures. *Annual Review of Public Health, 29*, 351–368. doi:10.1146/annurev.publhealth. 29.020907.143420

Powe, B. D., Daniels, E. C., & Finnie, R. (2005). Comparing perceptions of cancer fatalism among African American patients and their providers. *Journal of the American Academy of Nurse Practitioners, 17*(8), 318–324. doi:10.111/j.1745-7599.2005.0049.x

Powe, B. D., Hamilton, J., & Brooks, P. (2006). Perceptions of cancer fatalism and cancer knowledge: A comparison of older and younger African American women. *Journal of Psychosocial Oncology, 24*(4), 1–13. doi:10.1300/J077v24n04_01

Rivera-Ramos, Z. A., & Buki, L. P. (2011). I will no longer be a man! Manliness and prostate cancer screenings among Latino men. *Psychology of Men & Masculinity, 12*(1), 13–25. doi:10.1037/a0020624

Shin, H., Kim, M. T., Juon, H. S., Kim, J., & Kim, K. B. (2000). Patterns and factors associated with health care utilization among Korean *American elderly. Asian American and Pacific Islander Journal of Health, 8*(2), 116–129.

Smedley, B. D, Stith, A. Y., & Nelson, A. R. (Eds.). (2003). *Unequal treatment: Confronting racial and ethnic disparities in health care*. Committee on Understanding and Eliminating Racial and Ethnic Disparities in Health Care, Institute of Medicine. Washington, DC: National Academies Press.

Sobralske, M. (2006). Machismo sustains health and illness beliefs of Mexican American men. *Journal of the American Academy of Nurse Practitioners, 18*(8), 348–350. doi:10.1111/j.1745-7599.2006.00144.x

Stevens, C. J. (2010). Obesity prevention interventions for middle school-age children of ethnic minority: A review of the literature. *Journal for Specialists in Pediatric Nursing, 15*(3), 233–243. doi:10.1111/j.1744-6155.2010.00242.x

Strecher, V. J., Greenwood, T., Wang, C., & Dumont, D. (1999). Interactive multimedia and risk communication. *Journal of the National Cancer Institute Monographs, 1999*(25), 134–139. doi:10.1093/oxfordjournals. jncimonographs.a024188

U.S. Bureau of Census. (2007). *2007 census of population. General population characteristics*. Washington, DC: U.S. Government Printing Office. Retrieved from http://www.census.gov

Varshney, A. (1983). Ethnic and religious conflicts in India. *Cultural Survival Quarterly Magazine*. Retrieved from https://www.culturalsurvival.org/publications/cultural-survival-quarterly/ethnic-and-religious-conflicts-india

Warnecke, R. B., Oh, A., Breen, N., Gehlert, S., Paskett, E., Tucker, K. L., ... Hiatt, R. A. (2008). Approaching health disparities from a population perspective: The National Institutes of Health Centers for Population Health and Health Disparities. *American Journal of Public Health, 98*(9), 1608–1615. doi:10.2105/AJPH.2006.102525

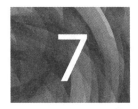

7

Ethical Considerations in Designing Intervention Studies

Dónal P. O'Mathúna

> A study of philosophy makes it more necessary, not less, to stand on your own feet, to be self-critical, and to be obliged to choose for yourself. It makes you more rational, more responsible, more of a human being. —*D. D. Raphael*

The primary goal of an intervention study is typically to determine the **efficacy** or **effectiveness** of an intervention. Other goals include establishing the intervention's safety, cost-effectiveness, or acceptability. The intervention may be an experimental drug or vaccine, a new piece of equipment, an educational program, a novel organizational system, or any other change whose impact can be measured. Intervention trials can be costly, time-consuming, and carry some level of risk. These costs and risks should be subjected to a careful ethical analysis to determine whether they are justified. Intervention trials can establish which intervention leads to the best outcomes for people and thus promote the ethical principle of beneficence. They can show which intervention is less harmful and thus promote the ethical principle of nonmaleficence (or *primum non nocere*; first, do no harm). Intervention studies also can demonstrate which intervention represents the best use of limited resources and, thus, promote the ethical principle of distributive justice. At the same time, interactions between all those involved in trials should be characterized by respect, honesty, compassion, and other ethical virtues based on people's dignity. These ethical foundations justify the huge investments made by individuals, organizations, and governments around the world in intervention studies.

Although the goals (or ends) of intervention studies may be ethical, this does not justify all the ways (or means) of achieving those goals. The ends do not justify the means. Unethical research does not become ethical just because some good comes from the results. In many cases, it leads to more ethical dilemmas, such as whether data obtained unethically should be published or used in decision making (Beecher, 1966). For example, medical research was carried out in Nazi concentration camps where people were forced to undergo horrendous procedures. Some claim these were so morally repugnant that any data obtained from them are ethically tainted and should never be used. Others claim that publishing such results is the best way to honor the subjects' sacrifice, avoid wasting important data, and prevent future violations. In the case of the Nazi experiments, the experiments lacked both ethical integrity and scientific rigor, leading some to reject their value on any count. The linking of ethical integrity and methodological quality is addressed further as follows.

Discussing the Nazi experiments or other well-known gross violations of research ethics carries the danger of suggesting that ethics violations occur only in the most extreme ways. Such cases are important to understand the origins of research ethics guidelines (see Table 7.1). They highlight how far researchers can fall from adhering to ethical standards. The gross violations should not distract attention from other ethical issues that are more commonly encountered in everyday research practice. Although the major violations have led to research ethics guidelines and codes, some are concerned that they have led to a bureaucratic approach to research ethics that can stifle research and scientific progress. The potential benefit can lead researchers to question anything that delays or prevents people from obtaining new interventions. Past tragedies and atrocities highlight the fact that precaution remains important in research, and ethical review is one way to encourage research that benefits everyone, reduces the risk of harm, and protects the dignity of research subjects.

TABLE 7.1 International Guidelines for Research Ethics

GUIDELINE	YEAR AND REVISIONS	ORIGIN	AVAILABLE AT
Nuremburg Code	1947	Nuremberg Military Tribunal	https://history.nih.gov/research/downloads/nuremberg.pdf
Declaration of Helsinki	1964, 1975, 1983, 1989, 1996, 2000, 2008, 2013	World Medical Association	www.wma.net/policies-post/wma-declaration-of-helsinki-ethical-principles-for-medical-research-involving-human-subjects
Belmont Report	1979	National Commission for the Protection of Human Subjects of Biomedical and Behavioral Research	https://www.hhs.gov/ohrp/regulations-and-policy/belmont-report
International Ethical Guidelines for Health-related Research Involving Humans	1982, 1993, 2002, 2016	CIOMS	www.cioms.ch
Code of Federal Regulations Title 21	1980 and yearly	U.S. Food and Drug Administration	www.accessdata.fda.gov/scripts/cdrh/cfdocs/cfcfr/CFRSearch.cfm?CFRPart=50
45 Code of Federal Regulations 46, The Common Rule	1981, 1991, 2005, 2009	U.S. Department of HHS	www.hhs.gov/ohrp/regulations-and-policy/regulations/45-cfr-46/index.html
Convention on Human Rights and Biomedicine	1997	Council of Europe	http://conventions.coe.int/Treaty/en/Treaties/html/164.htm

(continued)

TABLE 7.1 International Guidelines for Research Ethics *(continued)*			
GUIDELINE	**YEAR AND REVISIONS**	**ORIGIN**	**AVAILABLE AT**
EU Clinical Trials Directive 2001/20/EC and 2005/28/EC and Regulation EU No 536/2014	2001, 2005, 2014	European Commission	http://ec.europa.eu/health/human-use/clinical-trials
Universal Declaration on Bioethics and Human Rights	2005	UNESCO	www.unesco.org/new/en/social-and-human-sciences/themes/bioethics/bioethics-and-human-rights

CIOMS, Council for International Organizations of Medical Sciences; HHS, Health & Human Services; UNESCO, United National Educational, Scientific and Cultural Organization.

For some, however, ethics is seen as a hurdle to cross to get permission to conduct a study or gain regulatory approval for an intervention. Instead, ethics should be seen as an integral part of good research. Ethical considerations are involved in the inception of any intervention study, and ethical judgments are made at many stages during the conduct of an intervention study. **Ethical approval** is a process that can give an important input and direction to an intervention study. An **Institutional Review Board (IRB)** or Research Ethics Committee (REC) can identify ethical issues that researchers have overlooked, or suggest alternative ways to address ethical issues. In that way, the process aims to facilitate sound, rigorous research that is ethical, not to hinder research.

Much of what makes an intervention study ethical or unethical happens as researchers conduct the study when no one is watching. Many ethical decisions are made when researchers are alone with their consciences. This is often overlooked as research ethics becomes more highly regulated and monitored. Committees, policies, regulations, forms, and procedures play an important role in research ethics. Monitoring of ongoing studies can provide helpful ethical oversight. However, the most important determinant of ethical research is the researcher's ethics and personal integrity. Henry Beecher's 1966 article on the ethics of clinical research has been called the single most influential paper ever written on human subject research (Harkness, Lederer, & Wikler, 2001). Beecher stated that the most reliable safeguard to ethical research involving humans is "the presence of an intelligent, informed, conscientious, compassionate, responsible investigator" (Beecher, 1966, p. 1360). This should never be forgotten as an intervention study is designed and conducted.

THE MANY GOALS OF RESEARCH

> You can't get second things by putting them first; you can get second things only by putting first things first. —*C. S. Lewis*

The World Health Organization (WHO) has worked with the Council for International Organizations of Medical Sciences (CIOMS) since the late 1970s to provide ethical guidelines for health-related research with humans (see Table 7.1). Although acknowledging that such research is justified by its scientific and social value, the CIOMS guidelines declare that everyone involved in research has "a moral obligation to ensure that all research is carried out in ways that uphold human rights, and respect, protect, and are fair to study participants and the communities in which the research is conducted" (CIOMS, 2016, p. 1). More generally, the Universal Declaration on Bioethics and Human Rights states that "The interests and welfare of the individual should have priority over the sole interest of science or society" (see Table 7.1).

As noted earlier, intervention studies in healthcare aim to contribute to improving patients' health. Intervention studies in other fields aim to benefit those involved in the activities under study. However, researchers conducting intervention studies can have other goals that must be considered carefully at all stages of the research. Research is a means of advancement for researchers. Whether it is a graduate student seeking to complete a research degree, a new researcher looking for an early success, or an advanced researcher hoping to make a major breakthrough, the attraction of advancement can blur ethical boundaries. These have the potential to create conflicts of interest between what is best for researchers and the project and what is best for subjects. Add to this the financial stakes involved in today's multimillion dollar projects and the need to succeed can be blinding. Funding agencies insist on deadlines for project reviews and demonstrable outputs. In addition, individual researchers have their own targets for when they want their first or next publication, promotion, funded project, patent, or research team.

These goals may be perfectly compatible with good research, but they can raise ethical challenges. Personal interests can sometimes interfere with the interests of patients and research subjects. Researchers must remain aware of their own goals, desires, and pressures. Tensions may arise as researchers sense impending deadlines, deal with unexpected (or unwanted) results, and see that things are not working out as planned. How conflicts, pressures, and tensions are addressed point to the importance of researchers' personal integrity. Only as researchers identify the pressures they are under and consciously decide to keep subject well-being as their top priority will the research be able to remain ethical; sometimes it does not.

At the University of Oklahoma, a new vaccine to treat melanoma was being tested in an intervention study. The project was federally funded, approved by the university IRB, and led by a competent researcher. In early 2000, the project was shut down because of evidence that the vaccine was not being made or stored properly, ineligible subjects were enrolled, the informed consent form was overly optimistic, and patients' names were identifiable in a database in violation of confidentiality (Malakoff, 2000). When the patients enrolled in the study were contacted after it had been shut down, the letter stated only that further vaccination was not available because of great interest in the study. No mention was made of the protocol or safety violations.

It is unlikely that the principal investigator, J. Michael McGee, set out to conduct an unethical intervention study. Somehow, scientific and ethical standards were allowed to slip. The first deviations from the protocol may have been small, a tiny change here, a little shortcut there. Such "little changes" may be motivated by good goals. The biggest temptation may arise from a belief that we know what is going to help the most. According to the University of Oklahoma research nurse who first exposed the problems in this study, McGee was a good doctor and a decent man. "But he became a biased investigator. He thought he had found the cure for cancer. He really wasn't interested in running a clinical trial; he wanted to administer a drug" (Lemonick & Goldstein, 2000, p. 51).

Researchers make a large investment of time, energy, and resources, often because they believe their intervention will make a difference. Passion and persistence are important in research, but they can sometimes decline into bias. Intervention studies are justified when the best available intervention is not known, or there is debate over this question. Such a condition leads to what is called "a state of equipoise." Sometimes, it can be a struggle to remind oneself that the intervention is not proven until it is proven. The study must therefore be designed and conducted to the highest scientific standards. Future decision makers will use the findings in making decisions about these interventions. This is one reason why researchers have an ethical duty to be methodologically rigorous and precise in their research.

For example, as discussed in Chapter 5, random allocation of group assignment is crucial to conducting a valid, unbiased intervention study. Yet, researchers have admitted to going to great lengths to influence who gets assigned to which group. Envelopes have been held up to lights to decipher group assignments, central randomization offices have been called to deceptively uncover assignments, and offices ransacked to find the allocation list (Schulz & Grimes, 2002). Just about every method used to conceal allocation can be circumvented if people put their minds to doing so. Such actions may be maliciously motivated, but most often they are undertaken with a misplaced desire to ensure certain individuals get the "best" intervention. Regardless of the intention, they undermine the validity of the study, bias the results, and are unethical.

An IRB or ethics application form is unlikely to identify such problems (although they might identify a strong bias in the application and call attention to it). Such issues rely on the integrity of researchers and their commitment to using the highest standards in both research methods and ethics. Researchers must understand the methodological reasons for each step in their research and be ethically committed to conducting their research to the highest standards.

EQUIPOISE

As the "so what" questions are being addressed (Chapter 2), **equipoise** is important to identify. This concept is defined in various ways and has been the focus of heightened controversy in recent years (London, 2017). Much of this debate centers around whether a placebo group is ethically acceptable in intervention studies. When considering an intervention with a placebo group, this literature should be considered in more detail.

More generally, equipoise is an important ethical requirement in randomized intervention studies, although it is rarely made explicit in ethical guidelines. Literally, equipoise means we are equally poised regarding which intervention is best in a particular situation. Thus, equipoise arises "when there is uncertainty or conflicting expert opinion about the relative merits of diagnostic, prevention, or treatment options" (London, 2017, p. 525). When equipoise exists, randomization is ethically appropriate as a way to balance the duty to remove uncertainty about the best available evidence and the duty to respect and protect research participants. Reasoned deliberation is needed to decide if a particular project satisfied those ethical principles.

To know that equipoise exists, a thorough systematic review of previous research is necessary. This should ensure that the research question being addressed has not already been answered. If it has, conducting another project that will add little or nothing to our state of knowledge is an unethical use of limited resources. Replication of studies is important to confirm earlier results, but there comes a point at which further intervention studies are unnecessary, especially given the many research questions that always exist and require investigation. The importance of adequate review of previous research is increasingly recognized. Some funding agencies now require all funding proposals to be supported by the results of a systematic review or look more favorably on applications that justify their proposal with such results.

A thorough review of the literature also helps to identify challenges and limitations in the previous research. Careful attention to choosing the best methods for the research question is important, both scientifically and ethically. This should lead to higher quality research and reduce the incidence of mistakes. One study found that errors in treatment allocation occurred with surprising frequency, but were rarely disclosed in publications (Downs, Tucker, Christ-Schmidt, & Wittes, 2010). Research has been published where inappropriate methods were used, insufficient subjects enrolled without power calculations, wrong statistical tests conducted, or confounding factors ignored. Mistakes happen and they should be acknowledged when they occur so that others learn from these and other unexpected challenges.

During research design, competent researchers and reviewers should look for and correct errors to make the research as rigorous as possible. Although research ethics is not primarily about research methodology, an invalid research design leads to findings that are unreliable or invalid. Such projects are unethical because they waste limited resources and disrespect the subjects and the commitment made by others to the research enterprise. "Without validity, the research cannot generate the intended knowledge, cannot produce any benefit, and cannot justify exposing subjects to burdens or risks" (Emanuel, Wendler, & Grady, 2000, p. 2704).

SUBJECT SELECTION AND RECRUITMENT

An intervention may be intended for use by broad sections of the population (e.g., a dietary intervention) or by specific groups (e.g., those of a certain age or those with a particular illness). In either case, subjects should be chosen who are representative of the intended population for the intervention. Inclusion and exclusion criteria should be chosen for scientific reasons. This helps to ensure that selection is ethically fair and not based on convenience, prejudice, or irrelevant cultural criteria. Research studies have sometimes overrecruited some groups of people, such as prisoners or those in orphanages, whereas others have been excluded inappropriately, such as women from drug trials. Researchers may find it convenient to study an intervention in their own clinical practice. This may make access and cooperation more likely, which can be acceptable. However, if the subjects are thereby less appropriate for the goals of the research, convenience has been given a higher priority than the rigor of the project. Conducting an intervention study within one's own workplace raises other ethical challenges. Such studies may put undue pressure on colleagues or patients to participate, or lead them to fear some reprisal, however subtle, if they do not participate. To avoid such concerns and the potential bias they may introduce into the findings, it may be more appropriate to conduct the study at an alternative site.

Intervention studies in developing countries have highlighted the extreme end of this issue. Studies have been conducted in which subjects were more likely to agree to participate because of their lack of access to acceptable healthcare, not because they were good candidates for the intervention. They may thereby take on greater risks than they would otherwise accept. Such studies have highlighted the importance of "benefit sharing," in which those recruited to a study and who thereby bear its burdens and risks should also benefit from the results. Studies conducted among the poor who might never be able to afford the intervention, if it proves valuable, thereby become ethically questionable. This does not rule out studying poor populations. In fact, excluding the poor may be unethical if done for arbitrary reasons. For example, the impact of educational interventions on the proportion of fruits and vegetables in people's diets may fail to identify the impact of poverty if poorer people are not enrolled in the study. Here, poverty would be a variable to recognize in the study's design and take into account in subject selection, and not included for arbitrary or cultural reasons.

On the contrary, subjects may be inappropriately excluded because of challenges in subject recruitment. For example, studying an intervention that addresses teenage pregnancy might recruit only girls older than 18 years who could consent to the study as adults. The argument might be made that seeking parental consent for underage girls would add too many challenges to the project. It certainly would be challenging, but such is the nature of studying teenage pregnancy. Any teenage pregnancy intervention is likely to be used with girls younger than 18 years. The ethical challenges of recruiting underage girls would need to be addressed in the research so that the findings can be applicable to the real-world settings where the intervention will be used. Otherwise, the findings will be of questionable relevance and might be applied inappropriately.

SUBJECT RECRUITMENT

Once an appropriate set of criteria for subject selection has been determined, recruiting methods can raise ethical issues. Researchers sometimes assume that if they have access to people's personal data in their professional role, they can use this for recruitment. This may not be ethical on the basis of respecting people's privacy. This principle has been enshrined in data protection laws in many jurisdictions. The rule of thumb is that if a patient, student, or other person has provided personal information for the purposes of his or her healthcare, education, or otherwise, that information should be used only for that purpose. An employee may not use that information for his or her own purposes in recruiting research subjects or doing research on that data without first obtaining consent from the individual.

This can create challenges in recruiting subjects. Public advertisements and mass mailings are not the most effective in recruiting subjects because they lack a personal touch. However, data protection mechanisms help to preserve people's privacy and avoid placing undue pressure on fiduciary relationships. Otherwise, patients may feel their privacy has been violated if researchers were given details about their diagnosis or treatment. Students asked to be subjects in their instructors' own research projects may feel obligated to participate in case declining impacts their grade. Such conflicts may also arise for employers, supervisors, and others in positions of authority over potential subjects. These concerns can be addressed ethically. They can be avoided if researchers recruit subjects from a different clinic, class, or work setting. Those who hold private information (gatekeepers) can be asked to give people information about the research and how they can contact the researcher if they wish to participate. Then, private information is not disclosed to researchers, and the gatekeepers do not know who volunteers for the research. This approach both preserves privacy and helps to reduce sources of bias.

Respect for others should be the guiding ethical principle during subject recruitment and participation. This goes far beyond concern for privacy, confidentiality, and informed consent. In their seminal paper on clinical research ethics, Emanuel, Wendler, and Grady (2000) delineate five different ways potential and enrolled subjects should be respected:

1. Maintaining information about potential and enrolled subjects according to confidentiality rules
2. Permitting subjects to change their minds about enrollment without penalty
3. Informing subjects about new information gained during the study about the intervention or their own condition
4. Carefully monitoring subjects' welfare and responding appropriately to any adverse events or changes in their welfare
5. Providing subjects with information about what was learned from the study

All of these can be written into the study protocol and the information provided about the study. Mechanisms and guidelines can be put in place. However, the practical implementation of such factors often happens behind closed doors and points once again to the ethical character of researchers. Wolfe (2008) has described ways that researchers' attitudes can profoundly impact a research subject's experience of clinical research. Wolfe was a 36-year-old scientist working in clinical research when she was diagnosed with cancer. She was referred to a practice with a wonderful reputation and a strong emphasis on research. Her oncologist offered her a choice of three treatment regimens, one of which involved an intervention study. She met the research nurse to discuss the study details. Because of her own research background, Wolfe asked for detailed statistical information about the study drug but was provided with only generalities. The research nurse had no information beyond what was in the informed consent form, and some of her answers contradicted what the oncologist had said. Wolfe and her fiancé "felt belittled" after asking their questions and reported that they "began to question the validity of the information we were given and the expertise of the practice" (Wolfe, 2008, p. 39). They also felt pressured into joining the study, that "the nurse was trying to sell us one [trial], instead of helping us to consider our options" (Wolfe, 2008, p. 39). Wolfe decided not to participate, concerned that given her experience during recruitment, she would not be respected as an individual, but viewed as "patient #427 in a Phase III study" (Wolfe, 2008, p. 39). Although she remains a strong believer in the importance of research, she laments the lack of compassion and concern shown to her by this researcher.

Many others report positive experiences as research subjects. However, there is evidence that people's willingness to participate in clinical trials and recruitment rates are dropping, even while the number of subjects needed is increasing (Getz, 2008). The reasons for this are multifaceted, but trust is an important element. Trust is built on sound ethical character and the attitudes revealed in our interactions with others (O'Mathúna, 2009b). Such matters of character and attitude are rarely addressed in ethics training and will not be captured in research ethics applications. However, these attributes are crucial to respecting research subjects and providing them with the best possible experience during research studies.

RISK–BENEFIT RATIO

Wolfe was seeking clarification on the risks and benefits of her options. Assessment of risks and benefits is challenging and difficult but based on important ethical principles. Respecting people entails not exploiting them as mere research tools for the benefit of others. This involves reducing their risks in line with the ethical principle of nonmaleficence and enhancing their benefits according to the ethical principle of beneficence. Individual judgments regarding what counts as a favorable risk–benefit ratio will vary. The informed consent process is one means of taking account of this ethically by giving people enough information to decide for themselves. However, researchers also have an ethical duty to design the study in ways that make the ratio as favorable as possible for everyone. Ethical review can contribute here as reviewers' multidisciplinary backgrounds may highlight ways to improve the risk–benefit ratio by bringing to researchers' attention items they may not have seen or overlooked for various reasons.

Risk reduction can be achieved by finding ways to collect outcome data using procedures scheduled within clinical care rather than adding additional procedures. In educational contexts, replacing a focus group with individual interviews may be more time-consuming, but with some topics may reduce the risk of embarrassment, bullying, or discrimination. A questionnaire could be made completely anonymous to reduce the risk of violating confidentiality. Similarly, benefits may be enhanced by providing subjects with the results of tests or procedures carried out on them in the study. After the study is completed, all subjects could be provided with the most effective intervention so that those who received the less effective intervention during the trial would benefit later.

Some of the benefits of research accrue to society, not the individual. If a study is unlikely to personally benefit subjects, an appeal to altruism can be made. Potential benefits should not be invented or exaggerated. One of the problems with the University of Oklahoma study was an overly optimistic description of the vaccine's potential benefits. This optimism carried over to where even after the study was shut down and the subjects informed of its problems and violations, some subjects pleaded to continue to receive the vaccine (Lemonick & Goldstein, 2000).

This highlights what has been called "therapeutic misconception." The misconception is that the research is a form of individualized treatment. This issue arises when subjects have an unrealistic appraisal of the likelihood they will benefit personally from participation in a study. For example, if they enroll in an intervention study with a placebo arm, they should understand that they may receive a placebo. The only resulting benefits may be that they avoid the experimental intervention if it turns out to have more adverse effects. Misconceptions also can arise from believing that group assignment would be based on their individualized needs, rather than on random methods. Therapeutic misconception is particularly prevalent when people have serious illnesses with no good standard of care or when people see research studies as their only means to access any form of healthcare. This places an ethical obligation on researchers to clearly and accurately present the risks and benefits of an intervention study. Although no approach is foolproof, an ethically appropriate process involves more than providing potential subjects with long, complex information sheets.

Although typically discussed in clinical settings, a therapeutic misconception can exist in other fields of research. For example, in an educational study, students may believe that they are more likely to benefit from an innovative intervention than the traditional approach. They may seek out the new intervention or be more positively disposed to it if it appears novel or be dissatisfied at receiving the standard intervention. Such perceptions can impact outcomes, especially subjective ones, and raise challenges for randomization and blinding. They also point to the importance of researchers' attitudes as they describe the interventions' risks and benefits. They must carefully assess how they communicate about each of the interventions to avoid portraying one as more beneficial than the other.

The risks and benefits to subjects are widely acknowledged as are the potential benefits to society, but there also are potential risks to society. Research that is wasteful, invalid, or unethical runs the risk of undermining public confidence in research. Each study that is discredited for ethical violations adds to the risk of society becoming less tolerant of the research enterprise. This will delay the development and testing of new interventions and consequently any benefits these may provide society. Each study with ethical violations will not make national headlines, but each one risks undermining confidence and interest in research in its immediate environs.

> Wisdom is to know, that you do not know. —*Socrates*

Part of the challenge with risk assessment is the uncertainty inherent to research. Low-risk studies may bring few individual benefits to subjects. However, risk assessment should not be limited to examining direct physical harms but must explore the potential for indirect harms of various types, including psychosocial and spiritual risks. For example, a study involving an alternative therapy of spiritual or religious origins should inform potential subjects of these roots in case they would offend the subject's own spiritual beliefs. The researchers may see no potential harm, but the subjects should make this decision. As the risks of a study increase, the benefits should remain proportionate. Even when subjects are likely to receive no personal benefit, they may take on significant risks, so long as they make an informed decision to do so. In such cases, the benefits to society may justify individual risks. Although there is no straightforward calculus to permit the calculation of risk–benefit ratios, this is a crucial dimension in assessing the ethics of an intervention study and in evaluating how well it is ethically implemented.

INFORMED CONSENT

Research ethics discussions have, appropriately, emphasized informed consent. A study may have an ethical design and researchers may conduct themselves ethically, but if people do not freely choose to enroll as subjects, the study is unethical. Informed consent has been stressed because of the extreme violations seen in the Nazi medical experiments in which coercion was involved and the Tuskegee Syphilis study in which information and treatment were withheld from subjects to keep them enrolled. Informed consent is based on the ethical principle of autonomy and respecting people by allowing them to decide whether to enroll in research. The procedures should remind researchers that people are not required to be research subjects, but volunteer to be subjects. This should lead to an attitude of gratitude for the irreplaceable contribution subjects make to assist researchers in achieving their goals. At the very least, they deserve to be given the opportunity to make a fully informed decision about their participation.

Much has been written about how **informed consent** is an ongoing process of communication and dialogue, not a once-off signing of a form. The essential features of informed consent are enumerated differently, but five main components are involved:

1. Potential subjects should be competent, alert, and oriented to where they can understand the information presented.
2. A reasonable amount of information should be provided regarding the study's goals, design, risks, benefits, alternatives, the expectations on subjects, and their rights.
3. Subjects should have the opportunity to ask questions so that their understanding of the information presented is apparent.
4. Coercion and manipulation (from researchers, family, or others) should be avoided, and deception used to the minimal degree possible as approved during ethical review.
5. Authorization should be obtained and documented, using the most appropriate method for the subjects.

Each of these stages involves multiple decisions in practice. The precise information to be presented, how sufficient understanding is established, or how coercion is avoided will vary with each study. Research on incompetent patients or children can be important and ethical, requiring different mechanisms to obtain consent. Although adolescents may not be permitted legally to give informed consent, their **assent** to participation should be obtained. All these details should be clarified during the design and ethical approval of the study.

Unfortunately, and unethically, informed consent can be seen as little more than a hurdle to be overcome. The recruitment process can be slow, with challenges appearing around every corner. Having committed much time and energy to finding potential subjects, the process of informed consent can appear tedious and obstructive. The temptation to get the form signed and get the person into the study quickly must be resisted. Pushing people into a study before they are ready will only backfire and is unethical. Although the ethics approval process can evaluate the general approach to informed consent, many aspects of the process depend on the interactions between researchers and subjects, as exemplified by Pamela Wolfe's story (2008). Informed consent policies and forms are an important safeguard for research subjects, but they will never be enough. Henry Beecher viewed informed consent as very important, but he also held that "A far more dependable safeguard than consent is the presence of a truly *responsible* investigator" (Beecher, 1966, p. 1355). Again, the question of ethics comes down to the ethical character of researchers.

Informed consent is addressed in more detail in Chapter 13. Another point is made here. Making a fully informed decision to participate in a research study has many challenges. Lack of familiarity with research and the specific protocol contribute to this issue. Once subjects have begun participation in a study, they will understand the details and requirements better and be in a better position to make an informed decision. For this and other reasons, subjects should be informed about any new relevant information and asked about their willingness to continue in the study. Although this may lead to some participants withdrawing, it reflects better the ethical importance of informed consent as an ongoing process rather than a once-off decision made before enrolling in a study.

ETHICAL APPROVAL

Finally, you might be thinking, we get to discuss how to obtain ethical approval. This might have been where you expected this chapter to begin. Ethics application forms sometimes read as if the applicants are first considering the ethical issues of their project after locating the form. Some appear to seriously consider the ethical issues only after receiving feedback on their initial application. In contrast, ethical considerations should be identified, examined, and addressed from the study's inception. At every stage of the research process, decisions are made about the study that have ethical dimensions (O'Mathúna & Siriwardhana, 2017). Ethics is not an appendage to be added onto a study once it has been designed and is ready to be implemented. The ethical issues involved at each stage of a study should be discussed among the research team as the project is being designed. When all these factors have been taken into account, it is time to apply for ethical approval. If this is done carefully and documented, completing the application form should go smoothly. It may take some time to formulate answers to the questions and defend the decisions made, but this should be a way of describing the ethical decision-making process already undertaken.

The research ethics approval process has problems, and changes are needed (O'Mathúna & Siriwardhana, 2017). At the same time (from observations made over many years spent on RECs in the United States and Ireland), many of the delays and frustrations researchers experience could be resolved rather straightforwardly. Ethical applications are sometimes submitted, whereas projects are still being developed. Sometimes ethics application forms read as if the research project was developed only in response to the questions on the application form. An IRB or REC should approve a study as it will be conducted, not when important details are yet to be decided. This seems to be a more frequent issue with applications from graduate students. Applications can be made too early in an effort to avoid delays while waiting for ethical approval.

Sometimes applications are submitted without due attention to important details. I have seen applications in which the stated goals could not be achieved with the proposed methodology, power calculations have been done incorrectly, conflicts of interest have been ignored, or patient information sheets would require a PhD to interpret. Some of these issues impinge on the ongoing debate over whether ethical approval should address questions of methodology. My own view is that study methodology is an ethical issue because an invalid or flawed study wastes time and resources. Methodological questions are often raised during review, not because the methods are questioned, but because the form is unclear or the methods proposed are inappropriate for the study's stated aims.

Such factors should be addressed before submission of the ethics form. This can take place within the research team, in which each applicant should have the time to comment on drafts. Graduate students and supervisors should work together here, with both viewing the ethics approval process as an important training exercise for the students. Students should give supervisors sufficient time to review draft application forms and to incorporate their feedback into the application. Good planning is crucial here.

When a study is ready for the ethics application process, the lead applicant should identify all the forms and deadlines for the IRB or REC. Committees differ in the way submissions are to be made and what forms are involved. Identifying all these details can save time and frustration later in the process. Much of this information is now on the relevant websites, but a phone call to the committee's administrator can ensure that the most recent updates are available. The deadlines are important to identify and adhere to, especially for committees that do not meet very regularly. In larger organizations, identifying to which committee(s) to apply is important. Knowing the application deadline, a timeline should be developed that permits the research team to complete each stage of the process. Make sure to incorporate some flexibility to account for the inevitable delays that will appear. Permission letters to access various sites may need to be included, so time should be allowed to gather these. A feasible schedule is crucial to avoid a last-minute rush that can take away from the quality of the application.

> During ten years of study of [ethical problems in research] … thoughtlessness and carelessness, not a willful disregard for patient's rights, account for most of the cases encountered. —*Henry Beecher*

One of the most disappointing aspects of reviewing ethics application forms has been the poor quality of some applications. Some applications forms are replete with spelling and grammar mistakes. An occasional mistake is understandable, and applicants are not expected to be literary scholars. However, some application forms are so poorly completed that they lead to questions about the researcher's willingness to give the necessary attention to detail that good research requires. Such carelessness also reflects poorly on the institution and other researchers represented by the research team.

These issues also can have direct ethical significance. Recruitment letters, patient information sheets, and informed consent/assent forms must be carefully composed and edited. Not only must these be complete and accurate, they should be written at a comprehension level appropriate for the subjects. This may take several drafts and warrant having people of different reading levels comment on their legibility. Sloppiness in this area reflects a poor level of respect for research subjects and the time they will be asked to commit to the study. Poorly written forms also are likely to lead to poor subject recruitment.

In applying for ethical approval, it is important to plan out the process and review draft forms carefully. This application should be done with the same rigor and care that is required with funding applications. Adhering to deadlines and word limits is important, as well as double checking that all parts of the application are submitted.

Finally, expect comments and questions from the committee. IRBs and RECs exist not only to protect research subjects but also to facilitate good research. Most members are committed researchers themselves; otherwise they would not volunteer their time for this work. They believe in research and want to improve research studies where possible. It is highly unlikely you will have designed a perfect study, so expect some comments and suggestions that are intended to help your study. If the committee has serious ethical problems with your study, humbly take that input under consideration. They may have helped you avoid a serious pitfall. If you disagree, you will have the opportunity to respond to the committee in defense of your proposal.

SUMMARY

Ethical issues arise at many, if not most, critical junctures in a research study. In deciding on a research topic, ethical considerations are involved along with other factors—whether to study an intervention that could impact a serious illness in a developing country or one that concerns only the wealthy raises ethical issues. Decisions about which outcomes to measure, and with which tools, will involve some degree of ethical consideration. At each step along the way, decisions should be made to promote the good of subjects and minimize harm.

Some ethical issues are common to all research studies, but others relate to specific types of studies. The focus here has been on the general issues, with little attention given to unique factors. These include studies with children, mental health patients, and other vulnerable populations. Research studies in developing countries and in humanitarian contexts raise their own ethical issues (O'Mathúna & Siriwardhana, 2017). Detailed information about specific study types can be found in the resources listed in Table 7.2.

Addressing ethical issues is important in the training for and conducting of intervention studies. Ethics training courses are now available for researchers and IRB members. Although regulations and ethical approval processes are valuable, they are not sufficient to ensure that intervention studies are carried out to the highest ethical standards. Ethical research requires ethical researchers, which points to the importance of character development in research training. Just as researchers must learn to be accurate and observant, they must learn to be respectful and grateful toward their subjects. The recommitment to keep subjects' well-being as the highest priority during research is an ethical obligation based on the researcher's character.

This issue raises questions about how such character development can be fostered. Although this is a topic of some debate, only a few tentative suggestions are made here. The first is that researchers must recognize the tension that exists to put results, fame, and profit above people. If this tension is not recognized and resisted, the battle may already be lost. Sensitivity to people's well-being takes work to maintain. One way to do this is through honest and open discussions among members of the research team or with a mentor. Good team leaders create environments where people can express and process the struggles they may be having with deadlines, setbacks, and unexpected results.

Literature is another way to both recognize ethical issues and how character is involved (O'Mathúna, 2009a). Watching a play or movie like *Wit* (2001) can highlight the ways that patients give informed consent to become research subjects, only to be turned into lab experiments for the good of science and someone else's career advancement. At the same time, the movie portrays how a nurse can restore the humanity of a research subject. A novel or a movie like *The Constant Gardener* (2005) can highlight the challenges of research in developing countries and the powerful political, economic, and cultural forces that create conflicts

TABLE 7.2 Resources for Research Ethics

GUIDELINE	ORIGIN	AVAILABLE AT
Guidelines for Specific Research Topics	Council of European Social Science Data Archives	https://www.cessda.eu/
Resources on Research Ethics	Fogarty International Center, National Institutes of Health	www.fic.nih.gov/ResearchTopics/ Bioethics/Pages/investigators-ethics-committees.aspx

of interest. The degree of fact or fiction in such literature is irrelevant. Engaging with such movies or novels within a research team and discussing them together can help to develope sensitivity to ethical issues and ways to address them. Much effort is needed to resist the pressures and demands that can desensitize us to ethical issues and the ultimate goals of research. In-depth reflection on ethics is challenging, particularly if it is to engage with ethical character issues. But the rewards can be profound. Research ethics, properly understood, should promote the well-being of research subjects, help researchers become more careful and caring in their work, and contribute to the evidence necessary to improve decision making in practice and policy.

Key Points From This Chapter

- Ethical issues pervade the whole research process and should be considered from the inception of the project.
- The primary ethical principle in research is the protection and promotion of the well-being of research subjects.
- Ethical policies, regulations, and review are important, but not sufficient to ensure research is conducted to the highest ethical standards.
- Some ethical issues arise from the researcher's moral character and point to the importance of personal integrity in research.

REFERENCES

Beecher, H. K. (1966). Ethics and clinical research. *New England Journal of Medicine, 274*(24), 1354–1360. doi:10.1056/NEJM196606162742405; reprinted in Harkness, J., Lederer, S. E., & Wikler, D. (2001). Laying ethical foundations for clinical research. *Bulletin of the World Health Organization, 79*(4), 365–372.

Council for International Organizations of Medical Sciences. (2016). *International ethical guidelines for health-related research involving humans.* Geneva: Author. Retrieved from https://cioms.ch/wp-content/uploads/2017/01/WEB-CIOMS-EthicalGuidelines.pdf

Downs, M., Tucker, K., Christ-Schmidt, H., & Wittes, J. (2010). Some practical problems in implementing randomization. *Clinical Trials, 7*(3), 235–245. doi:10.1177/1740774510368300

Emanuel, E. J., Wendler, D., & Grady, C. (2000). What makes clinical research ethical? *Journal of the American Medical Association, 283*(20), 2701–2711. doi:10.1001/jama.283.20.2701

Getz, K. A. (2008, September). Public confidence and trust today: A review of public opinion polls. *Monitor, 22,* 17–21.

Harkness, J., Lederer, S. E., & Wikler, D. (2001). Laying ethical foundations for clinical research. *Bulletin of the World Health Organization, 79*(4), 365–366.

Lemonick, M. D., & Goldstein, A. (2000, April). At your own risk. *Time, 159*(16), 46–55.

London, A. J. (2017). Equipoise in research: Integrating ethics and science in human research. *Journal of the American Medical Association, 317*(5), 525–526. doi:10.1001/jama.2017.0016

Malakoff, D. (2000). Clinical research. Flawed cancer study leads to shake-up at University of Oklahoma. *Science, 289*(5480), 706–707.

O'Mathúna, D. P. (2009a). *Nanoethics: Big ethical issues with small technology.* London, UK: Continuum.

O'Mathúna, D. P. (2009b). Trust and clinical research. *Research Practitioner, 10*(5), 170–177.

O'Mathúna, D. P., & Siriwardhana, C. (2017). Research ethics and evidence for humanitarian health. *Lancet, 390*(10109), 2228–2229. doi:10.1016/S0140-6736(17)31276-X

Schulz, K. F., & Grimes, D. A. (2002). Allocation concealment in randomised trials: Defending against deciphering. *Lancet, 359*(9306), 614–618. doi:10.1016/S0140-6736(02)07750-4

Wolfe, P. (2008, September). Forgetting individuality in patient recruiting. *Monitor, 22,* 37–39.

Minimizing Threats to Internal Validity

Jacqueline Dunbar-Jacob

> Think not of yourself as the architect of your career but as the sculptor. Expect to have to do a lot of hard hammering and chiseling and scraping and polishing. —*B.C. Forbes*

"Internal validity" refers to the design characteristics that allow us to have confidence in the findings of or inference from a study. This is most relevant to studies that attempt to show causation or that variable *a* (treatment) causes or creates a change in variable *b* (outcome). These studies are particularly important in validating theory and in evaluating interventions. The conclusions should be clear, without the question of whether other factors could account for the findings.

First, what are *not* causal studies. Causal studies are not correlational studies. There have been numerous examples of misinterpretation of correlational data showing causal relationships. The classical example is the story of storks and babies. Numerous sets of data have demonstrated a significant and positive relationship between the number of stork pairs and the birth rate in various European countries (Bell, 2008; Engel & Schutt, 2008; Matthews, 2000). If correlational data were interpreted as causal, one would surmise that, indeed, storks may bring babies. That theory is not plausible, however, and so demographers and others searched for yet a third variable that could account for the presence of stork pairs and birth rate. What could lead to an increase in the stork population as well as an increase in the birth rate? Numerous factors were examined, including economic conditions, expansion of the population, and temperature.

Examples of correlational data being interpreted as causal continue to exist. For example, the correlation between receipt of vaccines in early childhood and the diagnosis of autism in early childhood was discussed in a causal light until more recent data showed that to be a spurious correlation (Chu-Carroll, 2007). A second example is the correlation between hormone replacement therapy and risk of heart disease, suggesting a protective effect of estrogen (Bush et al., 1987). Many women began hormone replacement therapy. Subsequent randomized, controlled studies showed that there was no protective effect of estrogen on heart disease, and, indeed, it appeared to lead to increases in breast cancer (Beral, Banks, & Reeves, 2002). Correlational studies cannot be used to ascribe causation.

Studies that are designed to identify causal relationships in the clinical arena are often referred to as "efficacy studies." Even in these studies, causation is difficult to establish when studies do not control for potential threats to validity. That this happens is evidenced by the criticisms found in numerous systematic reviews. For example, in a recent state-of-the-science review of the research on the prevention of Alzheimer's disease and mild cognitive impairment, the panel concluded that there is insufficient evidence to support any conclusions about risk factors or to support any lifestyle or dietary preventive strategies. The quality of evidence was rated low. It was noted that "existing studies have been hampered by methodological issues" (Daviglus et al., 2011). Similarly, systematic reviews of studies designed to evaluate interventions to improve adherence to treatment regimen have not yielded recommendations for practice. Several systematic reviews have been carried out. Each has noted that many studies have poor methodological quality, including lack of randomization, small sample sizes, and variability in measurement and definitions (DiMatteo, Giordani, Lepper, & Croghan, 2002; Haynes, Ackloo, Sahota, McDonald, & Yao, 2008; McDonald, Garg, & Haynes, 2002; Peterson, Takiya, & Finley, 2003a, 2003b; Prendergast & Gaston, 2010; Takiya, Peterson, & Finley, 2004).

There are many examples of attempts to justify or translate interventions for which the data are limited or based on inadequately designed studies. Studies that are testing causal relationships need to be designed to rule out competing explanations for the findings. Study designs that control for these competing explanations for findings are said to have high internal validity. The strongest designs that control for competing interpretations are experimental or randomized controlled trials. This chapter addresses the factors that pose threats to internal validity, how the threats present in research designs, and strategies to minimize the threats.

INTERNAL VALIDITY

Internal validity refers to the degree of confidence that the outcome of an experimental study is caused by the independent variable and not by potentially competing factors. Unfortunately, there are many factors that, if unaddressed, can lower confidence in the findings. These factors are typically referred to as "threats to internal validity." Although there is not a perfect study, efforts are typically undertaken to control for threats to internal validity in experimental or intervention research. Indeed, high internal validity is a hallmark of the quality of a study. High-quality systematic reviews and meta-analyses exclude studies with poor internal validity (Jüni, Altman, & Egger, 2001; Moher et al., 1999). Thus, it is important in designing a study or in reviewing a study to be familiar with the threats to internal validity and the strategies to address them (see Exhibit 8.1).

Threats to Internal Validity
History
A significant threat, which needs to be controlled in causal research, is history. History refers to the external events that happen during the study, which could influence the outcome. These events are particularly problematic when they occur differentially between the groups. When individuals within the study have different experiences during the study that could influence the outcome, or dependent variable, the validity of the study is threatened.

EXHIBIT 8.1 Threats to Internal Validity

- History
- Maturation
- Mortality
- Testing
- Instrumentation
- Regression to the mean
- Selection
- Group contamination
- Compensatory intervention
- Compensatory rivalry
- Resentful demoralization
- Statistical conclusion validity

There are numerous situations where the validity of a study can be compromised by such events. For example, when each treatment group receives intervention from a different interventionist, making the experience different between groups, the question must be asked whether the outcome was caused by the intervention or by some characteristic of an interventionist. Providing both groups with exposure to multiple interventionists can serve to minimize the potential effect of distinct therapists by treatment on outcome. Unplanned events can also occur during the course of a clinical trial. For example, if during the course of a study testing the effect of a specific protocol on infection control, the hospital changes the type of cleaning solution used for some of the patient units, the ability to attribute outcomes to the experimental protocol is threatened by the effect of the new cleaning solution on infection rates for some but not all of the units. If the study is designed to compare unit infection rates, internal validity is threatened by virtue of differential exposure to the new cleaning solution. These problems can be helped through the use of random assignment to intervention and control conditions, as well as clearly articulated procedures during the trial.

Events may also occur that affect both groups and potentially impact outcome. For example, the criteria for diagnosing diabetes was changed in 1985, 1996, and again in 2010 (McCulloch, 2011). Studies of interventions to control diabetes during the period of change needed to consider the effect of these diagnostic changes on study outcome, considering the outcome criteria targeted by the study and the new criteria targeted by the clinical world. In this case, the investigators must determine the continuing criteria for recruitment or outcome. In most cases, staying with the original criteria will preserve the internal validity of the study.

History, or external events particularly differentially experienced by the groups, can pose a significant threat to internal validity. Investigators need to be alert to such events and their potential impact on the outcome interpretation. As noted, random assignment to groups and the use of a control condition will help control for such threats.

Maturation

A second potential threat to internal validity is maturation or changes in the research subjects themselves over time. These changes could include developmental changes, such as increased abstract thinking in adolescents; physiological changes, such as immune response to a viral exposure; or disease progression, such as cognitive decline in Alzheimer's disease. In the absence of a comparison group, it would be difficult to evaluate the impact of the intervention. In a study of self-management among 12-year-old children, could changes in self-management be caused by cognitive maturation or by the patient education intervention? Could the response to an experimental cold treatment be a result of the novel treatment or of the immune response to the viral exposure? Could the failure of a medication for Alzheimer's disease be the result of the progressive cognitive decline in the disorder? The design consideration that alleviates the threat of maturation is the inclusion of a control group. The comparison of outcomes between the intervention group and a control group, where maturation is similar between the groups, allows for the test of the effect of the intervention beyond the maturational changes within the subjects.

Mortality

Mortality refers to the occurrence of dropouts from the research. The overall loss of subjects poses a problem for the power of the study to detect differences. Thus, larger dropout rates are likely to bias the outcome in the direction of no effect. This has been noted to be a common problem across clinical trials (Wood, White, & Thompson, 2004). Dropouts may vary by type of intervention or by data collection procedures. For example, dropouts have been identified as a substantial problem in eHealth intervention studies (Eysenbach, 2005).

Differential dropout can lead to inaccuracies in the interpretation of outcomes in a trial. Higher dropout rates among subjects who experience adverse effects from participation may lead to a conclusion that the treatment is safe and tolerable. Higher dropout rates in one of the research groups could influence the conclusion of effectiveness.

Several strategies are useful in protecting against the threat of mortality. First among those is an intention-to-treat analysis (Lachin, 2000; Wertz, 1995). In this case, all subjects randomized are included in the primary outcome analysis at the end of the study, even if they have dropped out. There are numerous strategies to impute data for dropouts for utilization in the outcome analysis. This may include bringing the last value forward, using the baseline data, using the group mean, and projecting trend data among others (Donders, van der Heijden, Stijnen, & Moons, 2006). Intention-to-treat analysis generally provides conservative estimates of outcome. In addition to managing the threat to internal validity caused by mortality, the intention-to-treat analysis preserves the randomization scheme, supporting statistical assumptions for analysis. It is the recommended approach to analysis in the design of clinical trials.

Of course, the important strategy in reducing mortality is to prevent its occurrence in the first place. Several studies have looked at the predictors of dropout from clinical trials. In part, one needs to examine predictors within the type of clinical trial being conducted. Is it a community study, a multicenter clinical trial, an acute illness study, a prevention trial, lifestyle trial, or a chronic disease trial? Some general areas, however, seem to be important. One of those is the site from which the subject was recruited. For example, Snow, Connett, Sharma, and Murray (2007) reported that subjects recruited through mass mailings were less likely to drop out than those recruited through referrals and other methods. Moser, Dracup, and Doering (2000) and Inelmen et al. (2005) reported that employed participants were more likely to drop out than those who were not employed. One can speculate that the burden of participation may be heavier for the employed or that the need to be absent from work may interfere with the commitment to the trial. Other factors such as socioeconomic status, extent of disease, and treatment group assignment may affect the tendency to drop out (Roumen et al., 2011). Even the method of data collection may affect retention. For example, Childs et al. (2011) reported higher levels of nonresponse using web-based methods of collecting self-report data. Thus, there is some literature to assist in identifying those at risk for drop out.

If those at risk for dropout can be identified, strategies can be designed to prevent it. Some investigators have noted that the nature of the relationships between the clinical trial personnel and the participant is an important determinant of retention (Good & Schuler,

1997; Mor, Niv, & Niv, 2006; Penckofer, Byrn, Mumby, & Ferrans, 2011). Other factors such as a desire to prevent or contribute to the treatment of a specific condition or the desire to participate in research may also be motivators for participation. These offer avenues for reinforcement of motivation to participate. Other strategies include the use of appointment reminders, staff review of missed visits, early rescheduling of missed visits, and incentives such as money.

Even with the best of retention protocols in a study, subjects may still decide to leave a trial. There has been some work on dropout retrieval. Probstfield, Russell, Henske, Reardon, and Insull (1986) describe a successful systematic protocol to retrieve dropouts in a multicenter clinical trial. It is well worth the effort to retrieve dropouts in the interests of preventing the threat posed by mortality.

Testing

The testing process itself can also threaten the internal validity of a study. Testing poses a particular problem when it is repeated over time. The test itself may identify what the investigators are interested in. On repeat testing, the subjects may respond with what they believe the investigators want to hear. A second problem is that tests may teach the subjects. Changes in test outcomes may then reflect the learning that has taken place as a result of prior testing rather than a result of the intervention. Indeed, research in education supports the impact of testing on learning (McDaniel, Roediger, & McDermott, 2007). This phenomenon may also be referred to as "practice effects" or as "reactivity."

Single-group studies are particularly vulnerable to the effect of testing. Baseline assessment followed by intervention followed by follow-up testing raises the question of whether any changes in outcome were caused by the intervention or by the testing itself. One strategy to avoid this potential threat is to employ a control group that does not receive the intervention. If both groups improve, then the effect is likely a result of testing. If the intervention group improves but not the control group, then the intervention is likely to have contributed to the change.

Even with a control group, testing can pose a problem if the same test is used in repeated assessments. The learning effect on both the control and intervention group could mask the effects of treatment. Therefore, if testing is repeated over time, it is desirable to use alternative forms of the test. This is particularly important where study outcomes are knowledge based.

Instrumentation

The simple process of testing, or data collection, can influence the outcome. However, equally as important is the instrument itself that is used for data collection. Inconsistencies in the instrument can lead to erroneous conclusions about the study outcome. For example, instruments that are not stable over time can lead to assessments that are functions of the measure rather than the variable being studied. Several specific factors can contribute to a threat to internal validity posed by the instrumentation itself.

An instrumentation threat is posed when the measure does not have adequate reliability. The measure should be internally consistent and stable over the time period in which assessments are being carried out. Thus, one is assured that the control condition will have a stable estimate of the variable, and any difference between groups will be a result of the intervention or experimental manipulation. There are multiple methods of estimating the reliability of a test. Their generally accepted levels of reliability fall in the range of 0.80 to 0.90 (Anastasi, 1988). It is important to note that reliability is established within a population (Wilkinson & The Task Force on Statistical Inference, 1999). Reliability in one population does not generalize to another population. An instrument with established reliability should be used rather than a new instrument.

Reliability also needs to be considered when ratings or observations are being used. In these cases, the raters or observers ideally rate or identify the same characteristics in the same manner. The raters' or observers' data are correlated with the criteria for acceptability at the 0.80s to 0.90s level. Several factors can influence the level of reliability. First is the training of the raters to an acceptable level of consistency. Second is the concrete definition of the characteristic to be identified or rated. Third is the opportunity the rater has to actually observe the person in a situation where the characteristic or behavior occurs. In situations where a provider or caregiver is asked whether a patient has engaged in some behavior, such as following a treatment regimen, other data may be used to infer whether the behavior occurred, which may lead to inaccuracies and variability in the data.

Instrument decay over time may also influence the internal validity of a study. If the observer or interviewer begins to take shortcuts or attend to differing elements of the participant or the data collection, the data may change over time. Further, the observer's judgment may also decay over time. Equipment may begin to function less effectively or consistently. Each of these leads to inconsistencies in the data collected. Quality control procedures to ensure accuracy in measurement over time are important in reducing this threat.

Special consideration needs to be given to the reliability of self-report of behavior or symptom experience. Self-report may pose particular issues with stability of the measure. For example, self-reported adherence may differ from adherence reported by other measures (Garber, Nau, Erickson, Aikens, & Lawrence, 2004) and may vary depending on the interval of the report (Lu et al., 2008). Self-reports of pain may also vary over hours or days (Jensen & McFarland, 1993), yielding different estimates depending on the time chosen for assessment and the duration of days assessed. Reliance of diaries poses the problem of variability when the diary is completed, leading to recall errors or prospective accounting of behavior (Stone, Shiffman, Schwartz, Broderick, & Hufford, 2002). An examination of the self-assessment of height and weight compared with objective measures showed a systematic bias in the self-report, with heights being overestimated and weights being underestimated (Connor Gorber, Tremblay, Moher, & Gorber, 2007).

A further threat posed by self-report of health outcomes, functional status, or quality of life is the phenomenon of "response shift." Response shift refers to a change in one's self-evaluation of a particular construct or function because of changing internal standards, changing values, or changes in how one defines the particular construct (Sprangers & Schwartz, 1999). The problem has been found in both pediatric and adult populations with serious and chronic illness (Breetvelt & Van Dam, 1991; Brossart, Clay, & Willson, 2002). An important issue is to detect whether a response shift has occurred. One common method is to use the *thentest* (Visser, Smets, Sprangers, & de Haes, 2000). Subjects are given a pretest and after intervention are given a posttest and a retrospective test to evaluate how they felt in the time period the pretest was covered. The response shift is assessed by a comparison of the pretest scores with the *thentest* scores. Standard methods of analysis do not control for the bias of response shift, for example, posttest analysis, analysis of difference scores, or analysis of covariance (ANCOVA; Bray, Maxwell, & Howard, 1984). Bray et al. (1984) suggest analysis of posttest minus *thentest* scores, which also protects statistical power.

Also relevant to the stability or consistency of the instrument, particularly when measures are repeated in a study, is the use of consistent procedures during an assessment. Most standardized instruments have been developed and evaluated for use under a specific set of conditions of administration. Changes in those conditions can lead to changes in the results, whether one is talking about psychosocial measures or physiological measures. For example, blood pressure readings will vary depending on whether the patient is talking or sitting silently, or whether the patient has rested or been active just prior to the assessment (Pickering et al., 2005). Without standard procedures, the risk of use of different procedures for different subjects is high, leading to lack of consistency in data between subjects because of inconsistency in measurement procedures. In addition, completing measurement of one group and then measuring the other group can lead to biases because of decay on the part of the data gatherers or the instruments being used.

Standard measurement protocols are important in reducing the threat to internal validity through instrumentation. Equally important is a quality control protocol, which is implemented throughout the study (Hulley & Cummings, 1988). The quality control protocol for measurement would include regularly scheduled evaluation of measures and data collectors to determine functionality, as well as consistency and adherence to the measurement protocol.

Regression to the Mean

Regression to the mean also poses a threat to internal validity. Regression to the mean refers to the tendency of outcome scores to come closer to a population mean over time (Barnett, van der Pols, & Dobson, 2005). Thus, subjects who score low at baseline will drift upward and subjects who score high at baseline will drift downward. This tendency to drift to the mean may lead to a conclusion that treatment is effective when it is not or is ineffective when it may not be. Regression to the mean has led to overestimation of treatment effects in some intervention trials (Chuang-Stein & Tong, 1997). Similarly, safety concerns have been underestimated (Chuang-Stein & Tong, 1997). The problem is most likely when subjects are chosen who initially score at the extremes of the population distribution of scores. It is also more likely to occur in the absence of a control condition, for example, when examining the effect of an intervention that everyone receives in a clinical or educational setting, or the sample serves as its own control (Tinkelman & Wilson, 2004).

There are several methods to reduce the potential threat of regression. The first is to include a control condition. Presumably, the regression effect will be experienced by both groups and will be reflected in control group changes. A comparison of the group outcomes will be more likely to detect the impact of intervention because regression will be controlled for by the control group change.

The second method is to randomize subjects to the intervention and the control condition (Barnett et al., 2005). Randomization increases the probability that the groups are alike regarding known and unknown factors and therefore increases the probability that extreme scores will be equally distributed between groups. There are several randomization methods (Friedman, Furberg, & DeMets, 1998). One is simple randomization, where every participant has a prescribed chance of being assigned to a group. For large sample sizes, this is effective but may not ensure equivalence between groups for small sample sizes. A second strategy for randomization may be used—blocked randomization. In blocked randomization, according to Friedman et al. (1998), subjects are randomized within smaller groups at specified time intervals. For example, subjects may be randomized in sets of six according to when they are recruited. This way, one treatment is not composed of subjects recruited early and one of subjects recruited late in the study. A third strategy is to use stratified randomization. For example, randomization could be stratified on screening score so that equivalent numbers of subjects with high, middle, or low values are randomized to each group.

A third method to manage regression is to take multiple initial measurements and use either the average of the measures or the latest measure as the baseline or the selection criterion (Barnett et al., 2005; Chuang-Stein & Tong, 1997). Regression is related to the amount of measurement variability, which is lowered by this strategy. A fourth strategy is to adjust for regression in the analysis. One method is the use of ANCOVA (Barnett et al., 2005; Chuang-Stein & Tong, 1997). In this instance, the covariate used is the baseline value. Barnett et al. (2005) also suggest examining a scatter plot of the data, baseline with outcome, and determine whether change is more likely at the extremes of the baseline values.

This would suggest that regression effects are operative. And very important to controlling for regression effects is random assignment to groups. In this case, even with the choice of subjects at the extremes of the distribution, regression will occur in both groups and will be controlled in the analysis.

Selection

The threat to internal validity through selection of subjects refers to inconsistencies between the groups within the study. Lack of randomization to groups is the most common cause of this problem. Even with randomization, differences between groups can occur that affect the outcome. For example, if, in an educational intervention, one group has a greater reading ability than the other, and that group has a higher outcome score than the other group, it is not clear whether the educational intervention or the differences in reading ability accounted for the outcome. Investigators should assess the groups at baseline on those variables that could influence the outcome. For example, socioeconomic differences are frequently assessed at baseline, as health effects, prevention, literacy levels, and other behaviors are often different for different socioeconomic levels. Other variables may be relevant to the study such as duration of disease, past behavioral habits, and mental health status.

A way to prevent threats caused by group differences on potentially competing explanatory variables is to identify such variables during study design and to measure them. They should be examined before the analysis phase. If known, they can often be handled through adjustment in the outcome analysis. It may also be possible to use stratified randomization to ensure that the groups are equivalent on these key variables. And, lastly, some of these factors may be handled through the criteria for inclusion and exclusion. For example, in the hypothetical study mentioned earlier, reading level could be a covariate in the analysis, could be a stratification factor in randomization to groups, or a specified level of reading necessary to complete the intervention could be set as a criterion for inclusion.

Group differences, or selection, can interact with each of the other threats to internal validity, further compromising a study. Maturational factors may operate differently within groups if the groups are not equivalent at baseline. Testing may yield a further threat if the groups are different. For example, if one group reflects a more extensive family history of the disease of interest in the research, the pretesting may lead to greater attention to risk factor reduction outside of the study. The same could be said for the impact of differential changes in instrumentation. For example, if subjects are recruited over a long interval, the later subjects may be different from the initial groups recruited. Changes in measures would affect the group outcome measure differently. Significant problems arise if there is differential dropout or mortality between the groups related to different characteristics between the groups. And having a group with higher or lower scores on key variables can lead to differential regression effects within the groups.

Some of the threats can be controlled within the design of the study. For example, consistency in measurement over time would be critical. Assessment of the comparability of the groups at baseline is also essential. Also, where necessary, analyses may need to adjust for the potential threats.

There are several other sources of threats to internal validity through contamination of the control group. In these threats, differences between the intervention and control group may be reduced or exaggerated by the behavior of the control group. In these cases, the control group may be exposed to the treatment or an alternative treatment, may increase effort, or may reduce effort (Borg, 1984). Blinding of treatments and assessments is one strategy to control for these effects in intervention studies. Blinding refers to keeping the participants unaware of their treatment group assignment. Double blinding refers to the investigators also being unaware of the participant group's assignment.

Imitation of Treatment or Group Contamination

A problem that occurs within clinical trials occurs when the control or comparison group receives some form of intervention similar to that offered to the treatment group. This is most likely to occur when the groups are in contact with each other, are unblinded, or providers or family member, in a position to apply the intervention, have information about the intervention itself. A prominent example of this phenomenon occurred with the Multiple Risk Factor Intervention Trial (MRFIT; Szklo, 1983). The MRFIT was a large multicenter clinical trial of approximately 12,880 males at high risk for coronary disease. The study was designed to test the effect of a multicomponent intervention on cardiovascular risk factors, hypertension, smoking, and cholesterol using antihypertensive medications, smoking cessation, and low-fat diet with the intervention group. The study used a randomized controlled design but was unblinded. The control condition continued usual care from their personal physicians who received information on the study. After 7 years, the study found no difference between groups in mortality. Further, the control condition had better risk factor reduction than expected. It has been hypothesized that increased intervention by the primary physicians may have been a contributing factor (Szklo, 1983). In other words, the control subjects may have received an alternate treatment for their risk factors through their primary care physicians.

Similar kinds of events can occur when subjects themselves have the opportunity to interact with each other and discuss the treatments within the study. Subjects in control conditions may learn about the intervention and apply it themselves, wholly or partly, reducing outcome differences between control and treatment conditions. In both of these conditions, the threat can be better managed by limiting contact or communication between the subjects in different groups or between study and primary care personnel.

Compensatory Intervention

Outside intervention may occur in other ways. In the case of compensatory equalization of treatments, it appears that the intervention group is gaining some value that the control group is not. An alternative treatment is provided to compensate the control condition for not receiving the value offered by the experimental intervention. Indeed, this could also be an explanation for the improvement in the control subjects in the MRFIT study. That is, the primary care physicians may have wanted to compensate for the lack of intervention by the study because they perceived value from the intervention. Consequently, they may have stepped up their own efforts to provide risk reduction.

Compensatory Rivalry

In contrast, in the case of compensatory rivalry, the control subjects themselves may adopt strategies to influence the outcome in a way that is favorable to themselves. Returning again to the MRFIT study, it could be that the subjects, having received the informed consent form and knowing the intentions of the trial, influenced their physicians to provide prevention intervention or they may have adopted lifestyle interventions on their own through a competitive spirit. They worked harder to achieve as much risk reduction as the intervention group.

Resentful Demoralization

The control group, on the contrary, might feel so demoralized by not being selected for intervention that they stop personal efforts related to study outcome, with a decline in their outcome measures after baseline. In this case, group differences, when the intervention group performed better than the control group and the control group declined over the study, could not be linked clearly to treatment effects. Differences may be caused by control group decline.

Borg (1984) suggests that strategies to cope with these threats caused by control group behaviors can be handled by providing an alternate intervention for the control group. He recommends that the control condition receive an intervention designed to change a specified but unrelated outcome variable. The intervention would be of similar duration with similar demands and similar procedures and be perceived as valuable to the subject. An example would be providing the control group with a meditation program while the intervention group is receiving an exercise intervention, when the outcome for comparison is cardiovascular fitness.

All of these threats to internal validity are the standard threats that should be addressed in the design of intervention or experimental studies. Minimization of these threats directly influences the quality of the study—an essential component for the utilization of the research in support for evidence-based practice. A study with poor internal validity does not make a contribution to evidence-based practice because one cannot have confidence in the findings. Such studies will be excluded from high-quality evidence-based summaries, whether through meta-analysis, systematic reviews, or integrative reviews. Similarly, studies with poor internal validity should not be translated to practice because there can be no confidence that the intervention embedded in the study produced any effect. The ideal study is tightly controlled—that is, the potential for confounding through these threats to internal validity is well managed—leaving the major source of variability to be a random error. Only then will studies contribute to the evidence base needed for practice.

Statistical Conclusion Validity

Related to internal validity is statistical conclusion validity. The threats to statistical conclusion validity include low statistical power, multiple comparisons, and violation of the assumptions of the statistical tests (Farrington, 2003; Wortman, 1983). Low statistical power in randomized controlled trials has been identified in the majority of published trials with a negative effect (Moher, Dulberg, & Wells, 1994). Investigators should determine the optimal sample size while designing a study, using a clinically meaningful outcome, and should also report the statistical power when reporting the trial. Studies with low statistical power and negative findings may be misinterpreted as the treatment having no effect when indeed the lack of adequate power does not permit an interpretation (see Exhibit 8.2).

The opposite occurs—that is, false-positive findings—when multiple comparisons or multiple significance tests are made within studies (Tannock, 1996). Multiple tests result in some findings showing significance on chance alone. Although there are procedures for correcting for multiple comparisons, there are differences of opinion on their use. Overall, it is best for the predetermined primary outcome to be analyzed and used to determine the effect of treatment on outcome. Other analyses should be exploratory and hypothesis generating.

Violation of the Assumptions of the Statistical Tests

Statistical tests are designed to be carried out when certain assumptions are met. When those assumptions are not met, the interpretation of the results of the test is open to question. For example, the use of the analysis of variance (ANOVA) model to analyze differences

---

EXHIBIT 8.2 Statistical Conclusion Validity

- Statistical power
- Assumptions of the statistical test
- Appropriate test for the characteristics of the data

EXHIBIT 8.3 Causation in Nonrandomized Studies (Bradford-Hill Criteria)

---

1. Strength of the association
2. Consistency of associations in replications
3. Temporal relationship between variables
4. Coherence
5. Dose–response relationship
6. Support from randomized controlled trials

between groups depends on the assumption that the observations are independent or not correlated and on the assumption that the data from each group are normally distributed and that the group variances are the same or homogeneous (Kuzma, 1984). Specific tests may be more or less robust when these assumptions are violated. Nevertheless, studies should report whether the data have met the conditions for the analysis.

Nonrandomized Studies

This discussion has centered around the intervention or experimental study that is desirous of showing that a specific manipulation (independent variable) produces an effect on some specified outcome (dependent variable). There are instances where the randomized controlled study necessary for this evidence of causation is not possible. In those cases, causation is evaluated by other criteria. A commonly used method is use of the Bradford Hill criteria that include (a) strength of association; (b) consistency of associations in replications; (c) temporal relationship between variables, such that "cause" precedes outcome; (d) coherence with natural history and biology; (e) dose–response relationship; and ultimately (f) randomized controlled trials, which support the observational findings (Grant, 2009; Mente, de Koning, Shannon, & Anand, 2009). Even here, it should be noted, the strongest factor is the randomized controlled trial (see Exhibit 8.3).

SUMMARY

Studies of intervention or experimental effects have a particular requirement to support the assessment of *causal* relationships between the manipulation or independent variable and the outcome or dependent variable. These studies need to have strong internal validity. Yet, there are many threats to internal validity (see Exhibit 8.4). Rigorous control over these threats needs to be assured at the design phase of the study, and then the study must be carried out with consistency to the protocol. Many of the threats are controlled through the use of intervention and control groups and random assignment of subjects to the groups. Yet, numerous other considerations must be given to the control of potential threats. Events that happen during the course of the study, the equivalence of the groups on important factors at baseline, quality control procedures to prevent problems with instrumentation, attention to practice effects or reactivity, tracking changes in the subjects over time, attention to the selection of subjects, appropriate control group procedures to prevent unwanted behavioral change, ensuring necessary statistical power, and the selection of appropriate statistical procedures can complicate the interpretation of intervention research or controlled clinical trials. Attention to each dimension can ensure a study with a clear outcome that can contribute to science.

EXHIBIT 8.4 Checklist for Internal Validity

YES	NO	DON'T KNOW	STUDY DESIGN FEATURE
____	____	____	Comparison groups
____	____	____	Random assignment to groups
____	____	____	Equivalent conditions for groups during the study
____	____	____	Equivalence in baseline characteristics of the groups
____	____	____	Change in condition or development examined in control group
____	____	____	Low dropout rate
____	____	____	Dropout rate equivalent between groups
____	____	____	Intention-to-treat analysis
____	____	____	Evidence of practice effect from testing in control group
____	____	____	Quality control of measurement over time (testers and instruments)
____	____	____	Acceptable reliability of instruments
____	____	____	Evidence of bias in measurement
____	____	____	Evidence of response shift in self-report
____	____	____	Evidence of regression to the mean
____	____	____	Control for regression to the mean in data analysis methods
____	____	____	Adjustment for group differences in analysis
____	____	____	Control group exposed to a similar intervention (contaminated)
____	____	____	Adequate statistical power
____	____	____	Data meeting the assumptions/conditions for the analytic test used

Key Points From This Chapter

- Internal validity is central to the quality of a study asking a question on causation, such as whether an intervention "works."
- There are multiple threats to the internal validity of a study that can be controlled with careful attention to overall study design and procedures for conduct of the study.

- Studies with poor internal validity provide low confidence in the findings and so are not ready for translation or use in systematic reviews or meta-analysis.
- Causation can be inferred in observational studies that meet rigorous, established criteria.
- The foundation for establishing internal validity is the randomized controlled trial (RCT).

REFERENCES

Anastasi, A. (1988). *Psychological testing* (6th ed.). New York, NY: Macmillan Publishing.

Barnett, A. G., van der Pols, J. C., & Dobson, A. J. (2005). Regression to the mean: What it is and how to deal with it. *International Journal of Epidemiology, 34*(1), 215–220. doi:10.1093/ije/dyh299

Bell, G. H. (2008). Deceptive data and statistical skullduggery: Part II. Audience development. Retrieved from http://www.audiencedevelopment.com/node/2029

Beral, V., Banks, E., & Reeves, G. (2002). Evidence from randomised trials on the long-term effects of hormone replacement therapy. *Lancet, 360*(9337), 942–944. doi:10.1016/S0140-6736(02)11032-4

Borg, W. (1984). Dealing with threats to internal validity that randomization does not rule out. *Educational Researcher, 13*(10), 11–14. doi:10.3102/0013189X013010011

Bray, J. H., Maxwell, S. E., & Howard, G. S. (1984). Methods of analysis with response-shift bias. *Educational and Psychological Measurement, 44*(4), 781–804. doi:10.1177/0013164484444002

Breetvelt, I. S., & Van Dam, F. S. (1991). Underreporting by cancer patients: The case of response-shift. *Social Science & Medicine, 32*(9), 981–987. doi:10.1016/0277-9536(91)90156-7

Brossart, D. F., Clay, D. L., & Willson, V. L. (2002). Methodological and statistical considerations for threats to internal validity in pediatric outcome data: Response shift in self-report outcomes. *Journal of Pediatric Psychology, 27*(1), 97–107. doi:10.1093/jpepsy/27.1.97

Bush, T. L., Barrett-Connor, E., Cowan, L. D., Criqui, M. H., Wallace, R. B., Suchindran, C. M., ... Rifkind, B. M. (1987). Cardiovascular mortality and noncontraceptive use of estrogen in women: Results from the Lipid Research Clinics Program Follow-up Study. *Circulation, 75*(6), 1102–1109. doi:10.1161/01.CIR.75.6.1102

Childs, J. D., Teyhen, D. S., Van Wyngaarden, J. J., Dougherty, B. F., Ladislas, B. J., Helton, G. L., ... George, S. Z. (2011). Predictors of web-based follow-up response in the prevention of low back pain in the military trial (POLM). *BMC Musculoskeletal Disorders, 12,* 132. doi:10.1186/1471-2474-12-132

Chuang-Stein, C., & Tong, D. M. (1997). The impact and implication of regression to the mean on the design and analysis of medical investigations. *Statistical Methods in Medical Research, 6*(2), 115–128. doi:10.1177/096228029700600203

Chu-Carroll, M. C. (2007, January 25). Basics: Correlation [Web log comment]. Retrieved from http://scienceblogs.com/goodmath/2007/01/25/basics-correlation-1/

Connor Gorber, S., Tremblay, M., Moher, D., & Gorber, B. (2007). A comparison of direct vs. self-report measures for assessing height, weight and body mass index: A systematic review. *Obesity Reviews, 8*(4), 307–326. doi:10.1111/j.1467-789X.2007.00347.x

Daviglus, M. L., Plassman, B. L., Pirzada, A., Bell, C. C., Bowen, P. E., Burke, J. R., ... Williams, J. W., Jr. (2011). Risk factors and preventive interventions for Alzheimer disease: State of the science. *Archives of Neurology, 68*(9), 1185–1190. doi:10.1001/archneurol.2011.100

DiMatteo, M. R., Giordani, P. J., Lepper, H. S., & Croghan, T. W. (2002). Patient adherence and medical treatment outcomes: A meta-analysis. *Medical Care, 40*(9), 794–811. doi:10.1097/01.MLR.0000024612.61915.2D

Donders, A. R., van der Heijden, G. J., Stijnen, T., & Moons, K. G. (2006). Review: A gentle introduction to imputation of missing values. *Journal of Clinical Epidemiology, 59*(10), 1087–1091. doi:10.1016/j.jclinepi.2006.01.014

Engel, R. J., & Schutt, R. K. (2008). *The practice of research in social work.* Thousand Oaks, CA: Sage.

Eysenbach, G. (2005). The law of attrition. *Journal of Medical Internet Research, 7*(1), e11. doi:10.2196/jmir.7.1.e11

Farrington, D. P. (2003). Methodological quality standards for evaluation research. *Annals of the American Academy of Political and Social Science, 587,* 49–68. doi:10.1177/0002716202250789

Friedman, L. M., Furberg, C. D., & DeMets, D. L. (1998). *Fundamentals of clinical trials* (3rd ed.). New York, NY: Springer-Verlag.

Garber, M. C., Nau, D. P., Erickson, S. R., Aikens, J. E., & Lawrence, J. B. (2004). The concordance of self-report with other measures of medication adherence: A summary of the literature. *Medical Care, 42*(7), 649–652. doi:10.1097/01.mlr.0000129496.05898.02

Good, M., & Schuler, L. (1997). Subject retention in a controlled clinical trial. *Journal of Advanced Nursing, 26*(2), 351–355. doi:10.1046/j.1365-2648.1997.1997026351.x

Grant, W. B. (2009). How strong is the evidence that solar ultraviolet B and vitamin D reduce the risk of cancer? An examination using Hill's criteria for causality. *Dermatoendocrinology, 1*(1), 17–24. doi:10.4161/derm.1.1.7388

Haynes, R. B., Ackloo, E., Sahota, N., McDonald, H. P., & Yao, X. (2008). Interventions for enhancing medication adherence. *Cochrane Database of Systematic Reviews, 16*(2), CD000011. doi:10.1002/14651858.CD000011.pub3

Hulley, S. B., & Cummings, S. R. (1988). *Designing clinical research: An epidemiologic approach.* Baltimore, MD: Williams & Wilkins.

Inelmen, E. M., Toffanello, E. D., Enzi, G., Gasparini, G., Miotto, F., Sergi, G., & Busetto, L. (2005). Predictors of drop-out in overweight and obese outpatients. *International Journal of Obesity, 29*(1), 122–128. doi:10.1038/sj.ijo.0802846

Jensen, M. P., & McFarland, C. A. (1993). Increasing the reliability and validity of pain intensity measurement in chronic pain patients. *Pain, 55*(2), 195–203. doi:10.1016/0304-3959(93)90148-I

Jüni, P., Altman, D. G., & Egger, M. (2001). Systematic reviews in health care: Assessing the quality of controlled clinical trials. *British Medical Journal, 323*(7303), 42–46.

Kuzma, J. W. (1984). *Basic statistics for the health sciences.* Mountain View, CA: Mayfield.

Lachin, J. M. (2000). Statistical considerations in the intent-to-treat principle. *Controlled Clinical Trials, 21*(3), 167–189. doi:10.1016/S0197-2456(00)00046-5

Lu, M., Safren, S. A., Skolnik, P. R., Rogers, W. H., Coady, W., Hardy, H., & Wilson, I. B. (2008). Optimal recall period and response task for self-reported HIV medication adherence. *AIDS and Behavior, 12*(1), 86–94. doi:10.1007/s10461-007-9261-4

Matthews, R. (2000). Storks deliver babies ($p = 0.008$). *Teaching Statistics, 22*(2), 36–38. doi:10.1111/1467-9639.00013

McCulloch, D. K. (2011). Diagnosis of diabetes mellitus. In D. S. Basow (Ed.), *UptoDate.* Waltham, MA: UpToDate.

McDaniel, M. A., Roediger, H. L., III, & McDermott, K. B. (2007). Generalizing test-enhanced learning from the laboratory to the classroom. *Psychonomic Bulletin & Review, 14*(2), 200–206. doi:10.3758/BF03194052

McDonald, H. P., Garg, A. X., & Haynes, R. B. (2002). Interventions to enhance patient adherence to medication prescriptions: Scientific review. *Journal of the American Medical Association, 288*(22), 2868–2879. doi:10.1001/jama.288.22.2868

Mente, A., de Koning, L., Shannon, H. S., & Anand, S. S. (2009). A systematic review of the evidence supporting a causal link between dietary factors and coronary heart disease. *Archives of Internal Medicine, 169*(7), 659–669. doi:10.1001/archinternmed.2009.38

Moher, D., Cook, D. J., Eastwood, S., Olkin, I., Rennie, D., & Stroup, D. F. (1999). Improving the quality of reports of meta-analyses of randomised controlled trials: The QUOROM statement. Quality of reporting of meta-analyses. *Lancet, 354*(9193), 1896–1900. doi:10.1016/S0140-6736(99)04149-5

Moher, D., Dulberg, C. S., & Wells, G. A. (1994). Statistical power, sample size, and their reporting in randomized controlled trials. *Journal of the American Medical Association, 272*(2), 122–124. doi:10.1001/jama.1994.03520020048013

Mor, M., Niv, G., & Niv, Y. (2006). Patient retention in a clinical trial: A lesson from the rofecoxib (VIOXX) study. *Digestive Diseases and Sciences, 51*(7), 1175–1178. doi:10.1007/s10620-006-8028-5

Moser, D. K., Dracup, K., & Doering, L. V. (2000). Factors differentiating dropouts from completers in a longitudinal, multicenter clinical trial. *Nursing Research, 49*(2), 109–116. doi:10.1097/00006199-200003000-00008

Penckofer, S., Byrn, M., Mumby, P., & Ferrans, C. E. (2011). Improving subject recruitment, retention, and participation in research through Peplau's Theory of Interpersonal Relations. *Nursing Science Quarterly, 24*(2), 146–151. doi:10.1177/0894318411399454

Peterson, A. M., Takiya, L., & Finley, R. (2003a). Meta-analysis of interventions to improve drug adherence in patients with hyperlipidemia. *Pharmacotherapy, 23*(1), 80–87. doi:10.1592/phco.23.1.80.31921

Peterson, A. M., Takiya, L., & Finley, R. (2003b). Meta-analysis of trials of interventions to improve medication adherence. *American Journal of Health-System Pharmacy, 60*(7), 657–665.

Pickering, T. G., Hall, J. E., Appel, L. J., Falkner, B. E., Graves, J., Hill, M. N., … Rocella, E. J. (2005). Recommendations for blood pressure measurement in humans and experimental animals: Part 1: Blood pressure measurement in humans: A statement for professionals from the Subcommittee of Professional and Public Education of the American Heart Association Council on High Blood Pressure Research. *Circulation, 111*(5), 697–716. doi:10.1161/01.CIR.0000154900.76284.F6

Prendergast, M. B., & Gaston, R. S. (2010). Optimizing medication adherence: An ongoing opportunity to improve outcomes after kidney transplantation. *Clinical Journal of the American Society of Nephrology, 5*(7), 1305–1311. doi:10.2215/CJN.07241009

Probstfield, J. L., Russell, M. L., Henske, J. C., Reardon, R. J., & Insull, W., Jr. (1986). Successful program for recovery of dropouts to a clinical trial. *American Journal of Medicine, 80*(5), 777–784. doi:10.1016/0002-9343(86)90615-7

Roumen, C., Feskens, E. J., Corpeleijn, E., Mensink, M., Saris, W. H., & Blaak, E. E. (2011). Predictors of lifestyle intervention outcome and dropout: The SLIM study. *European Journal of Clinical Nutrition, 65*(10), 1141–1147. doi:10.1038/ejcn.2011.74

Snow, W. M., Connett, J. E., Sharma, S., & Murray, R. P. (2007). Predictors of attendance and dropout at the Lung Health Study 11-year follow-up. *Contemporary Clinical Trials, 28*(1), 25–32. doi:10.1016/j.cct.2006.08.010

Sprangers, M. A., & Schwartz, C. E. (1999). Integrating response shift into health-related quality of life research: A theoretical model. *Social Science & Medicine, 48*(11), 1507–1515. doi:10.1016/S0277-9536(99)00045-3

Stone, A. A., Shiffman, S., Schwartz, J. E., Broderick, J. E., & Hufford, M. R. (2002). Patient non-compliance with paper diaries. *British Medical Journal, 324*(7347), 1193–1194. doi:10.1136/bmj.324.7347.1193

Szklo, M. (1983). Heart disease: The MRFIT test. *Journal of Public Health Policy, 4*(1), 5–7. doi:10.2307/3342181

Takiya, L. N., Peterson, A. M., & Finley, R. S. (2004). Meta-analysis of interventions for medication adherence to antihypertensives. *Annals of Pharmacotherapy, 38*(10), 1617–1624. doi:10.1345/aph.1D268

Tannock, I. F. (1996). False-positive results in clinical trials: Multiple significance tests and the problem of unreported comparisons. *Journal of the National Cancer Institute, 88*(3–4), 206–207. doi:10.1093/jnci/88.3-4.206

Tinkelman, D., & Wilson, S. (2004). Asthma disease management: Regression to the mean or better? *American Journal of Managed Care, 10*(12), 948–954.

Visser, M. R., Smets, E. M., Sprangers, M. A., & de Haes, H. J. (2000). How response shift may affect the measurement of change in fatigue. *Journal of Pain and Symptom Management, 20*(1), 12–18. doi:10.1016/S0885-3924(00)00148-2

Wertz, R. T. (1995). Intention to treat: Once randomized, always analyzed. *Clinical Aphasiology, 23*, 57–64.

Wilkinson, L., & The Task Force on Statistical Inference. (1999). Statistical methods in psychology journals: Guidelines and explanations. *American Psychologist, 54*(8), 594–604. doi:10.1037/0003-066X.54.8.594

Wood, A. M., White, I. R., & Thompson, S. G. (2004). Are missing outcome data adequately handled? A review of published randomized controlled trials in major medical journals. *Clinical Trials, 1*(4), 368–376. doi:10.1191/1740774504cn032oa

Wortman, P. M. (1983). Evaluation research: A methodological perspective. *Annual Review of Psychology, 34*, 223–260. doi:10.1146/annurev.ps.34.020183.001255

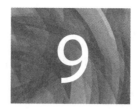

9

Minimizing Threats to External Validity

Wanda K. Nicholson

> Do you believe that someone else doing the same trial in the same
> kinds of patients would get the same result? —*Meinert C.,*
> *Conduct of Clinical Trials_1 (Meinert, 1986)*

Assessing **external validity** is a crucial step in the design and conduct of high-quality clinical trials (Tunis, Stryer, & Clancy, 2003). **Randomized controlled trials** (RCTs) are considered to be the most reliable method of determining the effects of treatments (e.g., behavioral interventions, drugs therapy, procedures) for populations with or at risk for disease. RCTs must maintain **internal validity**, but to be clinically relevant and policy valuable, the results must be generally applicable to a specified group of patients in a particular clinical or organizational setting. Intervention research is critical for the primary prevention of disease as well as secondary prevention of disease complications in children, adolescents, and adults. Minimizing threats to external validity in the conduct of RCTs provides high-quality evidence to clinicians and health decision makers that can facilitate the translation of these findings into daily clinical practice (Tunis et al., 2003).

EXTERNAL VALIDITY: DEFINITION AND RELEVANCE TO INTERVENTION RESEARCH

External validity, or as it is commonly termed, generalizability, is an assessment of whether the results reported from a clinical study of an intervention or treatment can be reasonably applied to the broader population in various clinical settings or routine practice (Meinert, 1986). External validity has garnered relatively little attention in the past. In fact, much of the focus of clinical trialists has centered on internal validity (see Chapter 8). Although internal validity is crucial to research integrity, the ability to operationalize the findings from RCT settings is predicated on the applicability of the results into broad clinical settings. Within the context of the current healthcare environment, the focus on translating clinical trial results into daily practice by health decision makers, funders, and clinicians demands greater consideration of external validity in the design and reporting of clinical trials.

There is increasing recognition of the gap between research findings and recommendations for preventive care in systematic literature reviews, evidence reports, and practice guidelines (Glasgow, Magid, Beck, Ritzwoller, & Estabrooks, 2005). Health decision makers and clinicians alike are constantly faced with the paucity of high-quality evidence to support clinical and policy choices for healthcare. Behavior change intervention research is a critically important area of research in the current fight against chronic disease in adults and children. Yet, there is a lack of study design considerations for external validity. Systematic reviews of behavior research targeting multiple behavior changes in adults and childhood obesity reveal flaws in study design that limit external validity (Glasgow, Bull, Gillette, Klesges, & Dzewaltowski, 2002; Klesges, Dzewaltowski, & Glasgow, 2008). As such, these design flaws can hinder the implementation of proven and broadly applicable interventions. In the sections shown subsequently, we review the threats to external validity and discuss strategies to address these threats. Also, we examine the use of the reach, effectiveness or efficacy, adoption, implementation, and maintenance (RE-AIM) framework and **Consolidated Standards of Reporting Trials (CONSORT) guidelines**, two well-established models for assessing external validity in the design and reporting of RCTs (Glasgow, Dzewaltowski, Estabrooks, Klesges, & Bull, 2002; Glasgow, Magid et al., 2005; Moher, Schulz, & Altman, 2001b). We conclude with a summary of strategies for investigators and funders to ensure external validity in future research.

Minimizing Threats to External Validity

Common threats to external validity in intervention research include patient selection, the setting in which the trial is conducted, characteristics of the clinicians and staff/interventionists providing the intervention, choice of the comparative or alternative intervention, and selection of clinical outcomes (see Table 9.1). In this section, we discuss each of these potential threats using illustrative examples from ongoing or completed behavioral RCTs.

Recruiting a Diverse Study Sample

Participant recruitment and retention are essential to the success of RCTs, but they also can be burdensome to trial recruiters and staff. Investigators often derive restrictive inclusion and exclusion criteria in an effort to readily recruit and retain study participants. As a result, RCTs often include participants who are highly motivated, relatively homogeneous, and with few comorbid conditions. Such criteria help to reduce variance and maximize the chances of detecting an intervention effect (Rothwell, 2005a). However, these criteria may also bias the study results or response to the intervention and result in a falsely elevated effect size between groups. A highly selected sample that is not representative of patients seen in community practice or organizational settings may render results that cannot be replicated in real-world settings in routine practice. For example, the Diabetes Prevention Program (DPP) screened more than 158,000 patients to select and randomize 3,819 participants (Diabetes Prevention Program Research Group, 2002). With this volunteer group who had impaired glucose intolerance, those in the lifestyle modification group achieved a 7% reduction in weight compared with a 5% weight loss in the metformin and control groups. Although the study findings demonstrate the effectiveness of the lifestyle intervention, such a highly selected population in RCTs can produce results that are difficult to replicate in multiple settings. In the time period since the initial DPP trial results were first published, the DPP lifestyle program has been successfully translated into several broad community-based settings, including community health centers, health departments, and community establishments (e.g., Young Men's Christian

TABLE 9.1 Threats and Solutions for External Validity	
POTENTIAL THREATS	**DESIGN SOLUTIONS**
Characteristics of study participants	■ Enroll a diverse study population by developing broad inclusion criteria. ■ Limit the number of exclusion criteria as appropriate. ■ Plan for subgroup analyses on key variables before starting the trial.
Trial setting and selection of centers and clinicians	■ Recruit from various practice settings. ■ Incorporate trials into medical organizational settings, such as HMOs or MCOs. ■ Include a detailed description of the setting and why it is appropriate for the generalizability of the study findings. ■ Select a representative group of clinicians and staff to provide the intervention. ■ Describe the characteristics of the personnel delivering the intervention. Report how their characteristics compare with those delivering the intervention in real-world settings.
Intervention arms	■ Compare clinically relevant alternative interventions. ■ Consider the use of alternative experimental designs, such as a wait list control group.
Clinical outcomes	■ Measure a broad range of relevant patient-centered outcomes that extend beyond disease states or morbidity. ■ Plan for collection of data on QoL, quality-adjusted life-years, economic outcomes, and client satisfaction. ■ Consider longer length of follow-up to adequately capture short-term and long-term outcomes of the intervention.

HMOs, health maintenance organizations; MCOs, managed care organizations; QoL, quality of life.

Source: Adapted from Rothwell, P. M. (2005a). External validity of randomised controlled trials: "To whom do the results of this trial apply?" *Lancet, 365*(9453), 82–93. doi:10.1016/S0140-6736(04)17670-8

Association [YMCA]). However, the percentage of weight loss and level of physical activity attained in the original trial has not been consistently replicated in these multiple settings with a more diverse participant population (Ackermann, Finch, Brizendine, Zhou, & Marrero, 2008).

Strategies to promote external validity include the recruitment of a more diverse study population. It is important to enroll patients in your trial with characteristics that reflect the range and distribution of patients that will be observed in everyday clinical practice settings. Broad inclusion criteria and fewer exclusion criteria can improve external validity. This approach can address the concerns about the application of results from studies with restricted eligibility criteria. Including a more diverse sample with a broader severity of symptoms also can ensure that higher risk patients who are likely to receive the greatest benefit from interventions are not excluded from clinical trials. Recruitment of such varied populations may increase the variance of results and therefore require larger study samples to demonstrate statistically significant differences but will increase the external validity of study results.

To enhance external validity, recruit study samples with different levels of symptomology or disease states. Another example of how restricting the study sample can reduce external validity is the absence of sufficient numbers of postpartum women with glucose intolerance in pregnancy that were included in the DPP trial (Diabetes Prevention Program Research Group, 2002). A separate analysis of participants with a prior history of gestational diabetes was performed and demonstrated some success in weight loss, but the findings did differ moderately from the general sample (Ratner et al., 2008). Although the results of this subgroup analysis are useful, the participants were relatively remote from the delivery at the time they were enrolled in the trial. The time frame from the diagnosis of gestational diabetes and trial enrollment also varied among participants. A useful strategy in the original DPP trial would have been to enroll a sufficient number of postpartum women within 6 to 12 months of delivery or women who had undergone postpartum glucose tolerance testing at 6 weeks and with results consistent with persistent glucose intolerance. In this fashion, subgroup analysis of specific moderating variables could have been performed and used for translation into primary and obstetrical practice. There are currently funded studies that are assessing the effect of the DPP lifestyle intervention on diabetes prevention in women with recent gestational diabetes. These findings, if deemed successful, can then be translated into perinatal practice.

Aligning the recruitment process with clinical practice can also promote generalizability (Rothwell, 2005a). Participants in an RCT reflect the diverse patients in clinical settings. Incorporating recruitment and selection processes that parallel the approach used by clinicians in daily practice to identify patients for intervention also maximizes external validity.

Ensuring the appropriate collection of participants' demographic and clinical characteristics confirms the recruitment of a diverse study sample and potential subgroup analyses on key characteristics that can influence outcomes (Rothwell, 2005b). Participants' characteristics, including race/ethnicity, education and income levels, and pretrial lifestyle behaviors, can also affect the external validity of study findings. In recruiting and enrolling a diverse study sample, investigators should plan to collect key clinical and lifestyle data that can have a direct effect on the outcome of interest. Planned subgroup analysis on key characteristics should be included in the research methods. A critical appraisal of the seven currently published RCTs of behavioral interventions for postpartum weight loss demonstrates how the absence of important moderating variables hinders subgroup analysis and limits generalizability (Kinnunen et al., 2007; Leermakers, Anglin, & Wing, 1998; Lovelady, Garner, Moreno, & Williams, 2000; McCrory, Nommsen-Rivers, Molé, Lönnerdal, & Dewey, 1999; Østbye et al., 2009; O'Toole, Sawicki, & Artal, 2003). Only one study specifically collected data on moderating variables that could influence postpartum weight loss for subgroup analysis. Analysis of potential moderators (e.g., race/ethnicity, parity, lactation status, prepregnancy body mass index [BMI], depression history) would be useful in extending the science by elucidating the circumstances under which proposed interventions work best (Østbye et al., 2009). Only two studies included a substantial number of nonwhite women to facilitate subgroup analysis by race/ethnicity (Østbye et al., 2009; O'Toole et al., 2003). Only one RCT was conducted in a diverse study sample recruited from a broad community-based setting (Østbye et al., 2009). As such, there are substantial differences in the study results with greater weight loss achieved in the study samples with relatively homogeneous samples compared with results obtained from the trial by Østbye et al. (2009) with diverse participants (National Health and Nutrition Examination Survey IV, 1999–2002). The difference in adherence to in-person and group sessions is of particular relevance, which was substantially lower in the RCT with the diverse study sample compared with the trials in homogenous study samples.

Recruiting From Diverse Trial Settings

RCTs can be conducted in various clinical settings although many are conducted in tertiary care centers or clinics affiliated with a university setting. Concerns about the generalizability of trials performed in such large centers compared with primary care practices, health departments, or community health centers are often noted by clinicians and public health officials (Rothwell, 2005a). There are core differences in the clinical infrastructure of tertiary care centers compared with community-based institutions (i.e., hospitals, health centers, health departments) that can affect external validity. Participants in RCTs at major medical centers may differ demographically, economically, and clinically from patients in community settings. Tertiary care centers often provide care to the most complex patient groups from various demographic and economic backgrounds because of their broad clinical expertise. In many instances, tertiary care centers provide specialty care to a broad range of individuals referred in from community settings, contributing to a degree of heterogeneity that may limit generalizability. In line with their teaching mission, large tertiary centers, for example, often provide care to lower income families, uninsured, and underinsured individuals from various social and economic backgrounds, all of which may contribute to biases in study results. Such biases may contribute to moderate differences between intervention groups or alternatively may reduce the effect size between intervention arms. Patients and staff at primary care settings are largely from one geographical region and may be more homogeneous with respect to demographic and economic characteristics. Moreover, studies conducted in primary care settings should garner results that are more applicable to other primary care settings.

There also may be variations in the number, characteristics, and experiences of study staff at community care settings compared with hospital-based settings or tertiary centers, which can affect external validity (Tunis et al., 2003). The Multicenter Trial of Nutritional Counseling in Mild Gestational Diabetes is an example of a tertiary care-based behavioral intervention, which was conducted in diet-controlled gestational diabetics as part of the National Institute of Child and Human Development Maternal Fetal Medicine Research Units (Landon et al., 2009). Gestational diabetes is associated with maternal hyperglycemia, excessive maternal gestational weight gain, and infant birth weight. In this trial, 958 pregnant women with gestational diabetes attending 14 tertiary care centers in the United States were randomized to receive nurse-administered nutritional counseling compared with usual care. Both the BMI and gestational weight gain from enrollment until delivery was lower among women in the treatment compared with the usual care group. Infants born to women receiving the intervention compared with those born to women receiving usual care had lower birth weights (3,302 vs. 3,408 g) and less frequency of large-for-gestational-age infants (7.1% vs. 14.5%). The nutritional intervention was administered by research nurses working with the Maternal Fetal Medicine Research Unit (MFMRU) network. The characteristics, experience, and delivery of the intervention by these research nurses likely differ substantially from nurses working in clinics in real-world settings. Moreover, study samples of gestational diabetics in tertiary care settings may differ substantially from those attending offices or practices in local communities. In designing and implementing interventions in diverse settings, it is important to develop protocols to measure and ensure the integrity of the intervention. The work experiences of the research nurses administering the intervention in the trial of mild gestational diabetes may have promoted integrity of the intervention and quality control (i.e., internal validity), but the experiences of these research nurses are likely to differ substantially from those of nurses in the community, particularly given the daily clinical demands of community-based practices. Clinical trials can improve external validity by including a wider range of physicians and settings to which the study will be applicable. Only a small proportion of patients with a specific disorder participate in a particular trial. Although this can be a concern for external validity, it is acceptable as long as the patients randomized in the participating centers are representative of the general population for whom the results will be applied.

Investigators should recruit and conduct RCTs in community-based settings, primarily general clinics and physician offices at which the primary activity is clinical care. Enrolling patients from a more diverse group of practice settings also allows for some variability in how the study intervention and associated clinical care will be provided. The ancillary care that these patients receive is more likely to reflect the average care patients would receive outside the research context. Moreover, RCTs conducted in community settings would ensure that the study sample represented the patient population typically observed in general practice.

With the conduct of RCTs in multiple settings, physicians and policy makers can be confident that the reported outcomes in this study are likely to predict results that will be observed across a wide range of practice settings. This eliminates a common barrier to physician implementation of clinical research findings. Although the translation of evidence-based interventions into multiple settings is crucial to broad dissemination, there is the challenge of ensuring it is delivered consistently across various clinical settings. Data on clinician and staff behaviors become increasingly important to assess adequate implementation of the intervention by patients and staff. Measures of intervention process and implementation become increasingly relevant to the effectiveness of the intervention.

Selecting Comparative Strategies

Investigators are constantly faced with the challenge of designing efficacy versus comparative effectiveness clinical trials. In efficacy trials, the expected outcome differences are likely to be moderate between the active intervention and control (placebo) groups. The expected differences between two active therapies are likely to be considerably smaller than the differences between a treatment and placebo. Trials designed to demonstrate such differences will require large sample sizes and may be expensive. It is important for investigators to choose alternative strategies that parallel clinical practice and can be fully implemented into multiple clinical settings. There are multiple behavioral interventions that have been supported as efficacious. Therefore, current trials are designed to determine the effectiveness of who administers the intervention, alternative delivery strategies, or different levels of intensity of the intervention. As such, several trials compare electronic versus web-based interventions versus traditional in-person, high-intensity services versus low-intensity services (Glasgow, Nutting et al., 2005).

An example of the challenges of comparative effectiveness research is demonstrated in Project Sugar 1. This RCT was a four-arm trial that evaluated nurse case manager, community health worker, and combined nurse case manager and community health worker interventions to improve diabetic control. The results of this initial trial demonstrated that the nurse case manager/ community health worker team community-based intervention produced a promising decline (0.8%) in hemoglobin A1C (HbA1c) and moderate improvements in lipids and blood pressure, compared with usual care, but small numbers limited the statistical power to fully assess outcomes in this intervention arm. In response, investigators designed Project Sugar 2 (Gary et al., 2004). The objective of this larger scale trial was to determine the effectiveness and cost-effectiveness of primary care and community-oriented interventions in improving diabetes control. Specifically, the trial compared two intervention strategies: (a) usual care plus minimal telephone intervention implemented by a trained lay health educator and (b) usual care plus intensive intervention implemented by a nurse case management/community health worker team.

Conducting comparative effectiveness trials also can be burdensome from an economic perspective. Trials designed to demonstrate differences between two active interventions require large sample sizes and may be expensive. Project Sugar 2, for example, was designed to recruit more than 500 participants from one organizational setting (Gary et al., 2009). One potential alternative is to conduct an equivalence trial (Djulbegovic & Clarke, 2001). In this fashion, a study is designed to demonstrate that there are no important differences in effectiveness between two active treatments. Equivalence trials have been used to compare drug treatments of HIV but are not widely used (Albrecht, Wilkin, Coakley, & Hammer, 2003). Additional discussions and frameworks are needed before the use of equivalence trials are fully considered in behavioral intervention research.

Measuring Relevant Clinical Outcomes

The external validity of an RCT also depends on whether the measured outcomes are clinically relevant to the patient, clinician, and healthcare decision makers. There has been an increasing recognition of the need for a broad range of relevant healthcare outcomes in clinical trials. Traditional outcomes in well-established clinical trials such as DPP and PREMIER supported by the National Institutes of Health (NIH) have included prevention of type 2 diabetes and hypertension in addition to disease complications and mortality as measured in Diabetes Control and Complications Trial (The Diabetes Control and Complications Trial Research Group, 1993; Diabetes Prevention Program Research Group, 2002; Svetkey et al., 1999). In 2001, the Institute of Medicine called for an expansion of clinical outcomes to include patient-centered outcomes including quality of life (QoL), symptom severity from disease or treatment, patient satisfaction, and cost-effectiveness (Institute of Medicine, 2001; Sox & Greenfield, 2009). Decision makers are increasingly turning to QoL measures, especially quality-adjusted life years, as a common measure to evaluate the results of interventions or treatments for a range of conditions. An advantage of using quality-adjusted life years is that this provides a common metric that can be used to compare outcomes across different interventions, conditions, and settings.

As recommended by Tunis and Glasgow, including measures of QoL and satisfaction is a critical step in the efforts to transition from medically centered to patient-oriented centered outcome research (Glasgow, Magid et al., 2005; Hill-Briggs, Gary, Hill, Bone, & Brancati, 2002; Tunis et al., 2003). The goal of behavioral research investigators is to develop interventions that are efficacious, translatable, and sustainable in multiple settings (Tunis et al., 2003). As such, economic outcomes are critical to long-term sustainability of interventions. Specific economic data are beyond the scope of this chapter but may include cost-effectiveness analysis (e.g., cost–benefit, cost–utility, and return on investment) from multiple perspectives (e.g., societal, patient, health plan, and government; see Chapter 21).

Selection of the outcomes to be measured should be based on the most important anticipated effects of the intervention, taking into account those outcomes of greatest relevance to clinicians and decision makers. As a result, the study end points collected in RCTs will include a broad range of functional outcomes, including QoL, symptom severity, satisfaction, and costs, as well as more traditional end points, such as mortality and major morbidity. In Project Sugar 2, trial investigators broadened the extent of patient-centered outcomes to include healthcare use (primary care and specialty visits), emergency room visits, frequency of glucose monitoring, and costs. Inclusion of economic outcomes in clinical trials provides information that has a significant impact on clinical and policy decisions. It may be that a particular intervention is more costly, but that the total costs of care may not differ if the higher cost intervention decreases healthcare use and promotes patient satisfaction.

Investigators should consider a longer follow-up period compared with traditional clinical trials to better reflect more of the natural history of a disease. This is particularly important in behavioral intervention research as it takes time for patients to move through the stages of behavioral change. In addition, many behavioral interventions have different results in the short term than in the long term. For example, interventions for type 2 diabetes may show short-term changes in HbA1c and longer-term changes in weight and fitness. In conducting Project Sugar 2, trial investigators extended the follow-up period to 24 months (increase from 1 year in Project Sugar 1) to better measure the effects of the interventions on diabetes control and to facilitate collection of important relevant healthcare use end points. Longer follow-up periods also provide important insight on longer-term outcomes, which could influence the wide adoption of interventions into primary care settings.

Additional Methodological Challenges to External Validity

Conducting clinical trials in diverse settings creates several methodological and ethical challenges that will need to be addressed. First, as indicated in the earlier sections, there can be substantial cost and participant burden when recruiting in diverse and multiple settings, which will require investigators to make difficult decisions regarding sample size and data collection of multiple outcomes. Because ancillary patient management may not be standardized, there are likely to be clustering effects at the levels of physicians and organizations that will require specialized methods to facilitate analysis or randomization at the organizational level. Such study designs pose some unusual methodological challenges that will require additional attention to refine.

Intervention studies typically compare different interventions and delivery strategies. As such, several trials compare new versus old technology and high-intensity versus low-intensity services. For example, there are multiple RCTs comparing in-person interventions to web-based interventions. Other RCTs are comparing high-intensity individual sessions with interval group sessions. In some instances, there may be concerns about whether some participants are being denied optimal services. Appropriate, well-developed consent procedures are required to ensure informed consent and to eliminate preferences in treatment.

Clinical trials with a control (placebo) group often raise ethical dilemmas for investigative teams. One potential alternative approach is the wait list control group design. A wait list control group is a group that is assigned to a waiting list to receive an intervention after the active treatment group gets the intervention. A wait list control group serves the purpose of providing an untreated comparison for the active treatment group while allowing the wait-listed participants an opportunity to obtain the intervention at a later date. A wait list control group is often thought to be preferable to a no-treatment control group in cases where it would be unethical to deny participants access to a treatment.

Frameworks for Assessing External Validity

The RE-AIM framework and CONSORT guidelines are two well-established models to help assess the extent and reporting of external validity (Altman et al., 2001; Glasgow, Lichtenstein, & Marcus, 2003). The ability of intervention trials to affect change within communities depends on translation of the findings from clinical research into real-world settings (NIH, 2004).

The RE-AIM Framework

The RE-AIM model includes four dimensions for evaluating health promotion interventions: *RE-AIM*. *Reach* refers to the characteristics of the population that are intended to receive the intervention. *Efficacy* refers to the inclusion of positive and negative clinical, behavioral, and satisfaction outcomes. *Adoption* refers to the diversity of settings in which the intervention is implemented. *Implementation* refers to the extent to which the intervention was delivered as intended, including participant follow-up or adherence to the intervention, and *maintenance* evaluates long-term behavioral change, both at the individual and community level, and the extent to which the intervention is integrated into the routine structure of an organization.

Applying the RE-AIM Framework Using an Urban African American Feasibility Study in a Community Setting

The four RE-AIM dimensions allow for a standard set of evaluation parameters that can be used to quantitatively evaluate each project. These four dimensions can be used to guide the planning and development of intervention or other types of clinical trials to promote generalizability. Investigators can further enrich the RE-AIM categories by adding specific program innovations/novel approaches and challenges as they relate to their target population, recruitment and outreach, efficacy, adoption, implementation, and maintenance. Figure 9.1 presents a sample feasibility study where the dimensions of the RE-AIM framework are used to assist investigators in the planning phase.

The Weight Loss Interventions after Delivery (also known as "First WIND") project was a feasibility study conducted among African American women in West Baltimore to promote postpartum weight loss. Our goal was to adapt the components of PREMIER, a well-established NIH-funded trial for adults with Stage 1 hypertension, for postpartum African American

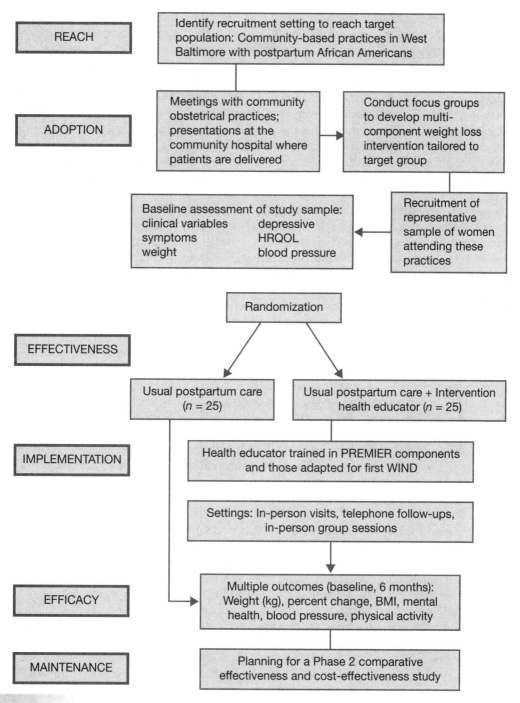

FIGURE 9.1 **Applying the RE-AIM framework to the planning phase of a pilot community-based trial.**

BMI, body mass index; HRQOL, health-related quality of life; RE-AIM, reach effectiveness or efficacy, adoption, implementation, and maintenance; WIND, weight loss interventions after delivery.

Source: Adapted from Gary, T. L., Hill-Briggs, F., Batts-Turner, M., & Brancati, F. L. (2005). Translational research principles of an effectiveness trial for diabetes care in an urban African American population. *Diabetes Educator*, *31*(6), 880–889. doi:10.1177/0145721705282254

women. In Phase 1, a pilot trial was planned and conducted in preparation for a larger scale comparative effectiveness trial. As shown in Figure 9.1, the target population for First WIND was postpartum African American women living in West Baltimore City. Statewide data had shown large disparities in overweight and obesity in Baltimore City compared with other areas of Central Maryland and particularly large disparities in obesity and the associated morbidities in African American women in the area. A series of focus groups were conducted with pregnant and postpartum African American women to effectively adapt the components of PREMIER to this specific population. Planning for the feasibility study included multiple meetings with community-based obstetrical practices in the West Baltimore area. Additional discussions were held with the chief of obstetrics and gynecology at the community-based hospitals in which labor and delivery services took place. The investigative team presented the final plans for the study at the community hospital's monthly grand rounds, where clinicians were able to make additional suggestions and modifications to the research plan. Fifty postpartum women were randomized to the adapted intervention (First WIND) or usual care. Women randomized to the usual post-partum care plus intervention ($n = 25$) received a 6-month postpartum intervention, consisting of five individual sessions with a health educator and 10 group sessions facilitated by the health educator in a community setting. The health educators had previously undergone training in participatory methods and received additional sessions on implementing the adapted compo-nents to postpartum women. Several outcomes were assessed at 6 months, including weight, systolic and diastolic blood pressure, mental health, and weekly minutes of physical activity. Analysis included comparison of outcomes between the usual care and intervention groups. Process outcomes including logistical barriers to intervention implementation, participant adherence to study protocol, and staff and participant behaviors were assessed. Because the objective of external validity is to demonstrate the extent to which treatments can be delivered successfully in broad representative settings, we included an assessment of staff behaviors and perceptions and participant perceptions through a series of postintervention focus groups. Assessment of clinical and process outcomes is the next step in planning for a larger comparative effectiveness study and cost-effectiveness analysis. Cost-effectiveness analysis will be included in the Phase 2 study. Therefore, methods to collect economic data will be incorporated into the planning for the larger study using process measures garnered from the feasibility study.

CONSORT Statement

The report of an RCT should clearly convey the target population of the research and the methods and protocols taken to ensure robust external validity. The CONSORT guidelines, originally written in the mid-1990s by an international group of clinical trialists, statisticians, epidemiologists, and biomedical editors were designed to guide transparent reporting of the methods of recruitment, follow-up, and analysis of RCTs (Moher, Schulz, & Altman, 2001a). The CONSORT statement consists of a checklist and flow diagram for reporting an RCT. For convenience, the checklist and diagram together are simply referred to as CONSORT. The checklist pertains to the content of the title, abstract, introduction, methods, results, and dis-cussion. The flow diagram depicts the passage of participants through the four stages of a trial (enrollment, intervention allocation, follow-up, and analysis). The guidelines are intended pri-marily for use in writing, reviewing, or assessing reports of simple two-group parallel RCTs, but multiple revisions have been made of particular relevance to external validity in the dis-cussion portion of the checklist, which outlines the requirements for the interpretation of study findings and the generalizability of the findings. Although a detailed summary of the CONSORT guidelines are outside of the scope of this chapter, it is important for intervention trial researchers to understand the components of CONSORT while in the planning stage of clinical trials. The CONSORT statement has gone through several revisions since the original publication based on insight and input by trial expertise in the United States and worldwide. This iterative process makes the CONSORT statement a continually evolving instrument that can be adapted in parallel to the adjustments made to the conduct of RCTs and ensure that the steps taken to maintain generalizability are adequately included in the reporting of RCTs.

SUMMARY

Conducting intervention trials with robust external validity is challenging. The competing demands of a rigorous study design combined with the necessity to recruit and retain a diverse study group from various clinical settings can be a daunting task. Moreover, the ability to collect data on a broad range of outcomes, such as patient satisfaction and cost, increases the effort and cost to implement RCTs. Clinicians and healthcare decision makers recognize the need for high-quality evidence to guide their decisions about which services to provide to optimize the public's health. A systematic and rigorous approach to intervention research is critical to determine what treatments are most effective and to whom the results apply.

Key Points From This Chapter

- External validity, or generalizability, is an assessment of whether the results reported from a clinical study of an intervention or treatment can be reasonably applied to the broader population in various clinical settings or routine practice.
- Common threats to external validity in intervention research include patient selection, the setting in which the trial is conducted, characteristics of the clinicians and staff/interventionists providing the intervention, choice of the comparative or alternative intervention, and selection of clinical outcomes.
- Consider recruiting a diverse sample from various practice settings to enhance external validity and use random sampling when possible.
- The report of an intervention study should convey the target population of the research and the methods and protocols taken to ensure robust external validity using the CONSORT guidelines.

REFERENCES

Ackermann, R. T., Finch, E. A., Brizendine, E., Zhou, H., & Marrero, D. G. (2008). Translating the Diabetes Prevention Program into the community. The DEPLOY pilot study. *American Journal of Preventive Medicine, 35*(4), 357–363. doi:10.1016/j.amepre.2008.06.035

Albrecht, M. A., Wilkin, T. J., Coakley, E. P., & Hammer, S. M. (2003). Advances in antiretroviral therapy. *Topics in HIV Medicine, 11*(3), 97–127.

Altman, D. G., Schulz, K. F., Moher, D., Egger, M., Davidoff, F., Elbourne, D., … Lang, T., for the CONSORT Group. (2001). The revised CONSORT statement for reporting randomized trials: Explanation and elaboration. *Annals of Internal Medicine, 134*(8), 663–694. doi:10.7326/0003-4819-134-8-200104170-00012

The Diabetes Control and Complications Trial Research Group. (1993). The effect of intensive treatment of diabetes on the development and progression of long-term complications in insulin-dependent diabetes mellitus. *New England Journal of Medicine, 329*(14), 977–986. doi:10.1056/NEJM199309303291401

Diabetes Prevention Program Research Group. (2002). The Diabetes Prevention Program (DPP): Description of lifestyle intervention. *Diabetes Care, 25*(12), 2165–2171. doi:10.2337/diacare.25.12.2165

Djulbegovic, B., & Clarke, M. (2001). Scientific and ethical issues in equivalence trials. *Journal of the American Medical Association, 285*(9), 1206–1208. doi:10.1001/jama.285.9.1206

Gary, T. L., Batts-Turner, M., Bone, L. R., Yeh, H. C., Wang, N. Y., Hill-Briggs, F., … Brancati, F. L. (2004). A randomized controlled trial of the effects of nurse case manager and community health worker team interventions in urban African-Americans with type 2 diabetes. *Controlled Clinical Trials, 25*(1), 53–66. doi:10.1016/j.cct.2003.10.010

Gary, T. L., Batts-Turner, M., Yeh, H. C., Hill-Briggs, F., Bone, L. R., Wang, N. Y., … Brancati, F. L. (2009). The effects of a nurse case manager and a community health worker team on diabetic control, emergency department (ED) visits, and hospitalizations among urban African Americans with type 2 diabetes mellitus: A randomized controlled trial. *Archives of Internal Medicine, 169*(19), 1788–1794. doi:10.1001/archinternmed.2009.338

Gary, T. L., Hill-Briggs, F., Batts-Turner, M., & Brancati, F. L. (2005). Translational research principles of an effectiveness trial for diabetes care in an urban African American population. *Diabetes Educator, 31*(6), 880–889. doi:10.1177/0145721705282254

Glasgow, R. E., Bull, S. S., Gillette, C., Klesges, L. M., & Dzewaltowski, D. A. (2002). Behavior change intervention research in healthcare settings: A review of recent reports with emphasis on external validity. *American Journal of Preventive Medicine, 23*(1), 62–69. doi:10.1016/S0749-3797(02)00437-3

Glasgow, R. E., Dzewaltowski, D. A., Estabrooks, P. A., Klesges, L. M., & Bull, S. S. (2002). Response from the Behavior Change Consortium Representatives and Translation Work Group: The issue is one of impact, not of world view or preferred approach. *Health Education Research, 17*(6), 696–699.

Glasgow, R. E., Lichtenstein, E., & Marcus, A. C. (2003). Why don't we see more translation of health promotion research to practice? Rethinking the efficacy-to-effectiveness transition. *American Journal of Public Health, 93*(8), 1261–1267. doi:10.2105/AJPH.93.8.1261

Glasgow, R. E., Magid, D. J., Beck, A., Ritzwoller, D., & Estabrooks, P. A. (2005). Practical clinical trials for translating research to practice: Design and measurement recommendations. *Medical Care, 43*(6), 551–557.

Glasgow, R. E., Nutting, P. A., King, D. K., Nelson, C. C., Cutter, G., Gaglio, B., … Whitesides, H. (2005). Randomized effectiveness trial of a computer-assisted intervention to improve diabetes care. *Diabetes Care, 28*(1), 33–39. doi:10.2337/diacare.28.1.33

Hill-Briggs, F., Gary, T. L., Hill, M. N., Bone, L. R., & Brancati, F. L. (2002). Health-related quality of life in urban African Americans with type 2 diabetes. *Journal of General Internal Medicine, 17*(6), 412–419. doi:10.1046/j.1525-1497.2002.11002.x

Institute of Medicine. (2001). *Crossing the quality chasm: A new health system for the 21st century.* Washington, DC: National Academies Press.

Kinnunen, T. I., Pasanen, M., Aittasalo, M., Fogelholm, M., Weiderpass, E., & Luoto, R. (2007). Reducing postpartum weight retention: A pilot trial in primary health care. *Nutrition Journal, 6,* 21. doi:10.1186/1475-2891-6-21

Klesges, L. M., Dzewaltowski, D. A., & Glasgow, R. E. (2008). Review of external validity reporting in childhood obesity prevention research. *American Journal of Preventive Medicine, 34*(3), 216–223. doi:10.1016/j.amepre.2007.11.019

Landon, M. B., Spong, C. Y., Thom, E., Carpenter, M. W., Ramin, S. M., Casey, B., … Anderson, G. B. (2009). A multicenter, randomized trial of treatment for mild gestational diabetes. *New England Journal of Medicine, 361*(14), 1339–1348. doi:10.1056/NEJMoa0902430

Leermakers, E. A., Anglin, K., & Wing, R. R. (1998). Reducing postpartum weight retention through a correspondence intervention. *International Journal of Obesity and Related Metabolic Disorders, 22*(11), 1103–1109. doi:10.1038/sj.ijo.0800734

Lovelady, C. A., Garner, K. E., Moreno, K. L., & Williams, J. P. (2000). The effect of weight loss in overweight, lactating women on the growth of their infants. *New England Journal of Medicine, 342*(7), 449–453. doi:10.1056/NEJM200002173420701

McCrory, M. A., Nommsen-Rivers, L. A., Molé, P. A., Lönnerdal, B., & Dewey, K. G. (1999). Randomized trial of the short-term effects of dieting compared with dieting plus aerobic exercise on lactation performance. *American Journal of Clinical Nutrition, 69*(5), 959–967.

Meinert, C. (1986). *Clinical trials: Design, conduct, and analysis.* New York, NY: Oxford University Press.

Moher, D., Schulz, K. F., & Altman, D. G. (2001a). The CONSORT statement: Revised recommendations for improving the quality of reports of parallel-group randomised trials. *Lancet, 357*(9263), 1191–1194.

Moher, D., Schulz, K. F., & Altman, D. G. (2001b). The CONSORT statement: Revised recommendations for improving the quality of reports of parallel-group randomized trials. *Journal of the American Medical Association, 285*(15), 1987–1991.

National Institutes of Health. (2004). *Proceedings from the conference: From clinical trials to community: The science of translating diabetes and obesity research.* Bethesda, MD: Author.

Østbye, T., Krause, K. M., Lovelady, C. A., Morey, M. C., Bastian, L. A., Peterson, B. L., … McBride, C. M. (2009). Active mothers postpartum: A randomized controlled weight-loss intervention trial. *American Journal of Preventive Medicine, 37*(3), 173–180. doi:10.1016/j.amepre.2009.05.016

O'Toole, M. L., Sawicki, M. A., & Artal, R. (2003). Structured diet and physical activity prevent postpartum weight retention. *Journal of Women's Health, 12*(10), 991–998. doi:10.1089/154099903322643910

Ratner, R. E., Christophi, C. A., Metzger, B. E., Dabelea, D., Bennett, P. H., Pi-Sunyer, X., … Kahn, S. E., Diabetes Prevention Program Research Group. (2008). Prevention of diabetes in women with a history of gestational diabetes: Effects of metformin and lifestyle interventions. *Journal of Clinical Endocrinology and Metabolism, 93*(12), 4774–4779. doi:10.1210/jc.2008-0772

Rothwell, P. M. (2005a). External validity of randomised controlled trials: "To whom do the results of this trial apply?" *Lancet, 365*(9453), 82–93. doi:10.1016/S0140-6736(04)17670-8

Rothwell, P. M. (2005b). Treating individuals 2. Subgroup analysis in randomised controlled trials: Importance, indications, and interpretation. *Lancet, 365*(9454), 176–186. doi:10.1016/S0140-6736(05)17709-5

Sox, H. C., & Greenfield, S. (2009). Comparative effectiveness research: A report from the Institute of Medicine. *Annals of Internal Medicine, 151*(3), 203–205. doi:10.7326/0003-4819-151-3-200908040-00125

Svetkey, L. P., Sacks, F. M., Obarzanek, E., Vollmer, W. M., Appel, L. J., Lin, P. H., … Laws, R. L. (1999). The DASH diet, sodium intake and blood pressure trial (DASH-sodium): Rationale and design. DASH-Sodium Collaborative Research Group. *Journal of the American Dietetic Association, 99*(Suppl. 8), S96–S104.

Tunis, S. R., Stryer, D. B., & Clancy, C. M. (2003). Practical clinical trials: Increasing the value of clinical research for decision making in clinical and health policy. *Journal of the American Medical Association, 290*(12), 1624–1632. doi:10.1001/jama.290.12.1624

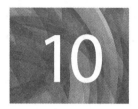

Measurement in Intervention Research

Dianne Morrison-Beedy & Bernadette Mazurek Melnyk

> Measure what is measurable and make measurable
> what is not so. —*Galileo (1564–1642)*

In intervention research, it is all about the outcome. Critical questions about **measurement** to ask yourself in preparing to conduct an intervention study are (a) What "so what" important outcome(s) do you want to change or influence with your **intervention?**; (b) How will you assess whether your intervention led to that change in outcome(s)? In intervention studies, you need to measure phenomena in a way that can then be analyzed statistically to determine whether your intervention made a difference in outcome(s) and, if it did so, was that difference beyond that expected by chance. You must measure variables of interest in a manner that allows you to determine true change in the **dependent or outcome variable** and what measures can accomplish this in a reliable and valid manner.

One of the first issues you must confront as an investigator is your choice of how detailed and specific your measures must be in order to adequately assess the constructs identified in your study. Every variable in your study must be defined, and its role within your model must be determined. These variables should be tied to key theoretical constructs and be measurable/observable. Before selecting your measures, you will need to operationalize your study variables (i.e., define how those characteristics in your sample can be measured and how they vary from subject to subject) and quantify them. These variables take two forms. **Independent variables** are those that precede or are antecedents to the dependent variable; they are also known as "predictor variables." The **dependent variable** is the variable of most interest in intervention studies and is measured to assess impact of the treatment; it is referred to as the "outcome" or "criterion variable."

TABLE 10.1 Determining Level of Measurement for Study Variables				
	NOMINAL	**ORDINAL**	**INTERVAL**	**RATIO**
Variable categories exclusive	Yes	Yes	Yes	Yes
Variable can be ordered/ranked	No	Yes	Yes	Yes
Intervals between categories equal	No	No	Yes	Yes
Absolute zero or absence of variable	No	No	No	Yes

LEVELS OF MEASUREMENT

One of the next decisions you will need to make is whether the variable should be measured using one of the four levels of measurement: (a) **categorical** variables, which are measured as unordered categories; (b) **ordinal variables,** which are measured as ordered categories with intervals that are not clearly equal; (c) **continuous variables,** which are ranked with quantifiable intervals; and (d) **ratio level variables,** which are continuous and have an absolute zero. Examples of categorical variables are one's profession (e.g., teacher, nurse, psychologist, physical therapist, social worker) and race (African American, White, Asian). Gender is an example of a categorical variable with only two answer options (male/female), known as a "dichotomous variable." Ordinal level variables might include degree of satisfaction (little, moderate, great) or perceived agreement with an issue (do not agree, agree somewhat, agree, strongly agree) and reflect a prioritization or leveling of answer responses, but the exact differences between each answer cannot be strictly quantified. Continuous variables do have both order and equally quantifiable distances between each category. Common examples include weight, pulse rate, milligrams of pain medication given or correct answers on an examination. Like continuous variables, ratio-level variables have both order and quantifiable intervals, but they also have an absolute zero point. Temperature is a common ratio-level variable. As scales progress from categorical to ordinal to interval levels, the measure of the construct becomes more precise. The end result of using scales with interval-level data is usually more ability to detect differences between groups in your intervention study. Even when categorical variables match well to the research question (e.g., studies examining whether an intervention leads to fewer patients diagnosed as obese), it is often best practice to measure the variable at a higher level, such as weight in pounds, and collapse the data later for analyses should you decide to do so. However, the collapse of data should be done with extreme caution as this consolidation of detail loses the very essence of differences between variable characteristics. Failure to quantify variables and quantify them at the highest level that is appropriate represents a lost opportunity to gather information that can help determine the impact of your intervention (see Table 10.1 for more examples of levels of measurement).

TOO MUCH OR TOO LITTLE: HOW MANY MEASURES ARE NEEDED?

One of the temptations you will face in conducting an intervention study is the often overwhelming urge to include as many measures as possible so that you do not "miss" collecting data that could reveal the "scientific find of a lifetime" (many scientists have been kept awake at night worrying about this very issue). Although you may want to measure multiple variables to assess change in outcomes, it is critical to prioritize which outcome is most important—in other words, what you are "going to hang your hat on." This being said, wise investigators often use multiple types of measures for their outcome (criterion) variable to ensure they can assess intervention efficacy or effectiveness while reigning in their use of multiple measures for every predictor (antecedent) variable. For example, in a study measuring the effect of a healthy lifestyles intervention on physical activity with teens, it would be wise to include both a self-report measure of activity along with an objective measure, such as data recorded by an actigraph of daily physical activity by the teens.

Clearly identifying your outcome variable is necessary to calculate power and determine sample size for your study. Conversely, not being selective with measures risks overwhelming your study participants, which can threaten your ability to collect data as you may risk losing several participants due to the burden you have placed upon them. You also need to determine measures for your study, balancing what is clinically important to assess with the actual logistics involved in each of the measures and the cost of the assessments. Therefore, measures used in intervention studies need to be (a) specific to the variable under study, (b) sensitive to change, (c) appropriate for the participants in the study, (d) cost effective, and (e) able to be collected in the minimum amount of time that the participant, researcher, and study sites can afford. Measures that are not psychometrically strong and lack evidence of validity or reliability place the investigator at risk for finding out absolutely nothing!

Many times interventions bring about very small changes in outcomes. Thus, outcome measures must collect data in a manner that can identify a small, but significant impact. In a HIV-prevention intervention targeted to adolescent girls, behavioral change would precede actual infection rates. Thus, pinning all hopes for intervention impact on measuring only HIV infections rates would minimize the impact of an intervention that successfully reduced sexual risk behaviors. When examining the appropriateness of measures, consider literacy levels, cultural tailoring, and developmental appropriateness. For example, studies of pediatric patients should not request long narrative responses to complex questions. The manner in which the measure is administered must be considered. Frail elderly participants asked to complete physically challenging measures might be unable to comply. Teenagers may be less likely to complete a diary requesting hourly information on symptoms or emotions. It may be difficult for participants to complete complex or open-ended questions in noisy waiting areas or public spaces. Measures also need to consume a reasonable cost within your budget. In addition, time and effort burden need to be considered for all persons involved in the study starting with those from whom you collect data to those collecting, coding, and analyzing them. Basically, you have to be thoughtful and judicious in your selection of measures in order to get the "best bang for your buck."

The basic premise of measurement in research is delineated with this question: Are you measuring the outcome construct that is most important to measure and are you measuring it consistently? Measures should be objective and not prone to fluctuations based on factors that are influenced by the investigator (e.g., data collection personnel or instrumentation). The theory of psychometrics underlies the principles of measurement, and, thus, the assessment of **reliability** and **validity** of instruments used in intervention research is termed the "psychometric evaluation" of measures. Validity and reliability are really a matter of degree, not an "all or none" issue. Thus, as an investigator, you must provide evidence of validity and reliability, not "prove" that the measure is psychometrically sound.

FORMS OF VALIDITY AND RELIABILITY

Validity and reliability go hand in hand. Assessing validity of a measure, that is, gathering evidence to conclude that your measure actually taps the construct you intend it to measure, is one of the two forms of psychometric evaluation. Reliability is the ability of an

TABLE 10.2 Forms of Validity and Reliability	
VALIDITY	RELIABILITY
Content Validity	Test–Retest Reliability
Construct Validity	Parallel Forms
Criterion-Related Validity	Inter-/Intrarater Reliability
	Cronbach's Alpha Coefficient
	Split-Half Reliability

instrument to consistently measure what it claims to measure. A measure cannot be valid if it is not reliable; that is, it cannot actually assess a construct if the measure cannot do so in a stable dependable manner. However, a measure can be reliable without being valid because it can be consistently measuring something other than the variable you may think you are measuring. For example, you may have a self-report measure of depression with very high levels of internal consistency (i.e., reliability)—it certainly measures "a construct" consistently; however, it could actually be assessing something other than depression, such as anxiety.

How can you determine whether your measure is valid or not? There are some established criteria used to judge validity, including **content validity, construct validity, and criterion-related validity** (see Table 10.2).

Content Validity

Content validity refers to the actual "meat" of the measure; specifically, whether it reflects the body of knowledge surrounding the construct. For example, a measure assessing parent–child communication might address all forms of communication—verbal, nonverbal, written—rather than assessing only one of these facets. A measure of "test anxiety symptoms" would include both physiological and psychological symptoms. Investigators determine content validity early in the process of instrument development. The congruence between the conceptual and operational definitions of the variable is assessed in content validity.

There are two basic approaches for determining **content validity**. The most common approach to assessing content validity is to use experts in the field who confirm that the measure is tapping what it is supposed to measure and to have individuals who actually are experiencing the construct of interest to evaluate the overall appropriateness of the measure under question. For example, if you wanted to measure stress in school-aged children using a questionnaire, your first step in determining the measure's validity would be to determine content validity by pulling together a group of "known experts" (e.g., school psychologists and nurses, counselors, and teachers) to review and critique the measure you have developed or selected. Their feedback on whether they believe the measure is assessing stress in school-aged children is used as one assessment of content validity. Interrater agreement between the experts on which items are pertinent can be used to provide evidence of content validity for the final items retained for the measure. Another approach to establish content validity is to ask individuals who "possess" the construct of interest (e.g., school-aged children experiencing high-stress situations or enrolled in stress-reduction programs) to provide feedback on whether the items on the measure reasonably assess or cover components of their experience. This approach of obtaining subjective feedback from participants is often referred to as **"face validity"** (Morrison-Beedy, Carey, Aronowitz, Mkandawire, & Dyne, 2002).

Construct Validity

A second form of **construct validity** assesses how well the measure meets the theoretical expectations of either converging or diverging with other related constructs. For example, if you are interested in measuring stress, you might also contend that individuals in your study who score high on your measure of stress would also score high on a measure of anxiety. Thus, scores on these two measures would be positively correlated and provide evidence of **convergent validity**. Similarly, participants who score high on your stress measure would, theoretically, score lower on your measure of calmness (which we hope at the time you are reading this chapter, you are also experiencing). Scores on these measures, stress and calmness, would be negatively correlated and serve as evidence of **divergent validity**. Both convergent and divergent validity are types of construct validity.

Another way to assess construct validity is through the statistical method of **factor analysis**. Factor analysis can be used to assess whether the items in a measure cluster into predetermined variable groupings. Usually, these groupings are theoretically driven. **Exploratory factor analysis** can be used to reduce and refine a group of items within a new measure. Factor analysis can also be used to confirm how multiple items conceptually "hang together"; that is, it can provide evidence for the items serving as a cohesive representation of the construct. For example, in developing a measure to assess HIV-related knowledge (Volpe, Nelson, Kraus, & Morrison-Beedy, 2007), 62 items were formulated based on subdomains identified as important—prevention strategies, testing and treatment, misconceptions, and transmission information. The goal was to develop an overall measure of HIV-related knowledge. Content validity was determined by experts in the field and at-risk populations. The expert feedback was used to reduce the items, based on redundancy or irrelevance. **Confirmatory factor analysis** revealed that the subscales reflected these predetermined areas, but the largest percentage of variance captured in the analysis supported that all of the items were relating to one large factor. The HIV Knowledge Questionnaire (HIVKQ) was construct validated using a statistically driven approach.

Validity can also be evaluated by comparing or contrasting measures on "known groups" with your intervention participants. For example, in the previously mentioned study, evidence for the validity of the measure was obtained by comparing total HIVKQ scores between groups (i.e., HIV experts, college students, and three community samples) with predictions made on which groups theoretically should have higher or lower HIVKQ scores (Volpe et al., 2007).

Construct validity can also be evaluated by conducting hypothesis testing. In this approach, you test assumptions about the variables in your study using hypotheses. If the testing supports this assumption, evidence for the construct validity of the measure is provided. For example, data were collected on the construct validity of the HIVKQ during intervention work that provided treatment-related evidence. We hypothesized that participants in a HIV-prevention program, which included an HIV-education component, would score higher on the HIVKQ than those in the control group. Mean scores on the HIVKQ were significantly higher for intervention versus control participants, thus providing evidence for construct validity of the measure (see Table 10.3).

Criterion-Related Validity

Finally, assessing whether a measure truly measures what you say you are measuring can be accomplished through **criterion-related validity**. This form of validity compares your selected measure with what is considered the "gold standard" for assessing that construct

TABLE 10.3 Forms of Validity Assessment and Examples		
Content	(Expert)	Example: Grief counselors and palliative care clinicians review a list of items on a questionnaire to determine whether the items tap a measure of the PELOC.
Content	(Face)	Example: Palliative care patients review the PELOC to determine whether items cover their areas of concern.
Construct	(Convergent)	Example: Scores on the PELOC are positively correlated with the measure *Worries in Terminally Ill Patients*.
Construct	(Divergent)	Example: Scores on the PELOC are negatively correlated with the measure *Situational Control*.
Construct	(Factor Analysis)	Example: Principal component analysis on the PELOC identifies one factor associated with 72% of the variance in the instrument's scores.
Construct	(Criterion)	Example: PELOC scores are correlated with a social worker's interview checklist of palliative care patients' fears and unmet needs.

PELOC, patient end-of-life concerns.

of interest. Therefore, if you have developed a wonderful measure assessing depression (let us call it the "WMAD"), you might chose to assess whether scores on your measure correlate positively with a well-validated measure, such as the Beck Depression Inventory-II (BDI-II; Beck, Steer, & Brown, 1996). If your measure is a valid measure of depression, you would expect that participants who score high on the BDI would also score high on your wonderful new measure. Data can be collected at (a) one time using both your predictor measure (WMAD) and gold standard criterion measure (BDI) or (b) at two different time points where the criterion measure is administered at some time after the predictor measure. These are termed "concurrent" and "predictive" validity, respectively.

RELIABILITY

When selecting measures for your intervention study, it is critical that they consistently assess your variable of interest. Assessing reliability can be thought of as determining the dependability or stability of your measure. Measures that are reliable are also considered accurate. In essence, any error within the measure itself is minimized. If you had a scale that at one time point gave you a weight of 150 pounds but a few minutes later gave you a reading of 145, you would not say the scale was reliable (although you might prefer the lower reading). Various forms of reliability measures are available that focus on the instrument's stability, equivalence, and homogeneity.

TESTS OF STABILITY

Test–Retest Reliability
Although there are several methods that can be used to assess an instrument's reliability, you need to be selective and targeted in your choice(s). Assessing the stability or consistency of a measure from one time to another is derived through test–retest reliability. In this approach,

you would ask the same participants to respond to the same measure at a specified time interval (e.g., 4 weeks apart). Although there are often standard assessment periods used commonly by investigators (e.g., 2-week test–retest interval for self-report measures), the time period has to make sense to you as an investigator. Calculating a reliability coefficient based on comparing the scores at both time periods for each participant provides a statistical measure of the instrument's stability.

Consider a situation in an intervention study where you might want to assess a participant's knowledge of pregnancy prevention methods using your newly developed "Contraception Information Scale." An important step in using your measure would be to pilot test it for usability, readability, completion time, and then assess its psychometric properties. For test–retest reliability, you might ask a group of women to complete your measure and record each woman's score for an overall assessment of their knowledge. You may then ask these same participants to retake the measure using a predetermined time interval (e.g., 2 weeks apart), one that would ensure participants were not simply responding from memory yet be within a time period that did not allow for a change in knowledge due to intervention or historical occurrence. You would expect that, without some type of educational intervention factor, such as a visit to a healthcare provider for contraception, the scores on your measure of contraceptive knowledge would be relatively (not necessarily exactly) the same from time 1 to time 2.

Equivalence
Inter- and Intrarater Reliability
The stability of a measure can also be assessed by comparing the scoring on instruments between at least two trained independent raters. In observational studies, this is referred to as **interobserver** or **interrater reliability**, and the scores of the two independent rater–observers are compared for equivalence, with higher levels of agreement or correlations indicative of a measure that can be used consistently regardless of the person conducting the assessment. When rater scores are compared to assess percentage agreement, a target of 90% or greater agreement between them should be met in order to ensure equivalence and fidelity of this measurement within your study. For example, in an observational study of maternal–infant interaction, two independent raters observed mothers and infants interacting with each other using a 16-item dichotomous scale that measured positive and negative interactions. Each rater checked "yes" or "no" for each of the 16 items on the scale (e.g., mother speaks quietly to the infant; mother quiets the infant by rocking). The raters' item-to-item responses were compared for equivalency, and the percentage of agreement was determined. Interrater reliability estimates comparability between different raters, whereas **intrarater reliability** assesses, in a similar manner, comparability or consistency in the same rater across multiple time points. Statistical results indicating 90% agreement or higher between or within raters provides evidence of the measure's reliability. Relying on correlational analysis for this reliability rating could result in scores with high correlations, yet the raters do not actually agree on specific item scoring. Throughout an intervention study, intermittent reassessment of interrater reliability should take place to assess rater drift in scoring. If drift has occurred, retraining of raters on the instrument is necessary until a 90% agreement is again reached. Reliability assessments also can take place within one rater conducting repeated scoring on the same measure; however, the items on the measure should be placed in random order for each completion.

Parallel Forms
Similarly, assessing the correlation between two versions of the same instrument is a measure of reliability using a coefficient of equivalence. Comparing **parallel forms** of a measure with one sample at one time point can provide evidence for the reliability of the measure.

To balance the impact of testing effects and fatigue, the measures should be administered in different order to participants; this approach is intended to reduce error rate. Oftentimes, the most common challenge encountered by investigators is that there are rarely true alternative forms of one measure available for use. These two instruments should have means and standard deviations that are approximately the same in order for the forms to be considered parallel. Acceptable correlations between the scores on both measures provide additional evidence for the reliability of the measure.

Tests of Homogeneity
Cronbach's Coefficient Alpha
Another method of assessing the reliability of a measure with multiple items is to determine its internal consistency by calculating a statistic called the **"Cronbach's coefficient alpha."** This statistic is by far the most common method for assessing homogeneity in a measure. We can quantitatively describe the consistency of how items within a measure relate to each other, that is "hold together" as one construct, using this analysis. If items within an instrument are not all related, or homogeneous, internal consistency will be reduced. For example, although a measure of locus of control may address the overall construct, the items may be heterogeneous and measure two aspects of the construct, internal and external locus of control. This statistic can be calculated for instruments that obtain continuous- or interval-level data. The Kuder–Richardson formula (KR-20) is a similar statistic used in the case of dichotomous data. This form of reliability is influenced by two forms of potential variance: the number of items in the measure and the interitem correlations between items. Increasing the number of items that correlate with the rest of the items will increase the reliability coefficient. However, savvy investigators always recognize that these modifications also increase participant burden, completion, time, and cost. These data can be used to refine your measure to capitalize on increasing the measure's reliability while balancing the aforementioned issues. Statistical packages will calculate a Cronbach's alpha as well as each item-to-total and interitem correlation. Scores on both measures can range from 0.00 to 1.00, with higher scores indicating greater consistency between items. Conventionally, Cronbach's alpha values of 0.70 or higher are considered satisfactory and acceptable as evidence of instrument reliability (Melnyk & Morrison-Beedy, 2012) although it is better to aim for using an instrument with an internal consistency reliability of 0.80 and above. A useful component of the analysis is the "alpha if item deleted" result. This function provides you with details regarding changes in alpha levels if each item in the scale was deleted. This strategy can help you to further refine your measure and eliminate redundancies. A word of caution in using this strategy—you, and not the computer, should be the judge on which items need to be retained even if the alpha might be increased slightly if certain items were removed.

Split-Half Reliability
Homogeneity within a measure can also be assessed using **split-half technique**. This method was used more commonly before computers made every investigator's life easier and is simply taking one-half of the items in a measure and correlating the scores between the two halves. Oftentimes, items are selected by the "odd-even" rule (of course, measures with odd-numbered items present their own challenge). These two "half" scores should correlate very highly if the measure is consistent. Reliable measures with more items will have higher levels of consistency than briefer versions based on the formula used to calculate the statistic. Spearman–Brown can be used to correct the lower alphas obtained simply because of the reduced number of items in each comparison measure.

TYPES OF MEASURES

The scientific literature is filled with a plethora of instruments that can be used to measure your study's variables. These can be classified into various categories which include, but are not limited to, self-report, biological, physiological, observational, and system measures. Knowing that you want appropriate, feasible, sensitive, and specific measures, the key is to be judicious in your choice of measures from an abundant "cornucopia" of choices. You will need to be selective and carry out a scientifically driven assessment of which instruments will best meet your needs for documenting change in your outcomes as well as antecedents. Evidence from pilot study data that supports the validity, reliability, and feasibility of your measures will do much to convince funding reviewers of their suitability for your intervention study.

The collection of self-reported data is extremely common in intervention research (e.g., ask the participants themselves if they liked the intervention, if they did the activities, if they felt stressed, if they have had angry outbursts, if they smoked a cigarette, if they love their mother). Much of intervention evaluation lies in these types of self-report responses. There are numerous mechanisms that can be used to collect this information; a few of the many options are presented here.

Self-administered questionnaires (SAQs) are surveys that are frequently used to gather information from participants. Many psychosocial constructs are assessed in this manner. These surveys can include those presented in paper/pencil format, administered through hand-held or laptop computer devices, or by cell phone. Audio computer-assisted self-interviews (ACASIs), computer-assisted self-interviews (CASIs), and computer-assisted phone interviews (CAPIs) are just a few examples of data collection methods that have been noted to increase the reliability and validity of information reported by participants (Morrison-Beedy, Carey, & Tu, 2006); these tools have become important options for researchers, especially when socially sensitive data, such as drug use, sexual behaviors, or criminal activity, need to be measured. Alternate methods for data collection can include interviews, conducted in person or by phone, where a research team member verbally presents the items to the participants and records their responses. Data collection may also involve the review of data already contained in written or computerized records; medical chart audits are a common example of this approach. System measures that assess constructs such as organizational change, quality, and conflict can be collected through electronic health system records, which are becoming more common in healthcare settings.

What can you do as an investigator if your participants are too young to tell you this information, if they cannot read or understand the language in which questions are written, if they are too ill or too frail to respond to questions, or if they are physically incapacitated and cannot write their responses? In these cases, data for your selected measures can be gathered using approaches that involve direct or indirect observation. Observational approaches can include filming and subsequent scoring of participant behaviors or activities. They also can include the use of checklists or other assessment measures completed by a research team member who is monitoring these behaviors or activities in-person, through a one-way mirror, or by review of audio or video tapes.

Physiological measures provide another option for measuring your study variables. Just about any aspect of human functioning can be quantified and measured although some approaches may be more costly than others. From the simple check of a participant's blood pressure, pulse, or weight to the cardiac output of a patient running on a treadmill, to the intensity of a baby's cry, assessing changes in physiological variables is a common measurement option. Measures that require the collection of biological specimens, such as cortisol, blood cells, genetic material, electrolytes, have become increasingly important ways to measure the impact of interventions. These measures oftentimes provide a more objective measure than other approaches and may be new to some investigators. Thus, we provide additional details about biological measurement in Chapter 11. Still, it must be remembered that not all variables *can* or *should* be measured using physiological or biological methods. Many variables of interest (e.g., respect, self-worth, risk taking, intentions) cannot be assessed using these types of measures. You, as the investigator, must determine the most appropriate choice for collecting data on each variable in your study.

TYPES OF SCALES

A second level of measurement decision making involves the selection of response or answer choice format or rating scales. Some commonly used scales in intervention studies with self-report or observational measures include open-ended questions, Likert-type scales, diaries, visual analog scales (VAS), multiple answer options, and observational checklists. These are but a few of the vast choices of measurement found in the scientific literature; each has its strengths and limitations. Characteristics of the participants, data collection setting, and resources must be considered when selecting one option of measurement over the other. Figures 10.1 to 10.3 contain examples of some common scales.

Likert-type scales often assess the respondent's agreement or belief in an item's statement (e.g., "never," "sometimes," "always"). These scales can be used to quantify behavior (just not to the detail of interval-level scales). A VAS measurement is a horizontal line with anchors at each end. The study participant places a hatch mark on the line closest to the preferred choice in the range. It is important to determine the appropriate levels of measurement of every study variable. Researchers desire the highest level of measurement that can be obtained; however, it must be relevant for specific participants. For example, in determining educational status, participants can be measured using a variety of levels of measurement depending on the detail you wish to achieve (see Figure 10.1). Educational level can be assessed using a variety of levels of measurement. For instance, a dichotomous measure might simply pose: "completed high school" and "did not complete high school." A categorical measure would state a wider range of choices such as "high school graduate," "some college," "college graduate." More detailed data on educational level could be obtained using an interval-level measure. For example, participants could be asked to circle the highest grade they have completed from the following choices: "7-8-9-10-11-12." Remember that it is easier to collapse data than to wish you had collected more detailed information during data collection time points.

Another important consideration in intervention research is to consider the order of administration of your questions. It is not uncommon for participants to have issues arise (e.g., feel ill, family member call, schedule conflict) that may prevent obtaining a completed survey. You may wish to avoid the more traditional order of "demographics, antecedents, and outcomes" and instead ask the participant to respond to "outcome" related items earlier in the battery of questionnaires rather than waiting until the end. This strategy helps to minimize the negative effect of participant fatigue. It also helps to increase the likelihood that you can collect outcome data even if the participant gets up and leaves. If participants decide they cannot complete the survey, then at least you have the core outcome data you seek to obtain.

Developing measures is a science unto itself and no easy task. Particularly for new investigators, selecting a measure that already exists with established validity and reliability enhances your chances of successfully designing, conducting, analyzing, and funding your intervention study. Try not to reinvent the wheel if at all possible—savings in time and effort should be considered. You also face the risk that your new measure will not be as useful or psychometrically strong as other current measures. Certainly, there are appropriate circumstances

THE NICU PARENTAL BELIEFS SCALE

Below are *18 statements* that relate to you and your baby's hospitalization. Hospital experiences differ for every parent. There are some parents who are not so sure about their baby's needs and how they can best meet them while they are in the neonatal intensive care unit (NICU), while other parents are more sure about how to help their baby through this experience. There are no right or wrong answers to the following statements. Please circle the number that best describes your agreement or disagreement with each statement.

1. I know what characteristics and behaviors are common in premature babies hospitalized in the NICU.

1	2	3	4	5
Strongly disagree	Disagree	Neither agree or disagree	Agree	Strongly agree

2. I am sure that what I do for my baby will be what is best to help him/her deal with being in the NICU.

1	2	3	4	5
Strongly disagree	Disagree	Neither agree or disagree	Agree	Strongly agree

3. I feel comfortable in caring for my baby in the NICU.

1	2	3	4	5
Strongly disagree	Disagree	Neither agree or disagree	Agree	Strongly agree

4. I know what characteristics and behaviors to expect in my baby while he/she is in the NICU.

1	2	3	4	5
Strongly disagree	Disagree	Neither agree or disagree	Agree	Strongly agree

FIGURE 10.1 Example of items from a Likert scale.

Source: From Melnyk, B. M. (1997). *The NICU parental beliefs scale.* Hammondsport, NY: COPE for HOPE.

Think of the person you know best who has the AIDS virus. How similar are you and this person in the way you live. Make a mark anywhere along this line which answers this question the best.

Not at all like me.   Exactly like me.

FIGURE 10.2 An example of a visual analog scale.

Source: From Morrison-Beedy, D. (1993). Self assessment of HIV risk in women: Functional and dysfunctional patterns of assessment (Doctoral dissertation, University of Rochester, NY). *Dissertation Abstracts International, 54*(5B), 2442.

THE INDEX OF PARENTAL BEHAVIOR IN NICU
Using the scale below, circle the number indicating whether you observed each
behavior or not during the 30-minute observation period. Circle "no opportunity"
if the parent did not have the opportunity to perform the behavior (Melnyk,
Feinstein, Fairbanks, & Small, 1998).

	No	Yes	No Opportunity
1. Parent makes at least one positive comment about baby.	0	1	2
2. Parent focuses on things/people in the environment more than on baby.	0	1	2
3. Parent stops an activity with baby when seeing that he or she is over-stimulated.	0	1	2
4. Parent speaks softly to baby.	0	1	2
5. Parent handles or repositions baby slowly and gently most all of the time.	0	1	2

FIGURE 10.3 Example of items from an observational scale.

Source: From Melnyk, B. M., Feinstein, N., Fairbanks, E., & Small, L. (1998). *Index of parental behavior in NICU*. Hammondsport, NY: COPE for HOPE.

when measures for the construct under investigation are not available or the state of the science indicates the need for such work. Such decisions always need to be weighed and carefully considered by the investigator.

MEASUREMENT ERROR

Measurement is not a perfect science, and all measures contain the possibility of error. The difference between the true value of a variable and the value obtained during data collection is the measurement error. Error can be classified as random, caused by chance, or systematic, a component of the measure itself. Researchers themselves may contribute to error in the measurement of a phenomenon. For example, participants may react to the researcher either positively (trying to please him or her during the course of the data collection) or negatively (not providing truthful or consistent responses because of fear or judgment). Common sources of error caused by the instrument itself include surveys with ambivalent or confusing questions, answer options that do not contain clearly delineated categories, or questions addressing sensitive issues that lead to response bias. Error in measurement can also occur because of environmental influences. Data collection that occurs in areas that are inconsistently lighted, noisy, or in temperature extremes can lead to error. Providing participants in the experimental intervention group with comfortable chairs and snacks while completing their assessments while placing your standard care control participants in a cold dark hallway for their data collection can contribute to measurement error. Finally, error can occur due to factors within the participants themselves—being in pain, fatigued, upset, or under the influence of substances—all contribute to subject error.

There are many ways in which to address these sources of error and increase the accuracy of measurement in your study. A fundamental approach is to use multiple measures for variables (e.g., self-report and observation), particularly those that target the primary outcome of interest. Data collection via blinded personnel who are not aware of which participants are assigned to which condition reduces the risk of differential bias. A critical component of conducting any research study, but often not on the mind or timeline of the investigator, is the need to standardize all study procedures and protocols, including standardization of measurement methods. Specific step-by-step instructions for all aspects of the study need to be documented. In particular, meticulous training of data collectors and assessing their competence prior to actual data collection in the field is imperative. This training can include observations by research team trainers or the principal investigator (PI), establishing inter- or intrarater reliability and mastery of equipment and mechanical devices. Strictly calibrated machines or instruments are essential as well as ongoing recalibration for standardization. In addition to using carefully trained data collectors, providing consistent environments for data collection is important. Meticulously editing, refining, and piloting instruments you may develop (or choose to use) to identify any items that are confusing, biased, incomplete, or too complex are critical to reducing measurement error.

SUMMARY

Selecting appropriate measures for an intervention study is the choice of the investigator. This choice can be both overwhelming (when there is a substantial array of measures for the variables of interest) and challenging (when the investigator must search extensively for even one appropriate measure). Developing a measure when one does not exist or when those that do are woefully inadequate is a science unto itself and requires intensive time and focus. Therefore, it is best to use already developed valid and reliable measures whenever possible. Remember, your intervention study will only be as good as the measures that assess study variables in a valid and reliable manner, so choose them carefully.

Key Points From This Chapter

- The investigator must decide which of the variables in his or her study is the primary outcome variable; power calculations and sample size are dependent on this choice.
- Levels of measurement (nominal, ordinal, interval, ratio) serve as the basis for type of statistical test used to evaluate intervention outcomes.
- A careful balance must be struck when it comes to selecting measures for your study—too few may leave you vulnerable to being unable to determine intervention effects; too many may increase participant burden as well as work for the research team.
- Specific, sensitive to change over time, appropriate, and feasible—these are all characteristics of useful measures in intervention work.
- Measurement error is both inherent and modifiable—careful attention must be paid to decreasing error related to researcher, instrumentation, environmental, and subject factors.
- Psychometrically sound measures are both reliable (consistently measuring constructs of interest) and valid (measuring the actual constructs of interest); evidence is needed to "support," not to "prove" validity and reliability.
- Scientific instruments including self-report measures, biological, physiological, observational, and system assessments abound; the key to success is judicious, scientifically driven selection by the investigator.

REFERENCES

Beck, A. T., Steer, R. A., & Brown, G. K. (1996). *Manual for BDI-II* (2nd ed.). San Antonio, TX: Psychological Corporation.

Melnyk, B. M., Feinstein, N., Fairbanks, E., & Small, L. (1998). *Index of parental behavior in NICU.* Hammondsport, NY: COPE for HOPE.

Melnyk, B. M., & Morrison-Beedy, D. (Eds.). (2012). *Intervention research: Designing, conducting, analyzing and funding: A practical guide to success.* New York, NY: Springer Publishing.

Morrison-Beedy, D. (1993). Self assessment of HIV risk in women: Functional and dysfunctional patterns of assessment (Doctoral dissertation, University of Rochester, NY). *Dissertation Abstracts International, 54*(5B), 2442.

Morrison-Beedy, D., Carey, M. P., Aronowitz, T., Mkandawire, L., & Dyne, J. (2002). An HIV risk-reduction intervention in an adolescent correctional facility: Lessons learned. *Applied Nursing Research, 15*(2), 97–101. doi:10.1053/apnr.2002.29530

Morrison-Beedy, D., Carey, M. P., & Tu, X. (2006). Accuracy of audio computer-assisted self-interviewing (ACASI) and self-administered questionnaires for the assessment of sexual behavior. *AIDS Behavior, 10,* 541–552. doi:10.1007/s10461-006-9081-y

Volpe, E. M., Nelson, L. E., Kraus, R. A., & Morrison-Beedy, D. (2007). Adaptation and refinement of the HIV knowledge questionnaire for use with adolescent girls. *Journal of the Association of Nurses in AIDS Care, 18*(5), 57–63. doi:10.1016/j.jana.2007.07.003

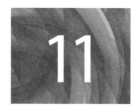

Biological Measures for Intervention Research

Rita H. Pickler & Cindy Munro

> To live a creative life, we must lose our fear of being wrong. —*Anonymous*

Adding biological measures to an intervention study is becoming a common practice, particularly when the study involves a biobehavioral phenomenon, as is true in many health-related research studies. There are a number of aspects to consider before adding biological measures to your study including the following: what biological component will be measured; whether you consider the biological measure an outcome, a mechanism of action, or a surrogate for either outcome or mechanism; the validity and reliability of the measure; the body substrate to be sampled; and how and when measurement will occur. Additional aspects to be considered are cost and resources needed to collect, store, process, and analyze biological samples. This chapter briefly addresses these issues, although a full discussion of the many considerations required when including biomarkers in an intervention study is beyond the scope of this work.

Before addressing the specific aspects of biological measurement, we define several parameters for our discussion. First, we limit our discussion to biomarkers. We further focus our discussion on recently identified "common data elements (CDEs)" proposed for inclusion in biobehavioral nursing studies.

BIOMARKERS

In 1998, the National Institutes of Health Biomarkers Definitions Working Group defined a biomarker as a biological characteristic that can be objectively measured and evaluated as an indicator of normal biological processes, pathogenic processes, or pharmacological responses to a therapeutic intervention (Strimbu & Tavel, 2010). Thus, biomarkers are *observable* characteristics indicative of a health state or surrogate measures for clinical end points that predict benefit or harm on the basis of epidemiological, therapeutic, pathophysiological, or other scientific evidence (Libby & King, 2015). Biomarkers differ from symptoms, which are *perceptions* of individuals about how they *feel*, and do not necessarily correlate with symptomatic perceptions. In fact, variations in biomarkers may be undetectable and without an observable effect on health. In addition, there are measurable biomarkers with such great variance among populations that they are unreliable predictors of a health condition or its absence.

The distinction between biomarkers and symptoms is an important one. Symptoms have dominated for some time as the most important measures of clinical research outcomes. Symptoms, which can also be considered clinical end points, are variables that reflect or characterize how a subject in a study or clinical trial feels or functions. Symptoms are, in other words, variables that represent a study subject's health and well-being from the *subject's* perspective. However, the use of biomarkers in basic and clinical research as well as in clinical practice has become more common. Thus, increasing numbers of researchers are using biomarkers as primary end points in clinical trials in addition to, or in place of, subject-reported symptoms. Moreover, a number of biomarkers have been shown to be predictive of a number of clinical outcomes across a variety of interventions and populations, thus acting as surrogates, or to explain the mechanism by which an intervention affects an outcome (Libby & King, 2015). It is important to remember, however, that a biomarker can be a valid and reliable indicator of a clinical outcome without being part of a causal pathway. For example, one antecedent may affect both a biomarker and the outcome of interest through two different, distinct mechanisms. Researchers need to be careful not to assume causation on the basis of a biomarker's correlational association with an outcome.

COMMON BIOLOGICAL DATA ELEMENTS

Use of CDEs has been touted as a way to improve efficiency and data quality across studies and populations, as well as to permit aggregation of data across studies. CDEs are defined as fundamental, logical units of data pertaining to one kind of information that are clearly conceptualized (Cohen, Thompson, Yates, Zimmerman, & Pullen, 2015). The use of CDEs may help a scientific area advance more quickly and, thus, have a positive effect on human health sooner. A work group composed of National Institute of Nursing Research–funded scientists has recently suggested that cytokines (i.e., interleukin [IL]–1b, IL-6, IL-10), hypothalamus–pituitary–adrenal (HPA) axis markers (i.e., free cortisol), select neuropeptides (i.e., brain-derived neurotrophic factor [BDNF]), and various genetics (i.e., single nucleotide polymorphisms [SNPs], epigenetics) could be useful for a CDE set for nursing science. Although not a comprehensive list of the biomarkers currently measured in any number of research studies, these suggested CDEs do represent a sufficiently broad spectrum of measureable biomarkers about which there is evidence for their usefulness in explaining how an intervention might work, acting as a surrogate for a clinical outcome, or serving as an outcome in intervention studies.

CHOOSING MEASURES

The selection of biological measures should be on the basis of a clear understanding of the biology of the biomarker. However, human biology is complex, with considerable interaction between body systems, such as that which exists between an inflammatory response and the

HPA axis. The role and importance of specific biomarkers may differ among health conditions and in the context of other biological characteristics such as sex. Levels of biomarkers frequently vary among different populations, over time of day, or other conditions. Moreover, human biological systems are affected by behavioral, social, and psychological factors. Thus, it is important to consider these potential factors when designing an intervention study that includes biomarkers. In general, there is much to think about when choosing biomarkers as they are generally influenced by many factors, some of which are not known and others that are not amenable to manipulation or control. Unless you are doing exploratory work, the measures you choose should have a known association with whatever variable or outcome you are studying.

To begin, it is necessary to identify factors that influence the biomarker you are considering. For example, many biomarkers are influenced by age, sex, genetics, and other characteristics and mechanisms that underlie normal biological variability. Knowing reference values appropriate to the sample is beneficial but these values are often not established; biomarkers that are not commonly used in clinical care (e.g., cytokines) are less likely to have established reference values. Seven criteria, based on clinimetrics, may help assess the suitability of a biomarker: universality, uniqueness, permanence, measurability, acceptability, performance, and circumvention (Feinstein, 1987). Universality requires that all subjects produce or possess the biomarker, whereas uniqueness requires that the biomarker be sufficiently different among individuals in the relevant population. Permanence relates to the manner in which the marker varies over time; biomarkers with permanence are reasonably invariant over time. Measurability or collectability relates to the ease of acquisition and measurement of the biomarker, whereas performance refers to the accuracy, speed, and robustness of technology used to measure the marker in the collected substance (e.g., serum, urine, sputum). Acceptability refers to how well individuals accept the technology used for collection and performance assessment such that they are willing to have their biomarker measured. Finally, circumvention refers to the ease with which a biomarker might be imitated using an artifact or substitute. No single biomarker meets all criteria. Thus, the researcher has to determine which criteria are most important to the study.

Validity and Reliability of Measures

The keys to a good biomarker are validity and reliability. The biomarker must demonstrate a plausible association with the disease process (i.e., reflects pathophysiology), be responsive to changes in symptomatology or disease progression, or importantly for clinical trials, be responsive to the intervention being tested to be considered valid. Note that a plausible association with a disease process does not require that the biomarker is causally related to a mechanism or outcome. Surrogate biomarkers, for example, may predict outcomes without being causally related (Libby & King, 2015). The "validity" of a measure is assessed through comparison with a reference standard or with simultaneous measurements of normal control samples and research samples. For example, serum cortisol remains the gold standard for measurement of cortisol. However, salivary cortisol is increasingly the biomarker of choice because it is easier to collect, has a higher acceptability among participants, and also has established norms that correspond well to serum cortisol.

Biomarkers must also be reliable, or, more accurately, they must have adequate sensitivity and specificity. Sensitivity and specificity directly affect a biomarker's validity. Sensitivity and specificity are statistical measures; sensitivity measures the proportion of actual "positives" who are correctly identified, whereas specificity measures the proportion of actual "negatives" who are correctly identified. For example, genetic biomarkers should correctly identify those with a particularly genetic predisposition to a health condition (specificity) while also eliminating those who do not carry the same genetic risk (sensitivity). A perfect biomarker would have 100% sensitivity (i.e., predict all people with the characteristic as having it) and 100% specificity (i.e., not predict anyone who does not have the characteristic as having it). However, nothing is perfect, and attempts to increase sensitivity may reduce specificity, and vice versa. Thus, the researcher needs to decide whether a biomarker has both sufficient sensitivity and specificity to make it useful in a particular research study.

In this chapter, we are limiting our discussion to biomarkers consistent with those identified as potentially important biological CDEs for nursing science—cytokines, cortisol, neuropeptides, and genetics. We define each biomarker type, discuss the use of the biomarker as an outcome or mechanism of action, provide any validity or reliability information, and identify ways to measure the biomarker including sample types and measurement timing.

Cytokines

Cytokines, originally called "interleukins" for their role in activating leukocytes to mount an immune response, are used to evaluate immune function. "Proinflammatory" cytokines, such as IL-1, IL-6, and tumor necrosis factor (TNF), are low-molecular-weight proteins produced in large part by cells involved in the innate or nonspecific immune response. These cytokines have local effects in cells and tissues that help to appropriately respond to and contain the offending event. Later, immune cells will produce "anti-inflammatory" cytokines, cytokine receptor antagonists, or soluble cytokine receptors, which block the effects of the proinflammatory cytokines and reduce the inflammatory response. These anti-inflammatory biomarkers include IL-10 and IL-1 receptor antagonist (IL-1RA). Proinflammatory and anti-inflammatory cytokines exist naturally in balance, and the relative amounts of each, pro or anti, underlie both natural healthy immune responses and abnormal pathological responses. With increased or more widespread production, proinflammatory cytokines enter circulation. Once there, cytokines act throughout the body to cause the classic signs and symptoms of acute illness including fatigue, myalgia, fever, and anorexia. They also increase hepatic production of acute-phase proteins, such as C-reactive protein (CRP), a classic nonspecific biomarker of inflammation. Under usual conditions, these responses are appropriate and are designed to mount a defense against acute illness; for example, fever may limit bacterial replication (Curfs, Meis, & Hoogkamp-Korstanje, 1997). Cytokines are not specific biomarkers of inflammation; rather, they are nonspecific biomarkers of the inflammatory response; this is an important consideration when choosing cytokines as biomarkers.

Although many disease processes involve increased production of proinflammatory biomarkers, other factors also affect their production (O'Connor et al., 2009; Zhou, Fragala, McElhaney, & Kuchel, 2010), including sleep deprivation and smoking. Given the strong relationship between sleep deprivation and inflammatory markers, unless the study is about sleep loss, subjects who report difficulty sleeping the night before a blood draw should have their sample collection time rescheduled. Diurnal rhythms also affect cytokines, notably IL-6, which increases in the late evening and during sleep and declines sharply in the morning. The diurnal rhythm is maintained even though circulating levels of cytokines increase with age and body weight. Blood should be drawn from all study participants at the same time of day to account for diurnal variations in cytokine production. The challenge for investigators is whether to control for these factors or any other factors known to influence cytokine production in the analysis plan or to narrow the subject inclusion criteria. Generally, research subjects should be instructed to refrain from exercise, high-fat intake, and caffeine for a minimum of 4 hours before samples are collected.

Probably the most important consideration when planning to include cytokines as biomarkers of the inflammatory response is the very short half-life of proinflammatory cytokines in the blood. Alternatively, cytokine antagonists, such as IL-1RA, sIL-6R, or sTNF-RII, which are produced as part of the antiinflammatory response, have a longer half-life and have a stronger association with symptom ratings than do serum levels of proinflammatory cytokines (Bower et al., 2011).

Proinflammatory cytokines can also be detected in saliva and urine. However, if urine is used, the concentration of the biomarker should be normalized to the total protein concentration in the saliva or urine. Urine levels are not sensitive to daily fluctuations in the production of these biomarkers, but can be used to track changes over longer periods of time, such as days or weeks. Before choosing a sample type, it is important to verify that the sample appropriately reflects the cytokines of interest. Cytokines tend to be compartmentalized in body fluids, so basal levels of many cytokines in saliva may not reflect those in plasma (Fernandez-Botran, Miller, Burns, & Newton, 2011; Williamson, Munro, Pickler, Grap, & Elswick, 2012). Levels of some cytokines do increase with exercise (Ives et al., 2011) and stress in healthy adults (Lester, Brown, Aycock, Grubbs, & Johnson, 2010). Salivary levels of some cytokines are increased in individuals with oral cancers, periodontal disease, and infections in the oral cavity. If the study is not focused on oral health outcomes, an oral health screening of potential subjects is warranted.

Cortisol

Cortisol, a steroid hormone, plays a significant role in regulating the availability of glucose to support cellular metabolism; it is a classic biomarker of chronic stress. Cortisol is secreted from the adrenal gland continuously; 90% of the cortisol in the circulation is bound to carrier proteins. Only free cortisol is able to interact with its receptors and is considered the biologically active fraction. Because cortisol can diffuse out of capillaries to reach its target tissues, unbound cortisol can also be measured in saliva or urine. Salivary cortisol is an accurate reflection of the unbound, biologically active cortisol circulating in the bloodstream at any given time point. Because only the unbound fraction of cortisol can be detected in saliva, salivary cortisol cannot be used to assess adrenal gland function including adrenal disease. However, salivary cortisol can be useful as a biomarker of HPA axis function and chronic stress. It should also be noted that less than 1% of unbound cortisol is excreted in urine; 70% is excreted as cortisol metabolites over the course of several hours, making urine cortisol an insensitive measure to changes in cortisol secretion during the course of a day.

In healthy individuals with normal circadian rhythm, circulating levels of cortisol are highest in the morning and lowest in the late evening. Measurement of morning levels must account for the surge in cortisol levels that occurs within 30 minutes of awakening, called the "cortisol awakening response" (CAR), after which levels decline to their nadir at night. The magnitude of change between morning and evening cortisol levels declines with age, as does the CAR. Infants do not have a detectable morning–evening rhythm until after 3 months of age, and circadian rhythms of cortisol secretion vary greatly in children younger than 3 years. A circadian rhythm of cortisol secretion similar to adults is evident by the age of 6 years.

Several factors influence the secretion of cortisol and need to be taken into account when designing a study using this biomarker. The normal circadian rhythm of cortisol secretion can be overridden by the central nervous system to produce an abrupt increase in cortisol secretion. This surge in cortisol secretion characterizes an acute stress response. Although the stress-induced increase in cortisol secretion in adults has been well characterized, there is sufficient evidence that it also occurs in infants and children in response to pain (Davis & Granger, 2009; McCarthy et al., 2009).

There is a substantial body of literature describing dysregulation of the HPA axis with chronic stress. This dysregulation is characterized by smaller stress-induced spikes in cortisol secretion, a smaller CAR, and a smaller difference (flatter slope) between morning and evening levels of cortisol. The dysregulation of the HPA axis is likely caused by changes in intracellular expression of glucocorticoid receptors so that elevated levels of cortisol fail to exert negative feedback on the HPA axis. Therefore, research to demonstrate that an intervention reduces stress in treated subjects compared with untreated subjects requires serial sampling of cortisol before and after the expected surge in cortisol secretion and comparison to basal levels on "normal" days in the same time frame of the circadian rhythm. Changes in circadian patterns of cortisol secretion require serial measures of cortisol levels over 24 hours before and after completion of the intervention. Changes in the circadian pattern of cortisol secretion can be examined by computing the difference between morning and evening cortisol levels (8 a.m. − 8 p.m.), the ratio of nocturnal to morning levels (8 p.m./8 a.m.), or as percent variation in cortisol levels ([8 a.m. − 8 p.m./8 a.m.] × 100).

When the study focus is on people with a chronic illness, the differential effects of psychoemotional distress on cortisol levels versus those of the disease process need to be sorted out. This can be challenging but necessary because research has demonstrated that aberrations in cortisol secretion in patients with chronic conditions including cancer and depression are mechanistically different (Andersen et al., 2010; Jehn et al., 2010; Weinrib et al., 2010). Research has also shown that cortisol is responsive to interventions (e.g., yoga) that improve mood and function (Curtis, Osadchuk, & Katz, 2011; Field, 2011), suggesting that cortisol is a sensitive biomarker of changes in HPA activity in populations with chronic illnesses characterized by dysregulation of the HPA axis.

Neuropeptides

Neuropeptides are small molecules (peptides) used by neurons to communicate with each other, providing signals that influence brain activity. Different neuropeptides are involved in a wide range of brain functions, including social behaviors and cognition. Neuropeptides are secreted from neuronal cells (particularly neurons) and signal neighboring cells (particularly other neurons) by acting on cell surface receptors. Many neuropeptides are coreleased with other small-molecule neurotransmitters; the human genome contains about 90 genes that encode precursors of neuropeptides. Neurons use many different chemical signals to communicate information; neuropeptides are unique among these cell–cell signaling molecules in several ways. First, neuropeptides are not recycled back into the cell once secreted, unlike other conventional neurotransmitters (glutamate, dopamine, serotonin). Second, after secretion, neuropeptides are modified by extracellular enzymes (peptidases), which may either inactivate biological activity or increase the affinity of the neuropeptide for a particular receptor while decreasing its affinity for another receptor. Thus, neuropeptides are complex and their use in intervention research is relatively new.

BDNF, which is encoded by the *BDNF* gene, is a neuropeptide related to nerve growth factor (NGF). BDNF acts on specific neurons in the central and peripheral nervous systems to encourage growth and differentiation of new neurons and synapses. In the brain, this activity is particularly common in areas necessary for learning, memory, and higher level thought. BDNF is particularly important for long-term memory. Deficiencies in BDNF are associated with neurodevelopmental disorders (Wang et al., 2017).

BDNF can be measured in a variety of substrates. However, most researchers have concluded that measurement is best done using serum. BDNF concentration in serum is higher than that in plasma levels because BDNF concentration in plasma is affected by handling of the sample because of the presence of platelets, which store BDNF and secrete it on degranulation. Serum BDNF is also more stable than plasma. Measurement of BDNF in saliva is not reliable (Vrijen, Schenk, Hartman, & Oldehinkel, 2017). A number of sociodemographic and other factors may affect serum levels of BDNF, including sex, age, body mass index (BMI), smoking status, and alcohol intake. The use of BDNF as a biomarker has been limited by the poor reproducibility of results, likely because of the variety of methods used for sample collection and BDNF analysis. An excellent review of measurement issues has been conducted by Polacchini et al. (2015).

Genetics

A genetic biomarker is "a measurable DNA and/or RNA characteristic that is an indicator of normal biological processes, pathogenic processes, and/or response to therapeutic or other interventions" (European Medicines Agency, 2007, p. 8). Genetic biomarkers may reflect the structure, expression, regulation, or function of genes. These can be useful at several stages of research, including assessment of risk, early detection of a condition, classification of subjects for intervention selection, and measurement of intervention effectiveness (Simon, 2011). Genetic biomarkers extend beyond human genetic material; for example, microbial genetic biomarkers are of exceptional interest in microbiome research.

SNPs, copy number variations (CNVs), and chromosomal abnormalities such as duplications, deletions, inversions, and translocations all reflect structural attributes of DNA. Although it is possible for structural attributes related to genes and chromosomes to change over time within an individual (e.g., as a result of DNA damage, or diseases such as cancer), genetic biomarkers on the basis of DNA sequence or gene copy number are relatively stable. Genetic biomarkers that reflect DNA structure tend to be more useful in the assessment of risk and classification.

Changes in expression, regulation, and function of genes can occur without any changes to underlying DNA sequence. DNA methylation, histone modification, RNA expression levels, and microRNA regulation are all examples of epigenetic processes that can serve as genetic biomarkers. Genetic biomarkers that reflect gene expression, regulation, or function vary over time. They represent complex genetic networks and can be affected by multiple environmental influences. Because they are malleable, they are generally better indicators of effects of interventions than are genetic biomarkers that reflect DNA structure.

Although genetic biomarkers have demonstrated important utility in oncology research, their application in chronic conditions and symptom science has lagged. Oncology research has focused on assessment of biomarkers found in tumors, rather than on genetic biomarkers present in the cancer patient's somatic tissues. There are multiple influences on genetics biomarkers in chronic conditions, including environment, lifestyle, and comorbidities; the confounding effects of these factors may be difficult to identify or account for in research studies.

Technology necessary for valid and reliable measurement of genetic biomarkers is continually advancing. However, current methodologies remain concentrated in well-equipped laboratories, require a high level of expertise, and are relatively costly.

RESOURCE CONSIDERATIONS

The inclusion of biomarkers in intervention studies requires appropriate resources. Researchers using biomarkers need laboratory space, equipment, reagents, personnel who have been well trained to run the particular assays proposed, and clear procedures for laboratory safety and reproducibility. If such resources are not available at the researcher's home institution, collaborations with other institutions or with other departments at the home institution are necessary.

The use of biomarkers should be pilot tested before study proposal. This allows the research team to optimize the protocol for the setting, study conditions, and population before beginning to collect samples from human subjects. A pilot study helps the researcher to establish acceptability of the biomarker in the population of interest. It also allows the researcher to assess time to laboratory and performance of the biomarker in the laboratory. A pilot study is also a good time to test the effects of storage conditions on the quality of the samples and reproducibility of the data.

Researchers will also need to be sure that the persons conducting the statistical analysis are knowledgeable about the various ways in which biomarker data are managed and manipulated. The statistician will need to see the data obtained during the pilot work to determine the best analysis plan and sample size needed to test the study hypothesis. Often, biological measures are positively skewed requiring data transformations, which can make interpretation of the data more complicated. Moreover, if repeated biomarker samples are collected, data analysis should include methods of hierarchical linear modeling, which will control for the nonindependence of multiple observations nested within the individual, and for missing data points.

Key Points From This Chapter

- The selection of biologic measures should be based on a clear understanding of the biology of the biomarker.
- The keys to a good biomarker are validity and reliability.
- Researchers using biomarkers need laboratory space, equipment, reagents, personnel who have been well-trained to run the particular assays proposed, and clear procedures for laboratory safety and reproducibility.
- Including biomarkers in intervention research may improve understanding of the biological mechanisms by which interventions affect outcomes.
- Use of biomarkers may provide meaningful intermediary or proxy indicators for outcomes that are difficult to measure.

SUMMARY

Including biomarkers in intervention research may improve understanding of the biological mechanisms by which interventions affect outcomes. Use of biomarkers may also provide meaningful intermediary or proxy indicators for outcomes that are difficult to measure for a variety of reasons. However, researchers need to choose biomarkers carefully; they need to be aware of the specific measurement, storage, and analytic concerns associated with the biomarkers they choose. Finally, researchers should use theoretically and empirically important biomarkers in their work to further advance nursing science.

REFERENCES

Andersen, B. L., Thornton, L. M., Shapiro, C. L., Farrar, W. B., Mundy, B. L., Yang, H. C., & Carson, W. E., 3rd. (2010). Biobehavioral, immune, and health benefits following recurrence for psychological intervention participants. *Clinical Cancer Research, 16,* 3270–3278. doi:10.1158/1078-0432.CCR-10-0278

Bower, J. E., Ganz, P. A., Irwin, M. R., Kwan, L., Breen, E. C., & Cole, S. W. (2011). Inflammation and behavioral symptoms after breast cancer treatment: Do fatigue, depression, and sleep disturbance share a common underlying mechanism? *Journal of Clinical Oncology, 29,* 3517–3522. doi:10.1200/JCO.2011.36.1154

Cohen, M. Z., Thompson, C. B., Yates, B., Zimmerman, L., & Pullen, C. H. (2015). Implementing common data elements across studies to advance research. *Nursing Outlook, 63,* 181–188. doi:10.1016/j.outlook.2014.11.006

Curfs, J. H., Meis, J. F., & Hoogkamp-Korstanje, J. A. (1997). A primer on cytokines: Sources, receptors, effects, and inducers. *Clinical Microbiology Review, 10,* 742–780.

Curtis, K., Osadchuk, A., & Katz, J. (2011). An eight-week yoga intervention is associated with improvements in pain, psychological functioning and mindfulness, and changes in cortisol levels in women with fibromyalgia. *Journal of Pain Research, 4,* 189–201. doi:10.2147/JPR.S22761

Davis, E. P., & Granger, D. A. (2009). Developmental differences in infant salivary alpha-amylase and cortisol responses to stress. *Psychoneuroendocrinology, 34,* 795–804. doi:10.1016/j.psyneuen.2009.02.001

European Medicines Agency. (2007). *Definitions for genomic biomarkers, pharmacogenomics, pharmacogenetics, genomic data and sample coding* (EMEA/CHMP/ICH/437986/2006). Retrieved from http://www.ema.europa.eu/docs/en_GB/document_library/Scientific_guideline/2009/09/WC500002880.pdf

Feinstein, A. R. (1987). *Clinimetrics.* New Haven, CT: Yale University Press.

Fernandez-Botran, R., Miller, J. J., Burns, V. E., & Newton, T. L. (2011). Correlations among inflammatory markers in plasma, saliva and oral mucosal transudate in post-menopausal women with past intimate partner violence. *Brain, Behavior, and Immunity, 25,* 314–321. doi:10.1016/j.bbi.2010.09.023

Field, T. (2011). Yoga clinical research review. *Complementary Therapies in Clinical Practice, 17,* 1–8. doi:10.1016/j.ctcp.2010.09.007

Ives, S. J., Blegen, M., Coughlin, M. A., Redmond, J., Matthews, T., & Paolone, V. (2011). Salivary estradiol, interleukin-6 production, and the relationship to substrate metabolism during exercise in females. *European Journal of Applied Physiology, 111,* 1649–1658. doi:10.1007/s00421-010-1789-8

Jehn, C. F., Kühnhardt, D., Bartholomae, A., Pfeiffer, S., Schmid, P., Possinger, K., … Lüftner, D. (2010). Association of IL-6, hypothalamus–pituitary–adrenal axis function, and depression in patients with cancer. *Integrative Cancer Therapies, 9,* 270–275. doi:10.1177/1534735410370036

Lester, S. R., Brown, J. R., Aycock, J. E., Grubbs, S. L., & Johnson, R. B. (2010). Use of saliva for assessment of stress and its effect on the immune system prior to gross anatomy practical examinations. *Anatomical Sciences Education, 3,* 160–167. doi:10.1002/ase.161

Libby, P., & King, K. (2015). Biomarkers: A challenging conundrum in cardiovascular disease. *Arteriosclerosis, Thrombosis, and Vascular Biology, 35,* 2491–2495. doi:10.1161/ATVBAHA.115.305233

McCarthy, A. M., Hanrahan, K., Kleiber, C., Zimmerman, M. B., Lutgendorf, S., & Tsalikian, E. (2009). Normative salivary cortisol values and responsivity in children. *Applied Nursing Research, 22,* 54–62. doi:10.1016/j.apnr.2007.04.009

O'Connor, M. F., Bower, J. E., Cho, H. J., Creswell, J. D., Dimitrov, S., Hamby, M. E., … Irwin, M. R. (2009). To assess, to control, to exclude: Effects of biobehavioral factors on circulating inflammatory markers. *Brain, Behavior, and Immunity, 23,* 887–897. doi:10.1016/j.bbi.2009.04.005

Polacchini, A., Metelli, G., Francavilla, R., Bai, G., Florean, M., Mascaretti, L. G., & Tongiorgi, E. (2015). A method for reproducible measurements of serum BDNF: Comparison of the performance of six commercial assays. *Scientific Reports, 5,* 17989. doi:10.1038/srep17989

Simon, R. (2011). Genomic biomarkers in predictive medicine. An interim analysis. *EMBO Molecular Medicine, 3*(8), 429–435. doi:10.1002/emmm.201100153

Strimbu, K., & Tavel, J. A. (2010). What are biomarkers? *Current Opinion in HIV and AIDS, 5,* 463–466. doi:10.1097/COH.0b013e32833ed177

Vrijen, C., Schenk, H. M., Hartman, C. A., & Oldehinkel, A. J. (2017). Measuring BDNF in saliva using commercial ELISA: Results from a small pilot study. *Psychiatry Research, 254,* 340–346. doi:10.1016/j.psychres.2017.04.034

Wang, R., Yan, F., Liao, R., Wan, P., Little, P. J., & Zheng, W. (2017). Role of brain-derived neurotrophic factor and nerve growth factor in the regulation of neuropeptide W in vitro and in vivo. *Molecular and Cellular Endocrinology, 447,* 71–78. doi:10.1016/j.mce.2017.02.040

Weinrib, A. Z., Sephton, S. E., Degeest, K., Penedo, F., Bender, D., Zimmerman, B., … Lutgendorf, S. K. (2010). Diurnal cortisol dysregulation, functional disability, and depression in women with ovarian cancer. *Cancer, 116,* 4410–4419. doi:10.1002/cncr.25299

Williamson, S., Munro, C., Pickler, R., Grap, M. J., & Elswick, R. K. (2012). Comparison of biomarkers in blood and saliva in healthy adults. *Nursing Research and Practice, 2012,* 246178. doi:10.1155/2012/246178

Zhou, X., Fragala, M. S., McElhaney, J. E., & Kuchel, G. A. (2010). Conceptual and methodological issues relevant to cytokine and inflammatory marker measurements in clinical research. *Current Opinion in Clinical Nutrition & Metabolic Care, 13,* 541–547. doi:10.1097/MCO.0b013e32833cf3bc

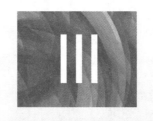

Implementing
Intervention Studies

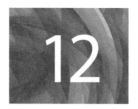

12

Developing the Budget for Intervention Studies

Steven Pease & Barbara Smith

> Ability is what you're capable of doing. Motivation determines what you do. Attitude determines how well you do it. —*Lou Holtz*

Individuals who work in research administration often hear investigators groan that there are not enough funds to complete the proposed research. It is crucial that the principal investigators (PIs) and research administrators work together *from the very beginning* to construct a budget that reflects the overall scope of the grant, includes accurate estimates of the percent effort for key personnel, and provides appropriate justification to avoid this dilemma and to ensure that the study can be completed on time and on budget. Although the budget and budget justification are critical to the successful execution of the project, it is often the last thing the PI completes prior to submission and frequently it is completed hastily by the research administrator who knows little about the science. Remember, the National Institutes of Health (NIH) and other sponsors ask those reviewing your grant to consider "whether the budget and the requested period of support are fully justified and reasonable in relation to the proposed research" (NIH, 2018). This chapter addresses preaward budget considerations, primarily for NIH-type grants, along with special issues and postaward budget management. Figure 12.1 is an example of a timeline, including budgetary priorities, used to help investigators, department chairs, and others to keep on schedule prior to submission. It reminds investigators of critical aspects of the grant that need to be completed, including the budget. You may wish to adapt this timeline to fit your own institution's policies and practices.

PRINCIPAL INVESTIGATOR: ASSIGNED TO: DUE DATE TO SPA: TO SPONSOR:

University of Maryland School of Nursing Pre-Award Checklist for Grants and Contracts

ACTION	TIME LINE	DATE	GA INITIALS	PI INITIALS
Did you receive approval from Dept Chair?	Before Director is notified			
Have you identified a biostatistician and reviewed aims?	Before Director is notified			
Notify the Director Office of Research of submission	2–3 months before grant due			
Director assigns project to Grant Administrator	1–3 days after Director notified			
Deadline dates given to PI and their support staff	1 week after Director notified			
Does PI have eRA commons account?	1 month before due			
Will project require additional space, equipment, or computers not budgeted?				
Meet with assigned Grant Administrator to begin budget process	1 week after Director notified			
Identify Key Personnel on the project	1 week after Director notified			
Include costs for biostatistician's effort in budget per policy	1 week after Director notified			
Deviations from the policy must be approved by Assoc or Asst Dean Office of Research				
If subcontracting, provide contact information to Grant Administrator 1 week after Director notified				
Review aims with Center members or a senior researcher	1 month before due			
Mock review or external review plan presented to Assoc. Dean	1 month before due			
Review near final project with Department Chair	15 days before due			
Provide purpose, aims, and either objectives, hypotheses and, or research questions; budget; and budget justification				
Director will send email to Chair (copying the PI and Grant Administrator) to confirm that the project is approved for routing on this date				
DATE TO LOAD INTO COEUS FOR REVIEW AND ROUTING	**10 business days before due**			
Final budget provided to Grant Administrator				
Proposals with cost sharing or in-kind contributions need to include cost share form				
Proposals with other UMB Schools need to include participating department form				
Subcontracts must be finalized and include				
Budget items needed: letter from authorized official, budget, justification and statement of work				
Other items needed: biosketch(es) and facilities/resources				
All documents and narrative types provided to Grants Administrator				
Abstract, specific aims, research strategy, biosketch(es), facilities, support letters and all other narrative types should be close to final				
Director pre-review documents in Coeus prior to routing	10 business days before due			
ALL FINAL DOCUMENTS LOADED INTO COEUS	**5 business days before due**			
Two day window for eRA commons corrections no longer allowed after due date				
PI and/or Grant Administrator confirm receipt of proposal	As soon as possible after submission			
PI reviewed final assembled application in eRA commons	No more than 2 days after submission			

I was informed of the expected time line for this submission and will work within the timeframes above to complete the submission on time.

Director _____ Date _____   Principal Investigator: _____ Date _____

FIGURE 12.1 Example of a timeline for grant production.

PI, principal investigator.

PREAWARD

Most sponsors provide specific guidance on budget development in the form of a funding announcement. For example, the NIH periodically releases requests for applications (RFAs), requests for proposals (RFPs), other types of funding opportunity announcements (FOAs), and/or program announcements (PAs). The acronyms may change, but the point is that these documents provide the applicant with guidance about critical aspects of the grant application including the budget. The three most important activities needing to be completed early in the grant development process that are critical to developing a fundable grant and grant budget are to (a) read the grant announcement from beginning to end, (b) reread the grant announcement carefully, and (c) finally, reread the grant announcement a third time extremely carefully and then follow the instructions meticulously.

If after reading the grant announcement you still have questions or concerns, consult with your department's research administrator and then the institution's sponsored programs office if needed. These individuals have considerable experience with many types of grants. Remember, you are the expert in the science; they are the experts in grant submissions and management. Together, you make a powerful team. If you still have questions related to the budget, do not be timid about calling the financial/grants management officer at the sponsoring agency (e.g., NIH). This person is usually listed at the end of the grant announcement. Again, do not be shy. One call can sometimes be the difference in a funded or unfunded grant.

The Budget

Agencies, foundations, and industries expect the grantees to use vastly different formats to present their budgets. Because each budget format is very different, contact the agency to determine the format that is expected. Here, we describe the two different formats (modular and detailed) that are the most common formats for NIH budgets. The budget format used usually depends on the total direct costs requested, the activity code used, and the mechanism. That is, some mechanisms that may technically fall under the modular guidelines may require a detailed budget, so, again, *read* the FOA or NIH website.

Modular budgets typically are used when a domestic institution submits the grant and the direct costs of the proposed research are less than or equal to $250,000 in each year of your proposal. If *any 1 year* of your budget exceeds $250,000 in direct costs, then a detailed budget must be submitted. A subcontractor's facilities and administration (F&A) costs are excluded for the purpose of calculating the modular direct cost cap. One advantage of using the modular budget is that specific items of cost do not need to be justified. However, all personnel should be thoroughly justified, including key personnel, nonkey personnel, consultants, and other significant contributors, even if the contributors are at no cost. Consortium costs are rounded to the nearest $1,000 but, again, *only personnel* are justified. Another advantage is that your budget requests are made in increments of $25,000. For example, after building your institutional budget, *not* the NIH budget, if the direct costs are greater than $225,000, you will actually request $250,000. Any variation in the number of modules requested also must be explained.

As mentioned earlier, a *detailed budget* and justification must be used when the budget exceeds $250,000 per year in direct costs, or the FOA requires a detailed budget. Major cost categories include key/senior personnel, other personnel, equipment, supplies, travel, patient care, other direct costs, and indirect costs. Foreign institutions submitting grants must *always* use the detailed budget regardless of the funds being requested.

Review the grant announcement carefully for budget limitations. The grant announcement sometimes will limit applications by *total costs* and other times by *direct costs*. A proposal that is limited by total costs must take into account the institution's **F&A costs**, which reduce the available funding to conduct the study. For example, assuming your institution has a 50% F&A rate, a limit of $250,000 *total* costs means the F&A portion of your budget must be taken out of the $250,000. Assuming there are no exclusions to F&A, $250,000 divided by 1.50 is $166,667 direct costs plus $83,333 F&A costs. Conversely, a grant announcement that limits *direct* costs to $250,000 per year would actually mean $250,000 in direct costs plus an F&A cost of $125,000. Total costs would be $375,000 per year. The PI must decide if the grant announcement is appropriate for conducting the science he or she is proposing before using a particular grant announcement. Consult your department's research administrator if you need help in making this decision.

Finally, if any 1 year of the grant budget exceeds $500,000 in direct costs, then permission from the NIH to submit the proposal must be obtained 6 to 8 weeks before the grant's due date. Be certain to contact the project officer at the institute that will likely fund your proposal. If it is determined to be scientifically meritorious, a cover letter is required stating that permission was given by an authorized official at the specific institute that will likely fund the proposal. However, the agency's approval to submit the proposal does not mean that it will be funded.

Select Items of Cost
Senior/Key Personnel
It is essential that a strong team with the proper blend of scientific and technical experts be assembled to accomplish the aims of the proposed research for a project to be successful. The NIH defines key personnel as the PI and any other individuals "who contribute to the scientific development or execution of a project in a substantive, measurable way, whether or not salaries are requested" (Department of Health and Human Services, 2018, p. 21). These are usually individuals who have terminal degrees (e.g., PhD, MD, and DDS) and possess expertise that cannot be easily replaced. Biostatisticians are often key personnel and including them with committed effort in your budget will strengthen your overall proposal. Do not shortchange these members of your team because they are essential and the Center for Scientific Review (CSR) at the NIH is including one or two biostatisticians on most scientific review panels, and the feasibility of the biostatistician's proposed effort is coming under closer scrutiny.

Estimating effort for personnel is often difficult because priorities shift as the research progresses. In the early stage of building your budget, an easy way to think about effort is to estimate the number of days in a week that each person on the project team will be working to accomplish his or her tasks. One day per week committed to a project equals 20% effort. Although this does not meet the NIH's strictest definition of effort, it is a good rule of thumb to use in building a budget. When awarded, your research administrator will make sure that efforts comply with federal policy.

When you need someone on your grant on a periodic basis, determining effort can be complicated. Consider the biostatistician who is assigned 20% to your grant. In the grant preparation stage, he or she needs to be involved in developing the specific aims and the hypotheses, analytical plan, and sample size/power calculation. In the first weeks or months after a grant is awarded, the biostatistician, if not involved earlier, may be used to review your aims and be certain of the analysis plan. He or she may help set up databases and your random assignment schema, and help train data entry and data management folks. He or she may work 50% time on your grant for a period of time to accomplish these tasks. Once these tasks are completed, there may be some downtime for the biostatistician until the data start coming in. As data begin to be entered, you may want to have the biostatistician supervising personnel hired to manage the data, assess the quality of the data, and identify problems.

Believe it or not, cleaning the data set and ensuring the quality of the data are the most time-consuming tasks for a biostatistician.

With new requirements for more rapid dissemination of research results, many investigators are trying to get their preliminary data out much sooner. This takes time and the statistician often needs to run the analysis several times or several different ways. Also, do not forget those data-based abstracts that you want to submit for presentations at conferences. Someone needs to be conducting the analyses for those abstracts and assisting in the writing of the parsimonious results section of the abstract. This is another reason you do not want to shortchange the effort of your biostatistician. The PI and the biostatistician need to work closely and collaboratively to achieve this goal. At this stage, the biostatistician may again be working far more than 1 day per week.

The NIH now requires that effort is shown in terms of person months committed to the project and not as a percentage. An example of this is a faculty member on a 12-month appointment committing 20% effort to a project, which is 2.4 person months. We show both on our template spreadsheet (Figure 12.2) to clarify person months. A detailed description of this and a conversion spreadsheet can be found at grants.nih.gov/grants/policy/person_months_faqs.htm#1040

Other Personnel

Postdoctoral associates, graduate students, other professionals, and support staff are included under this category. Although some scientists believe that these personnel are essential, they are best not treated as key personnel because they could be replaced relatively easily. If you list these individuals as key personnel and they are named in the notice of award, significant changes to their effort will require prior permission from your NIH project administrator. Administrative staff, such as research administrators and administrative assistants (secretaries), is not an allowable cost on many types of grant applications. However, some large center grants and program projects do allow administrative core costs, so it is important to read the FOA thoroughly before ruling them out and trying to keep these costs to a minimum.

Fringe Benefits

These costs are included on the personnel line and vary from one institution to another. Institutions set their own policy on the costs, so confirm the proper rate to use with your institution's sponsored projects office.

Consultants are individuals who typically are experts in the specific field being studied and will provide their advice or services for a fee. Consultants are *not* normally employees of the institution submitting the application. In situations where a consultant is serving as both a consultant and an employee of the same institution, work closely with your sponsored programs office to establish written guidelines outlining the conditions for payment of consulting fees to avoid apparent or actual conflicts of interest. Consultants can be very cost-effective by adding significant strength to the project with minimal expense. They should provide strong evidence of their expertise and a scope of work for their service. Payment terms will be determined as either a daily or an hourly amount or by task/deliverable.

Consultants

Consultants may be considered key personnel if justified thoroughly. In the postaward period, your institution will likely require that a purchase order (PO) be set up prior to the consultant beginning his or her work and may ask investigators for a rigorous sole source justification. Therefore, be sure to justify the consultant's expertise and the level of payment for both the granting agency and your own institution.

PRINCIPAL INVESTIGATOR	DR. A
PROJECT TITLE	The Study of Interventions
Date	July 1, 2012 - June 20, 2014

Personnel	Current Salary	Salary (3%)	100,00% Base	% Effort	Person Months to Project	Salary Request	Fringe Benefits (30.0%)	YEAR 1 Total	YEAR 2 Total
Dr. A	150,000	154,500	154,500	20.0%	2.40	30,900	9,270	40,170	
Dr. B	100,000	103,000	103,000	20.0%	2.40	20,600	6,180	26,780	
Biostatistician	80,000	82,400	82,400	15.0%	1.80	12,360	3,708	16,068	
Project Supervisor	50,000	51,500	51,500	100.0%	12.00	51,500	15,450	66,950	
Research Assistant	30,000	36,050	36,050	100.0%	12.00	36,050	10,815	46,865	
YEAR 2									
Dr. A	154,500	159,135	159,135	20.0%	2.40	31,827	9,548		41,375
Dr. B	103,000	106,090	106,090	15.0%	1.80	15,914	4,774		20,688
Biostatistician	82,400	84,872	84,872	10.0%	1.20	8,487	2,546		11,033
Project Supervisor	51,500	53,045	53,045	100.0%	12.00	53,045	15,914		68,959
Research Assistant	36,050	37,132	37,132	100.0%	12.00	37,132	11,140		48,272
					Subtotal	151,410	45,423	196,833	190,327

Consultants

	Description	Unit Cost	# of Units	Total Cost			
	Dr. Z	100.00	10.00	1,000.00			
				0.00			
			Subtotal	1,000.00		1,000	1,000

Equipment

	Description	Unit Cost	# of Units	Total Cost			
	Centrifuge	15,000.00	1.00	15,000.00			
				0.00			
			Subtotal	15,000.00		15,000	0

Supplies

	Description	Unit Cost	# Units	Total Cost			
	Binders	5.00	50.00	250.00			
	Test tubes	1.00	1,000.00	1,000.00			
	Shipping boxes	5.00	20.00	100.00			
	Tape, gauze, misc	10.00	10.00	100.00			
			Subtotal	1,450.00		1,450	1,450

Travel

	Description	Unit Cost	# Units	Total Cost			
	Local	0.50	500.00	250.00			
	National	1,500.00	2.00	3,000.00			
			Subtotal	3,250.00		3,250	3,250

Patient Care Costs

	Description	Unit Cost	# Units	Total Cost			
	Blood tests	100.0	100.00	10,000.00			
				0.00			
			Subtotal	10,000.00		10,000	10,000

Other Expenses

	Description	Unit Cost	# Units	Total Cost			
	Subject incentives	100.00	10.00	1,000.00			
	Subject parking	100.00	5.00	500.00			
	Courier	10.00	100.00	1,000.00			
	Publication	100.00	10.00	1,000.00			
	Service contract	500.00		0.00	year 2 only		
			Subtotal	3,500.00		3,500	4,000

Consortium/Contractual Direct Costs

					Subtotal	50,000	50,000

Consortium/Contractual F&A Costs

					Subtotal	25,000	25,000

TOTAL DIRECT COSTS		306,033	285,027	591,060
F&A BASE		231,033	225,027	456,060
F&A COSTS	50%	115,517	112,514	228,030
	GRAND TOTAL	421,550	397,541	819,090

FIGURE 12.2 Detailed budget for a 2-year grant application.

F&A, facilities and administrative costs.

Equipment

Although each institution can establish its own definition of equipment, the NIH provides guidance: The definition for equipment, as stated in 45 CFR Parts 74 and 92, is an article of tangible nonexpendable personal property having a useful life of more than one year and an acquisition cost of $5,000 or more per unit. However, consistent with recipient organizational policy, lower limits may be established (45 CFR Part 74.2 and 74.34 and NIHGPS; NIH, 2010). Only equipment needed for the project should be included in the budget. If equipment already exists at your institution, upgrading it to meet the needs of your proposal is a good way to lower cost to sponsor and demonstrate good financial stewardship.

Supplies

Consumable materials and supplies directly related to the execution of the study should be budgeted. Examples of this would be a study binder for each subject enrolled, specimen containers, test tubes, tape, gauze, and shipping boxes, just to name a few of the incidentals needed. Any special software needed for subject testing and encryption software to keep subject files secure are necessary and are often forgotten in budgets. Also, include anything that you or your research administrator might call "equipment," but falls under the $5,000 NIH definition of equipment, such as a rodent or human treadmill.

Travel

Costs for travel to study sites and travel related to dissemination of results at national or international conferences should be budgeted. International travel will be highly scrutinized and, therefore, should be thoroughly justified. Travel costs are much easier to estimate because mileage can easily be obtained using a mapping site found on the Internet. Flight and hotel costs can be obtained readily as well. First-class air travel is not allowed.

Patient Care Costs

Both inpatient and outpatient costs for laboratory tests should be included. Try to negotiate a "research rate" for all physiological testing from your institution and make sure to get it in writing. Often, the research rate will not include interpretation of the test results, so make certain you have a contingency plan if an interpretation is needed. For example, you may need a graded exercise test with continuous electrocardiogram (ECG). If you have an exercise physiologist, a cardiac nurse practitioner, or a cardiologist as a member of your team, he or she can interpret the test.

Other Expenses

When purchasing equipment, the manufacturer will often include a 1-year service agreement or warranty, so remember to include these costs in future years to cover annual renewal of the service contracts. A log book should be kept of all users for shared equipment, so an estimated proportion of a service contract and equipment depreciation can be budgeted. Incentives for enrolling subjects into the study and parking costs for them also should be included. Do not forget to include courier costs for getting fresh samples to the laboratory. Publication costs are another important item to include in the budget because many publishers charge the author per page and may add costs for color images.

Subcontracts

Experts in the field are often needed from other institutions. A consortium arrangement is needed between the two institutions to properly account for their effort costs and each institution's F&A. Any costs related to this portion of the proposal must be allocated to the subcontract. When using the modular budget format for an NIH proposal, a subcontractor's F&A costs are not included in the $250,000 direct cost cap.

Indirect Costs

Each institution negotiates its own F&A rate (indirect costs or overhead) with a funding agency. With biomedical research, the funding agency is often the Department of Health and Human Services. The NIH proposals use modified total direct costs to calculate the amount of funding that will be provided for your F&A. The first step in calculating this amount is to determine your F&A base. The F&A base is your total direct costs minus costs budgeted for equipment, patient care, tuition, and consortium costs over $25,000. Once the base dollar amount is calculated, multiply it by your F&A rate as shown in Figure 12.2.

There are different, usually lower F&A rates for projects that are conducted primarily off-site from the institution. Contact your sponsored program office for your institution's rate and to discuss whether you are applying the definitions of "off-site" appropriately. Institutions also have different F&A rates for industry-sponsored projects, but these rates, which are usually lower, are on the basis of total direct costs without the exclusions listed earlier. Because each institution negotiates its own rate periodically, make sure to check with your sponsored project office for the most current rates before building your budget.

Unallowable Costs

Many investigators would like to include costs for items such as renovations to facilities, honoraria, food, and excessive travel. Although not absolutely unallowable, these items will be scrutinized and need to be thoroughly justified.

A 2-year detailed budget is presented in Figure 12.2. Salaries in the additional years are normally inflated at 3%, but each person's effort may vary depending on the needs of the project. Significant variations should be well justified. Please note how quickly the costs add up, and this inflation factor may push your budget to more than the $250,000 limit for a modular budget. Some institutions attempt to keep salaries constant over the years of the grant to avoid the need for a detailed budget. However, if that is the case, the investigators may be doing the same amount of work on the grant but their percentage effort decreases. If the effort is declining, that is not a problem, but you must justify the reduced effort.

A spreadsheet like in Figure 12.2 can be used to estimate costs for an industry/ commercially sponsored intervention as well. Some differences are that the costs to the sponsor are usually presented on a per subject basis and may include additional funds for start-up such as effort-related protocol development and review.

Budget Justification

The budget justification is a critical component of your grant application. Each item in the budget for a grant application must be appropriately justified. Remember, justify, justify, and justify! An example of a budget justification for a funded NIH grant is included in Exhibit 12.1.

POSTAWARD BUDGET MANAGEMENT

After funding decisions have finally been made by the sponsor, you now need to get down to business and actually begin the proposed study. That is when a PI may say, "The good news is that I got the grant, and the bad news is I got the grant." In terms of the budget, the majority

(text continues on page 199)

EXHIBIT 12.1 Budget Justification for COPE/Healthy Lifestyles for Teens:
A School-Based RCT[a]

PERSONNEL

Bernadette Mazurek Melnyk, Principal Investigator, PhD, RN, CPNP/PMHNP, FAANP, FNAP, FAAN

2.40 person months in all project years

Dr. Melnyk will serve as the PI for this study. She is a seasoned pediatric nurse practitioner/child–family psychiatric nurse practitioner and a nationally recognized expert in child and adolescent mental health as well as RCTs and evidence-based practice.

Dr. Melnyk founded and provides the leadership for the NAPNAP KySS Campaign, a national initiative to improve the mental health of children and adolescents. In her role as director of this campaign, she spearheaded major national interdisciplinary initiatives to improve child and adolescent mental health, such as (a) conducting a 24-state survey to assess the mental health knowledge, attitudes, and needs of teens, parents, and primary healthcare providers; (b) chairing a national mental health summit that convened more than 70 leading experts in pediatrics/adolescence and mental health; (c) editing the recently published *KySS Guide to Child & Adolescent Mental Health Screening, Early Intervention and Health Promotion*; (d) implementing the KySS Institute for primary care and school-based providers that assisted interdisciplinary healthcare providers in learning how to better screen and intervene early for children and teens with mental health problems; and (e) spearheading the HRSA-funded KySS Fellowship Program, an online faculty-guided child and adolescent mental health continuing education program for nurse practitioners and physicians. Dr. Melnyk has been PI for a series of 10 RCTs over the past two decades, including two NIH-funded multisite experimental studies with an oversight of large interdisciplinary research teams. She also recently served as a member of the American Academy of Pediatrics' Mental Health Task Force and is a member of the U.S. Preventive Services Task Force.

Dr. Melnyk will ensure the scientific quality of the proposed study and assume the lead responsibility for oversight of the planning and conduct of the project. She will share responsibility for the data analytic strategy and data interpretation with her coinvestigators. She will have the primary responsibility for most reports, presentations, and manuscripts that are outcomes of the project. The NIH salary cap is being used for Dr. Melnyk.

Mary Z. Mays, PhD, Coinvestigator, Associate Professor

0.63 person month academic year and 0.21 person month summer in year 1; 0.90 person month academic year and 0.30 person month summer in years 2 to 3; 1.35 person months academic year and 0.45 person month summer in year 4

Mary Z. Mays, PhD, is a research associate professor and a biostatistician in the Office for Research and Scholarship. She will be a coinvestigator for the proposed study. Her extensive experience as a psychologist and seasoned biostatistician on federally funded studies and research-training grants ensures that she has in-depth knowledge and skills in conducting RCTs as well as performing complex statistical analyses. Dr. Mays has had a long-standing interest in health promotion interventions with adolescents, particularly those conducted in primary care and school-based settings. Her current research program includes community-based interventions addressing depression and substance abuse among American Indian and Hispanic adolescents. Dr. Mays will assist Dr. Melnyk with the planning, administration, and management of the proposed study and take the lead in designing the database for the study, data management, and conducting the planned statistical analysis. She will be a coauthor on all reports, presentations, and manuscripts that are outcomes of the project.

(continued)

EXHIBIT 12.1 Budget Justification for COPE/Healthy Lifestyles for Teens:
A School-Based RCT[a] *(continued)*

Flavio Marsiglia, PhD, Coinvestigator, Distinguished Foundation Professor of Cultural Diversity and Health/Center Director

0.90 person month academic year and 0.30 person month summer in all project years

Dr. Marsiglia is the distinguished foundation professor of Cultural Diversity and Health. He has demonstrated a sustained, high level of productivity, expertise, research accomplishments, and contributions to the field. He serves as PI of the Southwest Interdisciplinary Center, supported by both the NIH/NIDA and the Arizona Board of Regents. In addition, Dr. Marsiglia has been and is a PI and co-PI in other studies funded by the NIH/NIDA and CDC. He is a recognized leader in the field of culturally grounded prevention with expertise in minority populations and special needs populations, including his work as professor within the school of social work. Dr. Marsiglia participates actively in training/mentoring future researchers. The National Hispanic Science Network recently awarded him the National Mentorship Award for his "outstanding mentorship in the area of Hispanic drug abuse research to Hispanic graduate students and new investigators." Demonstrating a consistent record of outstanding research productivity, including program research funding and record of publication of scientific reports, such as publication of influential research papers or seminal theoretical papers, Dr. Marsiglia's recognition as a leading scientist has been reinforced by his ability to develop and maintain a high-quality environment for rigorous scientific investigations and the development of evidence-based practices throughout his areas of expertise. He has conducted numerous school-based intervention studies with Hispanic populations, including training teachers from 65 schools in Arizona to deliver his substance use prevention intervention, which will be invaluable to the proposed project. Dr. Marsiglia and Dr. Melnyk, along with their faculty researchers, have a close interdisciplinary working relationship already established from multiple collaborative research initiatives. Dr. Marsiglia will work with Dr. Melnyk and the research team to ensure that the interventions and interpretation of study findings are culturally sensitive. He will assist in training members of the research team on cultural sensitivity and work with them to address potential confounding variables in school-based settings. He will be a coauthor on reports and publications that stem from the findings. Dr. Marsiglia also will assist in forming and spearheading the community advisory board that will be assembled to address any issues of potential distrust, particularly as part of recruitment and ethics among a historically disadvantaged population. He has a long history of working with community advisory boards in his research.

Judith O'Haver, PhD, CPNP, Investigator, Assistant Professor

0.90 person month academic year and 0.30 person month summer in all project years

Dr. O'Haver is a seasoned pediatric nurse practitioner who recently completed her PhD at the University of Arizona and assumed an assistant professor position. She has been a part of Dr. Melnyk's team for the past 2 years in conducting their latest pilot intervention study (preliminary study #4) testing the COPE program with Hispanic high school teens. In her role on preliminary study #4, she delivered the attention control intervention to the high school teens. She will assist in training the teachers who will be delivering the attention-control interventions, monitor the integrity of the study, and also oversee data entry and verification for the proposed study.

Gabriel Q. Shaibi, PhD, PT, Coinvestigator, Assistant Professor

0.45 person month academic year and 0.15 person month summer in all project years

Dr. Shaibi is an assistant professor of nursing and exercise physiology. He has extensive experience working with overweight minority youth in both research and clinical settings. He completed his doctoral degree in biokinesiology and physical therapy at the University of Southern California with a focus on cardiorespiratory fitness, exercise, and metabolic disease risk in minority youth. Dr. Shaibi is a certified strength and conditioning specialist who has developed and assessed exercise programs for diverse populations. In addition, he has previous research experience assessing cardiorespiratory

(continued)

EXHIBIT 12.1 Budget Justification for COPE/Healthy Lifestyles for Teens: A School-Based RCT[a] *(continued)*

fitness, strength, and insulin resistance in overweight youth and has published several manuscripts on the subject. Prior to graduate studies, Dr. Shaibi was a public school teacher in Los Angeles and has worked on several school-based research projects. Dr. Shaibi has been a member of Dr. Melnyk's research team for the past year and an integral part of a recent study that tested the efficacy of the COPE intervention delivered in the context of a three-credit course to college freshmen. He designed and monitored the physical activity component during each COPE session and will do the same for the proposed study.

Leigh Small, PhD, RN, CPNP, Coinvestigator, Assistant Professor

0.45 person month academic year and 0.15 person month summer in all project years

Dr. Small is currently an assistant professor in the tenure track. She has been mentored throughout her doctoral program and early research career by Dr. Melnyk, and the two investigators are currently continuing their collaborative research projects together that are focused on theory-based interventions to improve health outcomes in high-risk children and adolescents, with a strong focus on the prevention and early treatment of overweight children and teens. Dr. Small is the PI of a NIH-funded R15 grant award to pilot test the efficacy of a primary care intervention for preschoolers who are overweight or at risk for overweight and their parents, with Dr. Melnyk as a coinvestigator. Dr. Small has been a coinvestigator on the preliminary studies for the proposed project and coauthor on several of Dr. Melnyk's publications. She will specifically assist in monitoring the integrity of the COPE intervention sessions being delivered in the study and assist Dr. Melnyk in training the teachers for the study. She will be a coauthor on reports and publications that are outcomes of the project.

Michael Belyea, PhD, Investigator/Statistician, Research Professor

0.27 person month academic year and 0.09 person month summer in year 1; 0.45 person month academic year and 0.15 person month summer in year 4

Dr. Belyea is currently a research professor. He is a nationally recognized statistician who has been a coinvestigator on numerous federally funded research projects where he has planned and conducted the statistical analyses. Dr. Belyea is an expert in structural equation modeling and hierarchical linear modeling who has taught courses on regression, the analysis of experimental designs, longitudinal methods and analysis, and structural equation modeling. He has a doctorate in sociology from North Carolina State University and a biostatistics postdoc from the University of North Carolina, where he specialized in medical sociology and statistics. Before joining the College of Nursing, he taught doctoral statistical courses and consulted in the Research Support Center at the School of Nursing at University of North Carolina. Dr. Belyea will assist Dr. Mays in planning and conducting the structural equation modeling and hierarchical linear modeling of study data in years 1 and 4.

OTHER PERSONNEL

Diana Jacobson, MS, RN, CPNP, Part-Time Project Co-Coordinator and Investigator

6.00 person months in all project years

Diana Jacobson is a seasoned master's-prepared pediatric nurse practitioner and doctoral candidate, with more than 15 years of practice experience in pediatric primary care practice. She joined Dr. Melnyk's research team as project coordinator in January 2005 and has been responsible for detailed oversight of the research assistants and detailed processes for two pilot RCTs that tested Dr. Melnyk's COPE/Healthy Lifestyles TEEN program with adolescents in two inner city high schools and also with a three-credit course for college freshmen testing the COPE program. She also was trained on administration of the COPE program and provided the intervention at one of the study sites. Ms. Jacobson will meet regularly with Dr. Melnyk and members of the research team, including the intervention research assistants and the data collectors. She will assume the following responsibilities: assist in the initial and ongoing

(continued)

EXHIBIT 12.1 Budget Justification for COPE/Healthy Lifestyles for Teens: A School-Based RCT[a] *(continued)*

training of study staff, organize the timing of the subject contact points over the course of the study, organize and track incoming data, create the majority of the databases and data code book for the study, maintain data files and records, and organize measures and materials prior to and following their completion. She also will assist in training the teachers on COPE and monitoring the integrity of the intervention as it is delivered in the high schools. Ms. Jacobson will assist in conducting the initial review of lab results from the adolescents' blood work as well as cleaning data and assisting with the conduct of preliminary analyses under the direction of Dr. Mays. Because of the size of this intervention trial and involvement of several participating classrooms at various high schools located in separate districts, outstanding oversight and coordination are required. With the extent of data collection, it is necessary to have a FTE of a project coordinator who will be shared between Ms. Jacobson and Ms. Kelly.

Stephanie Kelly, MS, RN, FNP, Part-Time Project Co-Coordinator and Investigator

6.00 person months in all project years

Stephanie Kelly is a family nurse practitioner with a research interest in adolescent overweight/obesity and currently a doctoral student. She joined Dr. Melnyk's research team during her PhD program and has been heavily involved in the pilot studies for this project. She recruited subjects and assisted in the delivery of the COPE intervention in preliminary study #4 and was involved in testing the efficacy of a lengthened version of the COPE program as a three-credit course with college freshmen. She will assume cocoordinator responsibilities as outlined for this project with Ms. Jacobson as well as provide assistance in the recruitment of subjects into the study and monitoring the integrity of the interventions. She also will assist in cleaning data and assist with the conduct of preliminary analyses under the direction of Dr. Mays.

Because of the size of this intervention trial and involvement of several participating classrooms at various high schools located in separate districts, outstanding coordination and oversight of this project are required. With the extent of data collection, it is necessary to have a full FTE of a project coordinator who will be shared between Ms. Jacobson and Ms. Kelly.

TBA, Data Input Operator

7.20 person months in years 1 to 3; 3.60 person months in year 4 (6 months)

Because of the large amount of data being collected, we are requesting a data input operator who will be responsible primarily for assisting with entering the large amount of data obtained from the subjects in this study.

TBA, Research Nurses

Two at 6.00 person months each in years 1 to 3; 3.00 person months each in year 4 (6 months)

These two individuals will be master's-prepared nurse practitioners who will be responsible for recruiting subjects into the study and assisting with the monitoring of the integrity of the intervention at the high schools. We will recruit for at least one of these research nurses to be a Hispanic bilingual Spanish speaker who will be able to communicate well with the Spanish-speaking parents in the study.

TBA, Data Collection Research Assistants

Two at 4.50 person months each academic year and 1.50 person months each summer in years 1 to 3; 2.25 person months each academic year and 0.75 person month each summer in year 4 (6 months)

These individuals will be nurse practitioner, psychology, or social worker doctoral students who will be responsible for collecting the baseline, immediate postintervention, as well as 6- and 12-month follow-up assessments on all participating adolescents and parents. They also will assist with data entry and verification of the study data. Dr. Melnyk currently has four doctoral students working with her research team, and there is an abundance of doctoral students in nursing, psychology, and social work throughout the university. The pay rate being requested is $25.00 per hour.

(continued)

EXHIBIT 12.1 Budget Justification for COPE/Healthy Lifestyles for Teens: A School-Based RCT[a] *(continued)*

SUPPLIES (TOTAL = $52,453)

Desktop computers, desktop printers, large-capacity printer, and printer supplies ($11,900): Three desktop computers (Dell OptiPlex 755 Minitower Intel Core 2 Duo Processor E6750, 2.66 GHz, 4M, VT, 1,333 MHz FSB, Genuine Windows XP Professional, DVD player/CD burner, and 19-inch UltraSharp 1908FP flat panel monitor) at a cost of $1,450 each, three desktop printers (HP Deskjet 6940) at a cost of $100 each, and one large-capacity printer (HP Color LaserJet CP3505n) at a cost of $850 will be used by the PI and research assistants to enter data and print the 16-session color intervention materials for the 600 teen participants, and the four-session color intervention materials for the 600 parent participants. Printer supplies in the amount of $1,600 are requested in years 1 to 4.

Laptop computers ($3,500): Two laptop computers (Dell Latitude D630 notebook, Intel Core 2 Duo T7300, 2.00 GHz, 4M L2 Cache, 800 MHz Dual Core, Windows XP Professional) at a cost of $1,750 each will be shared between the interventionists who will be delivering the PowerPoint presentations/interventions in every health class offered in the four high schools.

Filing cabinets ($1,750): Two locking four-drawer lateral filing cabinets at a cost of $875 each are necessary to store and secure the 1,200 completed, confidential questionnaires from both the teens and the parents in the study office.

Office supplies ($16,108): General office supplies will be drawn from the university's facilities and administrative costs. However, beyond this amount, we are requesting funding for the following designated items to be used specifically for this project:

Paper ($150 = 1 box = 5,000 sheets): The paper will be used for printing the study materials, such as informed consents, instrument packets, and the 16-session teen intervention materials.

Hanging file folders ($720 = $30/box × 24 boxes = 800 file folders): Each teen study participant will require coded hanging folders for completed study materials.

9 × 12 envelopes ($150 = $50/box × 3 boxes = 800 envelopes): Large mailing envelopes will be required to mail study questionnaires to the parent participants.

Labels ($1,200 = $80/box × 15 boxes = 60,000 labels): Labels are required to attach a coded identification number to each page of the consent/assent forms and the questionnaires.

Teen notebooks and dividers ($12,800 = $16/notebook × 800 teens): Teen notebooks with dividers are required for the teens to store their intervention materials as they are given to them at each of the 16 intervention sessions.

Facilitator notebooks and dividers ($1,088 = $34/notebook × 32 facilitators): Teachers will be given an entire notebook of intervention materials at the training sessions to be held at the beginning of the study.

Study instruments ($2,955): Research instruments will be purchased in the first year. The *BYI* is available for use only through purchase at Harcourt Assessment and comes with 25 in each packet (800 teen participants/25 BYI per packet = 33 packets × $85 per packet = $2,805). The manual of the BYI is required for data analysis ($150).

Physical measurement supplies ($1,680): Physical measurements of weight and height will be measured on each of the 800 participants at the eight high schools. Stadiometers (8 × $130 each = $1040) and scales (8 × $80 each = $640) will be required to collect these measurements.

Pedometers ($14,560): Pedometers (800 × [$17.95 + $0.25 freight] each = $14,560) will be given to each teen participant to directly measure physical activity throughout the study.

(continued)

EXHIBIT 12.1 Budget Justification for COPE/Healthy Lifestyles for Teens: A School-Based RCT[a] *(continued)*

TRAVEL (TOTAL = $28,042)

Travel for research team to the study sites for recruitment, monitoring integrity of the interventions, and data collection ($11,392): Funds are needed for reimbursement for local travel costs to and from the university for study recruitment (3 trips × 8 schools × 8 recruitments = $2,136); monitoring the integrity of the interventions (2 trips per week × 9 weeks × 8 schools = $6,408); and baseline, postintervention, as well as 6- and 12-month follow-up data collection (8 trips to 8 schools × 4 data collection points = $2,848). The distance for one round trip was estimated at 25 miles, and multiplied by the institution's current mileage reimbursement rate of $0.445 was used for the calculations.

Travel for conferences ($16,650): Funding for the PI and one coinvestigator to attend a professional conference for the exchange of information and presentation of papers is requested for years 1, 2, and 3 (2 trips × 3 years = $11,100). The PI and two coinvestigators will attend a professional conference in year 4 (3 trips × 1 year = $5,550). Estimated cost of conference travel for each person is $1,850, which includes conference registration, transportation, hotel, and meal expenses.

OTHER (TOTAL = $108,964)

Incentives for the teens and parents ($92,000): The study incentives, although minimal, will demonstrate the value of the teens' and parents' participation throughout the study.

Teen incentives: All teens will receive incentive department store gift cards for the completion of each set of study questionnaires. Total incentives for each teen participant = $55 over the course of the project ($55 × 800 teen participants = $44,000).

Parent incentives: All parents will receive incentive monies for the completion of their questionnaires at the beginning and end of the study. Total incentives for each parent = $60 over the course of the project. Parents will receive $30 for completing the first set of questionnaires, and $30 for an evaluation questionnaire at the end of the study on whether and how they think the program was helpful for their teens ($60 × 800 parent participants = $48,000).

Teacher training sessions ($9,700): Training for the teachers who will be delivering the intervention will take place during an intensive training session that will be offered four times during the summer prior to the beginning of the school year. We estimate that between the two school districts and eight high schools participating, 32 teachers will need to be trained in the intervention over the course of the 4-year study. Each teacher will be given a $250 incentive for his or her participation and training ($250 × 32 teachers = $8,000). The training will begin early in the day and continue until late afternoon. Therefore, catered food will be ordered for breakfast and lunch during the 4 days of training, at a cost of $425/day ($425 × 4 days = $1,700).

Postage ($7,264): Funds for postage are requested and will be used to send out reminder postcards to the teen participants (4 postcards × 800 teen participants × $0.27 postage per postcard = $864) and to send the questionnaire packets to the parents (4 packets × 800 parents × $2.00 postage per packet = $6,400).

[a]Principal investigator: Bernadette Melnyk. Funded by the National Institutes of Health/National Institute of Nursing Research (1R01NR012171.

BYI, Beck Youth Inventory; CDC, Centers for Disease Control and Prevention; COPE, Creating Opportunities for Parent Empowerment; FTE, full-time equivalent; HRSA, Health Resources and Services Administration; KySS, Keep your children/yourself safe and secure; NAPNAP, National Association of Pediatric Nurse Practitioners; NIDA, National Institute on Drug Abuse; NIH, National Institutes of Health; PI, principal investigator; RCT, randomized controlled trial.

of the costs for the project have been planned and discussed. A start-up meeting with your research administrator/financial manager is the best approach so you both have an idea of how the costs should be set up in your electronic financial system and continue throughout the course of the study. Managing a budget reduction, which is common in today's economy, is discussed in the section Special Issues.

Financial accounting systems used by institutions are almost as numerous as the number of institutions. Many systems do the job well, but can be confusing for some investigators; thus, many research administrators/managers develop their own shadow systems to assist investigators and their project managers in understanding budget, expenses, and balances available. Even though some investigators want to start spending quickly, you have to remember that the notice of grant award (NGA) does not provide an open checkbook. As stated in the beginning, it is time to read, reread, and read the grant announcement again. Your departmental administrator/manager will be able to interpret the language in the NGA, and his or her office is a good place to kick off your discussion of "I want." Personnel salaries and the associated fringe benefits are usually the highest expense of a proposal, so it is important to get these costs set up in the financial system and encumbered as soon as possible. This information may also feed into your institution's effort reporting system.

With NIH grants, it is often several months between submission and an award being made. Changes in personnel, their availability, and/or salaries may have occurred. Subcontracts, consultant, and equipment purchases should also be processed soon after the award is received and an active account is set up.

After the initial setup, monthly meetings with the investigator and his or her project manager are the best way to keep up to date with the budget. Although most want to know only how much they have left, there are numerous financial considerations that may affect the outcome of the study. Sometimes, the NIH awards 12 months of funding in a shortened first period. This may provide a windfall of funds left over from the first period. Also, be careful not to overhire initially because that may quickly lead to a budget shortfall in the continuing years.

We developed a postaward checklist in an attempt to keep on top of some of these issues (Figure 12.3). Although developed specifically for our institution's processes, the concepts are universal and can be adapted to your institution. There are budget components, such as cost sharing and subcontracts, that may prompt additional questions and can be discussed at these monthly review sessions. Again, these questions or issues will be specific to your institution and its processes.

Regular meetings provide the framework for an active resolution of problems and issues and can help the investigator understand the fiscal complexities involved in running a smooth grant. A good administrator/manager can guide the investigator through allowable costs and the complexities involved in making purchases. Issues identified in these regular meetings can preempt catastrophic consequences. Remember that the NIH has a 90-day rule regarding cost transfers (NIH, 2017); therefore, it is just as critical to keep on top of your budget as well as your science. As President Harry Truman said, "The buck stops here!" In his case, it meant the president's office; in this case, it means the PI's office.

CLOSEOUT

The NIH requires three reports to close out a grant: (a) a final progress report on the scientific accomplishments, (b) a final financial report, and (c) a final invention statement and certification (form 568 Health and Human Services [HHS]).

University of Maryland School of Nursing Postaward Checklist for Grants and Contracts

	YES/NO	DATE
Just in Time documents sent?		
Award notice received?		
Shadow set up with original budget/personnel loaded?		
Budget/personnel modified with PI after initial set up?		

	NUMBER
Project Identification Number assigned?	

	PAPER	ELECTRONIC
Annual Progress Report due		
Final Progress Report due		
Final Invention Report due		
Financial Report due		

Discuss and assign responsibilities for data required for report

YES/NO QUESTIONS	JUL	AUG	SEP	OCT	NOV	DEC	JAN	FEB	MAR	APR	MAY	JUN
Any significant changes to budget?												
Any significant change in scope of science?												
Any new sites?												
Any new personnel?												
Any personnel leaving?												
Any personnel status changes (eg. FT to PT)?												
Any personnel changing effort to project?												
Are there any budget variances?												
Is a budget modification needed?												
Is carry forward approval needed?												
Is prior approval from sponsor needed for any other reason?												
Did monthly meeting occur? If no, note reason below												
Any cost sharing?												
OPEN IF COST SHARING NEEDED												
Any subcontractors?												
OPEN IF SUBCONTRACTORS NEEDED												
Any consultants?												
OPEN IF CONSULTANTS NEEDED												
Any other large purchase orders?												
OPEN IF LARGE PURCHASE ORDERS NEEDED												
Principal Investigator's initials												
Issues noted												
Plan for corrections												

FIGURE 12.3 An example of a postaward checklist for grants and contracts.

Because you have been meeting regularly with your manager, closing out the grant should not present any surprises for you. The institution is given a specified time, usually 90 days, after the grant's end date to wrap up loose ends. Open encumbrances need to be reviewed to make sure the vendor has been fully paid and expense allocated to the grant. POs to consultants and subcontractors are usually the final expenses that need to be resolved before a final report can be completed. Subcontractors must be allowed time to capture all of their expenses in their financial system before they can send their final invoice. Then, the PI's institution can close out the PO. After all expenses are finalized, the institution's central authorized officials will ask for review and approval by the PI before they submit the final financial report to the sponsor. The final step is for the institution's authorized official to send in (or upload) the final reports to the sponsor.

SPECIAL ISSUES

Negotiating With the Sponsor

During the period between submission and the funding award, a PI may be contacted by the sponsor to negotiate the costs of the proposal. If the sponsor requests significant reductions to the budget, be careful not to accept the NGA until you have mutually agreed on reducing the scope of work or aims of project. Research is expensive, and in today's economy it is difficult for institutions to cover the additional costs for a project that has a significant budget reduction by the sponsor. Remember, once your institution receives the NGA and costs are charged to the project, the grant has in effect been "accepted" and the sponsor expects that you can accomplish the original aims of the proposal with the reduced budget. Negotiating with the sponsor prior to receipt of the NGA will make certain that all parties are in agreement before the work begins.

Cost Sharing

There are two kinds of cost sharing, involuntary and voluntary. An example of involuntary cost sharing is the NIH's salary cap. As of January 8, 2018, the NIH's salary cap is $189,600. So, if any of the personnel on your budget have a salary greater than this amount, you or your institution is required to pay for the difference between the cap and the actual salary using other sources, while keeping the person's effort the same. There also is voluntary cost sharing. The PI or institution agrees to provide effort or materials to the project without costs to the sponsor. It is often thought that this will give them a favorable consideration over the competition. However, despite this popular myth, proposing a cost-sharing (matching) arrangement where you request that the NIH supports only some of the costs of the project while your organization funds the remainder does not impact the evaluation of your proposal. Only a few selected programs require cost sharing and these programs will address cost sharing in the FOA.

In summary, budgets are one of the most important features of your proposal. Under the new criteria for NIH reviewers, "Reviewers will consider whether the budget and the requested period of support are fully justified and reasonable in relation to the proposed research" (NIH, 2016). Careful attention to the FOA before submission and then regular meetings with your financial manager postaward will make the business end of any grant an easy task.

Key Points From This Chapter

- Read the FOA carefully, paying special attention to allowable costs and instructions for completing the budget and budget justification.
- Establish a timeline for your grant.
- Discuss any questions regarding budget with experienced staff from your sponsored projects office.
- Justify, justify, justify all components of the budget.
- Negotiate any reductions in budget with the funding agency *before* accepting the notice of grant award.
- Monitor your budget often and carefully during the course of your grant so that your project can be successfully completed.

REFERENCES

Department of Health and Human Services. (2018). Instructions for grant application using PHS 398. Retrieved from https://grants.nih.gov/grants/funding/phs398/phs398.pdf

National Institutes of Health. (2010). Frequently asked questions: Equipment under NIH grants. Retrieved from https://grants.nih.gov/grants/policy/equipment_faqs.htm#2377

National Institutes of Health. (2016). Definitions of criteria and considerations for research project grant (RPG/R01/R03/R15/R21/R34) critiques. Retrieved from https://grants.nih.gov/grants/peer/critiques/rpg.htm

National Institutes of Health. (2017). NIH grants policy statement. Retrieved from https://grants.nih.gov/grants/policy/nihgps/html5/section_7/7.5_cost_transfers__overruns__and_accelerated_and_delayed_expenditures.htm

National Institutes of Health. (2018). Definitions of criteria and considerations for research project grant (RPG/X01/R01/R03/R21/R33/R34) critiques. Retrieved from https://grants.nih.gov/grants/peer/critiques/rpg.htm

Navigating the IRB for Investigators

Amanda A. Hastings, Cheryl L. Byers, & Barry B. Bercu

> Patience, persistence, and perspiration make an unbeatable
> combination for success. —*Napolean Hill*

The **Institutional Review Board (IRB)** provides an important function in that it is responsible for the review and oversight of research involving human participants, with the goal of ensuring that the rights and welfare of the participants (also called "**human subjects**") are protected from unnecessary risks or harm. This is the overarching mission of the IRB. The process of reviewing human subject research is guided by layers of statutes, regulations, and government-issued guidance documents, oftentimes leading to long or complex forms and questionnaires aimed at providing the IRB with all of the relevant information needed to render determinations on the appropriateness of a given study. Many investigators, when faced with the prospect of filing a research protocol with the IRB for review, question whether such a cumbersome bureaucratic process is necessary. Admittedly, this is not an unfair question. However, to frame this kind of query, it is important that we first understand the principles that led to the contemporary practices and processes of the IRB.

In addition to providing some of this foundational information, this chapter focuses on the details prevalent in the human subject protection field, and provides real-world examples and advice to aid investigators in working more efficiently with the IRB. Realizing that this is an evolving field, we also invite you to consider some of the prevailing philosophical arguments within the contemporary discourse surrounding the IRB, with the recognition that even this system, with its devotion to the protection of human research participants, is not without flaws.

HISTORICAL PERSPECTIVES

A look at the historical context leading to the formation of the IRB is required to begin our conversation. Table 13.1 provides a snapshot of the key historical influences that encouraged the 93rd U.S. Congress to enact the National Research Act of 1974 (The National Commission for the Protection of Human Subjects of Biomedical and Behavioral Research [The Commission], 1979). Among the key measures established in the Act was the formation of the National Commission for the Protection of Human Subjects of Biomedical and Behavioral Research (The Commission, 1979). "One of the charges to the Commission was to identify the basic ethical principles that should underlie the conduct of biomedical and behavioral research involving human subjects and to develop guidelines which should be followed to assure that such research is conducted in accordance with those principles" (The Commission, 1979, "Summary"). The document created by the Commission, today known simply as "The Belmont Report" (https://www.hhs.gov/ohrp/regulations-and-policy/belmont-report/index.html), provided the ethical cornerstones on which human subject research is now reviewed and approved. The Belmont Report identified three basic ethical principles that must be present in considering the appropriateness of a given research protocol: respect for persons, beneficence, and justice (The Commission, 1979). As we continue our examination of the IRB, we must do so with these basic principles in mind.

TABLE 13.1 Key Historical Events	
1938	Food and Drug Act is established, outlining the need for drugs to be shown to be effective prior to the marketing of the drug. Therefore, research involving human subjects was required.
1944 to 1974	Cold War human radiation experiments occurred where the U.S. government performed thousands of radiation experiments on U.S. citizens.
1947	The Nuremburg Code defining 10 points for the conduct of ethical human experimentation was published as a result of the Nuremburg Trials. The Nuremburg Trials occurred in Nuremburg, Germany, where 20 medical doctors were tried for medical experimentation on large numbers of individuals in the Nazi concentration camps. Individuals were coerced into participating in the experiments and were not provided the opportunity to consent to the research.
1932 to 1972	Tuskegee Study of Untreated Syphilis in the Negro Male (also known as the "Tuskegee Syphilis Study" or the "Public Health Service Syphilis Study") occurred in Tuskegee, Alabama. This research project was designed to study the natural progression of untreated syphilis in poor, rural black men. By 1947, penicillin was commonly used to treat syphilis; however, treatment was withheld from participants in this study until it was exposed in 1972.
1950s	Thalidomide experiments were implemented to study how thalidomide would affect a number of ailments during pregnancy. Women were not informed of the experimental nature of the drug as this was not standard practice at the time. The result was a number of deformities with the newborn infants.
1962	Kefauver-Harris Act was passed as a result of the thalidomide experiments that required researchers to inform individuals of the experimental nature of drugs.

TABLE 13.1 Key Historical Events *(continued)*	
1963 to 1966	Willowbrook Hepatitis Study was designed to study the natural progression of hepatitis. The study was conducted at a state school (institution) in New York for children with "mental retardation." Researchers intentionally infected children with hepatitis. Entry of children into the school was only through the program
1970s	Tearoom Trade Study involved a researcher posing as a "watch queen" while individuals engaged in anonymous homosexual behavior. He obtained their identities by gathering license plate numbers and went to their homes to conduct in-depth interviews. Many of the individuals were living heterosexual lives where exposing their homosexual lifestyle would be devastating to their families. These individuals were not informed that they were a part of a research project and the resulting publication contained information that could potentially identify the individuals.
July 12, 1974	National Research Act was signed, creating the National Commission for the Protection of Human Subjects for Biomedical and Behavioral Research. The National Research Act was primarily a result of the Tuskegee Syphilis Study that was exposed in 1972.
April 18, 1979	The National Commission published the Belmont Report that outlines the basic ethical principles for the protection of human subjects.
1981	U.S. DHHS and the FDA published similar regulations on the protection of human subjects.

DHHS, Department of Health and Human Services; FDA, Food and Drug Administration.

Having received the Commission's controversial report, the U.S. Department of Health and Human Services (HHS) and the Food and Drug Administration (FDA) began to work at establishing the regulations that first created, and now guide, the IRB (HHS, 2011b). These regulations, found first at 45CFR46, and later codified by 15 agencies (HHS, 2011b) to create the "**Common Rule**," apply distinctly to human subject research that is financially supported by agencies of the U.S. government (see Table 13.2). The regulations expressly define a human subject as "a living individual about whom an investigator (whether professional or student) conducting research obtains 1) Data through intervention or interaction with the individual, or 2) Identifiable private information" (Protection of Human Subjects, 2005).

Depending on the source of funding for the research, an IRB may expect to report to a large variety of federal and state agencies, in addition to adhering to the established policies and procedures of the institution. Although the regulations are intended to guide research that is federally funded, institutions may choose to apply these regulations to all research conducted at their sites or by their employees, regardless of the source of funding (Bankert & Amdur, 2006, p. 279). An institution's decision whether to apply the regulations solely to federally funded research or to all research under its purview is subsequently communicated to HHS, the agency primarily responsible for the oversight of human subject protections, via a mechanism known as "Federalwide Assurance" (FWA; Bankert & Amdur, 2006, pp. 278–279). The FWA is the institution's statement of **assurance** to the federal government that it intends to comply with the ethical principles outlined in the Belmont Report and the Code of Federal Regulations. It provides to HHS information regarding the specific IRB or IRBs on which the institution will rely for the review, approval, and oversight of the research it plans to conduct (Bankert & Amdur, 2006, pp. 278–279). Recent regulatory changes also require the registration of IRBs that will review and approve FDA-regulated research, utilizing the same registration mechanism as HHS.

TABLE 13.2 Agencies That Adopted the Federal Regulations—45CFR46
Department of Agriculture (7 CFR Part 1c)
Department of Energy (10 CFR Part 745)
National Aeronautics and Space Administration (14 CFR Part 1230)
Department of Commerce (15 CFR Part 27)
National Institute of Standards and Technology
Consumer Product Safety Commission (16 CFR Part 1028)
Agency for International Development (22 CFR Part 255)
Department of Housing and Urban Development (24 CFR Part 60)
Department of Justice (28 CFR Part 46)
Department of Defense (32 CFR Part 219)
National Institute of Justice
Department of Education (34 CFR Part 97)
Department of Veterans Affairs (38 CFR Part 16)
Office of Research Oversight
Office of Research & Development
Environmental Protection Agency (40 CFR Part 26)
Department of Health and Human Services (45 CFR Part 46)
National Science Foundation (45 CFR Part 690)
Department of Transportation (49 CFR Part 11)

CFR, Code of Federal Regulations.

Source: U.S. Department of Health and Human Services. (2011a). Federal policy for the protection of human subjects ('common rule'). Retrieved from https://www.hhs.gov/ohrp/humansubjects/commonrule/index.html

TYPES OF IRBs: HAS THE PENDULUM SWUNG TOO FAR?

Further adding to the complexity of the research review system is the variety of types of IRBs on which investigators and institutions may choose to rely. Moving away from reviewing research solely at a local level, some institutions and/or sponsors are now relying instead on central or commercial (or independent) IRBs, or are moving to a mixed model, relying on the local IRB for some research and a nonlocal IRB for others. Like local IRBs, other IRB types are required to adhere to the federal regulations, as applicable. There are, however, pros and cons to the use of these types of IRBs.

Among the pros for relying on a nonlocal IRB, being separated from the institution insofar as they are, it is conceivable that these IRBs may not hold the same propensity as a local IRB toward the potential influence of institutional goals. There are IRB composition mandates built into the regulations that serve to prevent this sort of institutional influence, requiring, for example, that nonaffiliated parties and members representing the community serve on the IRB; however, it is not rare to encounter instances of institutional influence on the board. As another example, using a central or commercial IRB for multicenter trials is especially attractive, as it streamlines the review process, allowing for all institutions to operate under the same approval, thereby eliminating site-specific nuances to the informed consent documents or requested protocol changes. Recognizing the benefits of this centralization, many pharmaceutical companies that conduct multicenter studies, often with upwards of 50 or more sites conducting a single study, will prefer to utilize a central or commercial IRB for reasons of both efficiency and economy. By way of example, the National Cancer Institute (NCI) has established a central IRB to undertake the review of certain Cooperative Group clinical trials for pediatric and adult oncology studies that are sponsored by the NCI (www.ncicirb.org). Some institutions will also choose to rely on a nonlocal IRB for the review of research in which it holds an actual or perceived institutional conflict of interest.

Of course, there are also cons inherent in utilizing a nonlocal IRB over a local one. For example, by removing the review from a local to a central or commercial IRB, there exists the potential for a lack of awareness about community context in the deliberations of the nonlocal IRB. This is especially important as it relates to indigenous peoples or other particularly vulnerable populations whose concerns may be unique to a given region. Another criticism of the central or commercial IRB process is in the composition of the boards. As discussed earlier, the regulations mandate a minimum composition as it relates to the boards. This mandate requires that each board be composed of at least five individuals, with "at least one member whose primary concerns are in scientific areas and at least one member whose primary concerns are in nonscientific areas ..., [and] at least one member who is not otherwise affiliated with the institution ..." (Protection of Human Subjects, 2005). The authors believe that most IRBs will even go beyond the minimums required per the regulations and will require, for example, that two or more lay people participate on the board to meet the regulations and maintain **quorum**. Quorum is achieved by a majority of the registered members of the IRB being present, which must include a minimum of one layperson (i.e., nonscientist). Those critical of nonlocal IRBs may question whether they go far enough to ensure that not only are the minimum requirements met by these IRBs but whether the boards are also sufficiently composed of experts, specialists, or other particularly knowledgeable individuals to allow a thorough review of the ethical issues involved. This argument is especially poignant as it relates to large, complex, and diverse organizations such as state or private universities that promote a research agenda.

As an investigator, it is important to weigh adequately the pros and cons of the different IRB types in determining the mechanism for review and oversight of a given protocol. We suggest relying on an IRB that has been accredited by the Association for the Accreditation of Human Research Protection Programs, Inc. (AAHRPP) to aid in this endeavor. As of May 2011, the AAHRPP has accredited 228 institutions' Human Research Protection Programs (HRPPs), made up of approximately 1,100 different IRB entities (AAHRPP, 2011a). As of May 2018, there were a total of 11,235 active IRBs registered with HHS (Office for Human Research Protections [OHRP], 2011). As "an independent, non-profit accrediting body, AAHRPP uses a voluntary, peer-driven, educational model to ensure that HRPPs meet rigorous standards for quality and protection. To earn accreditation, organizations must provide tangible evidence ... of their commitment to scientifically and ethically sound research and to continuous improvement" (AAHRPP, 2011b, para. 2). Relying on an accredited IRB fosters confidence in the quality of the review conducted, in that there is assurance that the IRB maintains a staunch commitment to the protection of human research participants.

INFORMED CONSENT: WHERE ARE WE TODAY?

The concept of **informed consent** is embodied within the Belmont Report's principle of respect for persons. In obtaining an individual's informed consent prior to beginning the research, it illustrates an investigator's commitment to respecting the participant's autonomy. So often, in discussions in IRB meetings, the conversation surrounds the informed consent document. Although the document is certainly important, it is essential to note that the entirety of informed consent does not begin and end with the document; rather, informed consent is a process by which the investigator (and his or her study staff) participates with the research subject in an ongoing exchange of information about the study (HHS, 2011a). In fact, according to the federal regulatory agencies, this process begins at the time of recruitment.

In other words, although the document is the mechanism by which an investigator may illustrate his or her commitment to respecting the right of the subject to his or her autonomous decision making, it does not embody the totality of the concept. In order for consent to be truly informed, the investigator must engage with the subject in a conversation about the protocol, allowing for plenty of time for the subject to consider the risks and any potential benefits associated with participation, and providing the opportunity for the subject to rescind his or her consent to participate. These conversations should take place in a manner that respects both the privacy and the **confidentiality** of the subject, taking into account the location of the discussion about the protocol and the ways in which information is recorded during the course of the conduct of the study. The investigator must also recognize cultural differences within the study population and work to ensure that the information is presented in a culturally sensitive manner, taking into consideration issues that are particular to individual groups (e.g., Native American populations, individuals with conditions subject to stigma, prisoners). This is not something that can be communicated strictly through the use of the informed consent document.

Furthermore, many of the informed consent documents currently in use in the United States, and even abroad, are decidedly lengthy, oftentimes greater than 20 pages. Although as an industry we are instructed to ensure that the document be constructed such that it may be understood by an individual with an average reading level, somewhere between sixth and eighth grades, the litigious nature of our American society and the general complexity of much of the research prove this to be increasingly difficult. In addition to the required elements of the informed consent document (see Table 13.3), many institutions and sponsors mandate that informed consent documents contain information such as injury statements, statements of liability, Health Insurance Portability and Accountability Act (HIPAA) authorizations, and the like, thereby increasing the length and convolution of the documents.

INFORMED CONSENT: WHAT SHOULD WE CONSIDER FOR THE FUTURE?

As an industry, this leads us to question the appropriateness of our status quo. Recent developments in international informed consent documents illustrate that there may be alternatives. As conversation turns toward concepts such as tiered consents, in which a subject may choose to participate in one part of a particular study while opting out of another, IRBs are beginning to take note of new options. Some consent forms are also now being designed with a newfound simplicity in mind. By including graphical representations of procedures or interventions to be performed, inserting information into tables rather than utilizing lengthy sentences to communicate important particulars about the study, or even including figures or pictures, it is intended that the document better serve as a tool for improving the understanding of the potential subjects at the onset of the study. There are also those investigators who will break down the required elements of a consent document into a one-sheet table that encourages the potential participant to read and agree to individual statements that would be otherwise presented in paragraph form, and are thereby designed to foster the subject's comprehension of the content. In short, as our understanding of the ethical conduct of research continues to expand, so, too, does our awareness that our current practices may yet be significantly improved, such that the consent provided by a potential subject is truly informed. In other words, the construction of the informed consent document as it is currently used in the United States today is not set in stone.

TABLE 13.3 Elements of Informed Consent—45CFR46.116

REQUIRED ELEMENTS

1. A statement that the study involves research
2. An explanation of the purposes of the research
3. The expected duration of the subject's participation
4. A description of the procedures to be followed
5. Identification of any procedures that are experimental
6. A description of any reasonably foreseeable risks or discomforts to the subject
7. A description of any benefits to the subject or to others that may reasonably be expected from the research
8. A disclosure of appropriate alternative procedures or courses of treatment, if any, that might be advantageous to the subject
9. A statement describing the extent, if any, to which confidentiality of records identifying the subject will be maintained
10. For research involving more than minimal risk, an explanation as to whether any compensation is available
11. An explanation as to whether any medical treatments are available if injury occurs and, if so, what they consist of, or where further information may be obtained
12. An explanation of whom to contact for answers to pertinent questions about the research and research subjects' rights, and whom to contact in the event of a research-related injury to the subject
13. A statement that participation is voluntary, refusal to participate will involve no penalty or loss of benefits to which the subject is otherwise entitled, and that the subject may discontinue participation at any time without penalty or loss of benefits, to which the subject is otherwise entitled

ADDITIONAL ELEMENTS

14. A statement that the particular treatment or procedure may involve risks to the subject (or to the embryo or fetus, if the subject is or may become pregnant) that are currently unforeseeable
15. Anticipated circumstances under which the subject's participation may be terminated by the investigator without regard to the subject's consent
16. Any additional costs to the subject that may result from participation in the research
17. The consequences of a subject's decision to withdraw from the research, and procedures for orderly termination of participation by the subject
18. A statement that significant new findings developed during the course of the research that may relate to the subject's willingness to continue participation will be provided to the subject
19. The approximate number of subjects involved in the study

INFORMED CONSENT: SPECIAL CONSIDERATIONS FOR TRANSNATIONAL POPULATIONS

It should be noted that in recognition of the Belmont Report's principles of justice and respect for persons, informed consent documents might require translations into multiple languages to ensure that those transnational populations that are anticipated to participate in the research are provided written information in a language that is understandable to them. When it is known that a large subset of the participants may speak a language other than English, investigators should make provisions for ensuring that an individual is available to respond to the subject's questions and to provide relevant study information.

In those rare instances in which individuals who speak languages that were not practicably anticipated by the researchers at the onset of the study become potential participants in the research, a document known as a "short form" may be used to document the informed consent process. In cases such as these, the investigator may rely on a witness who is conversant in both English and the language of the person from whom consent is being sought to provide the information about the study to the potential subject and to translate responses to subject queries. The witness will sign an attestation that states that what has been said to the subject matches a script that has been approved by the IRB. The witness, the subject, and the person obtaining consent will sign the short form, which states that all of the required elements of informed consent have been communicated and the subject is entering the research study willingly, to conclude the documentation of the informed consent process. The use of short forms, however, should be the exception rather than the rule. Furthermore, it is recommended that the investigator confer with the IRB prior to instituting a short form process, as not all IRBs currently allow this practice.

RESPONSIBILITY OF PRINCIPAL INVESTIGATORS: STUDY CONDUCT AND AUDITS

In addition to the responsibility for ensuring that the subjects on whom the research is conducted have provided their informed consent, it is of noteworthy importance that the **principal investigator** (PI) understands that at the end of the day, the entirety of the conduct of the research rests solely on the PI's shoulders. PIs may be asked to sign an attestation statement that is likened to a contractual agreement and describe his or her responsibilities as PI. In many well-funded studies or studies conducted at large academic or medical institutions, PIs will employ or be assigned a team of study staff. These staff members may include research coordinators who assist with the day-to-day operations of the study, other clinicians with whom the PI consults on the conduct of the study, phlebotomists, pharmacists, data abstractors or statisticians, laboratory technicians, bench scientists, and the like. In performing these duties, each of these individuals has been effectively delegated his or her respective responsibilities by the PI. Although the activity has been assigned to an individual other than the PI himself or herself, the culpability of the actions of the delegates remains with the PI.

EXPECTATIONS FOR AN AUDIT

The same is true at the time of an audit or monitoring visit. A number of entities, including governmental agencies (e.g., the FDA or HHS), the study sponsor, or the IRB, may conduct audits of a particular study on an either for-cause or random basis. During the conduct of an audit, the auditors will expect that the PI be intimately involved in the day-to-day operations of the research. They will anticipate the investigator's availability during the course of the audit, and will expect that he or she is willing and able to respond to questions that arise over the course of the visit. Many sponsors or contract research organizations (CROs) will also assign site monitors who are responsible for reviewing all study-related documents to ensure that the research is conducted in accordance with the regulations and with the sponsor's protocol. These visits, known as "monitoring" visits, are intended to ameliorate any issues with the conduct of the research throughout the study and serve to improve positive outcomes in an audit situation.

Many IRBs will also conduct audits; these audits, like monitoring visits conducted by sponsors or CROs, are intended to ward off regulatory or human subject protection issues and educate the research staff. In each of these situations, it is important to maintain an open line of communication with the individual conducting the visit. It is prudent to ensure that the study staff members to whom activities are delegated are appropriately trained in the conduct of research to help guarantee a successful audit. In so doing, it may be appropriate to seek out staff members who are certified in their particular discipline, or who are certified in the conduct of clinical research.

DISCLOSING CONFLICTS OF INTEREST

There are several different types of conflicts of interest, which are illustrated in Table 13.4. In 2004, HHS issued a final guidance document addressing the need for investigators to disclose financial conflicts of interest as a matter of protecting human subjects of research (Thompson, 2004). Within the document, HHS brings forth the recognition that merely holding a financial conflict of interest is not prohibited, or necessarily considered a negative (Thompson, 2004). HHS maintains that as a means of ensuring that human subjects are protected from coercion, undue influence, or other potential harms that may be derived from the investigator's conflict, the conflict of interest should be appropriately disclosed and/ or managed (Thompson, 2004). The document provides suggestions for IRBs to rely on addressing and ameliorating any potential risks to human subjects that may stem from the investigator's conflict (Thompson, 2004). During the time that this chapter was written, the federal regulations regarding financial conflicts of interest in research were in the process of being revised.

Each IRB may institute by policy its method for ensuring that disclosures of financial conflicts of interest are appropriately obtained, managed, and, when appropriate for human subject protections, disclosed to the potential research participants. As these policies and procedures may differ widely from institution to institution and from IRB to IRB, it is important to familiarize one's self with the expectations of the individual entity. Some institutions have committees designated to review financial conflicts of interest and provide management plans to the IRB; however, the final authority rests with the IRB. It is also worthy to note that some IRBs will, in addition, consider the financial arrangements of individuals aside from the PI, including, but not limited to, the study staff and immediate family members of the individuals conducting the research.

In addition to individual investigator conflicts of interest, HHS suggested that IRBs also maintain policies that identify the approach that will be taken to minimize potential conflicts of interest among their board members. As with investigator conflicts of interest, there exists the possibility that an individual IRB member may hold a conflict, whether financial, personal, or ideological, that would unduly influence his or her ability to maintain

TABLE 13.4 Types of Conflicts of Interest

TYPE OF COI	DESCRIPTION/EXAMPLES
Financial	Owning stock in the company that manufactures the test article; consulting, serving on the board of directors or in another capacity, and/or other relationships in which you are paid
Professional	Colleague or superior is the PI, which may result in a biased review of the research
Personal	Spouse or other family member is the PI or other study team member; also includes holding strong beliefs that would bias the research under review
Institutional	Institution where the research is taking place has a stake (i.e., owns stock) in the company or test article being studied

COI, conflict of interest; PI, principal investigator.

neutrality in rendering objective decisions for the studies in which the conflict exists. In these instances, IRBs will generally mandate that members with conflicts recuse themselves from the deliberations and not vote.

IRB REVIEW TYPES AND APPROVAL CRITERIA

IRBs are required per the federal regulations to review research according to certain specified categories (Protection of Human Subjects, 2005). Some minimal risk research may be considered "exempt," which allows the initial review to be conducted by the IRB or other designated individual or entity. Alternatively, some minimal risk research may be considered "expedited," which also allows for the chair or the chair's designee to review and approve the research. Research that does not meet the definition of minimal risk is generally required to undergo a "full board" review by the convened IRB. In short, each of the review types allows for a certain degree of relative risk, necessitating the type of review. Exempt research does not typically require subsequent or annual review; however, research protocols reviewed under expedited and full board procedures are required per the regulations to be reviewed on an at least annual basis (Protection of Human Subjects, 2005). Exempt procedures are generally reserved for research involving existing data or materials, with certain caveats (for a complete list of exempt categories, see Table 13.5) for the purposes of biomedical research. Given this fact, it is unlikely that any of the research described as "intervention" research would be reviewed under exempt procedures.

In order for a particular research study to be reviewed by the IRB under expedited procedures, as mentioned earlier, the research must first qualify as "minimal risk." Per the regulations, minimal risk research is such that "the probability and magnitude of harm or discomfort anticipated in the research are not greater in and of themselves than those ordinarily encountered in daily life or during the performance of routine physical or psychological examinations or tests" (Protection of Human Subjects, 2005). Following this determination, as with research that is reviewed under exempt procedures, studies that are reviewed under expedited procedures must also meet certain criteria as mandated per the regulations (for a complete list of expedited categories, see Table 13.6). Those studies that meet neither set of criteria are reviewed at the fully convened IRB meeting. As with the review category designation, research that is reviewed by the IRB must adhere to federally mandated criteria for approval (for a complete list of the federal criteria for approval, see Table 13.7).

TABLE 13.5 List of Exempt Categories—45CFR46.101(b)

1. Research conducted in established or commonly accepted educational settings, involving normal educational practices, such as:
   i. research on regular and special education instructional strategies, or
   ii. research on the effectiveness of or the comparison among instructional techniques, curricula, or classroom management methods.

2. Research involving the use of educational tests (cognitive, diagnostic, aptitude, achievement), survey procedures, interview procedures or observation of public behavior, unless:
   i. information obtained is recorded in such a manner that human subjects can be identified, directly or through identifiers linked to the subjects; and
   ii. any disclosure of the human subjects' responses outside the research could reasonably place the subjects at risk of criminal or civil liability or be damaging to the subjects' financial standing, employability, or reputation

---

(continued)

TABLE 13.5 List of Exempt Categories—45CFR46.101(b) *(continued)*

3. Research involving the use of educational tests (cognitive, diagnostic, aptitude, achievement), survey procedures, interview procedures, or observation of public behavior that is not exempt under paragraph (b)(2) of this section, if:
    i. the human subjects are elected or appointed public officials or candidates for public office; or
    ii. federal statute(s) require(s) without exception that the confidentiality of the personally identifiable information will be maintained throughout the research and thereafter.

4. Research involving the collection or study of existing data, documents, records, pathological specimens, or diagnostic specimens, if these sources are publicly available or if the information is recorded by the investigator in such a manner that subjects cannot be identified, directly or through identifiers linked to the subjects.

5. Research and demonstration projects that are conducted by or subject to the approval of department or agency heads, and that are designed to study, evaluate, or otherwise examine:
    i.   public benefit or service programs;
    ii. procedures for obtaining benefits or services under those programs;
    iii. possible changes in or alternatives to those programs or procedures; or
    iv. possible changes in methods or levels of payment for benefits or services under those programs.

6. Taste and food quality evaluation and consumer acceptance studies,
    i. if wholesome foods without additives are consumed, or
    ii. if a food is consumed that contains a food ingredient at or below the level and for a use found to be safe, or agricultural chemical or environmental contaminant at or below the level found to be safe, by the Food and Drug Administration or approved by the Environmental Protection Agency or the Food Safety and Inspection Service of the U.S. Department of Agriculture.

TABLE 13.6 List of Expedited Categories—63 FR 60364-60367

1. Clinical studies of drugs and medical devices only when condition (a) or (b) is met
    a. research on drugs for which an investigational new drug application (21 CFR Part 312) is not required (Note: Research on marketed drugs that significantly increase the risks or decrease the acceptability of the risks associated with the use of the product is not eligible for expedited review.)
    b. research on medical devices for which (i) an investigational device exemption application (21 CFR Part 812) is not required; or (ii) the medical device is cleared/approved for marketing and the medical device is being used in accordance with its cleared/approved labeling

2. Collection of blood samples by finger stick, heel stick, ear stick, or venipuncture as follows:
    a. from healthy, nonpregnant adults who weigh at least 110 pounds. For these subjects, the amounts drawn may not exceed 550 ml in an 8-week period and collection may not occur more frequently than two times per week; or
    b. from other adults and children, considering the age, weight, and health of the subjects, the collection procedure, the amount of blood to be collected, and the frequency with which it will be collected; for these subjects, the amount drawn may not exceed the lesser of 50 ml or 3 ml per kg in an 8-week period and collection may not occur more frequently than two times per week.

(continued)

TABLE 13.6 List of Expedited Categories—63 FR 60364-60367 *(continued)*

3. Prospective collection of biological specimens for research purposes by noninvasive means
   Examples:
   a. hair and nail clippings in a nondisfiguring manner;
   b. deciduous teeth at time of exfoliation or if routine patient care indicates a need for extraction;
   c. permanent teeth if routine patient care indicates a need for extraction;
   d. excreta and external secretions (including sweat);
   e. uncannulated saliva collected either in an unstimulated fashion or stimulated by chewing gumbase or wax or by applying a dilute citric solution to the tongue;
   f. placenta removed at delivery;
   g. amniotic fluid obtained at the time of rupture of the membrane prior to or during labor;
   h. supra- and sub-gingival dental plaque and calculus, provided the collection procedure is not more invasive than routine prophylactic scaling of the teeth and the process is accomplished in accordance with accepted prophylactic techniques;
   i. mucosal and skin cells collected by buccal scraping or swab, skin swab, or mouth washings;
   j. sputum collected after saline mist nebulization.

4. Collection of data through noninvasive procedures (not involving general anesthesia or sedation) routinely employed in clinical practice, excluding procedures involving x-rays or microwaves (Where medical devices are employed, they must be cleared/approved for marketing. Studies intended to evaluate the safety and effectiveness of the medical device are not generally eligible for expedited review, including studies of cleared medical devices for new indications.)
   Examples:
   a. physical sensors that are applied either to the surface of the body or at a distance and do not involve input of significant amounts of energy into the subject or an invasion of the subject's privacy;
   b. weighing or testing sensory acuity;
   c. magnetic resonance imaging;
   d. electrocardiography, electroencephalography, thermography, detection of naturally occurring radioactivity, electroretinography, ultrasound, diagnostic infrared imaging, doppler blood flow, and echocardiography;
   e. moderate exercise, muscular strength testing, body composition assessment, and flexibility testing where appropriate given the age, weight, and health of the individual.

5. Research involving materials (data, documents, records, or specimens) that have been collected, or will be collected solely for nonresearch purposes (e.g., medical treatment or diagnosis)

   (NOTE: Some research in this category may be exempt from the HHS regulations for the protection of human subjects. 45 CFR 46.101(b)(4). This listing refers only to research that is not exempt.)

6. Collection of data from voice, video, digital, or image recordings made for research purposes

7. Research on individual or group characteristics or behavior (including, but not limited to, research on perception, cognition, motivation, identity, language, communication, cultural beliefs or practices, and social behavior) or research employing survey, interview, oral history, focus group, program evaluation, human factors evaluation, or quality assurance methodologies

   (NOTE: Some research in this category may be exempt from the HHS regulations for the protection of human subjects. 45 CFR 46.101[b][2] and [b][3]. This listing refers only to research that is not exempt.)

(continued)

TABLE 13.6 List of Expedited Categories—63 FR 60364-60367 *(continued)*

8. Continuing review of research previously approved by the convened IRB as follows:
   a. where (i) the research is permanently closed to the enrollment of new subjects; (ii) all subjects have completed all research-related interventions; and (iii) the research remains active only for long-term follow-up of subjects; or
   b. where no subjects have been enrolled and no additional risks have been identified; or
   c. where the remaining research activities are limited to data analysis.

9. Continuing review of research, not conducted under an investigational new drug application or investigational device exemption where categories two (2) through eight (8) do not apply but the IRB has determined and documented at a convened meeting that the research involves no greater than minimal risk and no additional risks have been identified

Source: U.S. Department of Health and Human Services. (1998). OHRP expedited review categories (1998). Retrived from https://www.hhs.gov/ohrp/policy/expedited98.html

TABLE 13.7 List of Documents Required at Initial Review, as Applicable

Protocol	A description of how the study will be conducted: It includes inclusion/exclusion criteria, scientific rationale, and human subject protection information including how informed consent will be obtained, how the data and safety of subjects will be monitored, and how deviations or safety events will be communicated to the IRB.
Informed consent document	The explanation of the study given to individuals who participate in the research project: Subjects must receive a signed copy if HIPAA authorization language is compounded in the document.
IB	Scientific document that includes information regarding the composition of the test article under study and all previous animal and human studies that have occurred to date: Drugs and devices that have not been approved by the FDA or are undergoing studies for new indications should include this document with submission materials.
Grant application	Scientific rationale submitted to funding agencies in an effort to receive monies to conduct the research: The institution is responsible for ensuring congruency between the grant application and the research under review. Most institutions assign this task to the IRB.
Recruitment material	All flyers, brochures, and websites that provide detailed information related to the study: Letters and other notifications used to recruit potential subjects must be submitted for IRB review and approval. Doctor-to-doctor letters where investigators request colleagues to refer patients are not viewed as recruitment material.
Surveys, cognitive tests, or other materials used in the conduct of the research	All documents used to address your scientific question must be submitted to the IRB for review and approval.

FDA, Food and Drug Administration; HIPAA, Health Insurance Portability and Accountability Act; IB, investigator's brochure; IRB, Institutional Review Board.

It is important to note that although the term "expedited" seems to indicate that the research may be reviewed more quickly than a study that is sent to the fully convened board, this is not always the case because this refers only to its regulatory meaning. Depending on the volume at a particular IRB and the types of research it most often sees, the number of studies that are reviewed under expedited procedures may far exceed those seen by the fully convened board, especially in social and behavioral research. Ongoing dialogue between the designated reviewer and the PI may also lead to delays, and it is therefore advisable that the PI respond expeditiously to requests for additional information, even when the question seems extraordinarily simple. Furthermore, research reviewed under expedited procedures, as with what is considered at the fully convened board meeting, must also meet the overarching federal criteria for approval, as defined in the federal regulations. At their discretion, the IRB chairs may also choose for safety reasons to send a study to the fully convened IRB even if it technically qualifies for expedited review procedures. The authors encourage investigators to anticipate unforeseeable issues arising during the conduct of the review for planning purposes.

VULNERABLE POPULATIONS

The federal regulations make special provisions for those populations that have been identified as being particularly vulnerable. The Code of Federal Regulations outlines additional regulatory requirements for pregnant women, fetuses, and neonates (Subpart B), prisoners (Subpart C), and children (Subpart D). Although not exhaustive, Table 13.8 provides a list of additional populations that are generally considered to be vulnerable. In addition to those identified in this chapter, individuals who are not typically classified as vulnerable may become so when they are under duress or in the event of an emergency.

There is much to consider when planning research with these populations. In addition to assuring that the basic regulatory requirements are met, the investigator may expect that research that is proposed to include these particular subsets of society will be subjected to an even greater level of scrutiny than research conducted with normal, healthy volunteers or those not otherwise identified in the various subparts of the regulations. Although great attention is already paid to the informed consent process when the IRB considers a study that does not include these individuals, when vulnerable populations are included, one may anticipate that more details will be required by the IRB in order for the board to assure that the subjects are protected. The investigator should plan to provide a defense for the selection of these populations and be prepared to justify the decision.

TABLE 13.8 Vulnerable Populations

Prisoners[a]

Pregnant women and their fetuses[a]

Children[a]

Individuals with cognitive impairment

Individuals with low social, economic, or financial standing

Students, staff, or other individuals in a subordinate role

[a]Federal criteria exist for the review and approval of these vulnerable populations.

INTERACTING WITH THE IRB: PEARLS FOR THE NEOPHYTE

An investigator can expect to engage in multiple interactions with the IRB throughout the lifetime of a research study. Sometimes it is helpful to have an initial meeting with the IRB staff or chairperson prior to commencing the process. This is especially true in circumstances that are particularly revolutionary or complex to navigate the process more efficiently. This is an advantage of working with a local IRB and is supported at the authors' institution. That being said, it is wise to ensure that all correspondence with the IRB, even that occurring verbally, is documented in writing. Maintaining excellent documentation is the only way that an outside entity will know what has transpired. Although this may seem rather bureaucratic, it serves to benefit all of the parties involved.

At the time of initial review, an investigator will complete an application, describing the research in detail, to be used by the committee members during the course of the review. This application forms the basis of the regulatory record at the IRB. The initial submission will also include documents such as the official study protocol, informed consent document(s) and HIPAA authorizations, assent forms, and investigator brochure(s), as applicable (see Table 13.3 for a list of the required and other common elements of the informed consent document). Additional documents that would require IRB review include measurement tools, survey instruments, questionnaires, documentation of outside support, and laboratory specifics, among others. Given the scope of the required documentation, it may be prudent to create a checklist of to-do items, if it is not already supplied by the IRB.

Depending on the sponsor of the research and whether an investigational drug, device, or other test article is intended to be used therewith, there may be additional documentation that the IRB will require during its initial review. A list of the documents, along with their descriptions, is illustrated in Table 13.7. The IRB will request this documentation to reconcile it with the verbiage presented in the protocol and informed consent documents. Some IRBs may also require ancillary or departmental approvals from the organizations or departments at which the research will be conducted. The IRB may, in addition, request evidence of a thorough, multidisciplinary scientific review having been completed prior to submission, recognizing that the IRB is the final arbiter of the scientific validity of the research in the context of protecting the human subjects from what may otherwise be an unsound query.

Many IRBs will undertake a prereview process prior to the study being reviewed by the designee or full board. During the course of this prereview process, an investigator may expect to receive preliminary questions or requests for revisions. These question and/or requests are generally designed to facilitate the formal review process and seek to address the basic regulatory concerns noted by the individual responsible for the prereview. Once the designee or the full board has reviewed the study, the investigator may expect an additional series of questions or requests for revisions. Generally, these subsequent requests are aimed at correcting issues that affect the approvability of the research, as designated in the federal criteria for approval (see Table 13.9). Throughout the course of these communications, to avoid frustration with the process, it is important for the investigator to remain acutely aware of their underlying cause: the IRB's commitment to the protection of the rights and welfare of the human subjects who will take part in the research.

Once the IRB has approved a study, the investigator may expect to remain in contact with the IRB for a variety of reasons throughout the course of the research. The federal regulations require that research that is reviewed under expedited or full board procedures must be re-reviewed at least annually. Although this is the regulatory mandate, however, it is important to note that some IRBs will reduce this time frame per policy, or on an ad hoc basis, especially for studies involving higher risks to the participants. At the time of continuing review, the progress of the study will be considered, including, but not limited to, the number of

TABLE 13.9 Federal Criteria for Approval—45CFR46.111

Risks to subjects are minimized: (i) by using procedures that are consistent with sound research design and that do not unnecessarily expose subjects to risk, and (ii) whenever appropriate, by using procedures already being performed on the subjects for diagnostic or treatment purposes.

Risks to subjects are reasonable in relation to anticipated benefits, if any, to subjects, and the importance of the knowledge that may reasonably be expected to result. In evaluating risks and benefits, the IRB should consider only those risks and benefits that may result from the research (as distinguished from risks and benefits of therapies subjects would receive even if not participating in the research). The IRB should not consider possible long-range effects of applying knowledge gained in the research (e.g., the possible effects of the research on public policy) as among those research risks that fall within the purview of its responsibility.

Selection of subjects is equitable. In making this assessment, the IRB should take into account the purposes of the research and the setting in which the research will be conducted and should be particularly cognizant of the special problems of research involving vulnerable populations, such as children, prisoners, pregnant women, mentally disabled persons, or economically or educationally disadvantaged persons.

Informed consent will be sought from each prospective subject or the subject's legally authorized representative, in accordance with, and to the extent required by, the federal regulations.

Informed consent will be appropriately documented, in accordance with, and to the extent required by, the federal regulations.

When appropriate, the research plan makes **adequate provisions for monitoring the data** collected to ensure the safety of subjects.

When appropriate, there are **adequate provisions to protect the privacy of subjects** and to **maintain the confidentiality of data**.

When some or all of the subjects are likely to be vulnerable to coercion or undue influence, such as children, prisoners, pregnant women, mentally disabled persons, or economically or educationally disadvantaged persons, **additional safeguards have been included in the study to protect the rights and welfare of these subjects**.

enrollments, drops and withdrawals, information from any safety reports, and the like. When completing the continuing review documents, the investigator should refer to the IRB's definitions of terms such as "enrolled," "dropped," and "withdrawn," for example, to ensure that the figures being reported to the IRB are accurate and in accordance with the IRB's expectations. During the course of this process, the reviewer is instructed to consider the research in its entirety as if it were being presented as a new study. This is important to note because, depending on the structure of the IRB, it is also conceivable that the designated reviewer or board undertaking the continuing review process may differ from that which reviewed and approved the research at the onset. Therefore, it is possible that issues that were missed in the initial review will be caught at the time of continuing review, and subsequent revisions may be necessary.

In addition to communicating with the IRB at the initial and continuing review stages, investigators may expect to periodically engage with the IRB during the course of the study. Given the mission of the IRB to protect the safety, rights, and welfare of the human subjects, the IRB maintains an ongoing interest in the conduct of the study, and expects to promptly receive information about unanticipated problems that may arise. Unanticipated problems involving risks to human subjects or others, sometimes known as "Unanticipated Problems Involving Risk to Human Subjects or Others" (UPIRHSOs), "Unanticipated Problems," or "UPs", are defined by the OHRP as follows: incidences, experiences, or outcomes that are unexpected, related to, or possibly related to the research and that suggest that the research places the subjects or others at a greater risk of harm than was known or recognized earlier (HHS, 2007). For the purposes of FDA-regulated research, the definition of an unanticipated problem differs slightly (see Table 13.10 for a comparison of the OHRP and FDA definitions of unanticipated problems, and links to their respective guidance documents on the subject). In either case, whether the OHRP or the FDA is the overarching regulatory authority over the research, there are reporting requirements for unanticipated problems that arise during its conduct. In addition to familiarizing oneself with the guidance documents provided by these entities, it is important to consult the individual IRB's policies on the topic, as some IRBs will apply more stringent requirements than those outlined by the OHRP or the FDA.

As a final action, once the study has been concluded and all data analysis has been completed, it is imperative that the investigator provide to the IRB a final report to formally close the study. It is also important that the investigator understand the requirements for record retention, as outlined by the sponsor, applicable regulatory agencies, the IRB, and the investigator's institution. The authors have provided a list of useful websites related to the topics discussed here, as well as otherwise noteworthy topics and relevant websites that fall outside of the scope of this chapter (see Tables 13.11 and 13.12, respectively) to guide the neophyte.

TABLE 13.10 Comparison of OHRP and FDA Definitions of UPIRHSOs and Links to Guidance Documents

OFFICE OF HUMAN RESEARCH PROTECTIONS (OHRP)	FOOD AND DRUG ADMINISTRATION (FDA)
Unexpected	Unexpected
Related or possibly related	Serious
Different or greater risk of harm	Implications for the conduct of the study
www.hhs.gov/ohrp/policy/advevntguid.html	www.fda.gov/downloads/RegulatoryInformation/ Guidances/UCM126572.pdf

UPIRHSOs, Unanticipated Problems Involving Risk to Human Subjects or Others.

TABLE 13.11 Useful Websites

Association for the Accreditation of Human Research Protection Programs, Inc. (AAHRPP)	www.aahrpp.org
Association of Clinical Research Professionals (ACRP)	www.acrpnet.org
Belmont Report	https://www.hhs.gov/ohrp/regulations-and-policy/belmont-report/index.html
CenterWatch	www.centerwatch.com
Clinical Trials Networks Best Practices (CTN Best Practices)	www.ctnbestpractices.org

(continued)

TABLE 13.11 Useful Websites *(continued)*

ClinicalTrials.gov	www.clinicaltrials.gov
Collaborative Institutional Training Initiative (CITI Program)	www.citiprogram.org
Drug Information Association (DIA)	www.diahome.org/DIAHome/Home.aspx
International Conference on Harmonization Good Clinical Practice (E6)	http://ichgcp.net
Public Responsibility in Medicine & Research (PRIM&R)	www.primr.org
Society of Clinical Research Associates (SOCRA)	www.socra.org
U.S. Food and Drug Administration	www.fda.gov
U.S. Department of Health & Human Services, Office of Human Research Protections	www.hhs.gov/ohrp

TABLE 13.12 Specific Benchmark Moments and Other Significant Websites

SIGNIFICANT BENCHMARK MOMENTS	AREA(S) OF CONCERN
Dan's Law (MN)/Dan Markingson	Vulnerable populations; informed consent
Guatemala syphilis experiments	Informed consent; transnational research; vulnerable populations
Havasupai Tribe of Arizona	Genetics research; informed consent; biobanking; vulnerable populations
Henrietta Lacks/The Immortal Life of Henrietta Lacks/HeLa cells	Informed consent; biobanking; vulnerable populations
Jessie Gelsinger	Conflicts of interest; informed consent
Myriad Genetics	Patents; intellectual property
University of Washington *vs.* Catalona	Ownership; biobanking
OTHER SIGNIFICANT WEBSITE DESCRIPTIONS	**WEB ADDRESS**
Biobanking: International Society for Biological and Environmental Repositories (ISBER)	www.isber.org
Current affairs related to the field of bioethics: Presidential Commission for the Study of Bioethical Issues	https://bioethicsarchive.georgetown.edu/pcsbi/node/851.html
Genetic Information Nondiscrimination Act (GINA) of 2008	www.genome.gov/24519851
Genome-Wide Association Studies Fact Sheet	www.genome.gov/20019523
Health Information Privacy & Health Insurance Portability and Accountability Act of 1996 (HIPAA)	www.hhs.gov/ocr/privacy

IRB MEETING DYNAMICS

Although it may seem to be an intuitive point, it is important to note that each individual IRB has its own personality, even when multiple IRBs are managed by a common entity or are chaired by the same person. Although the federal criteria for approval remain constant, given the depth and breadth of the ethical issues that may be presented to boards, and the fact that boards are made up of individuals with varying backgrounds and experiences, it is only natural that separate boards may arrive at different conclusions. As discussed earlier, this is undoubtedly the primary reason that entices sponsors that are initiating multicenter trials to utilize a commercial, independent, or central IRB. It is the experience of the authors that discussing ethical issues in the research takes the most time during the meetings. That being said, these ethical discussions should not be regarded as a hindrance to the process; rather, although these ethical debates may result in a more lengthy review time frame, they also add to the quality of that review and lead to a more meaningful, interesting, and dynamic process.

There are certainly particular controverted issues that are more commonly discussed than are others. For example, it is not uncommon for a board to discuss matters of subject compensation at length (to determine whether or not the compensation would unduly influence one's participation in the research), to consider the method by which subjects will be selected, or to debate about the use or exclusion of a particular subject population. Regardless of the content of the discussion, the outcomes are expected to be on the basis of the principles of respect for persons, beneficence, and justice outlined in the Belmont Report. As described earlier, IRBs will often rely on subject matter experts or outside consultants to assist with navigating the issues pertinent to the individual research study. There are stringent requirements for detailed minutes to be recorded during the conduct of the meetings to ensure that IRBs are remaining true to this reliance on the principles outlined in the Belmont Report, as well as the federal regulations.

PITFALLS AND RECOMMENDATIONS: FAMILIARITY AND CLARITY

Perhaps the simplest recommendation that the authors can make for new investigators is to become familiar with the published policies of the IRB to which the research will be submitted. Not only will this help the investigator to familiarize himself or herself with the federal regulations that govern human subject research, but it will also serve to set out the expectations of the individual IRB. The investigator may also reach out to the IRB chairperson or administration to request admittance to a convened IRB meeting to take this concept one step further. This will allow the investigator the opportunity before submitting an application to the IRB to feel out the process and to potentially interact with the IRB staff and chair after the meeting has concluded.

Although many IRBs are moving to electronic submissions to improve efficiency and save costs, this does not substitute for the benefits gained from human interaction. Attending a convened IRB meeting will allow the investigator to witness firsthand the ways in which the IRB members utilize the application, whether paper or electronic, and will shed light on the overall review process, which will hopefully translate into a more well-written application by the neophyte. A well-written protocol and application are the surest ways to ensure an expeditious review. Given that many of the individuals who participate as IRB members are also scientists and academicians, it is important that investigators be cognizant of grammar and semantics when composing the documents that will be submitted for review. Assure that the appropriate homonym is used in your document, for example, in describing oneself as the "principal investigator" rather than the "principle investigator." Ultimately, simply remember that if the message is unclear to the reviewers, then they will not understand what it is that the investigator is attempting to convey, which will result in frustration and will ultimately slow down the process.

MULTISITE HARMONIZATION

There are occasionally instances in which an investigator may need to work with more than one IRB to implement a study, for instance, when the single investigator will be recruiting subjects at more than one institution, or when the study will take place at a correctional or educational facility. In these cases, insofar as it is possible, it is prudent for the investigator to attempt to work with his or her home institution in setting up a reliance agreement with the secondary facility, thereby creating a structure that allows for the investigator's institution to act as the primary IRB of record for the study. This will effectively provide that the investigator's institution is the sponsor of the study. Although the details of creating an agreement such as this fall outside of the scope of this chapter, the primary message to carry forward is that ample, ongoing communication with the IRB will serve to improve the investigator's overall experience.

In those instances in which secondary IRB approval is not required, despite the investigator's engagement in the research at an organization not affiliated with the investigator's institution, the IRB will generally require some acknowledgment from the outside organization that provides permission for the research to be conducted. When this occurs, it helps to obtain clear, unambiguous, and hopefully brief documentation of the legal agreement. Although not every situation requires a legal document, most cases will require formal permission from the person of authority that allows the use of the organization's resources in the research. This is another excellent example of a situation in which communication with the IRB at the onset of the research proposal will ensure a smooth process, as some IRBs may assist the investigator with this endeavor by providing sample language or templates.

IRBS IN THE "SUNSHINE"

No discussion about IRBs is complete without a brief mention of the pros and cons of working with IRBs that operate "in the sunshine." In an age such as this, in which full disclosure and transparency are the heralded concepts of the moment, investigators must be cognizant that there are certain IRBs that are held to a standard that requires open access to the records held therein. IRBs that are operated by public institutions may be subject to **sunshine laws,** which allow for the public to make formal information requests. The obvious benefit of these laws lies in the supposition that institutions subject thereto will maintain an especially high level of integrity. The downside of sunshine laws is in the potential loss of confidentiality. Regardless of the existence or absence of these laws, however, investigators and sponsors may rest easy with the understanding that these laws do not require that information deemed proprietary be disclosed during the course of responding to an inquiry. Where there is proprietary information involved, institutions may exercise a certain level of discretion in redacting the documents prior to their delivery to the interested party.

AN INVITATION

The authors conclude this chapter much as it was begun: with an invitation. It is a fact that even the best IRBs will on occasion make mistakes. Even those IRBs with electronic systems and a devotion to exemplary customer service will experience inefficiencies. This is only natural; IRBs are bureaucratic by nature and design, and are made up of individuals with varying backgrounds, experiences, and resultant opinions. Although it may be prudent for one to question the resources that are expended and the economic burden of the regulatory process, investigators who are new to research may rest easy in knowing that they may be a part of the solution. The first step that a new investigator may take in this course is to become well educated in the processes, procedures, and foundational concepts that drive the IRB, and engage in continuing education on the responsible conduct of research. The next step is then to become involved. Much as the continuation of scientific research relies on willing participants, IRBs cannot subsist without plentiful volunteers willing to donate their time to the protection of this valuable resource. Even the neophyte to this research world can have a profound impact and provide insights to improve the bureaucratic IRB process. Herein lies the invitation to participate in the discourse and advance the field of human subject protections.

ACKNOWLEDGMENTS

The authors would like to acknowledge those individuals who choose to participate in clinical research as subjects, without whom the advancement of medical science would be greatly hindered.

DISCLOSURES

All authors of this chapter are void of conflicts of interest to disclose.

Key Points From This Chapter

- Early and frequent communication with the IRB serves to streamline the process and improve turnaround times.
- Obtaining informed consent is the PI's exhibition of his or her commitment to the Belmont Report's principle of respect for persons. Individuals are autonomous beings and should be treated as such. Conducting research is not a right, but, rather, should be looked upon as a privilege.
- The PI is always the party who is ultimately responsible for the conduct of the research.
- The field of human subject protections is an evolving one. As science advances and cultural norms and mores progress, modifications to the regulations and guidance documents that frame the review process are to be expected.
- Even the neophyte can have a profound impact on the conduct of research in his or her community. Consider becoming involved by volunteering to participate as an IRB member.

ADDENDUM

On July 26, 2011, while this chapter awaited final publication, HHS issued an announcement and request for comment regarding proposed changes to the Common Rule. Prompted by the 2010 discovery of research studies that took place in Guatemala contemporaneously with the syphilis studies in Tuskegee, Alabama, President Barack Obama issued a presidential order that created the Presidential Commission for the Study of Biological Issues. The basic charge to the Commission was to review the current human subject protection regulations in force to ensure that they adequately protect human subjects of research (a review of the Commission's proceedings may be found at https://bioethicsarchive.georgetown .edu/pcsbi/node/851.html). The issuance of these proposed regulations is a derivative of the work done by the Commission. The notice may be found in PDF form at www.gpo.gov/ fdsys/pkg/FR-2011-07-26/pdf/2011-18792.pdf. Summary information, including FAQs, regarding these proposed changes may also be found at: www.hhs.gov/ohrp/humansubjects/ anprm2011page.html. The authors would like to recognize the downstream effects that these proposed changes will have on the conduct of interventional research studies, and thereby on the content of this chapter.

REFERENCES

The Association for the Accreditation of Human Research Protection Programs, Inc. (2011a). Accredited organizations. Retrieved from http://www.aahrpp.org/learn/find-an-accredited-organization

The Association for the Accreditation of Human Research Protection Programs, Inc. (2011b). Our mission, vision, and values. Retrieved from http://www.aahrpp.org/learn/about-aahrpp/our-mission

Bankert, E. A., & Amdur, R. J. (2006). In K. Sullivan, A. Sibley, K. Crowley., & S. Schultz (Eds.), *Institutional review board management and function* (2nd ed.). Sudbury, MA: Jones & Bartlett.

The National Commission for the Protection of Human Subjects of Biomedical and Behavioral Research. (1979). *The Belmont Report: Ethical principles and guidelines for the protection of human subjects of research.* Washington, DC: Government Printing Office.

Office for Human Research Protections. (2011). *Office for Human Research Protections (OHRP) database for registered IORGs & IRBs, approved FWAs, and documents received in last 60 days.* Washington, DC: United States Department of Health and Human Services. Retrieved from http://ohrp.cit.nih.gov/search/ search.aspx?styp=bsc

Protection of Human Subjects, 45 C.F.R. pt 46. (2005).

Thompson, T. G., Office for Human Research Protections. (2004). *Final guidance document: Financial relationships and interests in research involving human subjects: Guidance.* Washington, DC: United States Department of Health and Human Services. Retrieved from https://www.hhs.gov/ohrp/regulations-and-policy/ guidance/financial-conflict-of-interest/

U.S. Department of Health & Human Services. (1998). OHRP expedited review categories (1998). Retrived from https://www.hhs.gov/ohrp/policy/expedited98.html

U.S. Department of Health and Human Services. (2007). Guidance on reviewing and reporting unanticipated problems involving risks to subjects or others and adverse events. Retrieved from http://www.hhs.gov/ ohrp/policy/advevntguid.html

U.S. Department of Health & Human Services. (2011a). *Federal policy for the protection of human subjects ('common rule').* Washington, DC. Retrieved from http://www.hhs.gov/ohrp/humansubjects/commonrule/ index.html

United States Department of Health and Human Services. (2011b). *Informed consent—FAQs.* Retrieved from http://answers.hhs.gov/ohrp/categories/1566

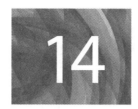

Participant Recruitment and Retention

Dianne Morrison-Beedy & Constance Visovsky

> Keep your dream bigger than your fears and persist
> through all of the character builders until it comes
> to fruition. —*Bernadette Mazurek Melnyk*

The most valuable of all resources in intervention studies are the participants who agree to take part in the project. Advances in intervention research involving human subjects have been made possible because of the participation of research participants who dedicate their time and efforts to the success of the study. Recruitment refers to the process used to select study participants. Although actual recruitment begins with the researcher or research team member approaching eligible persons with information about the study in efforts to consent sufficient numbers to meet the required sample size (Hulley et al., 2001; Keith, 2001), much forethought and planning is required prior to the actual identification of potential participants. The process or means by which investigators keep participants engaged in the study is known as "retention" (Patel, Doku, & Tennakoon, 2003). Despite the fact that a study cannot be successfully conducted if no one consents to participate, recruitment and retention of research participants are often considered of secondary importance as compared to the research design and, thus, may be given limited attention in the preparation of research scientists. However, successful recruitment and retention are vital to the validity and generalizability of study findings (Given, Keilman, Collins, & Given, 1990). Exactly how participants are recruited and/or retained in studies often is not sufficiently explicated. In a cross-sectional review of 172 randomized controlled trials (RCTs) reported in four high-impact medical journals from April 1999 to 2000, few provided adequate information concerning the recruitment process (Gross, Mallory, Heiat, & Krumholz, 2002).

Recruitment (the process by which study participants are screened and selected) and retention (keeping participants engaged throughout the duration of the study from enrollment to completion) of research subjects into intervention studies pose many challenges for which the principal investigator (PI) and research team must anticipate and prepare. In recent years, the Health Insurance Portability and Accountability Act (HIPAA) imposed barriers to identifying eligible study participants such that, generally speaking, the investigator is prohibited from directly contacting the potential participant. Instead, within healthcare settings, determination of eligibility and the first information concerning potential research study participation occurs through the healthcare provider. Whether they are MDs, RNs, physician assistants (PAs), therapists, or other clinicians, these providers may have limited understanding and investment in the research or are often too busy to consistently identify and refer eligible study participants (Aitken, Gallagher, & Madronio, 2003; Sullivan-Bolyai et al., 2007). In addition, shortened clinic appointment times and increasingly brief admission cycles make initial contact and relationship building between researcher and potential participants more difficult. The research training of the healthcare provider, along with the provider's general opinion of the value of the intended research, may influence participant referral to these intervention studies (Newberry et al., 2010). Similarly, in community-based settings or schools, the frontline contact to participant recruitment again may be individuals whose primary focus is not on the success of the research study. Thus, researchers are increasingly compelled to incorporate strategies that maximize potential participant contact opportunities and establish a trusting relationship while attending to the legal requirements of the informed consent process. In designing intervention studies, consideration of the time it takes to develop rapport and trust, screen and confirm eligibility of participants, and successfully recruit and retain subjects are vital to the success of the research.

RECRUITMENT ISSUES AND OBSTACLES

Although the RCT is considered the gold standard for experimental design, recruitment and successful randomization of study participants can pose significant challenges to a trial's success. In many cases, recruitment of individuals to clinical trials may be slower than anticipated. The assumption of the number of available study participants may be on the basis of prevalence of the targeted outcome (e.g., disease, educational dropout rate, incarceration rates) and fails to consider other factors that can impede study participation. Just as distressing for the investigator is successful recruitment and consent of individuals to participate in a study followed by higher-than-expected attrition rates.

Several factors may hamper the recruitment of eligible participants into intervention studies. These factors include the patient, the provider, the intervention itself, and the study design. Patient-related factors such as discomfort with randomization because of treatment preferences, distrust of the research process, impact of illness or health concerns, and the demands of daily life are barriers to research participation reported by patients (Mills et al., 2006; Ross et al., 1999). Depending on the purpose of the research, patients may have definitive preferences for one intervention over another, and, thus, be reluctant to agree to the randomization process. Participants have also reported feeling unclear about the personal benefits gained from research participation. Yet subjects have reported participating in research studies as a future benefit to others (Bill-Axelson, Christensson, Carlsson, Norlén, & Holmberg, 2008). Providers and staff can serve as the gateway to participant access. Issues surrounding workload or the environment in which providers and staff must function can affect their engagement in the research process and accessing participants. They may also believe that their role is to "protect" their patients and clients and may somewhat misconstrue research as a stressor from which to protect the patient. Even interventions that are very low risk may appear more daunting simply because of the extensive information and consent requirements that accompany intervention research. Very complex study designs that require extensive and prolonged contact or study activities may overwhelm potential participants if not clearly explained by research staff. It is helpful for staff to discuss concerns and brainstorm with potential participants leading to potential problemsolving that addresses such issues.

As a researcher, you must consider the perceived burden associated with any intervention. By nature, an intervention requires the study participant to *do* something. Researchers need to ask if the intervention is actually feasible considering the social, physical, psychological, or developmental state of the individual and the setting where the intervention and data collection are conducted. If recruitment efforts are not well planned, lower-than-expected recruitment rates may result, leading to a loss of statistical power impacting the ability to determine intervention effects. Barriers to recruitment are also present on the clinician side. Busy individuals needed to support the study—who are not employed as a research team member—often report lack of time, staff, and inadequate research training as barriers to research participation; the result is often poor recruitment (Oude Rengerink et al., 2010).

STRATEGIES TO ENHANCE RECRUITMENT

Recruitment of Eligible Participants

The first major issue faced by most investigators is the estimation of the available pool of potential study participants. Often, researchers tend to overestimate the availability of potential participants on the basis of the prevalence of a disease state or demographic characteristics in the recruitment area (Gul & Ali, 2010). The research team should establish productive relationships with the personnel at the designated research site to overcome potential barriers to recruitment. Likewise, if the research is to take place within a community setting, becoming familiar with the area, stakeholders, and any earlier successful recruitment strategies should be considered in the planning stage of the research. The PI must provide an accurate description of the research to be conducted and the responsibilities associated with participation while balancing the need to market the study so that it is appealing and pertinent to the target population. Face-to-face recruitment, although time-consuming, builds rapport and trust with potential participants and provides a purpose or context for their participation, even if they themselves are unlikely to benefit. A designated individual dedicated to recruitment at each research site to identify eligible participants and provide referral of persons willing to have the research team contact them is a key to successful recruitment.

Oftentimes, the first level of participant recruitment takes place at the targeted agency. Getting those employees "on board" is a requisite first step prior to study participant recruitment. The PI should consider training of referral staff and providing study materials (e.g., a notebook of study purpose, eligibility criteria, and scripted study information) for their reference. A laminated 3 × 5 card with the study title, purpose, study eligibility, and research personnel contact information that could be carried in a lab coat pocket is also recommended to offer quick referral for those persons being relied on to promote study participation. Providing referral staff with an introductory letter containing an introduction to the research staff that can be given to patients who express interest is a helpful, cost-effective recruitment strategy. The researcher should not underestimate the value of even small reimbursements or gestures of appreciation to providers and community stakeholders for their assistance in identifying and referring eligible study participants. These can range from monetary to continuing professional education, to coffee and donuts, or to handwritten thank you notes. If study participants provide positive feedback following their participation, relaying this input back to agency personnel (anonymously) is also an important way to maintain agency personnel commitment to recruitment.

Recruitment materials need to be consumer (i.e., participant) friendly, brief, and eye-catching yet contain sufficient information to describe the study. A recruitment poster that says "Make an easy $100—join our study!" may gain the attention of potential participants but would be unlikely to receive the institution review board (IRB) approval. Balance is needed between appealing and coercive approaches. Participants who consent for the study incentive alone often drop out of the study because they were not really invested in it. Remember that these "consenters" will be retained for data analysis in an intent-to-treat approach and must be reported on the Consolidated Standards of Reporting Trials (CONSORT) table. Beyond the recruitment materials themselves, investigators must make the overall study appealing and beneficial to improve recruitment rates.

Alternative Methods

Some methods shown to be effective in increasing recruitment to randomized trials are using telephone reminders to those who do not respond, or implementing "opt-out" as opposed to "opt-in" procedures. Recruitment strategies using open, unblinded designs have been used to increase recruitment. However, when designing studies, the investigator must consider the potential drawbacks of these alternative strategies that can influence generalizability. Newer strategies such as providing study information via video also have been recommended, but the influence of some of these practices on study sample results is not known. Other recruitment strategies that often are used for studies include study brochures made available at local hospitals, community centers, senior housing, health fairs, and healthcare provider offices or clinics. Posters of study information can be used and displayed in much the same manner as study brochures. It is important to check with the IRB because any advertising material requires prior approval and authorization before use. Online study recruitment has received increasing application in research studies with varying success rates noted between paid and unpaid efforts as well as differences in regard to sample demographics depending on delivery and dissemination route and visual presentation (Musiat et al., 2016). Broader health behavioral interventions in different clinical settings used social media. Conducting formative work with the population of interest prior to full-scale recruiting may identify unique targeted methods for recruitment of that particular group (Morrison-Beedy, Carey, Aronowitz, Mkandawire, & Dyne, 2002; Seibold-Simpson & Morrison-Beedy, 2010).

The development and implementation of the CONSORT guidelines to improve the reporting in clinical trials (Schulz, Altman, Moher, & CONSORT Group, 2010) require the investigator to carefully track study recruitment and attrition (Figure 14.1). Many journals now require the use of the CONSORT guidelines in the presentation of study participant flow for publication. Weekly recruitment reports that contain the number of potential participants who were approached, consented, declined, or withdrew, and the reason for nonparticipation or withdrawal provide important study-related information to the research team. Software tracking programs explicitly for use in clinical trials are available through many companies. Investigator-developed tracking protocols and procedures specific to the population being recruited are also important. For example, Morrison-Beedy, Carey, Crean, and Jones (2010a) used various recruitment and participant tracking procedures developed specifically for the Health Improvement Project (HIP) for Teens study to investigate sexual risk behaviors in adolescent girls. First, a comprehensive recruitment manual was developed for use by the research team. The recruitment manual contained detailed procedures for identifying and recruiting eligible participants, including sample scripts for approaching potential participants, procedures for obtaining biological specimens, and methods for follow-up contacts (Seibold-Simpson & Morrison-Beedy, 2010). Study recruiters received many hours of documented training in all research procedures, including screening, obtaining informed consent, and data collection. Role-playing with peers and the PI was used to assess study-related competencies for all recruiters on an ongoing basis.

This detailed information about reasons for attrition at each stage of the research study will help in later interpretations as well as planning for future work. For example, if most attritions occur because participants are lost to follow-up, a more extensive tracking and

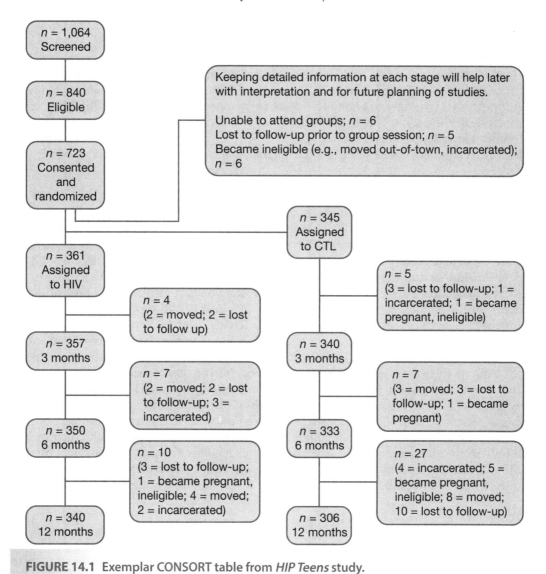

FIGURE 14.1 Exemplar CONSORT table from *HIP Teens* study.

CONSORT, Consolidated Standards of Reporting Trials; HIP, Health Improvement Project; PI, principal investigator.
Source: Morrison-Beedy, PI, funded by the National Institutes of Health/National Institute of Nursing Research #R01 NR0081994.

retention protocol needs to be developed. If most attritions occur because participants cannot arrange transportation, then including transportation should be considered for future work.

Some attrition-related factors may include death or increased severity of symptoms, which then prohibits participation. The investigator must consider if study inclusion criteria must be more restricted in future work or if, despite increased attrition risk and impact study, these at-risk participants are considered for inclusion.

Cost Associated With Retention

Often, little attention is given to the time and costs associated with recruitment of study participants. Expenditures can be associated with the actual costs of recruitment personnel, including salary, benefits, and training, or with the time allotted for nonfunded researchers to spend on recruitment efforts. Such recruitment and retention efforts account for considerable expense in conducting intervention research (Motzer, Moseley, & Lewis, 1997). In one study (Ott, Twiss, Waltman, Gross, & Lindsey, 2006), recruitment costs associated with a randomized trial intervention to decrease treatment-associated osteoporosis in women with breast cancer were estimated to be $480.00 per participant. A related problem associated with recruitment cost is the referral and follow-up of participants who do not meet eligibility criteria for study participation. The research team may spend unnecessary time in contacting and screening referred study participants, who on further examination are deemed ineligible, escalating recruitment costs (McMillan & Weitzner, 2003).

Retention Issues

Once study participants have been successfully recruited, strategies to ensure retention are needed. Similar to the consideration of recruitment, strategies for retaining study participants need to be considered in the study design phase. Failure to plan for and address retention could result in high study attrition that can result in bias and unanticipated study costs (Given et al., 1990). In longitudinal studies, attrition rates can vary from 16% to 50% (McMillan & Weitzner, 2003; Moser, Dracup, & Doering, 2000). Attrition can result from a host of issues including death of study participants, participants moving out of the area, intervention study requirements, length of the study, lack of time, burden associated with illness and treatment, participant dissatisfaction, and the result of randomization (participants not comfortable with group assignment; Cooley et al., 2003). Exact strategies used to decrease attrition will depend on the study population, the study site(s), and specific circumstances and health of the study participants. In a longitudinal study of quality of life in 250 women with breast cancer, McNees, Dow, and Loerzel (2005) found that making weekly visits to the cancer center, refocusing the timing of recruitment, obtaining renewed study commitment from referring physicians, providing referring physicians with a quick eligibility checklist, and formulating and distributing monthly enrollment were successful strategies that resulted in enhanced recruitment. Longitudinal studies need a cadre of participants who are motivated to perform the intervention for the required length of time and in the prescribed dose for the duration of the study.

Research Team Training

Significant time, effort, energy, and resources need to be directed to recruitment and retention activities. Much of this involves the research team members who will play key roles in these activities. The importance of training research team members responsible for recruitment and retention cannot be overstated. Determining the need for training begins with an overview of the specific job description or duties for each member of the research team and a complete review of the research project needs and responsibilities (Nelson & Morrison-Beedy, 2008). One technique that proves helpful is to review or practice recruitment, data collection, and the intervention with the research study staff acting in the role of the "study participant." This type of role-play by members of the research team in implementing the recruitment protocol is helpful in establishing consistency and confidence. In addition, training needs that may have been unidentified earlier may become apparent on the basis of feedback from the staff. In approaching recruitment, the use of standardized scripts for introducing and describing the study and developing a list of frequently asked questions and answers are strategies to lessen variability and ensure quality in recruitment efforts. In anticipation of personal scheduling conflicts or absences, cross-training of research personnel avoids gaps in absenteeism and scheduling conflicts that could result in the loss of potential participants. Research study personnel can fulfill more than one role, such as data collector and consenter, as long as the scientific integrity of the study is not compromised. For example, if the research study protocol calls for blinding of the data collector to group control or intervention group assignment, then the same individual cannot perform both functions. It is important not to overlook the training needs that are necessary at the sites of participant recruitment. Orienting all agency staff who may be involved in identifying eligible participants to the overall study is necessary. This type of research training helps to identify potential recruitment barriers and facilitates the conduct of the research (Nelson & Morrison-Beedy, 2008).

Rigorous training in obtaining informed consent is essential. In some institutions, members of the IRB provide training in an informed consent process to research project staff members. Such training provides additional assurance to the PI of compliance with IRB regulations and human subject protections. The PI or project manager should also be responsible for ensuring the integrity of staff in recruitment and retention protocols used in the study. A dedicated clinical trials manager and consistent personnel involved in the study are factors associated with successful recruitment (Campbell et al., 2007). Once participants have consented, frequent contact and reminders of "next steps" are invaluable to retention efforts. Similar to recruitment protocol manuals, documentation that clearly presents standardized approaches to follow-up and retention protocols are vital. The importance of putting effort "up front," prior to actual participant recruitment, by ensuring agency buy-in and a well-trained team sets the stage for successful recruitment and retention efforts.

RECRUITMENT AND RETENTION OF SPECIAL POPULATIONS

Dyad and Family-Based Research

Study designs that include dyads, such as parent–child, patient–caregiver, husband–wife, boyfriend–girlfriend, or teacher–student, pose unique challenges for conducting intervention research. Such study designs require informed consent from both individuals and both need to meet eligibility criteria. In cases of critical or terminal illness, the recruitment of dyads is even more difficult because families are overwhelmed and often feel too stressed to participate (Northouse et al., 2006). In a study of cancer pain in the palliative care setting, recruitment of patients and caregivers was poor because of high tension, depression, and strain related to the cancer diagnosis and demands of cancer pain management (Ransom, Azzarello, & McMillan, 2006). Often, the need for an extensive recruitment phase in studies of dyads is not given adequate consideration in the study design. The research team must take time to contact additional persons for consent and often must delay consent while dyads or family members consider and discuss potential research study participation. When determining the length of the recruitment phase, consider the special needs for assent and/or consent if the dyad or family in question includes children. Finally, the dissolution of family ties through separation or divorce can be a potential factor in study participant withdrawal (Motzer et al., 1997).

Research designs that include dyads or family members require greater organization and coordination for scheduling data collection. Keeping a spreadsheet for referrals, date approached, follow-up needed for delayed consent, and whether the dyad or family agreed to participate prevents reapproaching those who already declined. Developing a recruitment protocol is extremely helpful in attempting to recruit dyads or families. Northouse et al. (2006) designed a recruitment protocol for recruitment of prostate cancer patients and their partners. The research team provided the healthcare team with an introductory letter containing study information and research staff names to increase the likelihood that telephone calls would be answered and returned. Other strategies included rigorous research project staff training, role-playing response to questions about the study, and instruction in the informed consent process. In recruiting dyads or families for research, data collection at home or in conjunction with healthcare visits makes the study more appealing because of its convenience for minimizing additional travel and appointments.

Recruitment and Retention of Minority and Vulnerable Populations

Vulnerable populations are those individuals at risk for physical or psychological harm. Research studies that include pregnant women, neonates, children, and/or prisoners are considered to include vulnerable populations. Other populations that can be considered vulnerable are persons with cognitive impairment and those with terminal or life-threatening illness. In addition to specific populations, the notion of vulnerability can be expanded to include topics of an extremely personal or sensitive nature that would be considered stressful to the person involved (Lee & Renzetti, 1990). Finally, vulnerable persons may be socioeconomically stressed, dampening enthusiasm for research participation. The concept of vulnerable populations arose because of considerations that any research conducted may pose additional and/or unknown risks to these populations and as such may require additional safeguards. Protection of vulnerable populations considers factors related to potential exploitation in that the needs of the study participants are of the utmost importance, and secondary to study aims such as recruitment or retention. The American Nurses Association's publication *Ethical Principles in the Conduct, Dissemination, and Implementation of Nursing Research* serves as a guide for the ethical conduct of research. The second guiding principle specifically addresses research with vulnerable populations and requires the researcher to prevent or minimize harm and to promote good to all research participants, including vulnerable populations (Silva, 1995).

Consultation with the IRB in preparation for the conduct of research with vulnerable populations is recommended. The IRB can assist the PI with the institutional policies and procedures and help guide the design and implementation of critical safeguards for working with vulnerable populations. In all cases, the researcher must address all aspects for the ethical conduct of research including informed consent, ability to safely withdraw from the study without penalty, and the provision for confidentiality. Additional requirements may also be imposed by the organizational IRB to meet federal guidelines depending on the nature of the study and population to be recruited. As with most research recruitment efforts, a combination of strategies is recommended for recruiting and retaining minority and vulnerable persons for a study.

In 1994, the National Institutes of Health (NIH) initiated a policy requiring racially diverse ethnic and minority groups—women and children—in the conduct of research (NIH, 1994). However, because of experience with exploitative research conduct, the recruitment of African American persons to clinical trials remains a challenge because of suspicion and distrust (Bonner & Miles, 1997). Having a culturally tailored approach to recruitment is a priority to assist potential participants in understanding the purpose and responsibilities of the research study. Consult with someone of the same culture or ethnic group to assist in planning and executing recruitment. Recruitment staff training should include cultural awareness and, if possible, using cultural peers because recruiters are a means of facilitating research participation in minority populations. A challenge that is often faced in recruitment, especially of vulnerable populations, is that of transient residence. Some vulnerable populations tend to be highly mobile, which will require primary and secondary means of contacting participants. Multiple phone numbers and addresses of close family and friends help reach participants who may move often. In some cases, providing small incentives for participants to update their contact information can prove invaluable to the research team. In a pilot study to prevent weight gain in a population of low-income, overweight, and obese African American and White mothers, Chang, Brown, and Nitzke (2009) used many diverse strategies to enhance recruitment, including emphasizing confidentiality, a DVD overview of the study, and training in cultural sensitivity for the research staff. Likewise, Rosal et al. (2010) used a strategic approach to recruitment of low-income Latinos into a randomized trial of diabetes self-care at five community centers. In this study, a bilingual research site coordinator was identified at each site; staff underwent rigorous training in recruitment and retention that included interview skills, problem solving, and role-playing; and strict oversight of the research sites by the project director and PI. Finally, one should never underestimate the power of a personal, face-to-face relationship in recruitment and retention in studies with minority or vulnerable persons (Chang et al., 2009; Rosal et al., 2010).

Recruitment and Retention of Older Persons

Recruitment of older persons into research studies poses several challenges. Ethical issues can arise when illness or social isolation may influence decision making regarding research participation (Locher, Bronstein, Robinson, Williams, & Ritchie, 2006). The research team must recognize that loneliness may influence older persons to engage in research. Obtaining informed consent can be the most crucial ethical issue because older persons may have conditions that impair judgment. Researchers can choose more stringent consent processes to ensure obtaining informed consent in the recruitment process. For example, one approach involved a two-step consent process. The first step was for a trusted healthcare provider to obtain consent for study referral only. Once the older person agreed to referral, the research team member meets with the older person to obtain informed consent. This process was thought to increase the autonomy of the older person in determining willingness to participate (Locher et al., 2006). Obtaining informed consent can occur at each stage of the study, or reconsent can be obtained at specific study intervals. The research team should plan for adequate time to present the research study and for any questions regarding the study to be resolved. The research team should remind the older persons that study participation is voluntary, and that they can withdraw at any time without penalty.

Recruitment of older individuals with cognitive impairment poses inherent difficulties because of the need for ensuring informed consent, and the need often for consent by proxy in this population. In fact, persons with cognitive deficits are often excluded from studies that require an expressed understanding of the treatment, alternatives, and risk. In such cases, participation in a research study is a commitment on the part of the individual and the caregiver. The caregiver, as well as the research participant, will require guidance regarding the study protocol and data collection schedule. Developing and maintaining a relationship with the caregiver will result in a higher success rate for enrollment and retention. The research team should plan to stay in touch with the caregiver of cognitively impaired persons to keep participants engaged in the study. Friendly reminders about data collection schedules, newsletters, and birthday cards are also helpful in maintaining contact and enthusiasm for the study. Another consideration is to remain flexible regarding the site for the intervention and/or data collection. In some cases, a home visit for intervention implementation or data collection may be the best solution to maintain study participation. In designing intervention studies for older persons, especially those with cognitive impairment, one can expect the IRB process to be more prolonged, and to contain additional safeguards regarding the risk–benefit ratio, adding to the study timeline (Knebl & Patki, 2010).

Recruitment and Retention of Persons With Acute Life-Threatening or Terminal Disease

Traumatic, acute onset of illness or a diagnosis of a potentially life-threatening disease creates special challenges in terms of recruitment and retention of research participants. Intervention research designs requiring data collection or implementation of an intervention near death or at the time of a critical event serve to increase the challenges to recruitment and retention. In a systematic review of end-of-life research, George (2002) identified several methodological barriers to recruitment and retention of research subjects, such as the uncertain nature of the dying trajectory—issues that affect sampling and attrition. When research is focused on investigations of critical or terminal events leading to death, potential study participants recruited from intensive care units or hospices tend to enter such settings when death is imminent, greatly limiting the opportunity for recruitment and retention. In such settings, obtaining a representative sample is restricted. Investigators should strive to obtain data from multiple sites or settings to maximize generalizability. Attrition from death is encountered and, at times, expected in such research investigations (Shields, Park, Ward, & Song, 2010). However, "functional attrition," where dying persons are unable to participate in data collection, is problematic (George, 2002). In such cases, the use of surrogate or proxy respondents is often used. Investigators must be certain to set forth rigorous criteria for the inclusion of surrogates and carefully describe the circumstances for using surrogate or proxy respondents in lieu of the patient.

Researchers also must contend with the changing landscape of patient care that needs to balance sudden events, such as medical or surgical treatments that may negatively affect study recruitment or ongoing participation. Eligible patients suddenly may become compromised and, thus, decline study participation or drop out, or may not be referred to the research team by providers who inadvertently make predeterminations about potential eligibility without consulting the research team (Steinhauser et al., 2006). The initial time of a specific diagnosis or critical event may be the recruitment opportunity that best fits the research intent or design. However, this time is considered extremely stressful by patients and family members alike, and consideration of participation in a research study appears excessively burdensome (Newberry et al., 2010). Strategies for recruiting study participants during this difficult time need to be carefully planned and executed to meet eligibility while being sensitive to the needs and preferences of patients and their families.

In a randomized intervention trial (Sharing Patients' Illness Representations to Increase Trust [SPIRIT] intervention) of end-of-life care and decision making for African Americans receiving dialysis, various recruitment strategies were used (Shields et al., 2010). First, a trusted member of the healthcare team—the social worker—made the initial contact to the patient and family members. The use of key contacts or trusted personnel who have authority to access patients is a means of increasing the potential research subject's consideration of study participation. The time lapse between speaking to eligible patients and contact by research study staff is important to consider. The research team for the SPIRIT intervention contacted eligible persons who agreed to discuss the study within 2 to 3 days of meeting with the social worker to maintain interest and recall of the study. Because the SPIRIT intervention included the recruitment of the patient's surrogate decision maker, having the patient inform his or her surrogate about the study was a key component in preventing issues around "cold-calling" of potential research participants. Procedures for obtaining consent included calling and speaking to the surrogate prior to leaving phone messages—even though calls had to be made multiple times and at different hours of the day (Shields et al., 2010).

Recruitment and Retention of Teens

Certain considerations for teens are important to consider. For instance, easy access to interventions is critical, especially because some individuals do not have their own transportation and thus may walk or use local transportation systems to attend sessions (bus, metro). It also is important to consider what time of day the intervention and data collection sessions will occur because school hours and late evenings are usually prohibitive for teen participation. Identifying preferred method of contacts, in many cases by texting or cell phone, will help to ensure continued communication with teen participants. Capitalizing on social media and technology as pathways to enhance recruitment and retention of teens can be quite valuable. Finally, the importance of offering snacks during recruitment, intervention, and follow-up components cannot be minimized when it comes to teens; as any parent or clinician knows, teens are almost always hungry and having food available may be an important recruitment and retention tool. Having childcare available, even during the recruitment process, may be a strong influence on the success of the recruitment process. This is particularly important to consider when potential participants are pregnant women and teen mothers.

RETENTION STRATEGIES

Many factors affect the recruitment and retention of study participants. Yet, despite the importance of obtaining and maintaining an adequate study sample, few publications specify strategies for retaining study participants. Retention of research participants is most challenging in studies with longitudinal intervention designs that require data collection over time. Interventions imbedded within longitudinal studies require an ongoing commitment on the part of the research participant to engage in the requirements of the specific intervention and measures over time. Often, significant others or family members may also be involved because of direct or indirect research study needs.

Retention of study participants needs to be a priority consideration beginning in the study design phase. Retention strategies to be considered are maintaining contact information, planning for follow-up, research study identification methods, training of research team members, plans for communication throughout the study, and acknowledgments and incentives. In one longitudinal study of coronary artery bypass patient–spouse dyads, retention strategies included a philosophy of caring for research participants, maintaining contact between the research team and study participants, and using a systematic means of follow-up (Killien & Newton, 1990). Various methods of contact should be included in retention protocols (e.g., phone, mail, text). Developing an algorithm that documents the entire retention protocol is extremely useful. It promotes consistency of approach and makes it easier for research team members to independently take appropriate steps when they encounter difficulty contacting a participant. Very little time should elapse when contact with participants is lost; research team members must be trained to follow a detailed protocol and document success or lack of success at each step. Figure 14.2 is an example of a detailed algorithm developed to retain at-risk urban adolescent girls enrolled in a year-long RCT (Morrison-Beedy et al., 2010a, 2010b).

Maintaining Contact Information

Following recruitment and subsequent informed consent, it is important to have multiple means of ensuring the ability to contact study participants over time for several reasons. First, a longitudinal design incorporates multiple intervention sessions or scheduled data collection that requires multiple contacts. Second, it is possible that the investigator needs to reestablish contact for additional measures, such as blood sample collection, or other types of secondary analyses that require reconsent from the participant. In requesting contact information, it is helpful to have both primary and secondary contacts. Primary contact information consists of name, address, email, and all phone numbers of the research study participant. In seeking secondary contact information, the research team requests similar information from additional (collateral) contacts outside of the participant's home such as a family member, close friend, or both. This strategy ensures the research team's ability to contact participants despite unforeseen circumstances such as seasonal relocation, unstable housing situations, or interrupted phone service. Figure 14.3 presents a portion of the complex locator information used during an RCT with at-risk urban adolescent girls to maintain contact with them throughout the course of the year (Seibold-Simpson & Morrison-Beedy, 2010). Establishing a detailed protocol from the time of consent throughout the study to ensure adequate contacts at appropriate intervals is invaluable. Hiring of specific personnel for tracking participants can be extremely valuable for retention efforts; the extensive time

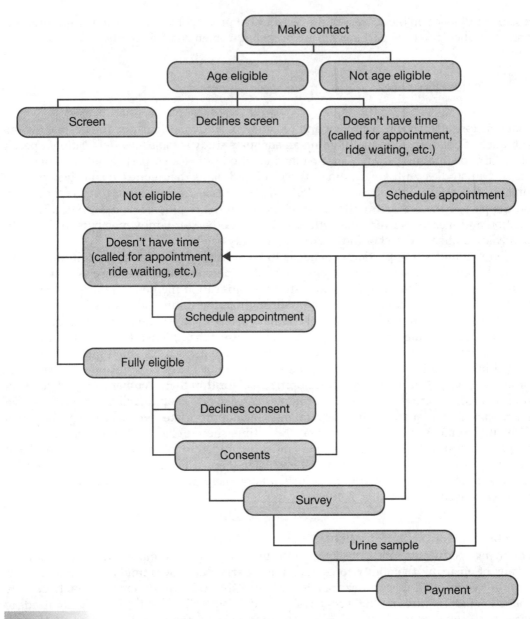

FIGURE 14.2 Flowchart of HIP Teen recruitment procedures.

HIP, Health Improvement Project; PI, principal investigator.
Source: Morrison-Beedy, PI, funded by the National Institutes of Health/National Institute of Nursing Research #R01 NR0081994.

required to both hire and train these team members is often not given sufficient consideration in the study timeline or in the budget.

Planning for Follow-Up

Once consent is obtained, provide study participants with a calendar or schedule of follow-up visits for intervention implementation and data collection to help research participants anticipate and plan for future appointments. Ideally, the data collector should remain consistent

STUDY ID#_____   RECRUITER_____

DATE ___/ ___/ ___   SITE_____

                                  HOW RECRUITED _____

**HIP TEEN
PROJECT LOCATOR FORM**

Once you are in the study, it's critical that we keep in contact with you! Without follow-ups with you, we won't know what helps girls stay healthy. Plus we need to make sure we can reach you about your lab test results if necessary. We will only get in touch with you the way you want–by phone, e-mail or mail, whatever is better for you. So please answer as many of these questions as you can.

1. Name: _____
          (First)   (Middle)   (Last)

2. Date of Birth: _____ / ___ / _____
                      (month) (day)   (year)

3. Are there other names or nicknames that you like to be called? _____

4. What is your address? *If living in a dorm, please give mailing address at school.*

_____
          (Street, Apartment #)

_____
          (City)   (State)   (Zip)

5. How long have you been living at this address? _____

6. Who do you live with?
      Full name: _____ _____
                    (First, Middle, Last)   (Relationship)

      Full name: _____ _____
                    (First, Middle, Last)   (Relationship)

      Full name: _____ _____
                    (First, Middle, Last)   (Relationship)

      Full name: _____ _____
                    (First, Middle, Last)   (Relationship)

7. If you live with your parents, will they know you are participating in this project?   Yes   No

8. Can we send you mail here?   Yes   No

      If no, where can we send you mail?

_____
          (Street, Apartment #)

_____
          (City)   (State)   (Zip)

      Whose address is this? _____

9. Is there any chance that you will be moving anytime soon?   Yes   No   Maybe

10. If so, when? _____

       Where to? _____

11. Home/Dorm phone: (____) _____

       OK to leave message?   Yes   No

       If no, why not? _____

       Best time to call: _____

       Does anybody at your house *not* speak English?   Yes   No

       If yes, who? _____

12. Cell phone: (____) _____ OK to leave message?   Yes   No

       Best time to call: _____

13. Pager: (____) _____

Page 1 of 2

FIGURE 14.3 HIP Teen Project Locator Form.

HIP, Health Improvement Project; PI, principal investigator.
Source: Morrison-Beedy, PI, funded by the National Institutes of Health/National Institute of Nursing Research #R01 NR0081994.

(continued)

14. Do you work?   Yes   No

     If yes where? _____

     How often? _____

     Work phone: (____) _____

          OK to call work?   Yes   No

          OK to leave message?   Yes   No

15. Which of the above numbers is the best way to reach you? 1st Choice: _____

                                      2nd Choice: _____

16. How do you want us to identify ourselves when we call you? (e.g. Health Improvement Project for Teens, HIP Teens, [recruiter's first name], University of _____)

_____

17. E-mail address:_____

     Is this a shared account?   Yes   No   OK to send e-mail?   Yes   No

     How often do you check your e-mail? _____

18. Please list three of your best friends that would know how to reach you

Full Name	Home Phone	Cell Phone	E-mail Address

19. Other contacts: Friends or relatives who usually know how to reach you should we have trouble contacting you for follow-ups. For example, best friends, relatives, people at work

    (1) Full name: _____ _____
                       (First, Middle, Last)   (Relationship)

    Address: _____
               (Street)

    _____
          (City)   (State)   (Zip)

    Phone: (____) _____   Cell phone: (____) _____

    Pager: (____) _____   Work phone: (____) _____

    E-mail address: _____

    Will they know you are participating in the study?   Yes   No

    Can we leave a message with this person for you?   Yes   No

    Can we send you e-mail here?   Yes   No   Can we send you postcards here?   Yes   No

Page 2 of 2

FIGURE 14.3 *(continued)*

for each study participant to build trust and maintain the integrity and consistency of data collection. After each visit, communicating appreciation for continued participation through a postcard, letter, or email maintains contact and helps solidify the relationship with the research staff (Northouse et al., 2006). This communication could also include a reminder for the next time a follow-up meeting is planned. Examples of intermittent contact cards from the HIP Teens trial are presented in Figure 14.4. The cards included brief motivational statements to facilitate study involvement.

HIP Teens Card Text

Appointment card (given to subject at enrollment if able to be placed directly in a Wave)

This confirms your next HIP Teen group meeting
On
_____, _____ at _____ pm
See you then!
Thank you for your contribution to learning how teens can stay healthy.

Thank you for enrolling (mailed to subject's home after enrolled)

Thank you for enrolling in the
Health Improvement Project for Teens.

You are essential to our project.
We will be contacting you soon about your group meetings.

Thank you card given at 1-week survey (given directly to subject with payment at the end of survey)

We appreciate all the time and effort you put into the HIP Teen Project.
You are helping improve the health of girls
just like you.

Thank you card given at 3 month reunion (given directly to subject with payment at the end of 3-month reunion session)

Thank you for being part of HIP Teens.
We look forward to meeting with you
again in 3 months.
Your participation is crucial to
our goal of keeping teens healthy.

FIGURE 14.4 Examples of participant contact cards from Health Improvement Program for Teens: HIP Teens Card.

HIP, Health Improvement Project; PI, principal investigator.
Source: Morrison-Beedy, PI, funded by the National Institutes of Health/National Institute of Nursing Research #R01 NR0081994.

Research Study Identification

In developing retention strategies, the research study team benefits from adopting strategies that permit research participants to self-identify with the proposed study. Just like marketing materials identify retailers in business, adopting an acronym and logo for the study could be considered. Moore et al. (2006) coined the term CHANGE (Changing Habits by Applying New Goals and Experiences) used in a 1-year randomized intervention trial to increase exercise maintenance following cardiac events. Acronyms could be helpful in conveying the main core concepts of the proposed study to healthcare personnel involved in study participant referral.

Another inexpensive means of providing study identification and creating a sense of belonging is the provision of laminated "study membership" business cards that contain the study logo, name, and research personnel's wallet-sized contact information card. If the research budget allows, small items associated with the research study prove useful in forming a study identity and sense of belonging. For example, a research logo placed on T-shirts or water bottles given to study participants in a study intervention involving physical activity could be considered. Such items can also serve as study incentives.

Acknowledgments and Incentives

It is important to remember that people who agree to participate in research are performing an important service in the name of science. They do so voluntarily and often with little compensation. Given et al. (1990) gave study participants a coffee mug with the study logo after the first data collection. Northouse et al. (2006) also provided study participants with a similar mug with the saying "Helping Others Through Research" imprinted on it to capitalize on the spirit of altruism many study participants report feeling. Providing small gifts as tokens of appreciation throughout the study is recommended. Other options for incentives include bookmarks, reading lights, water bottles, T-shirts, or tote bags imprinted with the study logo. Depending on what is required of participants in a study, monetary incentives may be appropriate. For example, $5.00 to $10.00 gift certificates to coffee houses, restaurants, grocery stores, or gasoline stations, or parking vouchers could be provided at each data collection appointment. If research funds are slim, providing this incentive at the final data collection point may be acceptable. On the other hand, there is the risk of attrition with this approach and, in some studies, the IRB may consider withholding payment to the end of the study to be coercive. Studies requiring more effort on the part of participants will require increased levels of incentives.

Determining appropriate levels of compensation can be aided by garnering information from similar projects and asking other investigators. Another route is collecting data that may be helpful in supporting planned incentive amounts. For example, in an RCT study of 15- to 19-year-old girls, appropriate incentive amounts for each 2-hour sexual risk reduction group meeting were determined by conducting preliminary survey work with similarly aged girls. In the survey, investigators assessed average hourly wages of girls on the basis of employment or babysitting activities and then investigators applied average wages that would be lost if the girls did not work but attended the research study instead (Morrison-Beedy et al., 2012). Gift cards are received very well by study participants but can be fraught with "challenges" for investigators related to documentation. Studies may also offer incentives such as mileage, parking costs, or research-related medical costs coverage for required study components such as lab work (although this is often only for costs above and beyond those covered by insurance). Documentation will be required from participants for any incentives, and institutions vary on the details needed in this documentation. The Internal Revenue Service (IRS) limits also exist for the yearly nontaxable amounts individuals can receive for research participation.

Research Team Training

Thorough and standardized research team training is critical to the ability to recruit and retain research participants. Potential barriers to remaining in intervention research need to be considered in the design phase of the study. Potential barriers to both accrual and retention in intervention studies include, among others, the time commitment required, complications of illness, and lack of perceived benefit from the intervention. Standardizing strategies for overcoming anticipated barriers as issues present themselves is vital. In spite of careful planning and problem solving on behalf of the research team, unanticipated issues arise related to remaining in intervention studies. Research team training carried out in small pilot studies is optimal. In such studies, recruitment, intervention, and retention strategy experience can be tailored in preparation for future, larger scale studies. Once barriers to retention have been identified, a standardized "script" or approach can be crafted for the research team to use that addresses these potential roadblocks. These scripts may include questions posed to participants such as: "Have you thought about how you will get to your appointment tomorrow?" or "How reliable is the babysitter you've been using; do you anticipate having any problems with child care for your session next week?" Scripts can also contain general problem-solving ideas for that question, for example, "Is there a bus route near your house?" "Can I text you directions?" "Do you have a friend or neighbor who could help out with child care?" Research team training can include techniques such as role-play with feedback and critique from the PI or from team members. Extensive time, often 40 hours or more, may be spent training team members prior to the implementation of such study protocols to ensure quality data.

MAINTAINING COMMUNICATION

Attrition during an RCT is unwanted but expected and is of particular concern in a longitudinal study. Maintaining communication with study participants has several advantages. First and foremost, participants become familiar with study personnel and begin to build a trusting relationship. These relationships become critical for ensuring commitment to the study intervention and procedures. Northouse et al. (2006) used deliberate retention strategies to retain cancer patients and their family members. Once recruited and after obtaining baseline data, letters were mailed to participants informing them of the result of the randomization process. The letter also included a timeline for data collection and the name of the intervention nurse or data collector who would contact them. Although blinded to group assignment, the same data collector would be responsible for all follow-up interviews to maintain consistency and foster a relationship of rapport with the research team member. Following each data collection cycle, study participants were mailed a personal thank you letter for their participation and encouraged to complete the following scheduled data collection.

If despite all proactive retention strategies participants voluntarily withdraw from the study, it is important to track the reason(s) for withdrawal. Discussing the reasons for withdrawal with the research team, as appropriate, and brainstorming about alternative approaches that can be instituted are helpful. In the final analysis, examining differential recruitment and retention rates between the intervention and control groups is imperative. Recruitment and retention strategies were assessed midway in a study of at-risk teens (Seibold-Simpson & Morrison-Beedy, 2010), and recruiters' experience (time in position), ability to provide home and cell phone numbers and leave messages at those numbers, as well as parental awareness of study participation were some of the key factors identified in recruitment approaches that increased the likelihood of study participation. Identifying such predictors of attendance can help participation and retention rates both in an ongoing study (if assessed early within the project) and in future planned studies that build on this intervention trial. Determining challenges to recruitment and retention, as well as reasons for attrition, serve to enhance future study endeavors.

SUMMARY

Recruitment and retention of participants remain— one of the "character builders" of intervention science, yet there are many well-tried approaches that should be used as "standard of care" for intervention study protocols. However, these measures may not be sufficient and it is up to you and your research team to think "out of the box" and continue to try new and innovative strategies that address the unique needs of your particular population. Some of your most relevant plans may come from your participants themselves—ask them for ideas as well as provide feedback on proposed approaches. Being able to recruit those participants who truly represent members of the target population and who will ultimately benefit from your intervention is paramount to study success. Once recruited, participants often need your help to continue study involvement; you, as the investigator, have the responsibility of devising strategies that enable this. As a research scientist, it is your responsibility to make good use of your funding agency or institution's financial and effort support. Retaining participants serves to strengthen validity and contributes to a rigorous scientific study. Intervention studies are strengthened further by intent-to-treat analyses; thus, minimizing attrition of participants is vital. CONSORT table requirements have provided a mechanism by which investigators can share detailed information about study participants—who did and who did not consent, who did and who did not attend the intervention and follow-up sessions. These data lead to increased understanding of generalizability and reproducibility of the intervention. Using a "multimethod" approach for identifying, enrolling, and maintaining participants throughout the course of your study requires persistence, dedication, and tenacity. Applying suggestions from this chapter to your intervention study will help you to recruit and retain that which is most precious to you—your sample.

Key Points From This Chapter

- Both recruitment and retention of participants take concerted effort and varied approaches on the part of all team members to ensure success.
- Loss of statistical power, the dilution of intervention effects, and threats to study validity are just a few of the harmful repercussions of participant attrition.
- Barriers to recruitment exist not only for participants but for recruitment site personnel as well.
- Maintaining enrollment requires a very detailed record of participant contacts using multiple venues (e.g., family, friends, cell phone, email, school, employer).
- Longitudinal retention of participants is facilitated by consistent contact by one team member.
- Developing an algorithm that documents the step-by-step retention protocol provides consistent procedures for research team personnel.
- Incentives for participation are an important component of successful intervention studies but should be tailored to each study on the basis of participation requirements.

REFERENCES

Aitken, L., Gallagher, R., & Madronio, C. (2003). Principles of recruitment and retention in clinical trials. *International Journal of Nursing Practice, 9*(6), 338–346.

Bill-Axelson, A., Christensson, A., Carlsson, M., Norlén, B. J., & Holmberg, L. (2008). Experiences of randomization: Interviews with patients and clinicians in the SPCG-IV trial. *Scandinavian Journal of Urology and Nephrology, 42*(4), 358–363. doi:10.1080/00365590801950253

Bonner, G. J., & Miles, T. P. (1997). Participation of African Americans in clinical research. *Neuroepidemiology, 16*(6), 281–284. doi:10.1159/000109698

Campbell, M. K., Snowdon, C., Francis, D., Elbourne, D., McDonald, A. M., Knight, R., … STEPS Group. (2007). Recruitment to randomised trials: Strategies for trial enrollment and participation study. The STEPS study. *Health Technology Assessment, 11*(48). Retrieved from http://aura.abdn.ac.uk/bitstream/handle/2164/179/Campbell2007.pdf?sequence=1

Chang, M. W., Brown, R., & Nitzke, S. (2009). Participant recruitment and retention in a pilot program to prevent weight gain in low-income overweight and obese mothers. *BMC Public Health, 9*, 424. doi:10.1186/1471-2458-9-424

Cooley, M. E., Sarna, L., Brown, J. K., Williams, R. D., Chernecky, C., Padilla, G., & Danao, L. L. (2003). Challenges of recruitment and retention in multisite clinical research. *Cancer Nursing, 26*(5), 376–384.

George, L. K. (2002). Research design in end-of-life research: State of science [Special issue]. *Gerontologist, 42*(3), 86–98.

Given, B. A., Keilman, L. J., Collins, C., & Given, C. W. (1990). Strategies to minimize attrition in longitudinal studies. *Nursing Research, 39*(3), 184–186.

Gross, C. P., Mallory, R., Heiat, A., & Krumholz, H. M. (2002). Reporting the recruitment process in clinical trials: Who are these patients and how did they get there? *Annals of Internal Medicine, 137*(1), 10–16.

Gul, R. B., & Ali, P. A. (2010). Clinical trials: The challenge of recruitment and retention of participants. *Journal of Clinical Nursing, 19*(1–2), 227–233. doi:10.1111/j.1365-2702.2009.03041.x

Hulley, S. B., Cummings, S. R., Browner, W. S., Grady, D. G., Hearst, N., & Newman, T. B. (2001). *Designing clinical research: An epidemiological approach* (2nd ed.). Philadelphia, PA: Lippincott Williams & Wilkins.

Keith, S. J. (2001). Evaluating characteristics of patient selection and dropout rates. *Journal of Clinical Psychiatry, 62*(Suppl. 9), 11–16.

Killien, M., & Newton, K. (1990). Longitudinal research: The challenge of maintaining continued involvement of participants. *Western Journal of Nursing Research, 12*(5), 689–692. doi:10.1177/019394599001200512

Knebl, J. A., & Patki, D. (2010). Recruitment of subjects into clinical trials for Alzheimer disease. *Journal of the American Osteopathic Association, 110*(9 Suppl. 8), S43–S49.

Lee, R. M., & Renzetti, C. M. (1990). The problem of researching sensitive topics. *American Behavioral Scientist, 33*(5), 510–528.

Locher, J. L., Bronstein, J., Robinson, C. O., Williams, C., & Ritchie, C. S. (2006). Ethical issues involving research conducted with homebound older adults. *Gerontologist, 46*(2), 160–164.

McMillan, S. C., & Weitzner, M. A. (2003). Methodologic issues in collecting data from debilitated patients with cancer near the end of life. *Oncology Nursing Forum, 30*(1), 123–129. doi:10.1188/03.ONF.123-129

McNees, P., Dow, K. H., & Loerzel, V. W. (2005). Application of the CuSum technique to evaluate changes in recruitment strategies. *Nursing Research, 54*(6), 399–405.

Mills, E. J., Seely, D., Rachlis, B., Griffith, L., Wu, P., Wilson, K., … Wright, J. R. (2006). Barriers to participation in clinical trials of cancer: A meta-analysis and systematic review of patient-reported factors. *Lancet Oncology, 7*(2), 141–148. doi:10.1016/S1470-2045(06)70576-9

Moore, S. M., Charvat, J. M., Gordon, N. H., Pashkow, F., Ribisl, P., Roberts, B. L., & Rocco, M. (2006). Effects of a CHANGE intervention to increase exercise maintenance following cardiac events. *Annals of Behavioral Medicine, 31*(1), 53–62. doi:10.1207/s15324796abm3101_9

Morrison-Beedy, D., Carey, M. P., Aronowitz, T., Mkandawire, L., & Dyne, J. (2002). Adolescents' input on the development of an HIV risk reduction intervention. *Journal of the Association of Nurses in AIDS Care, 13*(1), 21–27. doi:10.1016/S1055-3290(06)60238-0

Morrison-Beedy, D., Carey, M. P., Crean, H. F., & Jones, S. H. (2010a). Determinants of adolescent female attendance at an HIV risk reduction program. *Journal of the Association of Nurses in AIDS Care, 21*(2), 153–161. doi:10.1016/j.jana.2009.11.002

Morrison-Beedy, D., Carey, M. P., Crean, H. F., & Jones, S. H. (2010b). Risk behaviors among adolescent girls in an HIV prevention trial. *Western Journal of Nursing Research, 33*(5), 690–711. doi:10.1177/0193945910379220

Morrison-Beedy, D., Jones, S. H., Xia, Y., Tu, X., Crean, H. F., & Carey, M. P. (2012). Reducing sexual risk behavior in adolescent girls: Results from a randomized controlled trial. *Journal of Adolescent Health, 52*(3), 314–321. doi:10.1016/j.jadohealth.2012.07.005

Moser, D. K., Dracup, K., & Doering, L. V. (2000). Factors differentiating dropouts from completers in a longitudinal, multicenter clinical trial. *Nursing Research, 49*(2), 109–116.

Motzer, S. A., Moseley, J. R., & Lewis, F. M. (1997). Recruitment and retention of families in clinical trials with longitudinal designs. *Western Journal of Nursing Research, 19*(3), 314–333. doi:10.1177/019394599701900304

Musiat, P., Winsall, M., Orlowski, S., Antezana, G., Schrader, G., Battersby, M., & Bidargaddi, N. (2016). Paid and unpaid online recruitment for health interventions in young adults. *Journal of Adolescent Health, 59*(6), 662–667. doi:10.1016/j.jadohealth.2016.07.020

National Institutes of Health. (1994). NIH guidelines on the inclusion of women and minorities as subjects in clinical research. *NIH Guide, 23*(11). Retrieved from http://grants.nih.gov/grants/guide/notice-files/not94-100.html

Nelson, L. E., & Morrison-Beedy, D. (2008). Research team training: Moving beyond job descriptions. *Applied Nursing Research, 21*(3), 159–164. doi:10.1016/j.apnr.2006.09.001

Newberry, A., Sherwood, P., Hricik, A., Bradley, S., Kuo, J., Crago, E., … Given, B. A. (2010). Understanding recruitment and retention in neurological research. *Journal of Neuroscience Nursing, 42*(1), 47–57.

Northouse, L. L., Rosset, T., Phillips, L., Mood, D., Schafenacker, A., & Kershaw, T. (2006). Research with families facing cancer: The challenges of accrual and retention. *Research in Nursing & Health, 29*(3), 199–211. doi:10.1002/nur.20128

Ott, C. D., Twiss, J. J., Waltman, N. L., Gross, G. J., & Lindsey, A. M. (2006). Challenges of recruitment of breast cancer survivors to a randomized clinical trial for osteoporosis prevention. *Cancer Nursing, 29*(1), 21–31.

Oude Rengerink, K., Opmeer, B. C., Logtenberg, S. L., Hooft, L., Bloemenkamp, K. W., Haak, M. C., … Mol, B. W. (2010). IMproving PArticipation of patients in clinical trials–rationale and design of IMPACT. *BMC Medical Research Methodology, 10*, 85. doi:10.1186/1471-2288-10-85

Patel, M. X., Doku, V., & Tennakoon, L. (2003). Challenges in recruitment of research participants. *Advances in Psychiatric Treatment, 9*(3), 229–238. doi:10.1192/apt.9.3.229

Ransom, S., Azzarello, L. M., & McMillan, S. C. (2006). Methodological issues in the recruitment of cancer pain patients and their caregivers. *Research in Nursing & Health, 29*(3), 190–198. doi:10.1002/nur.20129

Rosal, M. C., White, M. J., Borg, A., Scavron, J., Candib, L., Ockene, I., & Magner, R. (2010). Translational research at community health centers: Challenges and successes in recruiting and retaining low-income Latino patients with type 2 diabetes into a randomized clinical trial. *The Diabetes Educator, 36*(5), 733–749. doi:10.1177/0145721710380146

Ross, S., Grant, A., Counsell, C., Gillespie, W., Russell, I., & Prescott, R. (1999). Barriers to participation in randomised controlled trials: A systematic review. *Lancet Infectious Diseases, 6*(1), 32–38.

Schulz, K. F., Altman, D. G., & Moher, D., CONSORT Group. (2010). CONSORT 2010 statement: Update guidelines for reporting parallel group randomized trials. *Annals of Internal Medicine, 152*(11), 726–732. doi:10.7326/0003-4819-152-11-201006010-00232

Seibold-Simpson, S., & Morrison-Beedy, D. (2010). Avoiding early study attrition in adolescent girls: Impact of recruitment contextual factors. *Western Journal of Nursing Research, 32*(6), 761–778. doi:10.1177/0193945909360198

Shields, A. M., Park, M., Ward, S. E., & Song, M. K. (2010). Subject recruitment and retention against quadruple challenges in an intervention trial of end-of-life communication. *Journal of Hospice and Palliative Nursing, 12*(5), 312–318. doi:10.1097/NJH.0b013e3181ec9dd1

Silva, M. C. (1995). *Ethical guidelines in the conduct, dissemination, and implementation of nursing research.* Washington, DC: American Nurses Association.

Steinhauser, K. E., Clipp, E. C., Hays, J. C., Olsen, M., Arnold, R., Christakis, N. A., … Tulsky, J. A. (2006). Identifying, recruiting, and retaining seriously-ill patients and their caregivers in longitudinal research. *Palliative Medicine, 20*(8), 745–754. doi:10.1177/0269216306073112

Sullivan-Bolyai, S., Bova, C., Deatrick, J. A., Knafl, K., Grey, M., Leung, K., & Trudeau, A. (2007). Barriers and strategies for recruiting study participants in clinical settings. *Western Journal of Nursing Research, 29*(4), 486–500. doi:10.1177/0193945907299658

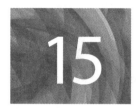

15

Maintaining Fidelity of an Intervention

Sandee McClowry & Sandra Gagnon

> Some people want it to happen, some wish it would happen, others make it happen. —*Michael Jordan*

Intervention fidelity, the extent to which an intervention is delivered as intended, is of growing concern in the fields of health, education, and psychology. An intervention cannot be deemed evidence based without having demonstrated fidelity (Bruhn, Hirsch, & Lloyd, 2015). Correspondingly, failure to achieve desired outcomes may erroneously be attributed to program ineffectiveness when instead it is a failure to implement the intervention with adequate fidelity (Gresham, Dart, & Collins, 2017).

The recent proliferation of evidence-based interventions challenges researchers and practitioners alike to pay careful attention to fidelity throughout the various stages of an intervention. Indeed, fidelity is a critical component of the design, implementation, efficacy testing, adaptation, and dissemination of an intervention. Although establishing and maintaining fidelity are critical (Gresham et al., 2017), it remains inadequately assessed in research studies and is even more rarely examined in applied settings (Reed & Codding, 2014).

In this chapter, we explore several facets of intervention fidelity. After the construct is defined, the current state of fidelity research is briefly discussed. Then, strategies for establishing and maintaining fidelity are offered, and remaining challenges within the field are acknowledged. Following that, the complexities of maintaining fidelity in new contexts are explored. To provide a practical example, we illustrate the procedures used to evaluate fidelity in a rural school district adaptation of an urban evidence-based intervention, INSIGHTS Into Children's Temperament. The chapter ends with five practical recommendations for establishing and maintaining fidelity of an intervention.

INTERVENTION FIDELITY DEFINED

Consensus on what constitutes intervention fidelity and how it should be measured is lacking. Even the terminology used to refer to the construct of intervention fidelity varies among and within disciplines. For example, "fidelity" has been used interchangeably with "treatment integrity," "process fidelity," "research integrity," and "adherence to protocol" (Bova et al., 2017; Gresham et al., 2017; Reed & Codding, 2014). Likewise, agreement on what constitutes fidelity is not universally accepted. In some reports, the focus of fidelity is on compliance, structure, and quality (Barrenger, Kriegel, Angell, & Draine, 2016) whereas adherence to protocol, competence of facilitators, and interactions between facilitators and recipients are discussed in others (Reed & Codding, 2014).

Several specific components of fidelity, however, are commonly addressed (Goncy, Sutherland, Farrell, Sullivan, & Doyle, 2015). **Exposure** is simply the number and frequency of treatment sessions. **Adherence** is the extent to which the intervention's components were delivered as outlined in the protocol. **Competence** is reflected in the procedural and interactive aspects of delivery. **Quality** of implementation refers to general characteristics and behaviors of facilitators. Some reports on fidelity add a more detailed assessment of the facilitators who conduct the intervention and the recipients. Treatment **understanding** is the level of the facilitator's comprehension of the intervention and its parts (Lakin & Shannon, 2015). **Responsiveness** refers to the degree of involvement and enthusiasm by facilitators and the participants (Goncy et al., 2015).

A recent conceptualization of fidelity ascribes to a multifaceted conceptualization of the construct that incorporates an intervention's core components or "active ingredients" (Abry, Hulleman, & Rimm-Kaufman, 2015). Core components are the essential parts of an intervention that are believed to promote the anticipated outcomes. From this broader perspective, fidelity is the extent to which an intervention's core components are implemented (Mendive, Weiland, Yoshikawa, & Snow, 2015).

THE CURRENT STATUS OF EXAMINING INTERVENTION FIDELITY

As discussed repeatedly in this book, multiple fields have reported a substantial increase in developing and empirically testing the efficacy of interventions. Dovetailing on the trend is the increasing demand by governmental agencies and foundations for fidelity assessments to be integrated within clinical and prevention trials (Reed & Codding, 2014). Likewise, applied settings are increasingly requiring that evidence-based interventions be adapted for their use.

Although the number of studies reporting fidelity data has increased, recent reviews of scholarly publications indicate that the rate of reporting is still disappointingly low. For example, a recent review of 79 schoolwide prevention programs reported that fidelity data were presented in only 46% of scholarly publications (Bruhn et al., 2015). Other reports, however, indicate a higher percentage of studies reporting fidelity. In a review of 65 evidence-based parenting programs, 75% of the studies reviewed assessed fidelity although only 45% demonstrated "high" fidelity (Garbacz, Brown, Spee, Polo, & Budd, 2014). Likewise, a meta-analysis of social and emotional learning programs found that 69% of studies provided fidelity information (Wigelsworth et al., 2016).

Several limitations are apparent in many published reports of fidelity. Researchers tend to provide a single index of fidelity for their programs (Bruhn et al., 2015) and offer little advice about how to use their fidelity data to inform practitioners' work in their settings (Bova et al., 2017). Without reliable data on intervention fidelity, practitioners' ability to critically evaluate and implement interventions with fidelity in their settings is compromised.

Yet, despite the relatively low and variable reports of fidelity in the literature, a number of notable examples of published studies that describe fidelity exist: programs that target parental diabetes education (Bova et al., 2017), substance abuse in incarcerated adolescents (Bassett, Stein, Rossi, & Martin, 2016), family-based treatment of anorexia nervosa with adolescents (Forsberg et al., 2014), parents of children and adolescents with externalizing disorders (Garbacz et al., 2014), middle school science (Lakin & Shannon, 2015), and bullying prevention (Goncy et al., 2015).

Two clinical trials are among the very few that have assessed the fidelity of both the treatment and control groups, which is recommended by Abry et al. (2015). Kelly, Oswalt, Melnyk, and Jacobson (2015) conducted a randomized clinical trial that compared the fidelity of the Creating Opportunities for Personal Empowerment Healthy Lifestyles (COPE TEEN) and Healthy Teens programs, which focus on improving physical and mental health and increasing knowledge of health topics, respectively. Mendive et al. (2015) conducted a randomized trial of A Good Start, a teacher professional development program for prekindergarten and kindergarten teachers.

The current state of fidelity research points to the need for more in-depth examinations of the construct. Likewise, greater attention to fidelity is needed both in research and practice. Still, a great deal of wisdom can be gleaned from what is already known about fidelity in interventions.

ESTABLISHING AND MAINTAINING FIDELITY IN RESEARCH AND PRACTICE

There are many methods for establishing and maintaining fidelity in interventions although a multimethod, multi-informant approach is considered best practice (Bruhn et al., 2015). Fidelity assessment, however, does not begin once an intervention is in place. Rather, many activities that promote fidelity should be taken prior to any implementation of an intervention:

Involve Key Stakeholders
Collaboration with key stakeholders during planning helps ascertain the feasibility of conducting an intervention and testing its fidelity in a particular setting (Kershner et al., 2014). Regardless of whether the intervention is in the early stages of development or whether the goal is to implement an existing evidence-based intervention, perceived acceptability, or buy-in, by stakeholders contributes to fidelity (Lakin & Shannon, 2015). A collaborative approach establishes ownership of the program and promotes adherence to the intervention's procedures, including the assessment of fidelity.

Barrenger et al. (2016) encourage the creation of a Community Advisory Board as part of the intervention team. Engaging stakeholders in an advisory board is advantageous because they possess insight into the community history and concerns. Furthermore, participants may be more inclined to trust those sharing their cultural backgrounds. The Community Advisory Board can also identify available resources, potential barriers, and anticipated challenges that may compromise fidelity and undermine intervention effectiveness (Barrenger et al., 2016; Mendive et al., 2015).

Develop a Clear Intervention Model
The next step in achieving the fidelity of an intervention is to establish a clear conceptual model, which often is presented graphically and depicts the intervention components and sequence of steps required to achieve the intended outcomes (Lloyd-Evans et al., 2016). Logic model mapping often involves illustrations, texts, and arrows to represent the relationships between intervention structures, materials, and outcomes (Holliday, 2014). Although the configuration of

the conceptual model will differ among interventions, it generally includes four components. **Intervention assumptions** explain the underlying theory that guides the intervention. The intervention **inputs** are the resources required to conduct the intervention and can include staff members, time, financial support, equipment, and community support. **Program activities** refer to the content of the intervention and other pragmatic issues such as the number of sessions and the location of services. **Outcomes** are the products of intervention activities, such as improved social or academic competencies. Logic models also can guide the evaluation of fidelity by connecting outcome data to each component of the conceptual model (Holliday, 2014).

Determine the Types and Frequencies of Fidelity Assessments

Prior to implementation, intervention teams need to determine the frequency and types of fidelity assessments they will use. The selection of measurement and fidelity tools should be guided by the logic model and be specific to the intervention's intended outcomes. Frequently used fidelity assessments are direct or video-recorded observations with detailed procedures and checklists, self-reports of facilitators' adherence to protocol, participant attendance and receipt of information, and permanent products (e.g., diaries, assignments) that result from the program (Gresham et al., 2017). In their review of 79 studies that reported fidelity data, Bruhn et al. (2015) found that permanent products and checklists were the most commonly used methods. Examples of the content included in checklists are time spent engaged with participants, number of sessions, content covered, and technical skills practiced (Bova et al., 2017).

As with the selection of any measurement tool, reliability and validity of fidelity assessments are of critical importance. Gresham et al. (2017) examined the reliability of direct observations, permanent products, and self-reports and found that each method demonstrated moderate to high reliability across raters and sessions. Self-reports demonstrated high consistency but did not correlate with either permanent products or direct observations. Direct observations were found to be the most reliable method. The authors, however, advise the use of all three methods.

Develop an Intervention Protocol

Another essential early component of fidelity planning is creating a protocol that details the procedures for conducting the intervention. Detailed program manuals should outline each session's content and materials, including training documents, videos, and participant handouts. The more detailed and user friendly the protocol, the better the intervention staff will be able to deliver the intervention with precision and consistency.

Some strategies for fidelity apply regardless of whether the intervention is in the development stage, part of a randomized clinical trial, or being implemented as an established evidence-based intervention in another setting. For example, a well-articulated and detailed protocol is important regardless of where on that continuum the intervention falls. Ideally, the same intervention manual can be used to train facilitators and fidelity reviewers (Garbacz et al., 2014). Of course, each subsequent iteration of the intervention will necessitate some edits to the manual. Other strategies apply when establishing and maintaining an intervention.

Select Staff Members Well Suited to Implement the Intervention

The selection of the intervention staff, including facilitators, fidelity reviewers, and other support personnel, plays a crucial role in the establishment and maintenance of fidelity (Reed & Codding, 2014). Facilitator characteristics, such as age (Barton, Whittaker, Kinzie, DeCoster, Furnari, 2017), level of education, experience with facilitating, and beliefs about the importance of fidelity, influence the extent of facilitators' buy-in, self-reports of fidelity, and attendance at training activities (Gagnon, 2014). Warmth, genuineness, and enthusiasm are other facilitator characteristics that influence fidelity (Jelalian et al., 2014). In fact, the facilitator's engagement with participants has demonstrated stronger effects than strict adherence to protocol (Low, Smolkowski, & Cook, 2016).

Moreover, facilitators who share the values and philosophical foundations of the intervention tend to report higher levels of fidelity (Cobanoglu & Capa-Aydin, 2015).

Provide Facilitators and Fidelity Reviewers With Adequate Training

Facilitators need to be well versed in the intervention's underlying framework and skilled in implementing its components. Direct didactic training of procedures is recommended although there is evidence that training through video simulations offers a promising alternative or addition (Barton et al., 2017). A combination of didactic training with weekly phone supervision and built-in "booster sessions" is recommended to support ongoing fidelity (Jelalian et al., 2014).

Before their training is completed, facilitators should be able to demonstrate all of the relevant intervention skills (Kershner et al., 2014). Procedural **competence**, however, is more strongly associated with participant responsiveness than procedural **adherence**, suggesting that the facilitators' relational competencies are essential (Goncy et al., 2015). For example, Kelly et al. (2015) observed higher fidelity in teachers who delivered an attention-control program than the group of teachers trained to implement the intervention being studied, which required the acquisition of new knowledge and skills.

In addition to the facilitators, fidelity reviewers should have a thorough understanding of the intervention and the strategies required for assessing its fidelity. They, too, should have didactic training and should practice until they demonstrate competence in evaluating the fidelity of the facilitators. Reliable reports by the fidelity reviewers can assist the program developer or project manager in supervising the facilitators and in knowing if they require additional training.

Determine the Extent of the Role of the Program Developer

Research exploring the benefits of developer involvement during program implementation is mixed, yet recent meta-analytic findings indicate no significant effects of developer involvement on the quality of implementation (Wigelsworth et al., 2016). The degree of developer involvement on intended outcomes appears to vary according to the outcomes measured. For example, studies of social and emotional learning programs in which the developer was involved reported changes in students' attitudes and emotional distress, whereas studies without developer involvement found an impact on social-emotional competence and conduct problems (Wigelsworth et al., 2016). The authors noted the possibility that the timing of the study may have moderated the associations between developer participation and effectiveness because involvement is expected to be higher during the initial stages of implementation. These mixed findings suggest that further research examining developer involvement is needed, but that there is value in having some level of involvement.

Provide Ongoing Supervision of the Whole Team

Continuing to examine the intervention's mechanisms for fidelity should continue throughout its course. Ongoing and frequent feedback to facilitators and regularly scheduled meetings with all members of the intervention team are recommended to avoid drift (Reed & Codding, 2014). Bruhn et al. (2015), however, found that most of the 79 studies they reviewed conducted fidelity assessments only once or twice per year. Only two studies reported daily assessments. Although frequent fidelity checks and feedback may be challenging in applied settings with limited resources, Gresham et al. (2017) achieved reliability in direct observations across raters and sessions after only four to five sessions, suggesting that with sufficient support, it is possible to collect fidelity data relatively quickly.

The impact on reducing the frequency of feedback, or fading, is not clear (Reed & Codding, 2014). Still, fidelity assessments during implementation can provide other collateral benefits.

Meetings with facilitators and fidelity reviewers can reveal problems with programming that might ultimately lead to changes in the intervention. For example, facilitators may be experiencing difficulties with certain parts of the protocol (Bruhn et al., 2015), or fidelity reviewers might observe that some parts of the intervention are not being relayed to the recipients. If identified during implementation, these issues may lead to improvements to the intervention or modifications of the protocol. Likewise, due to contextual differences, facilitators might recognize the need for modifications (Harn, Parisi, & Stoolmiller, 2013).

Randomized clinical trials that are conducted in natural settings, such as schools or hospitals, have particular challenges and opportunities. For example, drift is likely to occur when practitioners, such as teachers or nurses, attempt to juggle the multiple and often competing demands of participating in research along with their usual responsibilities. Advantages, however, can also occur. For clinical interventions that are not part of a randomized clinical trial but are intended as treatment, ongoing fidelity assessments can guide decisions about how long to continue an intervention for a particular client or student before increasing or decreasing the number of sessions or referring for other services.

CHALLENGES TO IMPLEMENTING INTERVENTIONS WITH FIDELITY

Despite its recognized importance, establishing and maintaining fidelity in efficacy studies involve a number of challenges. Even among studies reporting intervention effectiveness that were supported by high fidelity, authors have noted that fidelity assessments are costly and require a great deal of effort (Bova et al., 2017; Gresham et al., 2017). Moreover, they note that without the resources provided by partnering universities or supporting organizations, fidelity implementation would not have been manageable in clinical trials (Bova et al., 2017).

Additional fidelity challenges occur in practice settings. The mere selection of an evidence-based intervention for practice can be daunting. It is imperative that practitioners know how to interpret an intervention's outcomes and to assess whether its fidelity can be maintained in the setting. Issues such as inadequate financial and personnel resources and lack of control over environmental conditions can make it quite difficult, if not impossible, for practitioners to replicate the conditions adhered to in efficacy studies (Wigelsworth et al., 2016). For example, direct observations may be unacceptable in practice settings where confidentiality is a major concern. Consequently, evidence-based interventions are rarely applied as originally intended (Century, Cassata, Rudnick, & Freeman, 2012). Instead, it is imperative to strategically modify and adapt interventions so that they fit within the parameters of new settings.

MAINTAINING FIDELITY IN NEW CONTEXTS

Fidelity dilemmas are inevitable when "transporting" evidence-based interventions to new settings or implementing them with participants who differ from the original recipients (Wigelsworth et al., 2016). Culturally sensitive adaptations often warrant modifications to materials and format to better meet participant needs and maximize intervention outcomes. The intervention goals will not be achieved without ensuring that the program or service is sensitive to its context.

Balancing the fidelity of evidence-based programs with contextual constraints can promote ecological validity while maintaining experimental control (Barrenger et al., 2016; Reed & Codding, 2014). Challenges to fidelity should be taken into account to increase ecological validity, because they tend to interfere with strict adherence to protocol (Goncy et al., 2015). Modifications to protocol that address barriers to fidelity, such as logistical challenges (geography, adherence to timelines) and minimal community resources and support, allow the program to be sensitive to the culture of the organization and increase the likelihood of achieving desired outcomes.

A natural tension exists between fidelity and adaptations, a point well articulated by Ferrer-Wreder, Sundel, and Mansoory (2012), who comment that "fidelity lies at one end of a continuum and adaptation can be found at its other end" (p. 151). Adaptations are needed if an intervention is going to achieve a good fit with the new organization and/or the participants' characteristics. In contrast, too many modifications are likely to undermine the fidelity of the original program (Holliday, 2014).

Regardless of the philosophy used for conducting an intervention in a different context, a needs assessment should be carried out to ensure that the new setting is prepared for the intervention. Once again, engaging stakeholders is advantageous. With the participant community's involvement, the adaptation process includes reviewing the intervention's theory of change, core components, and intended outcomes. Explorations of the cultural appropriateness of the program are facilitated by interviewing and conducting focus groups with stakeholders. This approach is preferable because it provides an ecological context for the adaptation that can evaluate the social validity of the program. The constituents' feedback can be used to guide the next steps in systematically making the adaptations. It is possible that stakeholders' reactions may indicate that a program requires only minimal modifications to be considered acceptable by constituents. In the next section, a practical example for maintaining fidelity of an evidence-based intervention in a new context is described.

STRATEGIES USED FOR MAINTAINING FIDELITY IN *INSIGHTS INTO APPALACHIA*

INSIGHTS Into Children's Temperament is a comprehensive temperament-based intervention that was developed by Sandee McClowry in partnership with urban community stakeholders and cultural experts. The intervention teaches parents and teachers to use a temperament (personality) framework to support the individual differences of kindergarten and first-grade children. Parents and teachers also learn how to match behavioral management strategies to a child's particular temperament. The 2-hour, 10-session curriculum for the parent and teacher programs includes didactic content, videotapes, role-playing, discussion, and assignments. The children's version of *INSIGHTS* is a 10-week, 30-minute program conducted in the classrooms of participating teachers. Puppets with distinctively different temperaments and other curricula are used to foster empathy and problem solving. The logic model for *INSIGHTS* is shown in Figure 15.1.

The efficacy of *INSIGHTS* has been tested in three federally funded randomized clinical trials. The studies were conducted in public schools serving low-income Black and Hispanic children. For a detailed description of the intervention and its outcomes, see the reports written by McClowry and her colleagues (Cappella et al., 2015; McClowry, 2014; O'Connor, Cappella, McCormick, & McClowry, 2014).

An example of the transferability of *INSIGHTS* was explored in a pilot study conducted by a team of temperament researchers led by Sandra Gagnon at Appalachian State University. Based on its core assumptions (as listed in the left column of the logic model in Figure 15.1), the researchers regarded *INSIGHTS* as a promising program for prekindergarteners in a low-income, primarily Caucasian, school district in rural Appalachia. However, demographic characteristics of the rural community, which differed from the participants in the efficacy studies, raised concerns about the program's cultural and developmental appropriateness and acceptability in a rural setting. Perhaps some *surface* features might not resonate with the individuals in the geographically isolated, rural community, in which generations of families have had limited exposure to diverse individuals (e.g., racial minorities) and geographical areas (e.g., cities). For example, the intervention's content videos from the efficacy

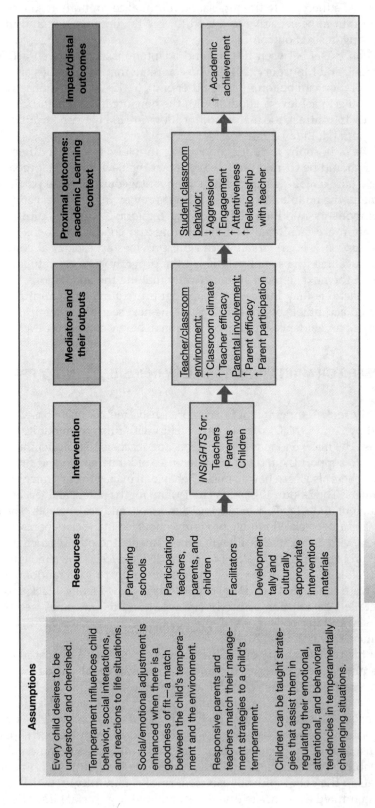

FIGURE 15.1 Logic model for *INSIGHTS into children's temperament.*

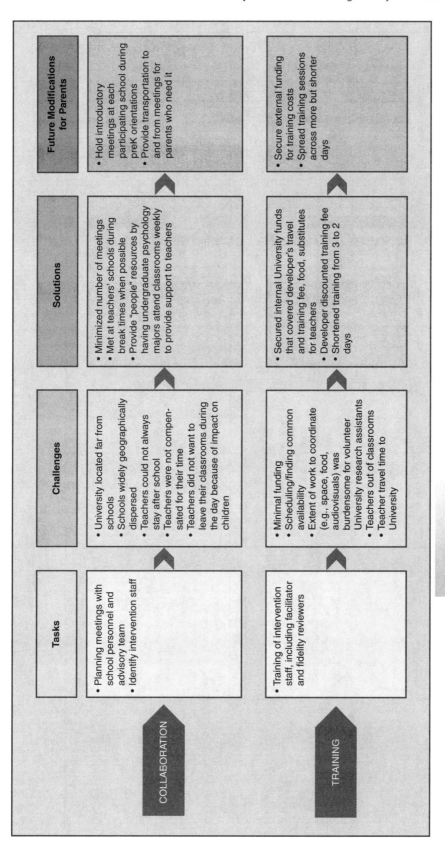

COLLABORATION			
Tasks	**Challenges**	**Solutions**	**Future Modifications for Parents**
• Planning meetings with school personnel and advisory team • Identify intervention staff	• University located far from schools • Schools widely geographically dispersed • Teachers could not always stay after school • Teachers were not compensated for their time • Teachers did not want to leave their classrooms during the day because of impact on children	• Minimized number of meetings • Met at teachers' schools during break times when possible • Provide "people" resources by having undergraduate psychology majors attend classrooms weekly to provide support to teachers	• Hold introductory meetings at each participating school during preK orientations • Provide transportation to and from meetings for parents who need it

TRAINING			
Tasks	**Challenges**	**Solutions**	
• Training of intervention staff, including facilitator and fidelity reviewers	• Minimal funding • Scheduling/finding common availability • Extent of work to coordinate (e.g., space, food, audiovisuals) was burdensome for volunteer University research assistants • Teachers out of classrooms • Teacher travel time to University	• Secured internal University funds that covered developer's travel and training fee, food, substitutes for teachers • Developer discounted training fee • Shortened training from 3 to 2 days	• Secure external funding for training costs • Spread training sessions across more but shorter days

FIGURE 15.2 INSIGHTS into Appalachian fidelity procedures.

(continued)

Tasks	Challenges	Solutions	Future Modifications for Parents
IMPLEMENTATION • Graduate student facilitator delivered program at district central office • University student attended for support and fidelity • University students collected data from all schools four times during school year • Teachers attended sessions after school hours • Teachers completed outcome measures	• Heavy burden on facilitator • No monetary compensation for travel costs for facilitator or teachers • Travel time for teachers and attendance after work hours with no monetary compensation for time or travel • Teacher absences due to outside commitments (family, medical) • Burdensome nature of completing outcome measures and no compensation • Extensive travel time and costs for data collectors with no monetary compensation for fuel or time	• Combined sessions 1 and 2 • Combined sessions 4 to 6 into one full-day training at University campus with lunch • Compensating teachers with on-campus training (suggested by Superintendent as a "day off/ break"), tour of University Library Instructional Materials Center, providing University library card and privileges; weekly classroom support by University interns (also to help teachers have time to complete outcome measures) • Continuing Education Credit for teachers • University Research Credits for interns and data collectors	• Funding for paid, community-based facilitator(s) • Transportation for parents to training sites • Child care for participating parents • Morning, lunch, and/or evening sessions to accommodate parents' schedules • Monetary compensation to incentivize parents to complete outcome measures • Funding for data collectors
FIDELITY REVIEW • University graduate students reviewed videos and completed fidelity coding sheets • Facilitator reviewed coding sheets and met with lead researcher to discuss concerns and troubleshoot	• Burden on graduate student fidelity reviewers (limited time to observe and complete coding sheets because of heavy workload) • No compensation for time or travel costs for fidelity reviewers • Time demands for facilitator to complete self-review of fidelity and meet with lead researcher	• University research credits provided to fidelity reviewers • Paid Graduate Research Assistantship for facilitator	• Contract between University and community to fund community-based facilitators, with eventual transition to ownership by district

FIGURE 15.2 (continued)

studies feature Black and Hispanic children and adults living in city apartments, whereas many of the Appalachian children were White and lived in homes located on difficult to access dirt roads.

Another concern was whether *INSIGHTS*, developed for kindergarten and first-grade children and their teachers and parents, was developmentally appropriate if used with prekindergarten caregivers. Those concerns prompted a pilot study of the teacher program with a sample of teachers who had sufficient cultural experiences and intimate knowledge of the community to be able to provide valid and reliable feedback on its relevance and feasibility. The adaptation process, presented in Figure 15.2, involved strategies that were similar to those employed in the efficacy studies: (a) initial collaboration with an advisory group of key stakeholders, (b) training and supervision of facilitators and fidelity reporters, (c) a manualized curriculum, and (d) video recording and reviewing implementation sessions.

Collaboration

Before developing the project, three steps were taken. First, the research team, which consisted of three psychology professors, consulted with the developer, who played an ongoing role throughout the program. Then, in keeping with *the* original community-based approach of *INSIGHTS*, an advisory group of key stakeholders from the district was formed, which included the district superintendent, an elementary school principal, and two prekindergarten teachers. The director of the University's Child Development Center was added to the team to enhance the connection between the university and the community.

Buy-in was easily established, and the school personnel were extremely excited to try *INSIGHTS*. It was fortuitous that the superintendent, who was born and raised in the community and extremely committed to his students, teachers, and families, embraced the project and took a lead role. He arranged for the team to present the project proposal to principals and teachers and also obtained approval from the school board. The advisory group understood the importance of fidelity, which, when combined with their extensive knowledge of their students, families, and community, allowed the team to adhere to protocol in a way that best fit their unique context and parameters. Finally, an intervention team that included several school psychology graduate students and undergraduate psychology majors were selected. Many of those students were responsible for managing and collecting data for the outcomes that were measured. Without the strong commitment and contributions of the program developer, advisory group, intervention staff, and data collectors, the project would not have been possible.

Training and Supervision

The intensive training requirements of *INSIGHTS* and detailed intervention manual provided the groundwork for adherence to protocol. The training requires 3 days of instruction for the intervention team, although as described in Figure 15.2, financial constraints led the Appalachian team to receive the training in 2 full days. In addition, facilitators must complete a "practice" implementation of the entire 10-week program to become certified. The facilitator for *INSIGHTS Into Appalachia* was a first-year school psychology graduate student and a former teacher. The comprehensive training ensured that the facilitator was well versed in the underlying temperament theory, the supportive research literature, and the mechanics of conducting the sessions, thereby increasing the likelihood of procedural fidelity. It was fortunate to have a facilitator with experience in early childhood education and development because she was familiar with the context of schools, understood the teachers' challenges, and interacted effectively with them.

Manualized Curriculum

The intervention manual provides detailed instructions and includes resources such as scripts, lists of required materials, explanations of handouts, brief descriptions of video content, and a structured fidelity checklist. The facilitator used the manual during each session, thereby increasing the likelihood of adherence to protocol. Although most of the content and methods are scripted, the manual provides flexibility for facilitators to respond to participants and guide discussions. A portion of a teacher session from the manual is included in Exhibit 15.1.

EXHIBIT 15.1 A Portion of a Teacher Session From the *INSIGHTS* Manual

---

TEACHER SESSION 3: TEACHER RESPONSES

Description

Session 3 introduces teacher responses that are optimal, adequate, and counterproductive.

Materials needed:

- Handout 3At: Teacher responses
- Handout 3Bt: Optimal parent responses
- Vignette 3.1t: The case of the missing math book

Additional materials:

- Sign-in sheet
- Cash receipts for incentives
- Session evaluation form

Time
2 hours

OBJECTIVES	ACTIVITIES
1. Review reframing. (25 minutes)	A. Welcome the teachers back. Allow 10 minutes for milling.
	1. Invite them to discuss past week's homework, Handout 2Et, so that they can demonstrate that they have learned to reframe their perceptions of their students. Use their comments to clarify and reinforce their perceptions.
2. Explain how teacher responses can be differentially effective (20 minutes)	A. Up until now, we have been talking about how children's temperament influences their behavior. In this session, we change the focus and talk about how we influence their behavior.
	1. Using Handout 3At, explain to the teachers that while children react, adults respond. Adult responses can be differentially effective.
	2. Using Handout 3At, define optimal, adequate, and counterproductive responses.
	3. Video 3.1t: The case of the missing math book. Coretta cannot find her math book and becomes disrespectful to her teacher. Coretta's teacher responds by yelling at Coretta. This vignette explores other ways Coretta's teacher can respond that might be more effective (3 minutes)

Video Recording and Review

The fidelity protocol for *INSIGHTS* requires that each session be videorecorded and evaluated by trained fidelity reviewers who also attended the 2-day training session. School psychology graduate students used the fidelity coding sheets of *INSIGHTS* (see Exhibit 15.2 for a sample coding sheet) to evaluate the facilitator's completion of the prescribed content, as well as any additions, changes, or omissions. The fidelity reviewers also noted observations about the facilitators' teaching style (i.e., didactic, interactive, or a balance of the two) and interactions with participants (e.g., appropriately posed questions, praised and validated participants, set limits). All feedback was reviewed by the facilitator, who also documented attendance, engagement, difficulties encountered during the session (e.g., absences, equipment problems), and the need for additional time on specific issues. When problems arose, the facilitator discussed concerns with the lead researcher, and, together, they developed strategies to address them.

Following the implementation of the intervention, the research team conducted a program evaluation to determine *the* cultural relevance, developmental appropriateness, and perceived feasibility of *INSIGHTS*. Teacher satisfaction was assessed by *the Teacher Satisfaction Survey* of *INSIGHTS*. The results indicated high levels of satisfaction that were consistent with those reported previously by teachers in urban areas. The teachers also participated in a focus group during which they enthusiastically endorsed the program for children and families in their schools.

In addition, after the program had been implemented with the teachers, a representative sample of parents participated in a focus group during which they received an overview of the parenting program and viewed one of the program's videos. The parents were excited by the program and indicated a strong desire to participate. Although specifically asked, they did not report concerns about cultural differences. Instead, they emphasized the universal nature of parenting challenges, regardless of race or community.

To begin adapting the classroom curriculum materials for prekindergarten, the developer delivered one session of the children's program to a class of kindergarten students. Not surprisingly, the puppets and activities were well received by the students and their teacher. All members of the intervention team, however, agreed that the children's program would need to be modified so that the teaching strategies matched the developmental needs of prekindergarten children.

The consensus among the teacher and parent participants, the advisory group, and the intervention team was that *INSIGHTS* holds promise for use in the district's rural schools. Implementing it on a larger scale would require more resources and would entail adapting it for prekindergarten children. Feasibility was a strong concern, as teachers and parents described potential barriers to implementation that could undermine fidelity. They also provided numerous practical suggestions for making it feasible. For example, teachers had difficulty staying after school to attend the 10 weekly sessions. Likewise, travel to the school would be a significant barrier for parents. Both teachers and parents agreed consolidating content into fewer sessions would reduce participant burden.

In conjunction with the American Academy of Nursing and the Robert Wood Johnson Foundation's Culture of Health initiative, representatives from the RAND Corporation observed the *INSIGHTS Into Appalachia* program evaluation activities and used the data for a case study on the intervention. Their recent report summarizes portions of the findings, including strengths, barriers, and challenges (Martsolf, Mason, Sloan, Sullivan, & Villarruel, 2017). Advancing a comprehensive culture of health is likely to capitalize on the very components that were discussed in the chapter: evidence-based interventions, collaboration with community stakeholders, adaptations for new settings, and, of course, fidelity.

EXHIBIT 15.2 A Sample Coding Sheet From *INSIGHTS*

SESSION 3: PARENTS AND TEACHERS ARE INTRODUCED TO ADULT RESPONSES THAT ARE OPTIMAL. ADEQUATE. AND COUNTERPRODUCTIVE

Prescribed Content: Activities completed; additions, changes, and omissions to material

		COMPLETED	ADDED TO	CHANGED	OMITTED	COMMENTS
Session 3 welcome	■ Welcome back ■ Discuss homework ■ Review reframing from previous ■ Clarify and reinforce their perceptions	✓				
Explain responses	Handout 3A					
	Child reacts/teacher responds					
	Define responses: optimal adequate counterproductive					
	Play Video 3.1 and summarize					

Key Points From This Chapter

- Stakeholders are invaluable. Include them in program planning, development of the intervention, implementation, and dissemination.
- Fidelity needs to be incorporated into the intervention protocol from the start and monitored throughout the implementation of an intervention.
- Detailed manuals are imperative for successful staff training and successful implementation of intervention protocols and regulations.
- Adaptations need to be made when interventions are conducted in new settings.
- Document fidelity issues to ensure procedures for consistent adherence to the intervention are closely followed throughout the duration of its implementation.

REFERENCES

Abry, T., Hulleman, C. S., & Rimm-Kaufman, S. E. (2015). Using indices of fidelity to intervention core components to identify program active ingredients. *American Journal of Evaluation, 36*, 320–338. doi:10.1177/1098214014557009

Barrenger, S. L., Kriegel, L. S., Angell, B., & Draine, J. (2016). Role of context, resources, and target population in the fidelity of critical time intervention. *Psychiatric Services, 67*, 115–118. doi:10.1176/appi.ps.201400108

Barton, E. A., Whittaker, J. V., Kinzie, M. B., DeCoster, J., & Furnari, E. (2017). Understanding the relationship between teachers' use of online demonstration videos and fidelity of implementation in MyTeachingPartner-Math/Science. *Teaching and Teacher Education, 67*, 189–201. doi:10.1016/j.tate.2017.06.011

Bassett, S. S., Stein, L. A. R., Rossi, J. S., & Martin, R. A. (2016). Evaluating measures of fidelity for substance abuse group treatment with incarcerated adolescents. *Journal of Substance Abuse Treatment, 66*, 9–15. doi:10.1016/j.jsat.2016.02.011

Bova, C., Jaffarian, C., Crawford, S., Quintos, J. B., Lee, M., & Sullivan-Bolyai, S. (2017). Intervention fidelity: Monitoring drift, providing feedback, and assessing the control condition. *Nursing Research, 66*, 54–59. doi:10.1097/NNR.0000000000000194

Bruhn, A. L., Hirsch, S. E., & Lloyd, J. W. (2015). Treatment integrity in school-wide programs: A review of the literature (1993-2012). *Journal of Primary Prevention, 35*, 335–349. doi:10.1007/s10935-015-0400-9

Cappella, E., O'Connor, E. E., McCormick, M., Turbeville, A., Collins, A., & McClowry, S. G. (2015). Classwide efficacy of INSIGHTS: Observed student behaviors and teacher practices in kindergarten and first grade. *Elementary School Journal, 116*, 217–241. doi:10.1086/683983

Century, J., Cassata, A., Rudnick, M., & Freeman, C. (2012). Measuring enactment of innovations and the factors that affect implementation and sustainability: Moving toward common language and shared conceptual understanding. *Journal of Behavioral Health Services and Research, 39*, 343–361. doi:10.1007/s11414-012-9287-x

Cobanoglu, R., & Capa-Aydin. (2015). When early childhood teachers close the door: Self-reported fidelity to a mandated curriculum and teacher beliefs. *Early Childhood Research Quarterly, 33*, 77–86. doi:10.1016/j.ecresq.2015.07.001

Ferrer-Wreder, L., Sundel, K., & Mansoory, S. (2012). Tinkering with perfection: Theory development in the intervention cultural adaptation field. *Child Youth Care Forum, 41*, 149–171. doi:10.1007/s10566-011-9162-6

Forsberg, S., Fitzpatrick, K. K., Darcy, A., Aspen, V., Accurso, E. C., Bryson, S. W., … Lock, J. (2014). Development and evaluation of a treatment fidelity instrument for family-based treatment of adolescent Anorexia Nervosa. *International Journal of Eating Disorders, 48*, 91–99. doi:10.1002/eat.22337

Gagnon, R. J. (2014). Exploring the relationship between the facilitator and fidelity. *Journal of Outdoor Recreation, Education, and Leadership, 6*, 183–186. doi:10.7768/1948-5123.1264

Garbacz, L. L, Brown, D. M., Spee, G. A., Polo, A. J., & Budd, K. S. (2014). Establishing treatment fidelity in evidence-based parent training programs for externalizing disorders in children and adolescents. *Clinical Child and Family Psychology Review, 17*, 230–247. doi:10.1007/s10567-014-0166-2

Goncy, E. A., Sutherland, K. S., Farrell, A. D., Sullivan, T. N., & Doyle, S. T. (2015). Measuring teacher implementation in delivery of a bullying prevention program: The impact of instructional and procedural adherence and competence on student responsiveness. *Prevention Science, 16*, 440–450. doi:10.1007/s11121-014-0508-9

Gresham, F. M., Dart, E. H., & Collins, T. A. (2017). Generalizability of multiple measures of treatment integrity: Comparisons among direct observation, permanent products, and self-report. *School Psychology Review, 46*, 108–121. doi:10.17105/SPR46-1.108-121

Hansen, W. B., Pankratz, M. M., Dusenbury, L., Giles, S. M., Bishop, D. C. Albritton, J., … Strack, J. (2013). Styles of adaptation: The impact of frequency and valence of adaptation on preventing substance use. *Health Education, 113*, 345–363. doi:10.1108/09654281311329268

Harn, B., Parisi, D., & Stoolmiller, M. (2013). Balancing fidelity with flexibility and fit: What do we really know about fidelity of implementation in schools? *Exceptional Children, 79*, 181–193. doi:10.1177/001440291307900204

Holliday, L. R. (2014). Using logic model mapping to evaluate program fidelity. *Studies in Educational Evaluation, 42*, 109–117. doi:10.1016/j.stueduc.2014.04.001

Jelalian, E., Foster, G. D., Sato, A. F., Berlin, K. S., McDermott, C., & Sundal, D. (2014). Treatment adherence and facilitator characteristics in a community based pediatric weight control intervention. *International Journal of Behavioral Nutrition and Physical Activity, 11*, 17. doi:10.1186/1479-5868-11-17

Keller-Marguilis, M. A. (2012). Fidelity of implementation framework: A critical need for response to intervention models. *Psychology in the Schools, 49*, 342–352. doi:10.1002/pits.21602

Kelly, S. A., Oswalt, K., Melnyk, B. M., & Jacobson, D. (2015). Comparison of intervention fidelity between COPE TEEN and an attention-control program in a randomized controlled trial. *Health Education Research, 30*, 233–247. doi:10.1093/her/cyu065

Kershner, S., Flynn, S., Prince, M., Potter, S. C., Craft, L., & Alton, F. (2014). Using data to improve fidelity when implementing evidence-based programs. *Journal of Adolescent Health, 54*, 529–536. doi:10.1016/j.jadohealth.2013.11.027

Lakin, J. N., & Shannon, D. M. (2015). The role of treatment acceptability, effectiveness, and understanding in treatment fidelity: Predicting implementation variation in a middle school science program. *Studies in Educational Evaluation, 47*, 28–37. doi:10.1016/j.stueduc.2015.06.002

Lloyd-Evans, B., Bond, G., R, Ruud, T., Ivanecka, A., Gray, R, Osborn, D., … Johnson, S. (2016). Development of a measure of model fidelity for mental health crisis resolution teams. *BMC Psychiatry, 16*, 1–12. doi:10.1186/s12888-016-1139-4

Low, S., Smolkowski, K., & Cook, C. (2016). What constitutes high quality implementation of SEL programs? A latent class analysis of second step implementation. *Prevention Science, 17*, 981–991. doi:10.1007/s11121-016-0670-3

Martsolf, G. R., Mason, D. J., Sloan, J., Sullivan, C. G., & Villarruel, A. M. (2017). *Nurse-designed care models and culture of health: Review of three case studies.* Santa Monica, CA: RAND Corporation.

McClowry, S. G. (2014). *Temperament-based elementary classroom management.* Lanham, MD: Rowman & Littlefield.

Mendive, S., Weiland, C., Yoshikawa, H., & Snow, C. (2015). Opening the black box: Intervention fidelity in a randomized trial of a preschool teacher professional development program. *Journal of Educational Psychology, 108*, 130–145. doi:10.1037/edu0000047

O'Connor, E. E., Cappella, E., McCormick, M. P., & McClowry, S. G. (2014). An examination of the efficacy of INSIGHTS in enhancing the academic learning context. *Journal of Educational Psychology, 106*, 1156–1169. doi:10.1037/a0036615

Reed, F. D., & Codding, R. S. (2014). Advancements in procedural fidelity and intervention. *Journal of Behavioral Education, 23*, 1–18. doi:10.1007/s10864-013-9191-3

Wigelsworth, M., Lendrum, A., Oldfield, J., Scott, A., ten Bokkel, I., Tate, K., & Emery, C. (2016). The impact of trial stage, developer involvement, and international transferability on universal social and emotional learning programme outcomes: A meta-analysis. *Cambridge Journal of Education, 46*, 347–376. doi:10.1080/0305764X.2016.1195791

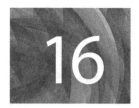

Study Implementation: An Example Using the *Madres Para la Salud* (Mothers for Health) Study

Colleen Keller & Barbara Ainsworth

> Quality is never an accident; it is always the result of high intention, sincere effort, intelligent direction and skillful execution; it represents the wise choice of many alternatives. —*William A. Foster*

Once a research study is initiated, but prior to participant recruitment, the important work of setting up the structure to frame the execution of the study begins. In many major research studies, implementation start-up can take as long as 6 months. Major tasks for the investigators include forming a study team, developing communication strategies among all team members and study participants, and training of study personnel. Training is required for every aspect of the study, including familiarity with recruitment and consent process, providing the intervention, and data recording and management. You must also obtain approval from the office that protects research subjects, monitor the study integrity as it progresses, and identify ways to manage potential conflicts that arise during study implementation. This chapter presents these issues and uses a National Institutes of Health (NIH)-funded randomized clinical trial to provide examples of each of these important research implementation steps.

The study example we use to illustrate study implementation is a 48-week prescribed program for walking activity, *Madres Para la Salud* [Mothers for Health]. This study sought to test a social support intervention—*Madres Para la Salud*—to explore the effectiveness of a culturally specific program using "bouts" of physical activity to effect changes on physical and psychological outcomes in sedentary Hispanic women. This innovative program has the potential to advance our understanding of the relationship between moderate increases in physical activity and specific health outcomes. The study aims were the following:

1. Examine the effectiveness of the *Madres Para la Salud* for reducing the distal outcomes in (a) body fat, (b) systemic and fat tissue inflammation, and (c) postpartum depression (PPD) symptoms among postpartum Hispanic women compared with an attention control group (at 6 and 12 months) after controlling for dietary intake
2. Test whether the theoretical mediators, intermediate outcomes of social support and walking, and environmental factor moderators affect changes in body fat, systemic and fat tissue inflammation, and PPD symptoms among postpartum Hispanic women at 6 and 12 months
3. Determine the relationship between the immediate outcome of *walking* (minutes walked per week) and change in the distal outcomes of (a) body fat, (b) systemic and fat tissue inflammation, and (c) PPD symptoms

A sample of 140 sedentary Hispanic women, 18 to 35 years of age, and between 6 weeks and 6 months following childbirth were selected as study participants. Participants were randomly assigned to the intervention or attention-control group. The intervention group received a 12-week didactic and practice social support intervention as well as weekly walking sessions and support interventions with *promotoras*. The attention-control group received health newsletters and follow-up phone calls. Data were gathered at baseline, 3, 6, 9, and 12 months using questionnaires, fat tissue biopsies, blood samples, and a subset sample for dual-energy x-ray absorptiometry (DEXA) body scans, as well as objective and self-report measures of walking adherence. The intervention's effectiveness was evaluated using a mixed model analysis of variance (ANOVA) comparing the two groups, structural equation modeling (SEM), and evaluating the relationship between walking and body fat loss. An overview of the study is presented in Figure 16.1.

The *Madres Para la Salud* theoretical framework, design, and approach were predicated on formative participatory work to refine the *Madres Para la Salud* intervention. We invited a study consultant who had funded research with young Latinas to share intervention development expertise and critique our intervention manual. We invited young postpartum Latinas who were interested in physical activity to join us in discussion and provide review and feedback, as well as expert consultants to guide the development of culturally relevant strategies needed to promote social support for walking. Young Latinas had the opportunity to incorporate their own experiences with physical activity, the ways in which group support might facilitate walking, and share strategies for walking initiation and maintenance in their individual lives, social networks, and neighborhood environments. In addition, postpartum Latinas participated in providing initial and ongoing feedback and refinement on the applicability and appropriateness of program materials, including language, reading level, and cultural equivalence (Keller, Coe, & Moore, 2014).

FORMING THE TEAM

The number and types of team members you will have for your study depend on the funding available. Federal grants often have a large enough budget to pay the investigators and to hire a paid project director (PD) and data collectors. Smaller studies with less funding may rely on student volunteers to collect data, and the principal investigator (PI) and/or coinvestigators may have to serve as the PD and/or data analysts. Forming the team requires investigators to determine, from the prestudy plans, what each team member will do. For example, a coinvestigator's tasks may be defined (from a budget justification) something like "Coinvestigator

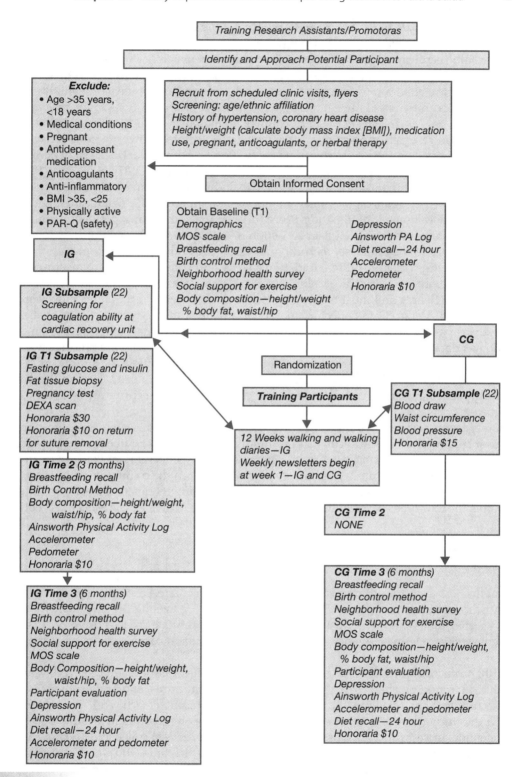

FIGURE 16.1 Overview of the *Madres Para la Salud* study design.

CG, control group; DEXA, dual-energy x-ray absorptiometry; IG, intervention group; MOS, medical outcomes survey; PAR-Q, physical activity recall questions.

Francis will participate in the hiring and orienting of project personnel, assist with developing recruitment materials and monitoring recruitment, work with the subcontract personnel to assure recruitment goals are being met, share responsibility for fidelity checks, and participate in interpretation and dissemination activities including writing the final report." As you pay close attention to forming the research team in budget development, this same information becomes useful in negotiating team members' contributions to the research implementation. For *Madres Para la Salud*, research team members included the identified investigators cited in research applications as primary investigators, coinvestigators, consultants, PD, research assistants, data collectors, data entry staff, and other identified study personnel.

One of the most critical members of the research team is the PD. The role of the PD is to flesh out all aspects of the study implementation including a recruitment plan, human subject approvals from the organization's Institutional Review Board (IRB), detailing activities for subcontracts, development of all study procedure manuals, including protocol manual and intervention manuals, making all data collection instruments suitable and orderly for collection and transfer to the database, recruiting and training both data collectors and interventionists, conducting fidelity and manipulation checks, and coordinating team meetings.

Data collectors are also critical members of the study team. They interact directly with the study participants and must assure that the data are collected accurately and according to the research design. Data collectors may be graduate students who are participating in the study as part of their graduate research experience, professionals employed by an organization as data collectors, or professionals from the community who are familiar with the culture, language, and key characteristics of the study participants. For example, in *Madres Para la Salud*, the data collectors are bilingual and bicultural and able to communicate with the study participants using a familiar language and incorporating culturally relevant values and customs.

Other team members being included more frequently on the research team are community members such as clinic directors and community health workers. In our study, Latina lay health advisors served as *promotoras* to implement the study intervention. *Promotoras*, literally translated as "developers," are lay health advisors who work in the community they serve. The *promotoras* provide the intervention that focuses on promoting moderate-intensity walking by delivering the four types of social support that underpin the *Madres Para la Salud* intervention.

COMMUNICATION

One of the best ways to communicate the implementation of a research study is through regularly scheduled team meetings. These meetings should be agenda driven. Our experience shows that agendas should follow the same order, with meeting minutes posted prior to subsequent weekly meetings. Agendas or topics for research team consideration may include:

- IRB: protocol approvals, changes, application renewals or issues, and their follow-up.
- Budget: report on charges, participant incentive expenditures, and budget changes.
- Recruitment and retention: the flowchart should be presented each week (see Figure 16.1 for the study flowchart) for research team information on recruitment locations, status of retention and attrition, reasons for attrition, and status of data collection. The flowchart should be updated weekly to reflect the number of participants who were recruited from each location, reasons participants were excluded from the study, why participants declined to enroll in the study, and reasons why participants dropped out of the study after enrollment.
- Other subjects to be discussed in this meeting include changes to protocol, strategies for trouble-shooting study flow, changes to data collection, and intervention personnel.

- Data collection and measures: changes with data collection, trouble-shooting, and status of data entry.
- Data analysis: a report from the research team statistician.
- Plans for publications and presentations and research team members responsible for aspects of dissemination.

Another form of communication is a manual of operation that describes methods and instruments used to complete each task. This includes a recruitment manual that records all procedures used and contacts made while recruiting and retaining the participants, with detailed explanations recorded for participants who drop out of the study. A quality assurance/ quality control manual is also needed, which describes training procedures to assure accurate data collection. An intervention manual that includes all study materials used in implementation of the intervention and the control group activities is also essential. These items should be placed in shared files for study team access, such as a password-protected website with access to data files restricted to the primary investigator and statistician. This avoids any potential surprises with the study data management and analyses and assures all members of the research team have access to the research materials that govern the conduct of the study. Exhibit 16.1 provides an overview of the types of information to include in the data study materials.

Communication among multicultural participants and team members is an essential component of studies that examine phenomena among diverse persons. In *Madres Para la Salud,* all of our manuals, scales, consent forms, and our telephone-answering messages are in Spanish and English. We employed bilingual, bicultural staff, and the translation of study materials were subject to review by persons with various Spanish-language experience in Spanish dialects and colloquialisms (all measures were translated into Spanish; all have been validated in Spanish language).

In this next section, we discuss processes we used to train the study staff and deliver the study as planned. This includes tasks referred to as "training the study staff" and "monitoring progress." Monitoring progress is described as the delivery fidelity, treatment design, treatment receipt, treatment enactment, and strategies to maintain adherence.

EXHIBIT 16.1   List and Examples of Data Study Materials for Research Study Implementation

---

Manual of operations

- Overview and equipment
- Recruitment
- Clinic examinations
  - Pre-exam activities
  - Examination guidelines
  - Interviews and questionnaires
  - Clinic examinations
  - Laboratory sample collection and processing
- Adverse events reporting
- Recording participant results
- Data management

Recruitment and retention manual

- Overview
- Recruitment contacts

(continued)

EXHIBIT 16.1 List and Examples of Data Study Materials for Research Study Implementation *(continued)*

- Eligibility criteria
- Screening/recruitment questionnaires
- Tips for recruitment calls
- Retention plans and materials
- Dropouts

Intervention manual

- Project overview
- Participant protection
  - Protection of participant rights—human subjects certification
  - Biosafety forms
  - Protection of participant rights—participant forms
  - CPR
- Randomization
- Intervention
  - *Promotora* training and evaluation
  - Intervention training and monitoring
  - Incident reporting and forms
  - Intervention fidelity
  - Intervention fidelity evaluation forms
  - Manipulation checks
  - Participant evaluation
- Administration

Quality assurance/quality control

- Quality assurance
  - Detailed protocols for data collection
  - Certified training of data collectors
  - Interrater reliability
  - Data collection logs
  - Outcome measures
  - Attendance and acceptability
  - Intervention attendance log
  - Questions and answers to possible questions
- Quality control
  - Monitoring protocol of field and clinic measures
  - Data collection quality check schedule
  - Data quality check schedule
  - Plan to resolve quality control problems

Ancillary study manuals

STAFF TRAINING

Training the PD and study staff, including interventionists and data collectors, with thorough and careful protocols is imperative because it produces fewer conflicts among team members and helps assure accurate data and a smooth protocol execution.

Project Director

The most critical team member is the PD. When developing this position and role, investigators need to have a clear idea about both the kind of person who might fill this role, as well as expectations for job duties and accountability. Many large studies require persons with doctoral degrees and research experience, whereas smaller studies rely on the PI and student workers for project direction. In *Madres Para la Salud*, we selected a bilingual and bicultural graduate-prepared PD with a Master of Social Work degree and with extensive research experience as a data collector in a large community intervention trial. We initiated training by making a work plan that addressed activities that (a) introduced the study aims and parameters (nature of the study), (b) addressed the tasks of the project as both a manager (human resource activities, clinical setting introductions and contacts, some budget activities including incentives and equipment purchases), (c) assured the scientific integrity of the project (meeting a science officer to learn the procedures for the human subjects and biosafety rules and application, data coding and spreadsheets, training data collectors and interventionists), and (d) instruction in the development of study procedure manuals and product fidelity procedures. The training and study work plan assured that the PD would accomplish in a systematic way the training and procedural processes needed to begin study implementation.

Data Collectors

Data collectors are trained in protection of human subjects' data collection instruments, their purpose, rigorous use, and in reliability of study measure procedures. The PD should train the data collectors systematically and reassess standards over time. Hiring the data collectors and introducing the study procedures and orientation to the measures, both written and physiological measures, and disposition of data are also important parts of study implementation procedures. In *Madres Para la Salud*, our data collectors were bilingual and bicultural. After the PD introduced the data collectors to the study aims and procedures, the study instruments (scales and physical measures) were reviewed, including practice sessions for collection. Next, the data collectors practiced with each other, and reliability assessments were performed by the PD. Finally, a "mock" data collection session occurred between a "model" participant and the data collectors. This session was observed, evaluated, and critiqued by the PD and PI. Data collection schedules are helpful in keeping data collectors on track and serve as a useful check for the PD monitoring study progress. *Madres Para la Salud* used a schedule of data collection time points as a general guide that included large artist drawing pads posted in the study office that displayed each participant's number and where she was in terms of scheduling for data collection during study implementation. For example, the charts displayed the participant's study number, anticipated data collection time and date, and actual data collection time and date. In this way, all team members could see each participant's status in the study flow. A checklist for supplies to be brought to each data collection event was developed, and data collection packets were prepared that were specific to each data collection time point. An example of the data collection schedule is shown in Table 16.1.

In *Madres Para la Salud*, we implemented the intervention using a *promotora* model that best addressed the criteria for validity that included stakeholders' views and concerns and ensured external validity by choosing interventionists who were long-term residents of the neighborhoods in the planned study settings (Ibrahim & Sidani, 2014). Two *promotoras* met our hiring preferences of self-reported Mexican descent, first generation in the United States, and of similar age to the study population. The *promotoras* received extensive training in the study protocol, completed certification in the protection of human subjects, and gained theoretical and practical knowledge and skills in how to build and maintain social support with the study sample. Practice and role-play were an integral component of training. Each *promotora* completed a minimum of 3 of the 12 social support intervention sessions while observed and evaluated by *Madres Para la Salud* investigators and Latinas from the target

TABLE 16.1 Example of a Staff Data Collection Schedule[a]

| | | ASSESSMENT PERIOD (MONTH) | | | | | |
DATA COLLECTION	FORM #	RECRUITMENT (−2)	BASELINE (0)	MID (3)	END (6)	FU 1 (9)	FU 2 (12)
SCREENING CHECKS							
Obesity (BMI)	1	A, B					
Safety (PAR-Q)	2	A, B					
Age, ethnicity	3	A, B					
Medication	4	A, B		A, B			A, B
PHYSICAL ACTIVITY							
SBAS	5		A, B				
Ainsworth PA Log	6		A, B	A	A, B	A	A, B
Accelerometer	7		A, B				A, B
Pedometer	8		A, B	A	A, B	A	A, B
DIET							
24R diet recall	9		A, B		A, B		A, B
BODY FATNESS							
Body composition	10		A, B	A	A, B	A	A, B
DEXA subgroup	11		C				C
Fat tissue biopsy (subgroup)	12		D				D
Blood draw	13		E				E
CHILD PRACTICES							
Breastfeeding	14		A, B	A	A, B	A	A, B
Birth control	15		A, B	A	A, B	A	A, B
SUPPORT							
Neighborhood	16		A, B		A, B		A, B
Social support ex.	17		A, B		A, B		A, B
DEPRESSION							
Medical outcomes survey	18		A, B		A, B		A, B

(continued)

TABLE 16.1 Example of a Staff Data Collection Schedule[a] *(continued)*

DATA COLLECTION	FORM #	ASSESSMENT PERIOD (MONTH)					
		RECRUITMENT (−2)	BASELINE (0)	MID (3)	END (6)	FU 1 (9)	FU 2 (12)
Postpartum depression	19		A, B		A, B		A, B
EVALUATIONS							
Participant evaluation	20				A, B		
Intervention manipulation check	21				A, B		

[a]Data collectors: A and B, data collectors; C, radiology technician; D, physician; E, nurse.
BMI, body mass index; DEXA, dual energy x-ray absorptiometry; FU, follow-up; PA, physical activity; PAR-Q, physical activity recall questions; SBAS, Stanford Brief Activity Survey.

population. A *promotora* manual was developed by the PD, with significant input from the *promotoras*. This manual (English and Spanish) included a cohort preparation checklist (what to take to each intervention session), blank forms for each cohort's contact information, pictures of stretching exercises, walking locations/settings and contact information for each site, the participant walking diary, goal-setting cards, pedometer instructions, and safety tip cards. Participant packets were made for each woman and provided on enrollment. These packets included study information, a copy of the informed consent, recruitment flyers, an example of health issue newsletters that were sent weekly, goal-setting cards, community resources, and walking safety tips for the intervention group members. An example of participant safety tip cards is shown in Figure 16.2.

MONITORING PROGRESS

Treatment Fidelity

Fidelity is defined as design and implementation strategies that ensure that a replicable treatment was delivered to all randomized study participants. To ensure delivery fidelity in *Madres Para la Salud* regarding the walking component, extensive activities were completed prior to the study implementation (Breitenstein et al., 2010). These activities included (a) *promotora* training for leading the daily walking sessions at the required walking intensity, (b) development and translation of the modified Ainsworth Physical Activity Diary used to identify the types of physical activity performed on a regular basis, (c) design of a walking calendar for participant recording of steps, (d) *promotora* training for participant accelerometer use to record the intensity and duration of walking sessions, and (e) identifying the key components for training participants in the walking intervention. Our training included close attention to treatment delivery—the strategies used to ensure that the intended treatment is delivered as planned. The *Madres Para la Salud* intervention required the *promotoras* to deliver a walking intervention and provide specific types of social support during each of the 12 intervention sessions. Treatment delivery fidelity is needed to address both walking and social support.

Madres Para la Salud
Safety Tips

There are safety and neighborhood issues to consider when walking, especially in Arizona. These are safety tips to prevent any injury when walking.

1. You should carry a picture ID when walking.
2. Wear a comfortable cotton blouse/top, loose and comfortable pants or shorts, socks that fit well and will not cause blisters, and walking shoes.
3. A water bottle is important to maintain hydration.
4. Sunscreen product with SPF 45 lotion to protect skin from the sun's burning UVA/UVB rays. Shake well before using.
5. Hat to protect your head if necessary & sunglasses to protect from the sun.
6. A watch or stop watch is optional.
7. Carry a cell phone if possible in case of an emergency.
8. A wet or dry towel or handkerchief to wipe off sweat is optional.
9. Avoid black clothes because it reflects and absorbs the sun.
10. Make sure that the places where you walk are not isolated and are well lighted at night.
11. If you've had a cold or the flu, wait until your symptoms are gone before you start walking again.

FIGURE 16.2 Example of safety tip cards (used with permission from *Madres Para la Salud*).

Fidelity of the social support component was as important as the walking component. Because the theoretical framework of *Madres Para la Salud* was social support, conceptual clarity regarding social support as a behavioral intervention required detailed specification. As a specific measure, a fidelity checklist consisting of the salient elements for each intervention session specifying the social support content to be provided for each of the 12 intervention sessions was developed. The checklist included a detailed assessment of each critical element of social support (e.g., emotional, appraisal, instrumental, informational). This fidelity checklist was used by a coinvestigator as he or she observed random intervention sessions for each *promotora*.

Treatment Design

Three important ideas underpin our selection of the treatment design in *Madres Para la Salud*. First is our conviction that the dose of social support is an instrumental facet in addressing a long-term (48 weeks) walking intervention. The second notion is that the walking "dose" or amount of walking performed at each session is instrumental in both adherence and outcome effects. Third, we believe that cultural tailoring in all aspects of the intervention is a critical component that impacts all aspects of treatment fidelity. Using top-down strategies, we used careful recording tools to identify social support at each treatment session. Logbooks, pedometers, and accelerometers were used to identify the minutes and frequency of walking (intentional physical activity) and the frequency and types of incidental (household, etc.) physical activity performed. Strategies that we used to ensure that our social support treatment was valid included preintervention interviews and focus/advisory group reviews for the cultural relevance of each social support component, and strategies to integrate the walking dose into daily activities that occur in the Latinas' lives.

Madres Para la Salud women were trained to walk at 20 minute/mile intensity, and they practiced this intensity at weekly sessions with *promotoras* and other group members. The moderate-intensity walking dose was monitored by a pedometer with a goal of taking 1,000 steps in 10 minutes. This cadence is based on recommendations of Tudor-Locke, Hatano, Pangrazi, and Kang (2008) on how to use a pedometer to assess moderate-intensity walking speeds. Women practiced walking 1,000 steps in 10 minutes, 2,000 steps in 20 minutes, and so on to assure a moderate intensity walking pace. At the completion of a walking session, the *promotora* audited the pedometer step counts to assure the women met their walking goals. Women who did not have the required steps-to-time ratio (i.e., 1,000 steps in 10 minutes) learned to increase their pace. During each of the 12 weeks of the social support intervention, the women walked together for intensity training. The *promotoras* monitored the cohort of women together once a week for their walking intensity by timing their speed of walking, assured the women recorded their step counts in an activity log, and wrote their incidental activity at three time points in the Ainsworth Activity Log. They also reviewed the weekly activity logs for cultural relevance. The cultural relevance was emphasized by review of the places selected for walking (e.g., neighborhoods assessed for safety) and how participants made time for walking by assessing their daily tasks, planned for walking, and used time management strategies to fit walking into schedules busy with family, jobs, and childcare.

For scheduled weeks during the study, women completed physical activity diaries for a 1-week period during each of five data collection sessions over the 48-week study, including accelerometer reports for incidental physical activity and weekly activity calendars recording pedometer goals and steps. The diaries were interviewer administered in the participant's preferred language (Spanish or English) and consisted of a 3-day recall of the primary activity performed every 30 minutes (e.g., walking, taking care of the baby, driving). The physical activity diaries provided a context for how participants integrate the intervention activities into their daily routines.

Treatment Receipt

Treatment receipt is evaluated as the ability of the participants to understand and perform treatment behavioral skills (Bellg et al., 2004). *Madres Para la Salud* women received the fidelity check and a manipulation check that ascertained that they understood and used the components of social support to enhance their walking regimen. This check was administered following the delivery of the 12-week social support intervention and at the end of the 48-week walking intervention. The manipulation check included 10 true/false or open-ended questions about social support while tapping the measurement domain for each of the critical elements. For example, the critical element of appraisal support was tapped as participants responded to the question of "If I set walking goals each week, I will be more committed to daily walking." Treatment receipt was measured at the end of each cohort's 12-session intervention, using the manipulation checklist.

Treatment Enactment

Treatment enactment is the ability of participants to perform skills in a real-life setting. Within the *Madres Para la Salud* intervention, participants were encouraged to specify how the critical elements of social support were applicable to their lives as young postpartum Latinas. For example, retention strategies were discussed during instrumental support sessions and participants were encouraged to dialogue about questions such as "What types of incentives are important to you?" and "What conditions are happening in your life that might influence your ability to walk?" An example of an opening question for emotional support discussions was "What do you do when your husband thinks you've been walking too much and you want to walk again?" Treatment enactment was measured through weekly

Promotora logs—field notes that were recorded by the *promotoras* after each cohort intervention session was recorded.

Strategies to Maintain Adherence to Madres Para la Salud

Madres Para la Salud provided incentives for participation to both the attention-control and the intervention groups. For the intervention group, these incentives included walking shoes, loan of strollers, and pedometers from study personnel; for both groups, health-related information was provided. Recruitment and retention materials included T-shirts, visors, water bottles marked with the study logo and Madres hallmark colors (hot pink and aqua). Recruitment materials were clearly marked "free" and "no identification required." Retention strategies were discussed during instrumental support sessions, and participants were encouraged to dialogue about questions such as "What types of incentives are important to you?" and "What conditions are happening in your life that might influence your ability to walk?" Additional retention methods included small incentives following the intensive week of accelerometer data completion and return, and gift bags with beauty products meeting weekly walking goals. Our preliminary work with Latinas showed that competition was a critical factor in sustaining participation and walking adherence. In *Madres Para la Salud*, we raffled iPods as part of incentives during the sustained 48-week walking protocol for women who met the protocol goals. Of course, without substantial funding, such incentives would not be possible. However, it is possible to provide incentives that are low cost or that can be donated from community merchants.

PREVENTING CONFLICTS

Conflicts are inevitable among any research team, and there are strategies that are helpful in conflict resolution. The sources of conflict, particularly among academic personalities, often stem from perceived ownership of data, ideas, and opportunities to present the data at scientific conferences and in publications. It is important to have a dissemination plan before any data are collected that all research team members understand and agree to follow. It is a good idea to have a data analysis application form that all persons complete who wish to analyze and present the data. The form includes the name of the publication team, title of the paper or presentation, the purpose of the paper, variables to be analyzed, and types of analyses proposed. This application is approved by a group of researchers sometimes referred to as a "steering committee" or a "publication committee." This group often includes the PI, statistician, and selected coinvestigators.

Other conflicts among the team may include inadequate communication, difficulty in reaching expectations, or inevitable family and personal problems that interfere with the execution of research project duties. Having regular weekly meetings often averts such conflicts. In cases where personnel issues that may threaten the success of the study arise, most worksites employ a personnel manager who can assist the PI and PD. A PD who "checks in" frequently with all staff on an individual basis can do much to avert negative responses, dissatisfaction, or strife among team members. Waiting until situations escalate into full-blown arguments or "melt downs" can often be averted by routine planned contact with staff. Conflict in implementing an intervention takes many forms; some conflicts occur within the communities between investigators and the execution of study procedures, and some conflicts may be out of the control of the study team. When our intervention launched as new immigration laws and procedures were implemented in Arizona, the latter of which received national attention, we quickly found out that the newly enacted laws did not solely affect undocumented aliens in our setting; women of

Hispanic origin who were legal residents were affected as well, and many feared for their safety. Our target population became invisible and exceptionally difficult to reach. Thus, the sociopolitical environment became an important element of intervention implementation (Keller, Vega-Lopez, et al., 2014).

Accordingly, our recruitment efforts became extraordinary, involving the gamut of resources, services, and merchants available for young Latina mothers. These included the Women, Infant, and Children (WIC) clinics, head start programs, elementary schools, health fairs, medical clinics, nonprofit organizations, Young Men's Christian Associations, grocery stores and shopping areas with primarily Spanish-speaking merchants, and neighborhood ministries. We placed recruitment advertisement on Spanish-language radio stations. In addition, our *promotoras* implemented two activities to help recruit and retain women in the study: (a) the use of telephone trees to alert women to immigration arrest "sweeps" that occur to detain suspected undocumented residents (public notice is released by the sheriff's department) and (b) maximizing neighborhood resources to assist women in maintaining their walking by using areas that do not coincide with law enforcement's planned activities or those that are located in hard to reach areas, such as along a neighborhood's many irrigation canals. With careful planning and problem solving, effective study implementation can be sustained throughout the course of a research project.

SUMMARY

The level of complexity in implementing a research study depends on the type of study; its size in terms of personnel, budget, and equipment; and the length of the study. Small laboratory studies may not require the number of personnel and resources used in *Madres Para la Salud*. However, all studies should use standard protocols for recruitment, planning study activities, training staff, delivering treatments, collecting data to assure quality control and assurance, intervention study fidelity, and evaluating the study outcomes. Intervention studies do not take place in a bubble—real-world situations, human nature, and the work environment all impact the implementation of intervention research. Hiring skilled staff, giving attention to rigorous training of team members, and having "detailed protocols and procedures" contribute much to successful intervention research.

Funding for this Study: Grant #1R01NR010356-01A2 *Madres Para la Salud* (Mothers for Health; C. Keller, PI).

Key Points From This Chapter

- It is critical to develop communication strategies among all team members and study participants.
- Training of study personnel, including familiarity with use of the data recording and management system, should be in place before a study begins.
- The PI must obtain approval from the office that protects research subjects before starting data collection.
- It is a best practice to monitor the study integrity as it progresses.
- The PI and study coordinator should identify ways to manage potential conflicts that may arise during study implementation.

REFERENCES

Bellg, A. J., Borrelli, B., Resnick, B., Hecht, J., Minicucci, D. S., Ory, M., ... Czajkowski, S. (2004). Enhancing treatment fidelity in health behavior change studies: Best practices and recommendations from the NIH Behavior Change Consortium. *Health Psychology, 23*(5), 443-451. doi:10.1037/0278-6133.23.5.443

Breitenstein, S. M., Gross, D., Garvey, C. A., Hill, C., Fogg, L., & Resnick, B. (2010). Implementation fidelity in community-based interventions. *Research in Nursing and Health, 33*(2), 164–173. doi:10.1002/nur.20373

Ibrahim, S., & Sidani, S. (2014). Strategies to recruit minority persons: A systematic review. *Journal of Immigrant and Minority Health, 16*(5), 882–888. doi:10.1007/s10903-013-9783-y

Keller, C. S., Coe, K., & Moore, N. (2014). Addressing the demand for cultural relevance in intervention design. *Health Promotion Practice, 15*(5), 654–663. doi:10.1177/1524839914526204

Keller, C. S., Vega-Lopez, S., Ainsworth, B., Nagle-Williams, A., Records, K., Permana, P., & Coonrod, D. (2014). Social marketing: Approach to cultural and contextual relevance in a community-based physical activity intervention. *Health Promotion International, 29*(1), 130–140. doi:10.1093/heapro/das053

Tudor-Locke, C., Hatano, Y., Pangrazi, R. P., & Kang, M. (2008). Revisiting "how many steps are enough?" *Medicine and Science in Sports Exercise, 40*(Suppl. 7), S537–S543. doi:10.1249/MSS.0b013e31817c7133

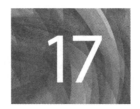

Considerations in Conducting Multisite Trials

Peter A. Vanable

> The extent and the complexity of the problem does not matter as much as does the willingness to solve it. —*Ralph Marston*

CONSIDERATIONS IN CONDUCTING MULTISITE TRIALS

An important consideration for researchers seeking to conduct an intervention trial concerns the question of whether the work can be achieved using a single study site or will benefit from a **multisite** study design. It can be difficult to obtain a sufficiently large sample size for large intervention trials by relying on a single hospital or community-based recruitment site. In such instances, studies can often still be conducted within a single city or region and with a single principal investigator (PI) by relying on multiple recruit settings. However, some research trials require a *multisite* design, with investigative teams residing in different regions of the country. A multisite intervention trial is defined here as a study that involves (a) at least two intervention sites that employ separate research staff, (b) a common data collection protocol that is shared across sites, and (c) a separate **data coordinating site**, where data are shipped, processed, and analyzed.

Multisite studies can provide an enormous boost to participant recruitment and can help to address specific design considerations (e.g., the need for a diversified sample). However, multisite studies are expensive and pose a number of unique challenges. This chapter provides a brief overview of considerations for investigators who are contemplating the possibility of conducting a multisite trial, as well as practical suggestions for implementing a successful multisite trial.

Included throughout the chapter are references to Project iMPPACS, a multisite trial sponsored by the National Institute of Mental Health (Hennessy et al., 2013; Romer et al., 2009; Vanable et al., 2009). Examples are included to illustrate a number of practical considerations that come into play in the context of implementing multisite trials. Project iMPPACS was conducted in four U.S. cities and involved investigators at six different research universities. The major goal of the project was to test the independent and combined impact of a small group intervention and a community-wide mass media HIV-prevention program for African American adolescents. The success of the project hinged in large part on the effectiveness of collaborations that were set up between four investigative teams at Syracuse University, Brown University, Emory University, and the University of South Carolina, as well as a data coordinating center at the University of Pennsylvania. Through intensive planning, the Project iMPPACS team was successful in recruiting more than 1,600 teens in less than 16 months to attend small group workshops and to provide 3 years of follow-up data.

CHOOSING TO CONDUCT A MULTISITE INTERVENTION TRIAL

The decision to initiate a multisite trial should be informed by careful consideration of the benefits and potential limitations of the approach. There may be a temptation for some investigators to implement a multisite trial simply because of a desire to work with valued colleagues at another institution. Such an interest should not serve as a primary rationale, as colleagues can easily engage in interdisciplinary and interinstitutional collaborations while maintaining a primary data collection site. Relatedly, researchers may be drawn to the appeal of conducting a large-scale multisite trial before such a trial is warranted. Scientific, methodological, and pragmatic considerations should be the primary basis for implementing such a trial.

Is a Multisite Trial Warranted Based on the Current State of the Science?

Like all areas of science, intervention research typically proceeds in stages (Rounsaville, Carroll, & Onken, 2001). Innovative approaches to intervention development often begin with clinical observations, followed by qualitative research and pilot intervention trials. Initial randomized controlled trials (RCTs) typically receive funding only with promising evidence from pilot research. A large-scale multisite trial is warranted only in instances where there is an accumulation of evidence across several smaller RCTs. In the case of Project iMPPACS, the team received funding after collecting extensive pilot data and by providing compelling evidence from smaller, single-city studies pointing to the promise of mass media as an innovative approach to motivating community-wide behavioral change in the context of HIV prevention.

Design Considerations

Research design considerations may necessitate a multisite trial for some projects. Project iMPPACS provides a clear example of such a case. Our group was interested in testing whether a mass media campaign involving television and radio ads could motivate behavioral change among at-risk adolescents. Although mass media campaigns have been evaluated using a single-city design (Agha, 2003; Alstead et al., 1999), such a design provides no comparison or "control" city on which to compare behavioral change over the same time for individuals who did not receive an intervention. Therefore, and because there was already promising evidence supporting the use of mass media to promote behavioral change from single-city studies, our research group chose to implement a multisite trial in which intervention condition (media or no media) was randomized by city, with two cities (Syracuse, New York and Macon, Georgia) receiving the mass media campaign and two other cities (Providence, Rhode Island and Columbia, South Carolina) serving as control cities.

A related design consideration concerns the question of **generalizability** of study findings. If a single-site RCT provides evidence that an intervention is effective, a multisite study may be appropriate to seek evidence that an intervention approach shows promise across multiple settings and in different regions of the country. Well-designed multisite interventions typically succeed in enrolling a greater diversity of patients, varying in both socioeconomic characteristics and clinical manifestations. Contextual factors within a given community or treatment setting may also influence intervention outcomes. A sufficiently powered multisite design can include analyses designed to detect site-specific differences, as well as differences in intervention response related to patient characteristics.

In addition, a multisite design often provides the opportunity for a stronger test of competing (or complementary) intervention approaches that have been tested individually but have not yet been subject to direct comparison. In the case of Project iMPPACS, we implemented a multilevel design in which we were able to test the independent and combined impact of a promising individual-level intervention (Stanton et al., 1996) along with an innovative mass media intervention. Project MATCH (Matching Alcoholism Treatments to Client Heterogeneity) provides an even larger scale example of a multisite design that was implemented to provide a comparison of multiple intervention approaches to treating alcohol dependence (Gordis & Fuller, 1999). It involved many sites, with patients randomized within site to one of several different intervention approaches. Such a design would not be possible to implement in a single setting.

There is an additional methodological benefit of the multisite study design. Results from single-site studies can sometimes be influenced by inadvertent biases when conducted by research teams that have a deep investment in a particular intervention approach. For example, in the context of pharmacotherapy trials, it may not be surpassing to find that researchers who are committed to drug-based interventions find that medication fares better than therapy-based interventions. Though unintentional, such sites may exert inadvertent biases on the basis of the selection of outcome measures or selective publications of findings, or by virtue of having less expertise in providing supervision and oversight of the therapy-based protocols (Kraemer, 2000). If, on the contrary, two sites that include investigators representing both behavioral and pharmacological approaches are brought together to study both intervention approaches, teams must agree on common intervention protocols, outcome measures, and data analytic approaches. As such, findings then might be assumed to provide the best available evidence. Because multisite studies require involvement of independent research teams that are charged with implementing a protocol-based intervention in a uniform fashion across research sites, the design can reduce such biases.

SUCCESSFUL IMPLEMENTATION OF A MULTISITE TRIAL

Although there are a number of benefits of a multisite design, implementation of a multisite trial poses a number of practical and methodological challenges that require careful consideration. In the remainder of the chapter, I review several important steps that should be taken to help ensure successful implementation of a multisite trial.

The Choice of Collaborators

The choice of collaborators is critically important to the success of a multisite trial. Investigative teams from participating institutions should possess the necessary skills to complete the proposed work. Research teams at each site also need to have an established, trusting relationship with the community in which the work will be completed and an established track record of success in recruiting the relevant patient population. If recruitment falters at one site, the success of the entire trial can be compromised. Likewise, the success of a project requires comparably skilled and trained staff, so that study implementation can be uniformly achieved at each site. Finally, each team will also need a highly competent scientist who can serve as site PI. The site PI must be capable of providing scientific leadership to ensure that the scientific integrity of the project is maintained, that data collection procedures are followed, and that human subject requirements are met.

In addition to choosing team members from each site who possess the requisite skill sets, it is also important to choose collaborators who work well together. Multisite trials require countless hours of meetings, conference calls, training sessions, and emails. Published reports describe the methods used for successful implementation of research trials. Left out of these reports are the disagreements and challenges that are sometimes encountered among collaborators. Some disagreements are inevitable for large research projects. Nonetheless, it is important to consider the "chemistry" among team members to ensure that competing perspectives, differences in approaches to collaboration, or past disagreements do not interfere with successful implementation of the project.

Importance of Pilot Data

Ambitious data collection plans can read well in a grant proposal, but are often met with skepticism from savvy grant reviewers. A central question that must be addressed prior to receiving funding for a multisite trial and prior to initiating data collection is whether each site is capable of carrying out the work as proposed. In addition to a team's past track record of success, pilot research can provide a powerful demonstration of each site's capacity to recruit participants and implement a proposed protocol. Pilot studies are not merely a "drill" that will help a team to get a project funded. To the contrary, pilot studies provide invaluable information to the research team regarding project feasibility and information regarding important changes that may need to be made to a project's approach and scope.

In the case of Project iMPPACS, pilot research proved to be essential, both for convincing reviewers that our teams were capable of carrying out the proposed research and in providing insight into challenges that we would face in conducing the work within each community.

Project Governance and Oversight

Prior to initiating a multisite trial, collaborators should develop a clear plan for project governance and oversight. One individual should serve as the overarching PI who is charged with overseeing all aspects of the project, including protocol development and refinement, scientific direction, and adjudication of disagreements among team members. The study PI is typically also charged with overseeing study documentation for the conduct of the trial and serves as a lead in communicating with the funding agency. In addition to the study PI, each site is overseen by a **site PI** who is charged with supervising the **site project coordinator** and other staff. The role of site PI requires considerable time, expertise, and dedication. The site PI is responsible for ensuring that the trial is carried out as planned within a given site, maintaining all correspondence with local institutional review boards, and serving as a liaison for the project within a given community.

Collaborators must come to a common understanding about the way in which decisions, both small and large, will be made. Commonly, projects appoint a **steering committee** to provide such scientific oversight. Membership in the steering committee can vary, but typically includes the study PI, site PIs, and the project statistician. At the outset of a project, the research team should establish a clear description of the steering committee's responsibilities, voting procedures, and methods for disseminating information to study team members.

Establishing an Authorship Agreement

Prior to the start of any multisite trial, steering committee members should reach a common set of expectations for authorship on papers derived from project data. An **authorship agreement** can be of tremendous value in helping to prevent misunderstandings and disagreements by providing a clear set of guidelines and expectations for the process of proposing, preparing, and submitting scientific publications. At a minimum, a written authorship agreement should establish a clear set of guidelines concerning who is eligible to be a lead or coauthor on papers, how eligible individuals earn authorship for a given paper, and how authorship order will be established. Typically, authorship agreements are built around well-established guidelines such as those that are published by the American Psychological Association.

In addition to establishing guidelines for authorship eligibility and order, the authorship agreement should also specify a process for submitting paper proposals. Multisite teams are often large, with literally dozens of coauthors listed on outcome papers. Study teams typically include senior-level investigators, junior colleagues, postdoctoral research associates, and graduate students. All team members can potentially benefit from involvement in the multisite trial. However, without strong senior leadership and fair authorship guidelines, opportunities for professional advancement among junior colleagues can be compromised. Therefore, it is important that procedures are put in place to allow opportunities for both junior and more senior members of the research team to take a lead and contributing role in preparation of scientific publications.

Establishing Community Advisory Boards

Intervention trials often involve sensitive health-related topics that are of importance to the community in which the research project is being conducted. It is often useful to establish a **community advisory board (CAB)** at each site to ensure that the project benefits from input from community members to facilitate successful completion of a multisite trial. Research should be conducted in such a way that it is mindful of the community-level sensitivities as well as practical concerns that could impact the success of the trial.

Typically, CABs serve in an advisory capacity to provide assistance and counsel concerning project goals, including: (a) informing study teams of local issues or concerns that might affect the implementation of the study; (b) ensuring that the research program is attentive to community concerns, needs, and priorities; (c) providing feedback regarding potential feasibility and implementation challenges faced by the study team and community partners; (d) advising investigators regarding how to improve recruitment and retention efforts; and (e) assisting with the dissemination of information to community members about the project to facilitate an understanding of the goals of the trial and the potential benefits to the community.

Although membership varies somewhat across cities, CABs often include representation from major community-based organizations in each city, as well as other community leaders and professionals in the human and health services fields. At the outset of a trial, research sites settle on a plan for CAB membership and frequency of CAB meetings. CABs provided critical input for radio and television ads that were produced for potential use as part of the HIV-prevention media campaign for Project iMPPACS. In some cases, ads that research teams feared might be too controversial were embraced by the CABs as appropriate and needed. In several instances, campaign spots were changed on the basis of CAB input. In other instances, CAB input corroborated feedback that the team received from teens about ads that were not well liked. Across all four cities, CABs also helped to publicize Project iMPPACS and to network among community leaders; their involvement was essential to fostering positive community response to the program.

Team Training and Establishment of Protocols

A final point about implementing multisite intervention trials concerns the importance of providing standardized training for each team and the need for a detailed, written protocol that reflects expectations for participant recruitment, assessment, human subject concerns, and intervention deployment. Although all behavioral intervention research projects require team training and written protocols, the importance of having a uniform approach to training and a detailed protocol is magnified in instances where the research is being conducted as a multisite study. Uniformity of training across research sites reduces the likelihood that research findings will be unduly influenced by cross-site differences in study implementation.

Typically, research teams participate in joint training sessions that are led by experts with relevant knowledge of the specific training needs of the project. Ideally, all levels of study personnel can participate in the training so that there is sufficient training depth and transportability of expertise to home sites. Research assistants and interventionists should be expected to be assessed for competence on completion of training, with regular opportunities for performance feedback.

Written protocols should provide a detailed description of every aspect of study implementation, including recruitment and assessment procures, intervention delivery, methods for monitoring fidelity of intervention delivery, and procedures for ensuring uniform monitoring of data integrity and ensuring adherence to human subject requirements.

SUMMARY

Multisite trials are not for the faint of heart. Implementation requires years of hard work, careful attention to the development of detailed training and data collection protocols, and care in ensuring uniformity of study implementation across research sites. Teamwork, collegiality, and a shared commitment to the project across study sites are essential to a project's success. With careful planning, well-trained staff, and outstanding scientific leadership, multisite trials can provide invaluable data on the effectiveness of interventions to promote health and wellness within a community.

REFERENCES

Agha, S. (2003). The impact of a mass media campaign on personal risk perception, perceived self-efficacy and on other behavioural predictors. *AIDS Care, 15,* 749–762. doi:10.1080/09540120310001618603

Alstead, M., Campsmith, M., Halley, C. S., Hartfield, K., Goldbaum, G., & Wood, R. W. (1999). Developing, implementing, and evaluating a condom promotion program targeting sexually active adolescents. *AIDS Education and Prevention, 11,* 497–512.

Gordis, E., & Fuller, R. (1999). Project MATCH. *Addiction, 94,* 57–59.

Hennessy, M., Romer, D., Valois, R. F., Vanable, P., Carey, M. P., Stanton, B., … Salazar, L. F. (2013). Safer sex media messages and adolescent sexual behavior: 3-year follow-up results from project iMPPACS. *American Journal of Public Health, 103*(1), 134–140. doi:10.2105/AJPH.2012.300856

Kraemer, H. C. (2000). Pitfalls of multisite randomized clinical trials of efficacy and effectiveness. *Schizophrenia Bulletin, 26,* 533–541. doi:10.1093/oxfordjournals.schbul.a033474

Romer, D., Sznitman, S., DiClemente, R., Salazar, L. F., Vanable, P. A., Carey, M. P., … Juzang, I. (2009). Mass media as an HIV-prevention strategy: Using culturally sensitive messages to reduce HIV-associated sexual behavior of at-risk African American youth. [Research Support, N.I.H., Extramural]. *American Journal of Public Health, 99,* 2150–2159. doi:10.2105/AJPH.2008.155036

Rounsaville, B. J., Carroll, K. M., & Onken, L. S. (2001). A stage model of behavioral therapies research: Getting started and moving on from stage I. *Clinical Psychology: Science and Practice, 8,* 133–142. https://doi-org.libezproxy2.syr.edu/10.1093/clipsy.8.2.133

Stanton, B. F., Li, X., Ricardo, I., Galbraith, J., Feigelman, S., & Kaljee, L. (1996). A randomized, controlled effectiveness trial of an AIDS prevention program for low-income African-American youths. *Archives of Pediatrics & Adolescent Medicine, 150,* 363–372. doi:10.1001/archpedi.1996.02170290029004

Vanable, P. A., Carey, M. P., Bostwick, R. A., Brown, L. K., Valois, R. F., DiClemente, R. J., … Stanton, B. (Eds.). (2009). *Community partnerships in adolescent HIV prevention research: The experience of Project iMPPACS.* Hauppauge, NY: Nova.

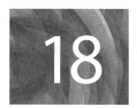

Considerations in Conducting Interventions in Specialized Settings

Interventions can take place in a multitude of places—global locations, long-term care facilities, public health and military settings, schools, and hospitals—the list is as varied as the people for whom we develop these interventions. Although many of the basic caveats for designing and conducting intervention studies hold true across these specialized settings, each brings with it unique challenges and nuances that can affect the ability to initiate and successfully carry out intervention work. In this chapter, we highlight just a few of these settings. This chapter also provides some commonsense advice and overall perspectives from investigators whose work has been conducted in these specialized settings with strategies that facilitate success.

18.1 Conducting Interventions in Global Settings

Carol M. Baldwin, Luis Gabriel Cuervo*, & Christine Hancock

> When it comes to global health, there is
> no "them" … only "us." —*Global Health Council*

Global health research is multifaceted. Researchers need to understand and respect regional, national, and international boundaries and contexts including lifestyles and habits, mores, laws, and political and religious beliefs to prevent disease, promote health and the quality of life of persons and communities, and address unjustified health inequities (e.g., de Cosío, Díaz-Apodaca, Ruiz-Holguín, Lara, & Castillo-Salgado, 2010). As people migrate from rural to urban areas, developing to developed regions, and from continent to continent, the advance of industrialized activities contributes to environmental and climate changes, new (e.g., Zika, chikungunya) and reemerging (e.g., Ebola, measles) infectious diseases, injuries, and chronic noncommunicable diseases (NCDs). The latter, especially, resulting from unhealthy lifestyle behaviors, combine to create a double burden of disease (Baldwin & Korniewicz, 2012). In addition, natural and human-made disasters (e.g., earthquakes, bioterrorism) can further complicate the ability to engage in research for human health.

> Open your arms to change, but don't
> give up your values. —*Dalai Lama*

Although the focus of this textbook addresses intervention research in nursing practice, resources, references, and information for this chapter are from diverse interprofessional orientations. It is incumbent on nurses, the largest healthcare delivery workforce worldwide, to develop collaborations with other professionals, policy makers, nongovernmental organizations (NGOs), as well as community dwellers to expand their understanding of these interrelated complex factors. This will allow nurses to assess, design, implement, and evaluate culturally and regionally responsive interventions that simultaneously address health equity and inform health policy locally to globally.

To delineate a comprehensive approach toward addressing research typologies, including interventions in global settings, this section uses the six objectives outlined by the Pan American Health Organization/World Health Organization (PAHO/WHO) Policy on Research for Health (PAHO/WHO, 2009) as heuristic devices for reviewing, understanding, and generating investigations, including intervention research for health no matter which global region is the focus of study. The six interdependent objectives on the Policy on Research for Health are intertwined and work in tandem with the five goals of the WHO Strategy on Research for Health: organizational, priorities, capacity, standards, and translation (PAHO/WHO, 2009; WHO, 2010).

* Dr. Luis Gabriel Cuervo's contributions to this publication were done on his personal time and do not necessarily reflect the decisions or policies of his employer.

> Research is to see what everybody else has seen, and to think what
> nobody else has thought. —*Albert Szent-Gyorgyi*

Objective 1: Generate Relevant, Ethical, Quality Research

Objective 1 focuses on developing tools to examine standards, indicators, impact, and cross-cutting issues, and identifying/resolving knowledge gaps in key areas (PAHO/WHO, 2009). As examples, Klingler, Silva, Schuermann, Reis, Saxena, and Strech (2017) posited that public health surveillance is not ethically neutral, yet training on the basis of comprehensive and clearly derived overviews of ethical issues for such programs is sparse. In their first-ever systematic review of ethical issues related to the topic of public health surveillance, Klingler et al. (2017) provide an ethics matrix for use in intervention and other research milieus to update guidelines, reports, policy, and strategy papers. These authors also incorporate educational tools and teaching/learning approaches for practitioners and the public.

In like manner, in their analysis of 36 multiproject research programs in 11 countries and two multicountries, Hanney, Greenhalgh, Blatch-Jones, Glover, and Raftery (2017) assessed the nature, research field, funding mode, time frame, and methods to assess impact of interventions and other research objectives, as well as the level of impact. Their analyses indicated widespread impact for some multi- and needs-led collaborative programs that could garner additional funding; however, improved standardized assessment methods could identify ways to improve research investment decisions (Hanney et al., 2017). Similarly, health systems guidance (HSG) are well-organized statements that support the development, evaluation, and reporting of evidence relevant to complex health systems; however, on the basis of a critical interpretive synthesis of the literature, no extant appraisal tools for HSG were identified (Ako-Arrey, Brouwers, Lavis, Giacomini, & AGREE-HS Team, 2016). On the basis of their review, these authors identified 30 concepts clustered into three domains (process principles, content, and context principles) that could serve as salient quality criteria in response to the evaluation of HSG (Ako-Arrey et al., 2016).

Health inequality and health inequity are important foci in research for health. "Health inequality" is a difference in health outcomes among individuals in a population, or between distinct groups, whereas "health inequity" is inequality that is unfair and avoidable (Whitehead, 1992). Systematic reviews are a salient approach to examine impelling and constraining forces for conceptual analysis that can foster ethical, quality intervention research and inform policy. The intent of the Preferred Reporting Items for Systematic Reviews and Meta-Analysis (PRISMA) checklist is to improve transparency of reporting systematic reviews (Welch et al., 2015b). Extending their PRISMA statement to include equity, these authors provide guidelines to enhance clear and complete reporting of health equity–centered systematic reviews. They argue that the enhanced reporting using equity-focused reviews can inform better policy and possibly reduce health inequity. Other significant developments are the growing number of agendas on research for health being developed by countries and to address regional and subregional health issues; nurses have influenced in different degrees the development of such agendas (Becerra-Posada, de Snyder, Cuervo, & Montorzi, 2014; Caribbean Health Research Council, 2011; Garcia, Cassiani, & Reveiz, 2015; Hotez, Bottazzi, Franco-Paredes, Ault, & Periago, 2008; PAHO/WHO, 2016).

Taken together, with training in evidence-based practice (EBP) and grounded in the exemplars for Objective 1, nurses with a passion for global health can perform systematic reviews on regional to global levels that can inform and promulgate research tools and that address relevant, quality intervention research, and influence research agendas. Garnering added training in policy development (DeMarco & Tufts, 2014) and developing collaborations with like-minded interprofessionals, nurses can make substantive contributions to ethical, high-quality interventions with a focus on low- and middle-income countries (LMICs) that also concentrate on health equity.

Objective 2: Strengthen Research Governance and Define Research Agendas

Objective 2 addresses the ability to build, support, and maintain health research systems by means of guiding research on the basis of past experiences, developing action plans, fostering and understanding the value of research from community to political levels, advocating for research resources, and stimulating regional to national ownership (PAHO/WHO, 2009). For instance, Bennett et al. (2017) identified 2015 as a banner year for global health with the anniversaries of the Global Alliance for Vaccines and Immunization; Global Fund to Fight AIDS, TB, and Malaria; adoption of the International Health Regulations; and formal entry into the Framework Convention on the Tobacco Control. These successes highlight the growth of global health diplomacy; however, they also noted chronic concerns regarding compliance, ongoing funding, and global health governance equity. The authors posited four themes consistent with Objective 2, including prioritizing within governance, identifying stakeholders, recognizing the relationship between behavior and health, factors critical to interventions, and the role of regulation and governance relevant to support at the global health level (Bennett et al., 2017).

In 2009, PAHO/WHO member states agreed to implement a Policy on Research for Health, the first of its kind, and was harmonized in its development with the subsequent WHO Strategy on Research for Health approved by the World Health Assembly in 2010 (WHO, 2010). Both the WHO and the PAHO are to monitor how countries and the organizations implement these policies and support countries in the process to ensure substantive progress is made with the six objectives so that all countries in the region have capacities in place to use research for health, and, when necessary, to develop research to address their public health needs. Pertinent to LMICs and health equity, despite reported advances in the health and life expectancy in Latin America and the Caribbean, inequality persists in this region (Villanueva, Abreu, Cuervo, Becerra-Posada, Reveiz, & Ijsselmuiden, 2012). These inequalities are frequently mirrored in the capacities of the countries to use research to inform their health policies and decisions, and to produce research that addresses their public health needs. In response to this need, members of the PAHO and the Council on Health Research for Development (COHRED) combined to develop an innovative web-based tool, HRWeb Americas (www.healthresearch web.org), to accelerate the promotion of a national health research system (NHRS) in this region that advances research and provides indicators to monitor and evaluate progress. Topics include governance and policies, research priorities, including culturally relevant interventions, ethics reviews, regulation, partners and funding, resources, and announcements by region and country (Villanueva et al., 2012). In addition, a series of regional debates pulled together the sectors of health and science and technology under the auspices of the Latin American Conferences on Research and Innovation for Health (LACRIH) to find ways of strengthening the NHRSs so that they effectively strengthen a national research health system in LMICs (www.paho.org/LACRIH). These conferences were the foundation for initial inputs to feed the health research website.

Another important aspect of Objective 2 is the improvement of research-reporting standards with the definition of standards and checklists for all kinds of research for health, whether basic, clinical, public health, or health systems research. This is reflected in the series of organized guidelines that are accessible through the Enhancing the QUAlity and Transparency Of health Research (EQUATOR) Network (www.equator-network.org) clearinghouse and the standards for leading publishers. An example is the guideline for the reporting of randomized controlled trials (RCTs) entitled Consolidated Standards of Reporting Trials (CONSORT), which also extended their guidelines to include equity-directed decision making (Welch et al., 2015a). A six-phase framework was used to create RCT guidelines, including equity-relevant trials, empirical evidence, methods and experts, feedback and prioritization, consensus on guidelines, and distribution and implementation of the equity-focused CONSORT extension. The authors indicate that operationalizing equity in RCTs can enhance practice, policy, research, and concomitant interventions in the social determinants of health, clinical care, public health and health systems, and global health milieus (Welch et al., 2015a).

Recently, Rodríguez-Feria and Cuervo (2017) reported that regulated and nonregulated clinical trial registration in Latin America and the Caribbean has made significant, but inconsistent progress. The authors recommend that legislation require all research be available on international platforms (e.g., WHO International Clinical Trials Registry Platform [ICTRP]) before funding, show proof of registration, facilitate good research governance, and enhance the use of the ICTRP. Notably, during the revision of this chapter, a global announcement was made indicating that major research funders and international NGOs agreed on new standards that require all their funded or supported clinical trials be registered; summary results of clinical trials are to be made available for free through open access registries within 12 months of study completion (WHO, 2017). Trial registration is a strategic component of research for health, including clarity and dissemination of findings, forming and informing research initiatives and interventions, and advising policy. The ICTRP provides definitions of and guidelines for clinical trials and their registration, as well as other resources, including internships (www.who.int/ictrp/en). Research registration is also extending to other research methods, including the International Prospective Register of Systematic Reviews funded by the National Institute for Health Research in the PROSPERO database (www.crd.york.ac.uk/PROSPERO), as well as observational studies increasingly being registered in the WHO ICTRP. (Guidance for trial registration can be seen at https://youtu.be/CeJm5deW50E?list=PL6hS8Moik7ku2Luc8YDsZfDzNkEv08Kow)

Objective 3: Improve Competencies of and Support for Human Resources in Research for Health

Objective 3 emphasizes work with interprofessional partners, legal sectors, and research institutions to improve competencies, capacity building, and engaging others who influence healthcare, systems, and governance. In addition, this objective encourages the development and retention of research groups, promotion of gender and underrepresented ethnic group equity, and strengthening of staff to use scientific knowledge and systematic reviews to promote research evidence that lead to plans of action for human resources for health (PAHO/WHO, 2009).

In 2009, the National Institutes of Health–National Heart, Lung, and Blood Institute (NIH–NHLBI) and the UnitedHealth Group teamed up to support a collaborative network of centers of excellence (COEs) in Argentina, Bangladesh, China, Guatemala, India (Bengaluru and New Delhi), Kenya, Peru, South Africa, Tanzania, Tunisia, and both sides of the United States–Mexico border. The goal was the generation of evidence to inform policy and to reduce and prevent the epidemic of NCDs (see Nabel, Stevens, & Smith, 2009, for a complete overview). Each center included a research institution in its developing region that was paired with one or more academic partners in a high-income country. Projects incorporated effective strategies used in other multicenter, international research programs (e.g., Aitken et al., 2008), including health surveillance, research dissemination, development of culturally appropriate policies, practices and intervention tactics, and community participatory activities to support local and national leadership.

Contributing to the global burden of NCDs is the observation that, as a country's economy develops, there is a concomitant increase in risky behavior, including smoking, change in diet, and increasingly sedentary lifestyles. Impediments to controlling this growth continue to include inadequate intervention research funding, failure to provide current evidence on disease burden to policy makers, health inequality, and academic programs that have yet to address chronic disease liabilities (Yach, Hawkes, Gould, & Hofman, 2004). On the basis of a set of targets issued by the WHO (2015), including a reduction in deaths from NCDs, GRAND

South (a network of 11 centers dedicated to research, capacity building, and advising on policy) developed a scorecard for tracking actions to reduce NCD burden (Roman, Perez, & Smith, 2015). Global experts developed a means to monitor progress from 23 high- to low-income countries on a 4-point scale (no to highly adequate activity) to assess four indicators (governance, risk factors, surveillance and research, and health system response). Findings show that NCD progress indicators vary and are relevant to country income and research structure. Future surveillance and outcome data will inform policy.

Most NCD-associated research addresses the behavioral factors of diet, physical activity, or smoking (e.g., Hughes, Hancock, & Cooper, 2012). Although these are essential factors relevant to health, frequently overlooked are the behavioral factors that contribute to poor sleep. Sleep disorders have been associated with several chronic NCDs, including cardiovascular disease, diabetes, mood disorders, overweight, and obesity (Stranges, Tigbe, Gómez-Olivé, Thorogood, & Kandala, 2012). Coauthor Carol Baldwin collaborated with the World Diabetes Foundation (WDF), PAHO, and academic programs, ministries of health, and NGOs along both sides of the United States–Mexico border. The outcome was a revised version of the NIH–NHLBI *Camino a la Salud: Su Corazon/Su Vida Manual para Promotoras y Promotores* (PAHO/WHO, 2014), which included the first session on sleep disorders and sleep health promotion in a manual of this type (Baldwin, 2014). Developed for lay health educators and promoters, the manual provides sleep health promotion and intervention information, as well as guidelines on diet, physical activity, diabetes, cardiovascular disease, and mental health to enhance health equity among underserved Spanish-speaking populations. The intent of the manual is to enhance training, competencies, and support for all persons engaged in human research for health. The Mexican Ministry of Health has since adopted training and interventions from *Camino al la Salud* for use throughout Mexico, primarily in rural areas to reduce the rates of diabetes. In addition, the bilingual sleep training is a component of the WDF-funded Certified Diabetes Educator program at the University of Guanajuato, Mexico; English versions train nurses regarding sleep and NCDs at academic institutions in the United States, and sleep health promotion and intervention strategies to community-dwelling adults. Many other examples emerge from collaborations in the Americas, such as the development of innovative approaches through collaborations to address chronic diseases in different environments of LMICs (Vedanthan et al., 2017) and to understand better context and variations (Bernabe-Ortiz et al., 2017; Miranda, Bernabe-Ortiz, Smeeth, Gilman, Checkley & CRONICAS Cohort Study Group, 2012).

Given the evidence of improved health of populations in LMICs, of growing importance are large-scale community health worker (CHW) programs. On the basis of their size and operational tasks, Perry et al. (2017) suggest that these programs require unique attention by policy makers, program implementers, and the global health community. For these reasons, Perry et al. (2017) cited a new online resource: Developing and strengthening CHW programs at scale: A reference guide and case studies for program managers and policy makers (see http://www.mchip.net/CHWReferenceGuide). This and other online resources cited in this chapter can lead nurses and their interprofessional colleagues involved in global health toward an improved understanding of the complexities of support and intervention training for human resources in research for health.

Objective 4: Enhance the Impact of Research via Useful and Strategic Alliances, Collaborations, and Encourage Public Trust and Engagement in Research

Objective 4 highlights interactions among multiple partners, opinion leaders, strategic alliances, WHO Collaborating Centres, and others for the purposes of innovation, sharing of ideas, and collaboration among various sectors (e.g., education, science, technology, non/for profits). The intent of this teamwork is to promote sustainable progress that addresses social determinants of health and facilitates equitable investment of resources to improve the health and well-being of populations (PAHO/WHO, 2009).

The work of coauthor Christine Hancock explicates Objective 4. She is the foundress-director of the nonprofit NGO C3 Collaborating for Health and works with international programs and organizations that are interested in preventing NCDs. C3 Collaborating for Health tackles the major risk factors of poor diet (including the harmful use of alcohol), physical inactivity, and smoking that contribute to cardiovascular disease, diabetes, respiratory disease, and some cancers. In 2010, a coalition consisting of C3, the International Council of Nurses (ICN), Pfizer External Medical Affairs, and the International Alliance of Patients' Organizations advocated for necessary social, economic, and political change regarding the global challenges of the lifestyle-related NCD epidemic. These organizations brought together a multinational group of stakeholders contributing different perspectives and expertise to explore a range of nurse-led options, ways to disseminate and implement evidence-based prevention interventions, and support personal health and well-being (C3 website; ICN, 2010). Hancock and colleagues also provide insight into the role the private sector can play, and describe a "business case" on NCDs for employees, consumers, and communities (Hancock, Kingo, & Raynaud, 2011). They provide a pragmatic and comprehensive review of ways in which business can work in partnership to make a difference for the better toward reducing NCDs and promoting health, thereby becoming part of the solution.

Another initiative coordinated by C3 Collaborating for Health, the "first 1,000 days," designed a blueprint for change that enables women to have a healthy pregnancy and for their children to have a healthy start in life. This includes access to appropriate nutrition, including micronutrients, as well as screening for and management of conditions such as gestational diabetes. In joining this effort, the partners acknowledge the need for positively influencing women's standing in society, including the cultural, family-related, political, and societal contexts set for maternal and child health. The development of interventions to promote health literacy among mothers and persons influencing their health will be an indicator for the long-term impact of these efforts and will be a key outcome of the partnership. The founding partners aim to build a wide consortium of like-minded partners and, using the existing evidence base, identify effective areas for intervention, and subsequently design and establish a large-scale pilot project in LMICs.

In addition to the developmental origins of health and disease, exposures to environmental toxicants, including heavy metal and endocrine-disrupting chemicals, are correlates of early life predisposition to disease risk in adulthood (Balbus et al., 2013). These authors underscore the need to comprehend in utero and early childhood experiences that may be risk factors for the development of NCDs separate from lifestyle choices made in adulthood. Social determinants of health, including poverty, gender inequality, education, and food insecurity, are factors of disadvantage in LMICs and should be incorporated into intervention research and have policy implications given that lifestyle choice necessarily reduces governmental and societal culpability (Balbus et al., 2013). These factors are essential to fostering strategic alliances and garnering public trust to address these issues, and open opportunities to develop sustainable capacities and human capital in research for health (Miranda et al., 2016). As well, to promote the understanding of research for health, and more specifically of the methods most frequently used in health technology assessment, Evans, Thornton, and Chalmers (2010) published a book geared toward the educated public that was later followed by a dedicated interactive website that includes the book now available in 14 languages (see http://www.testingtreatments.org).

A further example of practical research into interventions is the Community Interventions for Health (CIH) initiative, a program of the Oxford Health Alliance. This study focused on chronic disease prevention activities in select communities in developing country settings (India, China, and Mexico). It is comprehensive in its scope and design, including a combination of structural interventions, health education, and community coalition building as well as rigorous evaluation (O'Connor Duffany et al., 2011). An extensive analysis of each of the community's environmental assets and challenges is incorporated by including stakeholder analyses, policy analyses, and an environmental scan that assesses physical attributes (Wong, Stevens,

O'Connor-Duffany, Siegel, & Gao, 2011). The interventions take place simultaneously in schools, workplaces, healthcare settings, and the community at large, with the goal of addressing physical inactivity, tobacco use, and unhealthy diets. Although all sites are engaged in the same broad categories of interventions, they are culturally specific and tailored to each setting. For example, in Indian schools, baseline data revealed the importance of addressing cultural norms around girls and physical activity, so one intervention strategy was to provide bicycle training for girls. In Mexico, the major focus of interventions is physical activity in the community, primarily music and dance. The results of CIH will provide guidance and a road map as to what works—or does not work—in these different settings, and pave the way for future intervention research.

Tackling tobacco use is also a public health priority—as reflected in the Framework Convention on Tobacco Control, the first international treaty on a health issue. Globally, more than 1 billion people smoke and 80% of these smokers reside in developing countries (Jha, 2009). Deaths from smoking-related diseases are already at 5 million a year globally and this is projected to reach more than 8 million by 2020 (Shafey, Eriksen, Ross, & Mackay, 2009). The Tobacco Free Nurses Initiative, funded by the Robert Wood Johnson Foundation, aims to ensure that the nursing profession is also prepared to promote health actively by reducing nurses' barriers to involvement in tobacco control. It will equip them to assist with smoking cessation, prevent tobacco use, and promote strategies to decrease exposure to secondhand smoke. The Tobacco Free Nurses Initiative accomplishes its mission through (a) supporting and assisting smoking cessation efforts of nurses and nursing students, (b) providing tobacco control resources for use in patient care, and (c) enhancing the culture of nurses as leaders and advocates of a smoke-free society.

Objective 5: Foster Best Practices and Augment Standards in Research

Objective 5 concentrates on advocating for civil society to participate in research as a valued partner, provides access to and use of registries, systematic reviews, summaries, and briefs, works with local to international organizations to promote ethical review committees, and promotes indicators to assess effects of research, as well as standards and norms in line with research for health (PAHO/WHO, 2009). There are several advances in research that are of increasing interest to health policy and healthcare costs, including the use of comparative effectiveness research (CER) to inform the interaction of research and policy in developing countries, cost-effectiveness analysis of interventions to prevent NCDs, and operations research (OR).

The goal of CER is to improve health outcomes by developing and disseminating evidence-based information to patients, clinicians, and other decision makers, focusing on effective interventions for patients at individual and population levels (Chalkidou et al., 2009). Characteristics of CER include directly informing clinical or health policy decisions; comparing at least two alternatives, each with the potential to be best practice; results generated at population and subgroup levels; outcome measures that are important to patients; methods and data sources that are appropriate for the decision of interest (quantitative and/or qualitative); and studies conducted in real-world settings. Interventions may include medications, procedures, medical and assistive devices and technologies, diagnostic testing, behavioral change, and delivery system strategies.

As an example of CER to policy, Rubinstein et al. (2010) estimated cost-effectiveness ratios from six interventions, including salt reduction in bread, a media campaign to promote tobacco cessation, pharmacological treatment of hypertension, elevated cholesterol and tobacco cessation, and multidrug approach for Argentinians with an absolute risk estimate greater than 20% in 10 years. Results outlined in detail the cost savings in disability-adjusted life years, incremental cost-effectiveness ratios, and dollar amounts for pharmacological treatment. Findings from this research inform policy makers on resource allocation to reduce the cardiovascular disease burden in Argentina. The application of CER can help to determine the salience, cost burden, and other factors relevant to interventions.

OR uses advanced analytical methods to understand complex systems and making complex decisions. Methodology includes simulation not unlike the simulation labs used in nursing and medical schools, and Decision Theater, which brings together interprofessionals to manipulate various standards, norms, and factors involved in research for health. Bradley et al. (2017) performed a systematic search of the literature using OR in global health relevant to the theme of health equity. The three essential components identified for success in bridging OR and global health policy, interventions, and other research included collaboration with stakeholders, contextually appropriate data, and communication outlets for research findings. Having community members, thought leaders, and other stakeholders collaborate to determine the variables for study and altering such variables, OR holds enormous potential to determine the most feasible and cost-effective research for health approach for any given region. The use of research-reporting standards, like standards in other aspects of research, are essential to increase the value of research and reduce its waste (REWARD-EQUATOR Conference, 2015; *The Lancet*, 2014).

Objective 6: Disseminate and Utilize Research Findings

Objective 6 emphasizes the need to make visible regional to national research and disseminate the use of knowledge to improve health, equity, and development; work in cooperation with specialized centers and media to improve understanding of the value of research for health; participate in international intellectual property debates; and promote health via knowledge translation initiatives and tools (PAHO/WHO, 2009).

In addition to publishing original research, systematic reviews, opinion pieces, white papers, and policy briefs in professional journals, and as posters and papers at notable international conferences, various approaches are available to disseminate and apply research. The PAHO Evidence Informed Policy Network (EVIPNet), on the basis of the EBP synthesis and analysis methodology, facilitates knowledge transfer and translation of research into programs, policies, and law (Chapman, 2012; WHO, 2016). Cochrane is a predominantly online independent network of more than 30,000 mostly volunteer researchers, biostatisticians, professionals, patients/consumers, scientific communicators, and others providing informed decision making to promote global health (www.cochrane.org). The organization is based on and draws from the work of Archie Cochrane, who emphasized using research evidence to provide information that was more reliable than other forms of information; it emphasized the need of research fit for purpose (Cochrane, 1972).

The Patient-Centered Outcomes Research Institute (PCORI), established in the United States and authorized by Congress, is a private, independent, nonprofit institute that represents the needs and perspectives of the healthcare community, as well as acting as reliable information resource (Barksdale, Newhouse, & Miller, 2014). The PCORI funds CER that evaluates the risks and benefits of interventions, procedures, medical devices, and diagnostic tools; healthcare promotion; management and delivery programs; and other evidence-based strategies used to promote health and prevent, treat, and manage disease (Barksdale et al., 2014). Although the intent of CER is to promote cost-effective practice-based interventions that can inform the PCORI, a focus of CER is to implement interventions to improve health outcomes and reduce inequality in large, local, and global patient populations. Implementing CER requires the development, expansion, and use of a variety of data sources and methods to assess comparative effectiveness and disseminate the results.

Knowledge is not information, it's transformation. —*Osho*

One final topic area that crisscrosses all six of the PAHO/WHO objectives and is highly relevant to research and interventions in global settings is a brief commentary on "big data." The concept of big data can be defined as the collecting and storage of a large volume of information at an unprecedented speed in a wide variety of formats including structured traditional databases, as well as unstructured text files, audio/video information, and several types of transactions, the magnitude of which may pose management difficulties and the quality of which may vary, affecting accurate analysis (Tattersall & Grant, 2016). Software developers, including IBM, Microsoft, Hewlett Packard, and others, globally have developed a variety of solutions for use by governments, international development, manufacturing, modeling, education, media, online technology (e.g., Amazon, Google, eBay), science, healthcare, information technology for retail and real estate purposes, sports, and research activities (World Economic Forum, 2012).

For the purposes of this textbook section, the focus is on the pros and cons of big data in global research, including interventions. Big data studies have ranged from surveillance studies for the occurrence of the Zika vector on the basis of elevation as a proxy for transmission of the virus (Watts et al., 2017) to global maps of insecticide resistance risk for vector control (Coleman et al., 2017) to clinical trials applied to precision medicine (Weng & Kahn, 2016) to the use of big data for improving health in LMICs (Wyber et al., 2015). These topics alone suggest substantive and diverse applications of big data to global health issues.

There are, however, as many disadvantages as advantages to the global use of big data. For example, there are serious concerns regarding the confidentiality and security of personal health information in LMICs (as well as developed countries) that are intended to collect the use, cost, outcomes, and impact of health services at subnational and national levels (Beck, Gill, & De Lay, 2016; Salerno, Knoppers, Lee, Hlaing, & Goodman, 2017). Recently, a Framework for Responsible Sharing of Genomic and Health-Related Data, and outcome of the Global Alliance for Genomics and Health (GA4GH) have been posited as a more positive approach to address human rights from the privacy, nondiscrimination, fair access, and procedural impartiality to address the challenges of big data and the respect for human dignity (Salerno et al., 2017). Other issues that hamper the use of big data in global research are inherent in its definition, that is, different database structures, including coding of diagnoses, medications, laboratory results in structured data and clinical narratives in unstructured data, different terminology systems, timing of data collection, coding differences, as well as variations in analytical procedures that can converge to result in suboptimal levels of patient care, and hinder the development of evidence-based interventions. One approach to tackling these issues at the global level is that of a systematic emphasis on deriving models from smaller datasets to visualize ways in which the public, politicians, and policy makers can understand the value of big data as applied to big global health research (Mann et al., 2016).

Finally, in terms of clearinghouses and collections focused on addressing the public health questions, and the questions faced by policy makers, McMaster University has developed and maintained free access comprehensive databases that pull together, index, and curate systematic reviews, policy briefs, and policy documents from intergovernmental organizations. These databases offer free access (with registration) and can be found at www.healthevidence. org and www.healthsystemsevidence.org respectively. When it comes to emergency response, EVIDENCEAid, a spin-off of the Cochrane Collaboration, is an important resource of research evidence (www.evidenceaid.org). The development of these resources, as well as the subsequent distribution of indexed WHO (http://apps.who.int/iris) and PAHO documents (http://iris.paho.org), has changed the landscape enabling the public to identify better policies and priorities, and the relevant research evidence and policy options.

Key Points From Section 18.1 of This Chapter

- Designing and implementing culturally and regionally responsive interventions require an understanding and respect for boundaries, mores, laws, political and religious beliefs, as well as lifestyles and habits.
- Evidence-informed (or based) healthcare requires the integration of values and context with research; missing the considerations of values and context in which research is applied can result in unhelpful or harmful application of research findings (Evans et al., 2010; Sackett, Rosenberg, Gray, Haynes, & Richardson, 1996).
- The six interrelated PAHO/WHO objectives on the Policy on Research for Health are salient heuristics for understanding research intervention needs in global settings.
- Although many global interventions address new and reemerging infections, the need for transdisciplinary studies aimed at reducing and preventing NCDs associated with lifestyle will continue to increase.
- Cost-effectiveness research, eHealth, evaluating large datasets (big data), global clinical trials registration, information technology, OR, and knowledge transfer are important growing trends and technology relevant to interventions in global settings.

18.2 Conducting Interventions in Long-Term Care Settings

Debra Parker Oliver & Marlys R. Peck

Wisdom comes with winters. —*Oscar Wilde*

In the United States, 2.6% of the population older than 65 years—or 1.4 million people—reside in nursing homes. More than 3 million people receive services over the course of a year. In 2015, this included 2.6% of the population older than 65 years. Care is provided in more than 15,000 facilities participating in the Medicare and/or Medicaid program (Centers for Medicare and Medicaid Services [CMS], 2015). To manage these facilities and their vulnerable older populations, the government has been very active such that nursing homes are one of the most highly regulated industries in the United States.

The nursing home setting offers excellent opportunities for researchers interested in **gerontology**. Residents are most often older than 65 years (84.5%) and 7.8% are older than 95 years. Most residents are female (65.6%) and Caucasian (77.9%). The **CMS** have a three-part aim to improve the quality of care including better health for the population, better care for individuals, and lower cost through improvement (CMS, 2015). The goals of this plan are in support of intervention and implementation research projects whose purpose is to understand what works, identify barriers, and improve the lives of seniors residing in these settings ("Challenges in research and practice in residential long-term care," 2016).

UNDERSTANDING THE CULTURE OF LONG-TERM CARE

There are a variety of long-term care settings, but this chapter focuses on congregate housing in which residents require some degree of assistance with their activities of daily living. The skilled nursing facility, often being the last stop along the continuum, is a primary site that offers unique opportunities for intervention research and is the focus of this chapter.

Imagine a vertical hierarchy of **long-term care settings** based on real or pretended levels of acuity. Independent living with limited services is, by its own name, the least restricted environment. This is followed by residential care often regulated by state reimbursement agencies; assisted living that attracts private paying residents and is now the most popular setting in the United States; aging-in-place facilities, a relatively new concept that has the intent of caring for the person in the same place until he or she dies; and skilled nursing facilities (nursing homes) that care for those who often are much less independent and require significantly more assistance. Specifically, it is the ability to leave the facility and the need for 24-hour supervised professional care that differentiates the nursing home from the other living environments.

Although special rehabilitation and dementia care units can be found in most nursing homes, the number of residents receiving these services is usually small. Medicare-financed rehab services are usually provided to patients who have been discharged from hospitals, can withstand 3 hours of aggressive therapy sessions each day, 5 days per week, and who hope to be rehabilitated to the point of being able to return home; those who do not improve must pay for services with their own money or qualify for state Medicaid funds. If the resident is going to remain financially solvent during the entire stay in a nursing home, long-term care insurance can be a good option. Otherwise, a person can "spend down" depleting assets and qualify for Medicaid. He or she will discover that the quality of care is the same regardless of method of payment.

Another specialized service that is underutilized is **palliative care**. The needs of older adults with noncancer illnesses or comorbidity have not been identified in the literature. Frequently, knowing when to initiate palliative care for residents is often late in the disease progression. Medicare coverage and knowing when to initiate care are areas that need additional research (Neiman & Kovach, 2016).

Dementia care units for residents with **Alzheimer's disease** and related dementias are becoming more common in nursing homes and assisted care facilities. This is largely because of increased state and federal reimbursement for these services and the need to allow these residents greater movement within the facility. Although their minds are deteriorating, they often remain physically ambulatory. Sometimes referred to as "memory care units," they are locked so that residents will not wander into the larger nursing home, or, worse, wander outside the facility and endanger their lives.

Entering a nursing home for the first time can be an uncomfortable experience, not only for a first-time visitor but also clearly for a first-time resident, and it can be an ordeal for family members who have made the arrangements. "Promise me you won't ever put me in a nursing home!" is often a plea from the lips of an aging adult. The dream, of course, is to die peacefully in one's own chair or bed, a fitting end to a long life lived fully and independently. In a nation that worships youth and measures worth by activity, nothing so epitomizes a "failed old age" as admittance to a nursing home. This was the message introducing the book *The Human Factor in Nursing Home Care* almost 30 years ago (Oliver & Tureman, 1988). Little has changed. If anything, the challenges of nursing home living have become more complex and the need for interventions ubiquitous.

The drama of everyday living in the world of the nursing home encompasses many players, roles, and performances. A would-be researcher should take all into account before initiating any intervention, no matter how limited it may be in scope. The administrator, from whom approval must be gained, and the director of nurses, the second and sometimes the most important professional in the home, must be aware of and be supportive of the plan. The quality of nursing home care is directly linked to the number of consecutive years of employment in these two positions (Geletta & Sparks, 2013; Tellis-Nayak, 2010).

The physician and family members are very important, but it is typically the nurses' aides, housekeepers, and other frontline employees who are closest to the resident. They are at the center of all activity and life. If they failed to show up for work, there would be chaos in 15 minutes. They constitute at least 70% or more of the workforce at such a facility. Unfortunately, they experience the most stress and account for the highest degree of turnover in the facility. As pointed out:

> They are expected to clean butts, smile when bitten, be in two places at once, not talk back, stand in awe of supervisors who have more education, and get all the work done regardless of how "short" (understaffed) the floor, wing, or unit might be. ... They are indeed the most important yet the most vulnerable group in the nursing home drama. (Oliver & Tureman, 1988, p. 70)

It is not surprising that turnover rates for nurses' aides are the highest, and the lack of continuity of care can lead to poor quality (Castle, Engberg, & Men, 2007).

Mealtime can occupy up to 6 hours each day because of preparation, transportation to the cafeteria, and return to rooms. Baths, activities, and visitors often fill the remaining time. In all the hustle and bustle, and in the midst of all the stress, the frontline employees find time to establish a great rapport with those for whom they provide care. Clearly, the greatest satisfaction in nursing home care occurs in exchanges and relationships between residents and staff, and this is most pronounced for those who bathe, feed, share stories, and care for them on a daily basis. Nursing home culture promotes the acceptance of residents as they are and this is reinforced with these intimate and rewarding relationships.

CHALLENGES FACING INTERVENTION RESEARCHERS

As is the case with all intervention research, the setting and environment present challenges as well as opportunities. Long-term care, especially the nursing home setting, has unique challenges that arise from its culture as well. These challenges need to be understood, as they will impact the design and implementation of any intervention research agenda.

A study by Mentes and Tripp-Reimer (2002) divided issues in long-term care research into three categories. The first involves resident issues, focused primarily on their frailty, and low motivation to change and to participate in research. This is particularly challenging in light of the number of residents with impaired cognition or Alzheimer's and related dementia disorders (Jenkins, Smythe, Galant-Miecznikowska, Bentham, & Oyebode, 2016; Snyder et al., 2001). The second involves staff issues related to high turnover, high demand on time, and an inadequate number of staff. Finally, organizational issues related to the external inspections and other outside evaluations of quality are notable.

One of the most important considerations in nursing home intervention research is the unstable environment because of both resident and employee turnover. Data collection of multiple repeated measures for a prolonged time is required and, usually, the assistance of staff for both the intervention and data collection is a must. High turnover of residents and staff makes data collection problematic. This instability creates numerous challenges, including threats to both internal and external validity, which can have negative consequences (Buckwalter et al., 2009). Internal validity refers to the degree to which outcomes can be attributed to the intervention rather than other variables. External validity refers to the degree to which the results can be generalized. The concern in long-term care settings is that the culture itself creates instability in which extraneous events impact interventions, which then create alternative explanations for outcomes and limit the generalization of results to other settings. Specific threats to validity come with the high turnover rates of staff and management, the workforce issues created by diverse and changing staffing structures, the stability and quality of data sources (including the physical decline of participants), the varied organizational mission and structures, changes in ownership, and, finally, changes in legislative mandates (Buckwalter et al., 2009).

In addition to the instability, the culture has the additional impact that must be considered. The long lengths of time residents are in a facility can be beneficial for longitudinal data collection, but it can also present challenges. Residents develop close relationships with staff and, believing they know the residents' needs and abilities, staff may tend to make judgments about residents' capabilities. This may be in direct conflict with the change the intervention is designed to accomplish. As a result, staff can become protective and even angry, thus blocking the success of the intervention and derailing enrollment and participation (Phillips & Van Ort, 1995).

Another factor involves the power dynamics within the organization. Tremendous turnover in the organization, at all levels, results in the emergence of an informal power structure.

Longevity reins and the power of persuasion of a few individual staff members overshadows whatever formal power structure is outlined. The resulting conflict has the potential of creating problems for research when the intervention is supported by the formal structure but not by the persuasive players, or vice versa (Phillips & Van Ort, 1995).

Finally, there are ethical issues unique to nursing homes. Frail and vulnerable subjects, often with cognitive impairment and loss of physical function, have lost a tremendous amount of control in their environment. In addition, rules, routines, and policies abound in this setting and can result in a lack of resident decision making and choice. Furthermore, the lack of social support by an absent family can hinder resident autonomy. Thus, ethical issues facing intervention research in these settings include equity, informed consent, special protections, confidentiality, and resident rights (Maas, Kelley, Park, & Specht, 2002).

STRATEGIES FOR SUCCESSFUL INTERVENTION RESEARCH

Numerous researchers have published their secrets for success in the long-term care setting. These suggestions are summarized in Exhibit 18.2 and present an important opportunity for new researchers entering these environments. It has been shown that with effort and planning, the challenges can be minimized early in the design and implementation process.

Choosing the most appropriate facility for the study is a key success strategy. Every nursing home is unique; thus, selecting homes with the least "field noise" is important (Phillips & Van Ort, 1995). Exhibit 18.1 provides an outline for the assessment of nursing homes for intervention research. Asking critical questions and conducting homework on individual settings before finalizing an intervention plan will help reduce noise and threats to internal and external validity.

EXHIBIT 18.1 Elements for Environmental Assessment of Nursing Homes for Intervention Research

---

Create a spreadsheet for comparison of every facility under consideration in your study. Assess the following elements related to each facility. Consider the elements in terms of those that are unlikely to change during the course of the study, those that are likely to change, and changes that if they occurred could mean study failure (Buckwalter et al., 2009).

1. Assess the quality of care for any important variables using government reports on www.medicare.gov/NHCompare
2. Assess the ownership and mission of home (for profit, not for profit, private, chain, etc.).
3. Calculate the bed size of the home (potential sample size).
4. Calculate the length of time administrator and director of nurses have been in their positions in the nursing home.
5. Does the home have a quality improvement process they can articulate?
6. Calculate turnover rates in the home.
7. Are there any new changes planned or recently implemented in the home impacting the workforce or workflow?
8. Are there recent or planned changes in ownership?
9. Assess the status of home with compliance surveys. When is a survey expected? What were the recent survey results? Is there unusual pressure for plans of correction?
10. Identify potential legislative or policy changes that might influence the study.

Source: From Buckwalter, K. C., Grey, M., Bowers, B., McCarthy, A. M., Gross, D., Funk, M., & Beck, C. (2009). Intervention research in highly unstable environments. *Research in Nursing & Health, 32*(1), 110–121. doi:10.1002/nur.20309

EXHIBIT 18.2 Strategies for Facilitating Success in Nursing Home Intervention Research

---

1. Before selecting a site for research, complete a careful assessment of the nursing home environment under consideration and decide the cost–benefit of choosing an ideal facility for the intervention versus the ability to generalize results.
2. Design a pilot study for the intervention.
3. Create noncoercive incentives for recognition and appreciation of all stakeholders who support or are directly involved in the research.
4. Decide on the requisite characteristics of the research staff that will help them establish rapport and comfortable relationships with the nursing home staff, and outline training and orientation to include these aspects.
5. Consider the special needs and opportunities for residents with cognitive impairment.
6. Outline and plan for ethical dilemmas that may arise.
7. Obtain a written letter of support from administration. This is useful for many things, including education of any new administrators if the consenting one leaves.
8. Identify key informal leaders among the staff by assessing the tenure of employees. Ask who has been there the longest and who has the most influence; be sure they are included.
9. Communicate with key stakeholders so they have a clear overall understanding of the intervention and keep them informed on the progress of the research.
10. Build opportunities to facilitate relationships, both social and political, between research staff and nursing home staff.

A summary of success strategies is presented in Exhibit 18.2. The value of pilot testing an intervention in this setting cannot be overstated. Even a small-scale pilot study will allow the testing of feasibility, the pretesting of instruments, and refinement of an experience-based intervention protocol, including the recruitment strategy. Experience from a pilot study can help the researcher finalize the elements to include in a prestudy assessment. Finally, this experience can provide the orientation necessary for the research team in a larger study.

Given the shortage of staff and high turnover in these environments, the recognition of staff time and effort for the intervention is important. Noncoercive compensation can provide an opportunity to compensate for the time involved, show recognition and appreciation for the support, and build valuable bridges between subjects and researchers. Even if the "subject" in the intervention is a resident, the efforts and support of nursing home staff should not be overlooked. Compensation does not necessarily have to be monetary; in fact, it often is not. Continuing education credit, lottery drawings, gift certificates, prizes, and educational materials are all appropriate (Buckwalter et al., 2009).

Mentes and Tripp-Reimer (2002) suggest several important strategies for the training of the research team. Good team and nursing home staff relationships are critical. Attention to the selection, training, and support given to the research team is very important. Role-playing can be a valuable way to prepare researchers for interactions with the facility staff as well as the recruitment of residents. Allowing prestudy time for the research team to get acquainted and understand the culture of the home and become familiar with routines and policies can be very helpful. It will assist them to establish an identity within the home and build relationships that will be invaluable in data collection and continuing support for the study. In addition, the research team needs to spend extra effort to assure that staff and administration understand what the research is about, what will be required for success, and how they benefit. Prestudy meetings and allowing as much decision making as possible by the facility administration and staff will prove to be a valuable investment (Maas et al., 2002).

Snyder and colleagues offer some advice on working with cognitively impaired residents who have Alzheimer's disease or related dementia. They hold that investigators should not avoid persons with cognitive challenges, but rather embrace and plan for them. Weekly team meetings, regular communication between investigators, regular communication with the nursing staff, and a willingness to solve problems that arise are all necessary when intervention research involves this study population (Snyder et al., 2001).

Finally, the researcher needs to prepare for ethical dilemmas that may arise during the study. Considerations regarding the protection of subjects' rights, potential witnessing of abuse or neglect, and treatment errors need to be accounted for and reported. If a researcher is reported to a regulator for providing substandard care, it will have serious negative effects on the research and potentially bring the study to a close (Maas et al., 2002).

SUMMARY

Improvements in the quality of care delivered in long-term care settings have been recognized and supported by the federal government. These improvements provide a wealth of opportunity for intervention research. Before implementing interventions in these environments, it is critical that the researcher understands the diversity of long-term care settings, the culture, the basics of financing, and the regulation of care. Special considerations are needed to face the unique challenges presented in these environments. Specific strategies are required. Through detailed assessment, planning, and flexibility, nursing homes can provide many opportunities for improving the lives of older persons and their caregivers through tested innovative interventions.

Key Points From Section 18.2 of This Chapter

- Investigators face unique ethical challenges when working with frail, vulnerable, long-term care residents, including issues related to informed consent and confidentiality, residents' rights, and the need for special protections.
- Given the shortage of staff, high turnover, and workload in these environments, recognizing staff time, effort, and support is critical.
- Believing they know the residents' needs and abilities, staff may make judgments about residents' capabilities; the personnel may significantly influence residents' study participation and follow-through.

18.3 Conducting Interventions in Public Health Settings

LaRon E. Nelson & Dianne Morrison-Beedy

> The man who moves a mountain begins by carrying away small stones. —*Confucius*

INTERVENTION RESEARCH IN LOCAL PUBLIC HEALTH DEPARTMENTS

Overview of Public Health Departments

Public health departments represent a cornerstone of the nation's health system. They are also excellent venues for accessing participants and testing interventions that can have a broad impact on the health of the community. Understanding the overall mission and functions of public health departments, including their unique challenges, will increase an investigator's ability to successfully partner with them (Zahner, 2005).

The **local health department (LHD)**, the main focus of this section, is a staple of the healthcare system, providing a broad range of health services to diverse populations. These departments generally have access to large numbers of people on the basis of their mandate to serve the general public, including populations that experience barriers that oftentimes limit their access to private sector healthcare.

Although many LHDs provide clinical services, their main functions are structural, that is, to facilitate and maintain community-level conditions that promote health and prevent disease (National Association of County and City Health Officials, 2005).

In general, state-level health codes and statutory provisions guide local public health policies and practices. LHDs are funded through municipal (city or county) tax bases; however, many LHDs receive funding from state and territorial departments of health to support their core functions (Erwin, Greene, Mays, Ricketts, & Davis, 2011). At times, the **U.S. Centers for Disease Control and Prevention**—the federal-level public health authority—may provide supplemental funding directly to LHDs for specific health initiatives, or indirectly via grants directly to states/territories that are then subawarded to LHDs within their jurisdictions.

Understanding the Public Health Workforce and Environments

It is important to remember that public health agencies at the local, state, and federal levels are governmental entities. As such, the employees of these agencies are usually also governmental employees, and the role of the public health workforce is to implement public health policies. The work environments of public health employees exist along a spectrum from education—motivating volitional enactment of health-promoting behaviors—to regulation, which involves compelling health-promoting behaviors through legislation (Turnock et al., 1994).

This is an important nuance to keep in mind because it is the regulatory function of health departments that is most likely to require careful negotiation between the aims of the research and the government's mandated aims to protect the public's health. For example, when conducting sexually transmitted disease prevention research with patients, many health departments will require that the positive results be reported and that a public health investigation be initiated to locate a person's known sexual partners, so that the partners can be screened and treated. Thus, one may consider whether certain intervention research outcome measures may put participants at risk for this type of disease investigation.

Public Health Departments' Perspectives on Intervention Research

Public health has a long history of collaborative research, and LHDs tend to be especially interested in community-based research projects (Grimes, Courtney, & Vindekilde, 2001; Landry, Lee, & Greenwald, 2009) or projects with a potential for positive community-level impact versus those that will yield primarily individual-level impacts (Broderick, Dodd-Butera, & Wahl, 2002; el-Askari et al., 1998). Although there is a long history of public health–academic research collaboration that has yielded many evidence-based interventions, in the current era of dwindling resources, LHDs are under increased pressure to demonstrate impact of interventions on population-level outcomes. In recent times, LHD interest has shifted to a greater focus on understanding how to improve the use of evidence-based interventions among individuals and organizations within their communities to achieve population-level impacts in various health domains (Lobb & Colditz, 2013; Proctor, 2004; Proctor & Rosen, 2008). Research that focuses on either investigating the real-world effectiveness of interventions or the processes to improve intervention uptake will be increasingly viewed as more congruent with public health imperatives to demonstrate impact, rather than studies that focus only on establishing intervention efficacy. There is also an emerging scientific literature on hybrid trials which aims to integrate questions of intervention effectiveness and implementation within one study design (Curran, Bauer, Mittman, Pyne, & Stetler, 2012; Simmons et al., 2017). In the current environment and into the future, LHDs are likely to favor intervention research collaborations that can help them advance science while also being responsive to political pressure to the impact of interventions on the larger population level.

Research Relevance to Public Health Practice

As mentioned earlier, LHDs are typically funded with public (taxpayer) dollars. Thus, whereas public health leaders and workers will be interested in novel and innovative studies, those with the most immediate relevance to public health practice will have the greatest chance of resulting in a public health research partnership. Leaders in public health must be able to provide clear and sound justification for the importance of the project and how it will help advance the mission of the LHD. Unlike hospitals and, to some degree, community health centers, LHDs are accountable to the general public usually via an elected body of representatives such as city council or county legislature. Even if you are not familiar with the practice of public health, your willingness to learn how your research agenda can be complementary to public health practice will usually be appreciated and will likely facilitate a willingness among the public health staff to work with you on ways to make your project "fit."

Developing a Study With a Local Public Health Department

There is usually a clear chain of command within the LHD, and decisions about whether to embrace your research will likely have to receive approval by the director or deputy director of the department. When trying to get your ideas accepted by an LHD, a good approach is to always start with someone on the inside of the organization. This person can serve as an "ambassador" to champion your proposal within his or her division. The insider is also an important liaison who will help you understand how to balance your research interests/agenda with the interests/agenda of the LHD.

The investigator must remember the importance of being proactive. The staff at LHDs are generally keen to engage in research that they believe will help the communities and clients whom they serve. Start with a phone call directly to the division where you believe your research has the most relevance (e.g., maternal/child health, communicable disease, health education). In some cases, you will be able to talk with a division manager or supervisor on your first call, but in most cases you will need to schedule an appointment for a telephone or a face-to-face meeting. Face-to-face meetings allow you to use your full character and personality resources to convey your message to the LHD division manager or supervisor. Also, given his or her heavy workload, phone calls increase the likelihood that the manager/supervisor will be multitasking during your conversation, in which case full attention may not be given to you and/or understanding your proposal for a research partnership; however, if you have a time-sensitive need for the meeting, then you may want to opt for a telephone meeting.

Although the LHD manager/supervisor will have expertise on his or her own field of work, he or she may not be familiar with your program of research or the methods you use to explore your questions of interest. Thus, it will be important to provide the manager with a maximum of two articles (preferably articles on which you are the primary author) that offer background context to your current proposed study idea(s). It also is important to send these articles prior to your conversation with enough lead time for reading them. Nonetheless, be prepared to provide reprints of other articles if more information is requested about the research topic area. Please be aware that simply providing references to the manager/supervisor will usually not be helpful because LHDs often do not have broad access to research journals as in university libraries.

The Impact of Bureaucracy and Local Politics

Developing a study with LHD personnel is a very intense endeavor that involves the ongoing negotiation of agendas, interests, and positions. The first step in co-constructing a proposal is to clearly outline who is the person and organization that will be principally responsible for the research study. This decision has very important implications for the rest of the research proposal construction process. For example, research is not typically a core mission of LHDs, and, as such, it is difficult for managers, supervisors, or directors to justify diverting human or material resources away from essential public health services to contribute to and manage the development of a research proposal. This most often means that a very small number of LHD staff may be available to support the development of the proposal, which, in turn, will mean that the full development of the proposal may take longer than what may be expected at an academic institution.

The health director often does not always have the final authority with regard to submitting a research grant application. First, city or county legal departments will review the request to protect the interests of the municipality and must usually approve research grants. After legal approval, the research proposal will likely also be reviewed by someone in the office of the senior elected official to ensure that the grant submission (or award) will not have negative political ramifications. It will take time to navigate through the layers of bureaucracy; thus, you will need to budget sufficient time for these processes to occur. It is not uncommon for the approval process within county or city government to take weeks to months. Here again, ensuring that your project is clearly aligned with local health priorities may facilitate its processing.

Presenting a Funded Study to a Local Health Department

LHD staff members often learn about research studies taking place in their communities through serendipitous one-on-one conversations with the investigator or other persons involved in the study. However, this "chance encounter" is not the most efficient way to establish an academic–public health partnership; rather, a proactive approach with planned contact is needed. The major advantage to presenting a funded study to the health department is that much of the legwork has been completed without having to bear the intense political and litigation scrutiny embedded within governmental approval algorithms. The major drawback to presenting a funded study to the LHD is that there is a considerable risk that there is a mismatch between your research priorities and the priorities of the LHD. Also, it may be difficult to demonstrate "good will" if the proposal was developed, submitted, and funded without the active input from public health professionals. The LHD staff could view this as evidence that you are not genuinely interested in their public health expertise and may want only to use them to access potential subjects for your research. In general, even if you already have a funded proposal, it is important to still convey (in word and deed) that you desire and appreciate having LHD input to help shape the study protocol.

Identifying Research Opportunities
The most basic step in identifying potential research opportunities is meeting with LHD staff and learning about the work that they are doing. It is sometimes possible to arrange site visits to public health clinics or programs to observe their work. Equally, if not more, important is that public health staff understand your areas of research interest and know that they can contact you. Public health staff encounter situations daily that generate researchable questions, but often they do not have outlets to which they can funnel these questions for further exploration. By knowing how to contact you, the staff will be much more likely to keep you abreast of developments in public health, which will lead to research studies with immediate public health relevance. Many LHDs publish information regarding the local community health priorities. Although LHDs are particularly skilled at identifying population health needs, the development and implementation of interventions is an area where contributions from the academic sector can be particularly useful. Investigators should review local, regional, and state community health reports to identify current priorities. These reports will also list challenges faced by the health department in addressing population health needs. Remember, if you can position your research as addressing an identified or emerging health priority, you will have a greater chance for gaining LHD support for your study.

Potential Challenges (Anticipatory Guidance)
Academic and public health research partnerships can result in long-term research engagement to advance the health of some of the community's most **vulnerable populations** (Grimes et al., 2001; Landry et al., 2009). This can be a very rewarding experience; nonetheless, there are common challenges that you should take care to avoid. Most of these challenges, if encountered, can be resolved; however, the process of salvaging the relationship with the LHD will unnecessarily consume your scarce time and that of the LHD staff. Note that Table 18.1 lists common avoidable challenges with intervention research in LHDs, as well as guidance for avoiding most of them, and addresses the ones that you encounter.

Design Considerations
There are important issues to consider when designing a study to be conducted within LHD programs. One of the first considerations needs to be ensuring that there is equity in the logistical research burden and in the potential direct benefits for subjects participating in the research. Traditionally in intervention studies, people are assigned to conditions without attention given to the degree of need for the intervention. In public health settings, you will need to give attention to assessing the degree of need exhibited by potential research subjects and the amount of burden that will have to be assumed by some participants (given their

TABLE 18.1 Common Challenges to Avoid and Anticipatory Guidance

AVOIDABLE CHALLENGES	ANTICIPATORY GUIDANCE
Mismatch between research and public health priorities	■ Easiest challenge to avoid. Reports listing the current local public health priorities are usually posted online via the LHD website. ■ Ensure that your research ideas are clearly linked to current public health priorities and that you can articulate what the links are.
Failure to identify an LHD ambassador who can champion your research	■ Exhibit cultural sensitivity. Unless you have worked in a local public health system, it is possible that you will not be able to fully appreciate its culture or its internal dynamics and processes. ■ An ambassador can introduce you and your research to her or his division and help you establish trust and credibility among staff.
Poor display of appreciation for public health mission/goals	■ Be patient. Remember, public health workers have regular job responsibilities outside of your particular research project. ■ View things from the LHD perspective. Staff often have very defined scopes of work and are trying their best to balance your research with their mandate to provide services core to the public's interest.
Unwillingness to compromise between the academic and public health interests	■ Be clear. Public health departments are not laboratories. ■ You cannot do clinical research in public health settings without LHD support. Keep them on your side. ■ Find common ground. What is in the best interest of the community is not necessarily what will be in the best interest of your research.

LHD, local health department.

circumstances) that will not have to be assumed by other participants. The orientation toward fairness for marginalized and/or highest risk (highest need) groups is a reflection of public health's mission to improve the overall health status of populations, which is best achieved through improving the health status of subgroups within populations that have the poorest outcomes. Another important consideration is the inclusion of LHD staff and leadership in the collaborative design of the study. The researcher is likely to have expertise in intervention design; however, the LHD personnel will have expertise in the daily realities of working with the individuals, programs, and systems that will be involved in the study. A collaborative codesign approach will help minimize the risk of mismatch between the intervention itself, evaluation strategy and the LHD structure, operations and programmatic priorities. One final consideration relates to the feasibility of randomization. Although it is still possible to conduct randomized trials within LHD settings, it is unlikely that you will be able to assign LHD program participants to a placebo-controlled condition. The control condition will likely need to be the standard of care, whereas the experimental condition will be the proposed new or enhanced public health program.

Implementation

Unlike private practice, hospital, or community health settings, there are legislative statutes that actually direct the activities of the LHD department and its employees. One of the most important considerations to keep in mind is that LHD operations are almost entirely funded by taxpayers' dollars. Thus, projects that are considered low risk from a medical or ethical standpoint may be high risk from a political standpoint. For example, sexual risk reduction research for the prevention of pregnancy, HIV, and other sexually transmitted infections can be controversial regardless of the extensiveness of the evidence base to support the research. If there has not been sufficient relationship and support building within the health department and municipal (city or county) leadership structure, your research project could be vulnerable to political undermining, and city/county officials could be pressured to reduce or eliminate any direct or in-kind, taxpayer-funded resources that are being used to support your project. This all is largely avoided when careful attention has been given to understanding the match between your research and the local public health priorities and securing buy-in from leadership at the LHD.

Whereas core public health programs are funded via taxpayer-backed budgets, some programs are funded by grants from state and federal governmental agencies as well as private foundations, donors, or grantors. Grant-funded programs within LHDs are usually time limited, although renewals are usually successful as long as satisfactory performance in the previous grant period is documented. Nonetheless, there are times when grant funder priorities shift or resources diminish, which can lead to cuts or elimination of programs. If the program where your research is being conducted is not considered essential to the protection of the public's health, it is possible for it to be eliminated within any upcoming budget cycle. The risk of essential LHD programs being eliminated is very low. Hence, it is important to know the source of funding for the LHD program with which you want to partner to conduct your research. Moreover, find out for how many years they have received the funding. New programs with short histories of success are most vulnerable (Smith, Gunzenhauser, & Fielding, 2010).

The final implementation issue surrounds the use of human resources. Many public health departments operate under civil service systems, with extensive rules related to the use of governmental employees including public health department staff. These rules govern such things as pay ranges, pay raises, and promotions by persons occupying civil service job titles. When developing your grant proposal, you should be very deliberate about how you will use civil servants and what it will cost, and ensure that you budget accordingly. Also, make sure you understand if and which staff persons within the public health program are allowed to perform the activities that you need for your research. Civil service rules do not usually allow staff to work outside of their roles. It is possible for staff persons to temporarily assume roles outside of their function if your research grant assumes the costs for those roles. Sometimes, hiring staff outside of the local municipal system to perform the research functions within the public health setting can avoid the complexities of navigating civil service rules. One strategy for addressing the issue of resources is to include a cost-related component to the study. An LHD will be interested in studies of costs because it will provide evidence that will inform projections regarding the long-term sustainability of the intervention. Factors such as the amount of time it takes to deliver an intervention, the educational level of the person needed to deliver the intervention, space requirements, and intensity of follow-up will all have implications on the amount of resources needed to sustain an intervention program (Antonelli, Stille, & Antonelli, 2008; Proctor, Silmere, Raghavan, Hovman, & Aarons, 2011). Giving attention to studying aspects of the costs associated with your intervention is an important way to demonstrate to your public health officials that you are sensitive to the needs to be good stewards of limited public resources, human and financial—which can sometimes mean the difference between an LHD accepting or rejecting a research partnership opportunity.

Building Successful Research Partnerships With Public Health Departments

Public health research influences the health of the most vulnerable residents in our society and has a broad population reach. Despite the numerous words of caution, research in public health settings can be some of the most rewarding and most impactful that you can conduct. In closing, there are several important "tips for success" (Table 18.2) to keep in mind when developing your program of research with LHDs.

TABLE 18.2 Tips for Success	
TIPS FOR SUCCESS	**ANTICIPATORY GUIDANCE**
Know the local situation	■ LHDs are most concerned with what is happening in their jurisdictions. ■ Do your homework. If you do not know the local epidemiological situation, you are not prepared. Know what they are and acknowledge their importance.
Invest in relationship building	■ If all else falls apart, you will want to have a strong relationship. ■ Out of sight is out of mind. Be careful to maintain communications. ■ There are countless other ways that you can contribute. ■ Always ask what you can do to help. ■ Commit to do something that is meaningful to them and reasonable for you, and that you can accomplish on time.
No time for puzzles	■ Do not expect LHD staff or leaders to find the connection between your research and their priorities (because they will not). ■ Connect the "dots" for them. Make the links clear and visible.
Ask, don't tell	■ Ask them for their input and be open to different ways of knowing what the LHD staff will bring. ■ Make sure their contributions to the research are visible.

LHD, local health department.

Know the Local Situation

It is important to know the state and national epidemiology, but LHDs will be most concerned with what is happening in the local population. Ensure that you have a clear picture of the local distribution and impact of the target health issue. Also, obtain copies of the most recent health report to learn the local public health priorities. Even if your research does not match one of the published priorities, it is still beneficial to describe your research in the context of those priorities.

Invest in Relationship Building

When agreements fail and subcontracts are delayed, the only thing that will keep your research project alive will be the relationship that you have built with the LHD. Maintain regular contact with your LHD partners before, during, and between projects. Participating in the local public health task force or providing a research conference update at a staff meeting can show your commitment to LHDs beyond their ability to provide steady streams of subjects for your studies.

No Time for Puzzles

Be clear when communicating your message. You will not get many chances to present your case for research partnership, so please be very careful to show exactly the ways that you believe your research advances their efforts to address health priorities. LHD staff are very busy and will not have time to figure out what the links are between your research and their priorities. Connect the "dots" for them.

Ask, Don't Tell

You will encounter diverse ways of knowing in public health that will be related partly to the interdisciplinary composition of public health staff and partly to the staff's development of diverse cultural understandings of the world derived from their work within communities

(VanDevanter et al., 2003). Demonstrate your appreciation for LHD expertise by eliciting and incorporating their ideas into your research and ensure that their contributions are visible (not tucked in the back).

> **Key Points From Section 18.3 of This Chapter**
>
> - The regulatory function of health departments will require careful negotiation between the aims of your research study and the government's mandated aims to protect the public's health.
> - Public health employees are civil service employees whose pay ranges, pay raises, and promotions are regulated by the government; this should be taken into account when including them as study personnel.
> - Investigators must actively work at "partnering" with public health departments particularly because it may be difficult to demonstrate "good will" if the proposal was developed, submitted, and funded without the active input from public health professionals.
> - Even after receiving internal health department approval, your research proposal will likely be reviewed by someone in the office of a senior elected official to ensure that the grant submission (or award) will not have negative political ramifications.

18.4 Conducting Interventions in School Settings

Bonnie Gance-Cleveland

Research in the school setting is a complicated but fruitful endeavor. Because children aged 5 to 18 years spend most of their days in the school setting, it is a rich source of opportunity to intervene with children. This includes vulnerable groups such as impoverished children who might not be as easily accessible in other settings. In 2015, one in five children (21%) in the United States lived in poverty. Fifteen million children lived in poverty, resulting in associated health risks (The Annie E. Casey Foundation, 2015). Research exploring the relationship between poverty and health outcomes can be enhanced by conducting well-designed studies in the school setting. The school setting also offers a unique opportunity to evaluate interventions focused on prevention or community-based health conditions such as asthma, obesity, teen pregnancy, decreasing risky sexual behaviors, substance abuse including smoking, and accidents.

There are challenges, however, to conducting research in the school setting. A primary challenge is that the priorities and goals of the school setting focus on education and not health per se. Researchers should keep this in mind as they develop research proposals and include educational outcomes when possible. The educational services must take priority, and schools are faced with multiple projects that compete for their limited resources. This challenge is compounded by the fact that many health programs in the schools have very limited staff, which may consist primarily of volunteers. If the school setting has staff dedicated to health programs at all, they rarely have time for research. Finally, children in the school setting are viewed as vulnerable groups. School staff are very protective of their students, and both parents and staff may be suspicious of the researcher.

Key strategies for addressing these challenges should be considered. Establishing a relationship with the school and community during the grant-planning process is paramount to interest or success. This planning process takes longer than traditional approaches to research and requires "buy-in" from administration, teachers, counselors, and school health providers. Including the community in the planning process for the grant from the beginning, with strategies such as community-based participatory research (CBPR; described in the following text), may pay off in the long run. The investigator must plan to minimize the amount of work required of staff and compensate the staff or reward them for their contribution to the study. An important strategy to facilitate success is to link the **outcomes** of your intervention research to school achievement, academic success, or attendance whenever possible. Maintaining contact with the school partners throughout the research process to sustain the trusting relationship helps to ensure the success of the project. Finally, the investigator should provide follow-up at the end of the study to share findings and information that might be useful to the school or board of education.

CBPR is a methodology designed to overcome many of the challenges common to school-based research. The fundamental elements of CBPR are that it is a collaborative approach using participatory methods focused on a colearning process with the goal of community capacity building (Minkler & Wallerstein, 2008). The aim is to empower the community to address the needs that are of concern to them while balancing between the research and action. CBPR includes the school and community in all aspects of the research process and helps to obtain their commitment during the planning, implementation, and evaluation phases of the grant. Using CBPR in the school setting, the staff are a part of the research team and are included in grant team meetings held at their site and a time convenient for them. CBPR has been shown to improve recruitment and retention of participants in the school setting (Amed et al., 2015) because of the ongoing relationship that staff have with the students and parents.

Additional strategies to consider during enrollment include sensitivity to timing your approach to consent. Do not overwhelm the potential participant with information; instead, break the information into manageable pieces and highlight the major requirements for participation and screen for inclusion and exclusion criteria. Technology can be used to facilitate the enrollment process, including use of computerized screening, texting, or cellular phones to contact potential participants.

Working with participants in the schools presents additional logistics that should be considered. Additional challenges in recruiting school-aged children and adolescents include employment, after-school activities, transportation issues for students who take the bus, and unstable home environments that may prohibit participation by some high-risk students. A strategy for obtaining parental **informed consent** and participant **assent** will be required. Parents are not readily available at the school sight for obtaining consent. Strategies to consider are **passive consent**, sending consents home with children, and recruitment at school events such as school enrollment, parent–teacher conferences, school programs, or back-to-school night. It is important to work with your institutional review board (IRB) as well on the consent/assent approaches to garner their support.

Once recruitment has occurred, steps should be taken to minimize attrition. Maintaining a consistent contact person, preferably from the school with a similar ethnic background, is essential. Regular contact should be maintained by sending cards, text messages, or calling to remind children of appointments and for special occasions such as birthdays and holidays. Monetary incentives can be considered, but many IRBs consider cash for high-risk populations as putting the youth at risk. Gift cards are considered a better approach, providing an amount that compensates for their time but does not appear to be coercive. Maintaining long-term contact for high-risk populations can be facilitated by providing incentives for participants for notifying the study personnel of change of address. This process can be best achieved by maintaining a close relationship with school personnel. Access to school records requires special permission from parents and is governed by the Family Educational Rights and Privacy Act (FERPA) in addition to research regulations. FERPA is a federal law that protects the privacy of student educational records. The law applies to all schools that receive funds under an applicable program of the U.S. Department of Education. FERPA gives parents certain rights with respect to their children's educational records. These rights transfer to the student when he or she reaches the age of 18 or attends a school beyond the high school level.

School-based health centers (SBHCs) are also a rich source of data for intervention studies focused on health. The 2013 to 2014 census indicated there were 2,315 SBHCs in the United States serving preschool, elementary, middle, and high school–aged children in 49 of 50 states and the District of Columbia (School-Based Health Alliance, 2014). Most of the centers serve poor, underserved, and diverse populations and provide a rich source of data on these populations. Most recent data indicate that students in a school with an SBHC are predominantly members of minority and ethnic populations who have historically been underinsured, uninsured, or have experienced other health disparities. A survey conducted in the 2013 to 2014 school year indicated that 78% of the centers served a Title I school and nearly half of the centers reported that 76% to 100% of the students were eligible for free/reduced lunch. The ethnic profile of schools with an SBHC was 30.6% Hispanics, 31.7% Whites, 25.7% Blacks, 3.9% Asian/Pacific Islanders, 1.9% Native Americans, and 3% two or more races (School-Based Health Alliance, 2014).

A systematic review of school-based sexual health and relationship educational interventions reported that comprehensive interventions and those in school-based clinics were found to be effective in improving knowledge and changing attitudes, behaviors, and health-related outcomes (Denford, Abraham, Campbell, & Busse, 2017).

Although SBHCs are a rich source of data on an ethnically diverse, disadvantaged population, additional challenges may be involved in research with SBHCs. The health centers are frequently owned and operated by an entity other than the school, with only 12% sponsored by a school system (School-Based Health Alliance, 2014). SBHCs may be affiliated with local health departments or hospitals, universities, health maintenance organizations, or public or private health centers. Research conducted in these settings may require multiple layers of approval, and the research team should take this into consideration for planning their timeline.

EXEMPLARS

Collaborating With Community

An example of the CBPR method to collaborate with parents, teachers, coaches, school administrators, and middle school children is evident in the evaluation of a school-based obesity prevention program conducted in Arkansas. The Arkansas legislature passed Act 1220 in 2003 that created a Child Health Advisory Committee to coordinate statewide efforts to combat childhood obesity and related conditions to improve the health of the next generation of Arkansans. Act 1220 also mandated that Arkansas public school students must have an annual body mass index (BMI) assessment performed and reported to parents. The Act also required that the schools reduce elementary school students' access to food and beverage vending machines, report the monies received through food and beverage contracts, and convene a local advisory committee to incorporate physical activity and nutritional goals into the annual school plan. In order to meet these new legislative requirements, schools reached out to the school nurses across the state, including those at the school of nursing at a local university, and the CBPR collaboration evolved.

Faculty and student nurses collaborated with the school nurse to obtain the BMI measurements and to develop a plan to implement an obesity prevention curriculum for gym/health class. The prevention program consisted of nutritional education, exercise instruction, a physical activity component, and behavioral change strategies. Passive consent was attempted to obtain evaluation of the initial curriculum with low enrollment ($n = 78$; 26%). After pilot testing the curriculum with this small sample, a move to the CBPR method was made and focus groups were conducted with parents, teachers, coaches, and the middle school-aged children who had participated in the pilot classes to gather their feedback. Changes were made to adapt the curriculum to make it more culturally appropriate. After adapting the curriculum on the basis of community feedback, active consent was obtained at school registration with the research team sitting at the school nurses' table and answering questions about the study and obtaining consent. Recruitment dramatically improved with 226 students (87%) and parents providing assent/consent and the CBPR approach improved retention from 81% in Year 1 to 95% in Year 2. Results of the intervention indicated significant improvement in students' reports of healthy eating ($p < .0001$), family support for healthy eating ($p = .0044$), family discouragement for unhealthy behavior ($p = .0005$), peer encouragement for healthy eating ($p = .0001$), family participation in physical activity ($p = .0104$), and peer participation in physical activity ($p = .0016$), but there were no changes in physical activity or BMI (Wardbegnoche et al., 2009).

Comparative Effectiveness Trial in 24 School-Based Health Centers

A multisite trial with 24 SBHCs in six states was possible because of relationships with national organizations that promote school-based health including the School-Based Health Alliance, the National Association of Pediatric Nurse Practitioners, and SBHCs special interest group (Gance-Cleveland, Dandreaux, Aldrich, & Kamal, 2015). This comparative effectiveness trial evaluated outcomes of SBHC providers' participation in a virtual collaborative with web-based training on obesity with and without HeartSmartKids™ (HSK) decision-support technology. The providers reported high satisfaction with the web-based training and intention to change practice on the basis of participation in the virtual collaborative (Gance-Cleveland, Aldrich, Dandreaux, Otzel, & Schmiege, 2015). Chart audits reported significant improvement for both groups after training in documentation of BMI percentile (HSK 77.5%–98.6%, non-HSK 71.3%–91.5%; $p = .01$) and for blood pressure (BP) percentile (HSK 37%–56.7%, non-HSK 21.3%–32%; $p = .015$). The HSK group improved motivational interviewing (MI) counseling on diet (HSK 6.3–6.5, non-HSK 6.0–5.26; $p = .04$) compared with training alone (Gance-Cleveland, Aldrich, Schmiege, & Tyler, 2016).

SUMMARY

The school setting is an ideal place to conduct intervention studies that focus on community-based health problems of youth. With careful planning, successful research can be conducted, obtaining rich data from youth that might not be available in other settings. Capitalizing on the strengths of community-based participatory methods within the educational system increases the likelihood of successful intervention research in school-based settings.

Key Points From Section 18.4 of This Chapter

- Research conducted in the school setting provides a rich source of data on diverse populations of children.
- Schools are the ideal setting for prevention and community-based intervention studies.
- Research in the schools is complex and requires careful planning and buy-in from the school partners to navigate the multiple layers of permission.

18.5 Conducting Interventions in Palliative Care Settings

Kathryn B. Lindstrom

Palliative and **hospice** care are a national research priority led by the National Institute of Nursing Research (NINR) at the National Institutes of Health (NIH; NINR, 2011). The WHO describes palliative care as an interdisciplinary team approach that improves the quality of life of individuals and their families facing the problems associated with chronic disease and life-threatening illness through the prevention and relief of suffering by means of early identification and treatment of physical, psychosocial, and spiritual issues (WHO, 2002). Although patients and families receiving palliative care/symptom management are not necessarily in the last 6 months of life, palliative care research more often focuses on patients with incurable diseases and a limited prognosis (Whalen et al., 2007). Hospice, on the other hand, is an interdisciplinary team focusing on palliative care (symptom management) targeted for individuals in the last 6 months of life and their families (Fine & Davis, 2006).

Hudson, Zordan, and Trauer (2011) surveyed members of an International Palliative Care Family Carer Research Collaboration and found that research priorities in palliative care included (a) intervention development and testing, (b) underresearched caregiver groups, (c) access to services, (d) unmet needs, (e) bereavement, (f) experience and implications of the caregiver role, and (g) development of assessment tools. Unfortunately, there is a paucity of interventions for patients receiving palliative care and hospice services or their families because of complex methodological challenges related to this population. Complicating the development of interventions, researchers suggest that no single intervention will help all patients and families in palliative and hospice care (Hebert & Schulz, 2006; King & Quill, 2006). In addition, when recruitment strategies fail to recruit an adequate sample size, outcomes are affected as is the validity of the overall study (Williams, 2007). It is important to understand the challenges in end-of-life research for studies to be designed to ensure integrity of the research and responsibility to research dollars.

This section focuses on methodological aspects that should be considered when developing interventions for patients and families receiving palliative care and hospice services. Methodological aspects covered include (a) ethical issues, (b) feasibility pilot studies and RCTs, (c) cultural aspects, (d) recruitment issues, and (e) retention strategies.

METHODOLOGICAL DESIGN ISSUES

Ethical Aspects of Palliative Care Research

Although researchers have questioned whether patients and families receiving palliative care or hospice services are considered to be too vulnerable to be part of research endeavors, multiple studies suggest that patients and family caregivers are interested in helping others who also are having similar experiences (Casarett, 2005; Murphy et al., 2007; Pessin et al., 2008; Williams, Shuster, Clay, & Burgio, 2006). Murphy and colleagues found that caregivers wanted to participate in a study because they recognized they needed help and felt they deserved to receive the help. For example, a survey asking about benefits and burdens regarding research in a dying population was delivered to 68 dying persons with cancer (Pessin et al., 2008). These individuals identified that they participated in research because they wanted to help others, receive additional attention, and be able to discuss their disease process. Overall, most reported that participating in the research was moderately to highly beneficial with very little, if any, burden associated with participating. Pessin and colleagues concluded that terminal persons who are willing to participate in research will probably benefit from participating in end-of-life research and are unlikely to experience burden. Williams and colleagues found that almost half of the hospice patients and caregivers they surveyed preferred interview, survey, and therapeutic research. Younger hospice patients were more likely to favor survey and therapeutic research than hospice patients older than 75 years. Moreover, older hospice patients were as likely to participate in research as were the ambulatory senior citizens surveyed.

Casarett (2005) identified six ethical aspects on which researchers can focus when performing research with patients and families in palliative care. First, determining whether a study is "research" or "quality improvement" holds implications for study design and ethical standards that must be addressed. Second, determining potential benefits to patients and families has both methodological and ethical implications. Generally, if a study will be deemed potentially beneficial, then taking the next steps makes sense. Moreover, if a study does not have a theoretical framework justifying the problem and resulting intervention, the interpretation of the results will be negatively impacted. Third, maximizing the potential benefits of an intervention for patients and families through rigorous methodology will be important criteria for funding purposes as well as the ethical implications that must be addressed. Fourth, minimizing risks and burden to subjects is always important in intervention work. Casarett recommends conducting research with subjects who have decision-making capacity to decrease confounding results and ethical concerns. However, this can be challenging to accomplish when patients are too critically ill or are close to death and often leads to interventions being developed primarily for the caregiver (McMillan & Weitzner, 2003; Williams, 2007). Including family can also help to decrease family objections or "gatekeeping" of a patient, especially when family members may think their relative is too ill to participate (Williams, 2007). Finally, it is important for researchers to ensure that participation is completely voluntary and that participants are able to withdraw from the study at any time without consequences for the patient or family member. In summary, attending to these issues in hospice and palliative care interventions will increase ethically sound research and reduce the risk of violating ethical principles in a potentially vulnerable population.

An additional aspect of ethical concern is the aging patient and family. Palliative care and hospice patients are often older and, therefore, attention to how aging affects intervention design and implementation is necessary for human subjects' protection and optimal outcomes. As people age, researchers must be familiar with common aging issues such as changes in hearing or vision, fatigue, mobility, and cognition (McNeely & Clements, 1994). Adaptations to study protocols may be required to accommodate elders and increase the likelihood of recruiting this population. Furthermore, McNeely and Clements found that giving clear and simple explanations is important for human subjects' protection and may improve recruitment efforts. Studies with older people have also suggested that avoiding the word "research" can be beneficial when approaching older adults (Carter, Elward, Malmgren, Martin, & Larson, 1991). Instead, use of words such as "study" or "project" may counter any immediate negative perceptions.

Feasibility Studies and Randomized Control Studies

The development of palliative care and hospice research is relatively new and, as a result, few intervention studies exist (Lindstrom & Melnyk, 2009). Feasibility pilot studies are necessary as a precursor to RCTs to determine whether the research hypothesis is appropriate and whether it is feasible to conduct the study in the setting and population (Bowen et al., 2009;

Bruera, Willey, Cohen, & Palmer, 2008; Whalen et al., 2007). For example, although expressive writing has been shown to be effective in young and healthy persons, Bruera and colleagues found that it was not feasible in the palliative care population they studied and suggested that major methodological changes would need to be made before any further studies.

Feasibility studies also address whether a study can be designed to answer a specific problem related to the care of dying persons among the multitude of potential intervention needs (Whalen et al., 2007). Besides determining which populations should be included in the study, which multisites are appropriate to include, and which agencies to apply for funding, Whalen and colleagues found that selecting a primary end point for a RCT in a palliative care population was a challenge for their research team to determine. They suggested that methodological aspects of the study be addressed early in the design phase and that evaluation of methodological issues continue throughout the entire study.

Cultural Aspects

The lack of cultural diversity in palliative and hospice research affects numerous aspects of the study, including generalizability of the research. Hospice patients are predominantly White/Caucasian, compounding the problem of recruiting diverse racial and ethnic groups into studies (National Hospice and Palliative Care Organization [NHPCO], 2010). Although the REACH study was successfully conducted with patients who had dementia and cancer and with their caregivers, few palliative care and hospice studies include cultures other than the White/Caucasian population (Lindstrom & Melnyk, 2009). Recruitment methods as well as intervention components need to be culturally sensitive and purposeful to facilitate inclusion of diverse participants (Coon et al., 2004; Nichols et al., 2004).

Social marketing is a recruitment strategy that has been shown to assist researchers in developing interventions so they will be well received among community participants (Nichols, Malone, Tarlow, & Loewenstein, 2000; Nichols et al., 2004). This technique assists researchers in meshing the intervention with a community culture and to get "buy-in" from the community. These and other authors suggest collaborating to assess community attitudes, beliefs, behaviors, and ideology before beginning intervention development when previous descriptive research is lacking (Moreno-John et al., 2004). One technique is to present the study to key leaders in the community as well as professional leaders prior to the start of enrollment and continue public awareness strategies throughout the length of the study (Tarlow & Mahoney, 2000). This technique can help to provide the study with credibility and has been shown to increase rates of recruitment. Ultimately, the success of recruiting participants depends on the principal investigator's ability to build community partnerships (Eaves, 1999). Focus groups have also been successfully used to effectively develop appropriate and applicable components of interventions when descriptive research is scarce (Gagnon et al., 2002).

On the other hand, researchers suggest that no one type of intervention will be appropriate to everyone (Crawley 2005; King & Quill, 2006); thus, the need to tailor interventions is imperative. Theoretical frameworks help to guide intervention development by identifying key constructs influencing the intervention outcome. Prior to hospice services, the predominant theoretical framework used for family caregiver interventions was the stress and coping framework for psychoeducation and skills training interventions (Coon, Gallagher-Thompson, & Thompson, 2003; Gallagher-Thompson et al., 2003; Hebert, Prigerson, Schulz, & Arnold, 2006; Sörensen, Pinquart, & Duberstein, 2002). These studies often focused on the long trajectory of caring for a person with dementia and cancer. However, this framework may not effectively address the new and unexpected experience of family caregivers of a dying family member and researchers may need to think beyond traditional frameworks (Lindström, 2010). The impact of location of an intervention is important to consider, as palliative care and hospice settings present unique challenges.

Recruitment

Recruiting caregivers of palliative care and hospice patients and their caregivers can be challenging (McMillan & Weitzner, 2003). Poor recruitment of subjects can seriously impact components of a study, such as sample size, and therefore challenge research findings (Gallagher-Thompson et al., 2004). One of the major costs in research studies is associated with the recruitment of subjects, especially diverse groups (Patrick, Pruchno, & Rose, 1998; Tarlow & Mahoney, 2000). However, few researchers report the time and cost of recruitment nor do they report the processes of recruitment (e.g., How many participants were approached? Why they participated or why they didn't? Why they stayed in the study or why they dropped out? [McMillan & Weitzner, 2003]). McMillan and Weitzner (2003) point out that unless researchers report these details, researchers will be challenged to know how much time and money are needed to fund recruitment efforts.

Lingler et al. (2009) also suggested that researchers devise methods to evaluate recruitment processes to inform future research studies. They found that recruitment depended on the personnel at the site, flexibility in maintaining communication with the project director, study participants, and research assistants, and identification of a contact person at each site. Another issue in recruitment strategies is timing of recruitment. Lindström (2010) found that recruitment during the holiday season was unsuccessful in the hospice caregiver population. She suggested doing training and retraining during the fall season and conducting recruitment for caregivers of hospice patients and implementing the intervention between mid-January and early November. Sherman et al. (2005) tried ongoing recruitment strategies with palliative care patient–caregiver dyads to decrease attrition rates. However, high attrition rates were experienced because patients and family caregivers reported high levels of stress and/or the patient's illness was causing inability to participate. Recruitment can be impacted by change in patient–family relationships; family caregivers who must leave a dying loved one in an agency are less apt to participate in a study. Northouse et al. (2006) found that recruitment and retention patterns in patients and caregiver dyads differed by research site, recruitment strategies, and phase of the patient's cancer and caregiver dyads where recruitment took much longer than expected.

Kavanaugh, Moro, Savage, and Mehendale (2006) used a theory of caring as an innovative framework to recruit and retain vulnerable participants into a study. This theory was also used as a framework for developing their recruitment methods. Casarett, Kassner, and Kutner (2004) found that including screening questions about research into the hospice intake process was successful in identifying hospice patients who were willing to participate in research.

Retention Strategies

Inclusion and exclusion criteria for study participants are important for increasing the homogeneity of a sample, being able to compare subjects before and after an intervention, and decreasing attrition rates (Kazdin, 2003; Lindstrom & Melnyk, 2009). The most common reason identified for participant dropout in interventions using hospice patients and caregivers was patient death (Lindstrom & Melnyk, 2009). However, although many patients at end of life have a diagnosis of cancer, most hospice patients have a diagnosis of a chronic disease process (i.e., heart failure, chronic obstructive pulmonary disease [COPD], dementia; NHPCO, 2010). The impact of these health conditions on the ability to participate in a research study also represents a major threat to retention. Patients may also participate in the intervention or data collection sporadically because of symptoms related to these chronic conditions; this intermittent "participation" will influence the intervention dose received and the ability to obtain data at all collection time points. Therefore, researchers should give thoughtful consideration to inclusion and exclusion criteria for patients and family caregivers, as well as develop detailed plans for missing data and attrition.

The issue of using incentives (e.g., gifts or money) as a way to increase retention has been a controversial topic in research, primarily because it can be viewed as a form of coercion (Moore, 1997). Some researchers suggest that writing cards to the participants as well as giving monetary incentives or small gifts during visits is an appropriate way to increase retention and decrease attrition (Given, Keilman, Collins, & Given, 1990; Moreno-John et al., 2004). Low-income and disadvantaged persons may be more likely to participate in a study when they receive financial or material incentives (Moreno-John et al., 2004). Suggesting an altruistic motive—that is, participating to help others—increased recruitment in a study of Hispanic females with breast cancer after other methods failed (Naranjo & Dirksen, 1998). Developing novel ways for participants to feel connected to the research study, such as offering a magnet with the researcher contact information, was a successful method of increasing retention (Campbell, 2007). Ensuring confidentiality and paying attention to the needs of the participants is also a crucial part to retaining them during a research study. Whether a researcher chooses to use incentives or not, careful consideration to avoid coercion in recruiting these vulnerable participants is imperative and requires thoughtful protocol development. Certainly, both grant and manuscript reviewers will expect this issue to be addressed.

SUMMARY

Interventions are critically needed for patients, family members, caregivers, and agency personnel in palliative care and hospice settings. These patients and their significant others represent an extremely vulnerable population. Because of this status, astute focus on the ethical and legal implications needs to be woven into all aspects of recruitment and intervention approaches. Understanding the impact of agency personnel, who oftentimes are proxy family members, on a patient's decision to participate and stay enrolled in research studies should not be underestimated. As researchers, we understand that study participants from palliative care and hospice settings are more than data points or disease processes. They require our utmost attention and gratitude for helping to improve the science of their care during the most challenging time in their lives.

Key Points From Section 18.5 of This Chapter

- Hospice and palliative care are not one and the same; investigators must understand how prognosis and diagnosis differ between the two and consider how those factors may impact their intervention study.
- Patients in palliative care and hospice settings represent an extremely vulnerable study population; they and their caregivers are in need of targeted scientifically rigorous interventions.
- Investigators must devise well-articulated plans for missing data, attrition, and limited intervention dosing in studies targeting this population and these settings.

18.6 Conducting Interventions in Acute Care Settings

Cindy Munro

Acute care settings provide unique opportunities and challenges for intervention research. Perhaps, most importantly, research in acute care settings enables evaluation of the effectiveness of acute care interventions in the clinical context where they will ultimately be used. Translation of research findings is enhanced because many of the barriers to clinical implementation will have been identified and addressed as part of the research process. Some research questions require recruitment of subjects who are at a particular phase of illness or treatment. The acute care setting can offer unique access to certain populations such as critically ill or perioperative subjects. However, it is important to remain aware that research in acute care settings usually takes place within the context of clinical care, and thus the likelihood of success is enhanced when researchers recognize and develop their study with this at the forefront. In the acute care setting, potential subjects are first and foremost patients, and the principal concern of healthcare providers is delivery of care to attain individual patient goals. Several authors have noted that providers' advocacy for patients can extend to behaviors that create barriers for researchers (Chlan, Guttormson, Tracy, & Bremer, 2009; De Backer & Schortgen, 2014; Glickman et al., 2008; Wiegand, Norton, & Baggs, 2008). Recruitment of subjects, delivery of interventions, and data collection can be challenging in the acute care environment. Conducting research in the acute care setting also poses issues in analysis, such as control of confounding variables.

PREPARATION FOR INTERVENTION RESEARCH IN ACUTE CARE SETTINGS

The most important stage of intervention research is designing the project. Accomplishment of the research aims depends on careful planning prior to initiation. Attention to detail and a thorough understanding of the context in which the intervention will be delivered are crucial; this is particularly true in the acute care setting. The likelihood of success is enhanced when the researcher has a clear understanding of the clinical setting where the project will be conducted. Interventions are often evaluated against "usual care" or "standard of care," which are influenced by both formal and informal clinical activities. The investigator must have knowledge of written policies, **protocols**, and standards of care, but also appreciation of the workflow, informal practices, and unit culture (including receptiveness to research and to researchers). An understanding of the broader culture of the institution and its support (or lack thereof) of research is also important (Pattison, Arulkumaran, Humphreys, & Walsh, 2017). Active engagement with the clinical providers early in project planning can identify potential difficulties or areas of tension between care and research, which can be addressed proactively. For example, adjusting the timing of a research intervention to avoid periods of intense clinical activity, such as clinical rounds or change of shift, can increase providers' cooperation with the research.

In the planning phase, estimation of the number of potential subjects available and the effect size of the intervention will inform statistical **power** determinations. Statistical power is important in assessing **feasibility** of the study. Feasibility determinations should be honest and conservative; it is important not to overestimate either the ability to enroll eligible subjects or the robustness of the intervention. **Pilot** studies are a valuable way to gauge feasibility in the acute care setting and can be used to evaluate both the availability of subjects and the effect size of the intervention.

Specific information about targeted clinical areas is necessary to evaluate the pool of potential subjects. In addition to age, gender, race, and ethnicity, severity of illness and comorbidities are important considerations in planning for recruitment in acute care intervention research. The characteristics of acute care patients often differ among institutions in the same geographical area. Racial and ethnic mix of a particular institution is influenced by factors such as patient preferences and choices, transportation patterns, and availability of specialty care. Patient acuity levels also differ among institutions and even among units in the same institution. It is important to pay particular attention to targeted recruitment of elderly and minority subjects who tend to be underrepresented in acute care research (Glickman et al., 2008; Grap & Munro, 2003; Natale et al., 2017).

Access to potential subjects should be carefully considered. Several factors may complicate access to subjects. There may be multiple research studies recruiting from the same clinical area, and equitable access to subjects (for researchers) and to research participation (for subjects) can be difficult. In some instances, participation in one research study will make subjects ineligible for some or all other research studies. There has been concern expressed about subject burden associated with being approached for multiple studies, although Randolph (2009) found that potential subjects do not share the concern. Traditionally, equitable access of researchers to potential subjects has been accomplished through institutional policy and negotiation with clinical providers. The process of negotiating for access to subjects is improved if researchers build mutual respect and seek innovative solutions that benefit all parties. Researchers may work collaboratively to design research that can address multiple objectives in the same subjects. Innovative research designs such as factorial design or adaptive design, coenrollment, and clustered RCTs are among the appropriate methodologies to accomplish this goal (Cook et al., 2008; Cook et al., 2015; François, Clavel, Vignon, & Laterre, 2016; Randolph, 2009). A large study of clinical trials recently found that coenrollment did not influence either patient safety or the results of the coenrolled trials (Cook et al., 2015).

Extrapolations for enrollment numbers from institutional census data should be very conservative in acute care intervention research. Investigators tend to overestimate potential enrollment and enrollment time frames (François et al., 2016). Enrollment efficiency in RCTs, defined as the percentage of eligible patients enrolled, is generally around 20% in acute care settings. Subjects in acute care are more likely than subjects in other settings to be lost to attrition because of worsening of condition (including death) or conversely because of clinical improvement that changes their eligibility or continued involvement in the study.

In designing intervention research, there is a temptation to use data that are already being collected for patient care as research data. This is particularly the case in acute care settings, where large amounts of clinical data are collected and may be easily (often electronically) available. Caution should be used in this approach. The validity and reliability of many **clinical measures** is often not comparable or robust enough for research purposes, and variability in measurement cannot be well controlled. Rather, investigators should select measures on the basis of an evaluation of what measures best represent the variables of interest, psychometrics, and precision. In general, where a summative score (e.g., a severity of illness score) will be used in data analysis, each component element should be recorded rather than the calculated total score. Potential errors are reduced if the scores are computed electronically after entry into the study database rather than manually at the time of data collection. Data gathered in the acute care setting can be collapsed much more easily than expanded, and monitoring of data quality is easier with component data than with summative scores alone.

Prior to initiation of the project, a fully developed and very detailed study protocol should be developed. Pilot testing is essential to developing the protocol and to ensuring that unanticipated problems associated with the acute care environment and with the specific study sites have been addressed. The protocol must demonstrate adherence to all approval requirements of the study site and be attentive to institutional regulatory requirements. Acute care settings may have specific accreditation requirements, which may impact interventional research.

Investigators must garner adequate resources for the intervention study that do not depend on uncompensated efforts of clinical staff and do not shift costs of items used only for the research (extra laboratory tests, supplies, etc.) to clinical care reimbursement. Research personnel should be responsible for all aspects of the research (recruitment and enrollment, delivery of intervention, data collection), or staff should be compensated for their involvement. Compensation may be monetary, but investigators might compensate the clinical unit for assistance with the project by offering other services to clinical colleagues, such as continuing education, assistance with literature reviews, and mentoring in publication or evidence-based practice.

ISSUES RELATED TO CONSENT

In acute care, consent issues are consistently documented as the primary reason for eligible subjects not being enrolled (Crowley et al., 2008; Grap & Munro, 2003; Sole et al., 2017; Wiegand et al., 2008). Potential subjects' ability to comprehend information about the study and give **informed consent** may be influenced by many factors, including illness severity, medications such as analgesics and sedatives, interventions, and stress related to acute illness. In the acute care setting, it may be difficult for subjects to differentiate the clinical care they receive from research interventions, and the risk of therapeutic misconception is high.

Several strategies have been used to address consent issues in acute care. First, careful assessment of decision-making capacity must be conducted and documented. Fan et al. (2008) have published a widely used two-step process to assess consent ability in critically ill adults. In some instances involving subjects whose decision-making capacity is impaired, the use of a surrogate decision maker may be permitted by the IRB. Under the U.S. federal code 45 CFR 46, state law determines who may act as a surrogate decision maker for research. This law varies significantly from state to state; some states have very specific legislation regarding surrogate consent for research, whereas others are silent on the matter. The appropriateness of surrogate consent has generated much debate in acute care research, and research regarding surrogate decision making is ongoing (Burns et al., 2013; Burns et al., 2015; Hartog, Aneman, & Ricou, 2015; McBain et al., 2016). In a randomized trial comparing surrogate decision makers' experiences with MD versus non-MD approach for consent, Burns et al. (2015) found that personality and professionalism of the consenter were more important to surrogate decision makers than the consenter's profession; 85.7% of the surrogate decision makers indicated that they would prefer that physician time be focused on clinical care. The IRB may grant a waiver of consent under specific circumstances; for example, a waiver may be granted for appropriate emergency interventions or if the research intervention involves minimal risk.

ENGAGING CLINICAL STAFF

Intervention research in acute care requires engagement with the clinical setting and providers. It is helpful to remember that the primary concern of providers is provision of clinical care to individual patients. Clinicians may enthusiastically support the research but cannot be expected to put the research ahead of patient care.

Clinical staff need clear, concise, and complete information about the research. They want specific information about enrollment criteria and processes, what interventions are being tested, what data are being collected, how subject rights and welfare are protected, whether the research will interfere with their care activities, and what is expected of them related to the research.

Being regularly visible in the acute care setting is essential to building positive relationships with the clinical staff (François et al., 2016; Pattison et al., 2017; Wiegand et al., 2008). Both formal and informal interactions with staff are vital. Face-to-face time is important and should be supplemented with audiovisual and written materials. The research team will need to communicate with all clinical staff, which generally requires formal meetings with groups of staff not only during weekdays but also on evening and night shifts as well as weekends. Meetings should be conducted prior to initiation of the project and periodically throughout the involvement of the clinical site. This provides regular reinforcement of study information and ensures that new staff is informed. Posters summarizing the study and providing contact information for the research team, posted in areas where staff congregates, can provide additional visibility for the research.

INTERVENTION AND BEYOND

Acute care research interventions and data collection must fit around clinical care needs. Successful investigators incorporate information about the usual flow of care in the unit (e.g., if the protocol involves fasting laboratory work, knowing when breakfast is delivered is essential). Because the acute care setting is not always predictable, established rules should be developed to deal with foreseeable contingencies and a plan generated to deal with unforeseen circumstances. For example, how will the research team accommodate the subject being off the unit for a radiology exam when research intervention or data collection is scheduled? What will happen if the subject is discharged from the acute care setting before his or her planned involvement in the study is complete?

Ongoing assessment of enrollment patterns, **intervention fidelity**, and **data integrity** should be performed at regular intervals so that any problems can be addressed. Investigators who wait until the end of the study to assess processes may be unpleasantly surprised to discover that elderly or minority subjects are underrepresented, or that a critical data element was unavailable or not collected in most subjects.

Subjects in acute care intervention research have complex problems and variable illness trajectories and may differ from each other despite clear inclusion and exclusion criteria. Collection of extensive demographic and descriptive data is essential to assess equivalence of study groups. If groups are not equivalent before intervention, the statistical analysis must account for differences. Because acute care settings and the populations they serve are heterogeneous in many ways, care must be exercised in interpretation and generalizability of the findings.

SUMMARY

Intervention research in acute care offers exciting opportunities to improve patient outcomes. Careful planning is required to minimize difficulties presented by the acute care environment and high-acuity population. Recruitment of subjects in acute care is complex, and obtaining informed consent may be difficult. Building and maintaining a good relationship with clinical staff is essential for conducting successful intervention research in acute care.

Key Points From Section 18.6 of This Chapter

- Active engagement with the clinical providers throughout the project is essential to success.
- Pilot testing is crucial to developing the protocol and identifying potential problems.
- Obtaining informed consent in the acute care setting poses challenges.
- Ongoing assessment of enrollment patterns, intervention fidelity, and data integrity should be performed at regular intervals.

REFERENCES

Aitken, L. M., Pelter, M. M., Carlson, B., Marshall, A. P., Cross, R., McKinley, S., & Dracup, K. (2008). Effective strategies for implementing a multicenter international clinical trial. *Journal of Nursing Scholarship, 40*(2), 101–108. doi:10.1111/j.1547-5069.2008.00213.x

Ako-Arrey, D. E., Brouwers, M. C., Lavis, J. N., Giacomini, M. K., & AGREE-HS Team. (2016). Health systems guidance appraisal: A critical interpretive synthesis. *Implementation Science, 11*(9), 1–20. doi:10.1186/s13012-016-0373-y

Amed, S., Naylor, P. J., Pinkney, S., Shea, S., Mâsse, L. C., Berg, S., … Wharf Higgins, J. (2015). Creating a collective impact on childhood obesity: Lessons from SCOPE initiative. Canadian Journal Public Health,106 (6), e426–e433. doi:10.17269/cjph.106.5114

The Annie E. Casey Foundation. (2015). 2015 Kids count: Data book. Retrieved from http://www.aecf.org

Antonelli, R. C., Stille, C. J., & Antonelli, D. M. (2008). Care coordination for children and youth with special health care needs: A descriptive, multisite study of activities, personnel costs, and outcomes. *Pediatrics, 122*, e209–e216. doi:10.1542/peds.2007-2254

Balbus, J. M., Barouki, R., Birnbaum, L. S., Etzel, R. A., Gluckman, P. D., Grandjean, P., … Tang, K. C. (2013). Early life prevention of non-communicable diseases. *Lancet, 381*(9860), 3–4. doi:10.1016/S0140-6736(12)61609-2

Baldwin, C. M. (2014). Sesión 13: Los Trastornos del sueño y la promoción del sueño saludable (Sleep disorders and sleep health promotion). In *Camino a la Salud (Su corazón, su vida) Manual para Promotoras y Promotores.* Washington, DC: PAHO/WHO.

Baldwin, C. M., & Korniewicz, D. M. (2012). Are emerging infectious diseases the most significant global health concern for nurses? *Maternal and Child Nursing, 37*(5), 288–289. doi: 10.1097/NMC.0b013e31625ecd0f

Barksdale, D. J., Newhouse, R., & Miller, J. A. (2014). The Patient-Centered Outcomes Research Institute (PCORI): Information for academic nursing. *Nursing Outlook, 63*(3), 192–200. doi:10.1016/j.outlook.2014.03.001

Becerra-Posada, F., de Snyder, N. S., Cuervo, L. G., & Montorzi, G. (2014). Priority research agendas: A strategic resource for health in Latin America. *Revista Panamericana de Salud Publica, 36*(6), 361–367. Retrieved from http://www.scielosp.org/scielo.php?script=sci_arttext&pid=S1020-49892014001100002&lng=en

Beck, E. J., Gill, W., & De Lay, P. R. (2016). Protecting the confidentiality and security of personal health information in low- and middle-income countries in the era of SDGs and big data. *Global Health Action, 9*, 32089. doi:10.3402/gha.v9.32089

Bennett, B., Cohen, I. G., Davies, S. E., Gostin, L. O., Hill, P. S., Mankad, A., & Phelan, A. L. (2018). Future-proofing global health: Governance of priorities. *Global Public Health, 13*(5), 519–527. doi:10.1080/17441692.2017.1296172

Bernabe-Ortiz, A., Sanchez, J. F., Carrillo-Larco, R. M., Gilman, R. H., Poterico, J. A., Quispe, R., … Miranda, J. J. (2017). Rural-to-urban migration and risk of hypertension: Longitudinal results of the PERU MIGRANT study. *Journal of Human Hypertension, 31*(1), 22–28. doi:10.1038/jhh.2015.124

Bowen, D. J., Kreuter, M., Spring, B., Cofta-Woerpel, L., Linnan, L., Weiner, D., … Fernandez, M. (2009). How we design feasibility studies. *American Journal of Preventive Medicine, 36*(5), 452–457. doi:10.1016/j.amepre.2009.02.002

Bradley, B. D., Jung, T., Tandon-Verma, A., Khoury, B., Chan, T. C. Y., & Cheng, Y. L. (2017). Operations research in global health: A scoping review with a focus on the themes of health equity and impact. *Health Research Policy Systems, 15*(1), 32. doi:10.1186/s12961-017-0187-7

Broderick, M., Dodd-Butera, T., & Wahl, P. (2002). A program to prevent iron poisoning using public health nurses in a county health department. *Public Health Nursing, 19*(3), 179–183. doi:10.1046/j.0737-1209.2002. 19305.x

Bruera, E., Willey, J., Cohen, M., & Palmer, J. L. (2008). Expressive writing in patients receiving palliative care: A feasibility study. *Journal of Palliative Medicine, 11*(1), 15–19. doi:10.1089/jpm.2007.0112

Buckwalter, K. C., Grey, M., Bowers, B., McCarthy, A. M., Gross, D., Funk, M., & Beck, C. (2009). Intervention research in highly unstable environments. *Research in Nursing & Health, 32*(1), 110–121. doi:10.1002/ nur.20309

Burns, K. E., Rizvi, L., Smith, O. M., Lee, Y., Lee, J., Wang, M., … Mehta, S. (2015). Is there a role for physician involvement in introducing research to surrogate decision makers in the intensive care unit? (The Approach trial: A pilot mixed methods study). *Intensive Care Medicine, 41*(1), 58–67. doi:10.1007/s00134-014-3558-3

Burns, K. E., Zubrinich, C., Tan, W., Raptis, S., Xiong, W., Smith, O., … Cook, D. J. (2013). Research recruitment practices and critically ill patients. A multicenter, cross-sectional study (the Consent Study). *American Journal of Respiratory and Critical Care Medicine, 87*(11), 1212–1218. doi:10.1164/rccm.201208-1537OC

Campbell, C. L. (2007). Respect for persons: Engaging African Americans in end-of-life research. *Journal of Hospice & Palliative Nursing, 9*(2), 74–78. doi:10.1097/01.NJH.0000263528.91929.0d

Caribbean Health Research Council. (2011). Health research agenda for the Caribbean. Trinidad and Tobago. Retrieved from http://test.carpha.org/downloads/Health_Research_Agenda_for_the_Caribbean.pdf

Carter, W. B., Elward, K., Malmgren, J., Martin, M. L., & Larson, E. (1991). Participation of older adults in health programs and research: A critical review of the literature. *Gerontologist, 31*(5), 584–592. doi:10.1093/ geront/31.5.584

Casarett, D. (2005). Ethical considerations in end-of-life care and research. *Journal of Palliative Medicine, 8*(Suppl. 1), S148–S160. doi:10.1089/jpm.2005.8.s-148

Casarett, D., Kassner, C. T., & Kutner, J. S. (2004). Recruiting for research in hospice: Feasibility of a research screening protocol. *Journal of Palliative Medicine, 7*(6), 854–860. doi:10.1089/jpm.2004.7.854

Castle, N. G., Engberg, J., & Men, A. (2007). Nursing home staff turnover: Impact on nursing home compare quality measures. *Gerontologist, 47*(5), 650–661. doi:10.1093/geront/47.5.650

Centers for Medicare and Medicaid Services. (2015). Nursing home data compendium. Retrieved from https://www.cms.gov/Medicare/Provider-Enrollment-and-Certification/CertificationandComplianc/ Downloads/nursinghomedatacompendium_508-2015.pdf

Chalkidou, K., Tunis, S., Lopert, R., Rochaix, L., Sawicki, P. T., Nasser, M., & Xerri, B. (2009). Comparative effectiveness research and evidence-based health policy: Experience from four countries. *Milbank Quarterly, 87*(2), 339–367. doi:10.1111/j.1468-0009.2009.00560.x

Challenges in research and practice in residential long-term care. (2016). *Journal of Nursing Scholarship, 49*(1), 3–5. doi:10.1111/jnu.12270

Chapman, E. (2012). Evaluation of the evidence informed policy network (EVIPnet). Retrieved from http://www.who.int/evidence/EvaluationEVIPNetAmericas.pdf

Chlan, L., Guttormson, J., Tracy, M. F., & Bremer, K. L. (2009). Strategies for overcoming site and recruitment challenges in research studies based in intensive care units. *American Journal of Critical Care, 18*(5), 410–417. doi:10.4037/ajcc2009400

Cochrane, A. L. (1972). *Effectiveness and efficiency: Random reflections on health services.* London, UK: Nuffield Provincial Hospitals Trust.

Coleman, M., Hemingway, J., Gleave, K. A., Wiebe, A., Gething, P. W., & Moyes, C. L. (2017). Developing global maps of insecticide resistance risk to improve vector control. *Malaria Journal, 16*(1), 86. doi:10.1186/ s12936-017-1733-z

Cook, T. D., Cook, D. J., Blythe, D., Rischbieth, A., Hebert, P. C., Zytaruk, N., Menon, K., … Meade, M. O. (2008). Enrollment of intensive care unit patients into clinical studies: A trinational survey of researchers' experiences, beliefs, and practices. *Critical Care Medicine, 36*(7), 2100–2105. doi:10.1097/CCM.0b013e31817c00b0

Cook, T. D., Cook, D. J., Ferguson, N. D., Hand, L., Austin, P., Zhou, Q., Adhikari, N. K., … Canadian Critical Care Trials Group. (2015). Coenrollment in a randomized trial of high-frequency oscillation: Prevalence, patterns, predictors, and outcomes. *Critical Care Medicine, 43*(2), 328–338. doi:10.1097/CCM.0000000000000692

Coon, D. W., Gallagher-Thompson, D., & Thompson, L. W. (Eds.). (2003). *Innovative interventions to reduce dementia caregiver distress: A clinical guide.* New York, NY: Springer Publishing.

Coon, D. W., Rubert, M., Solano, N., Mausbach, B., Kraemer, H., Argüelles, T., … Gallagher-Thompson, D. (2004). Well-being, appraisal, and coping in Latina and Caucasian female dementia caregivers: Findings from the REACH study. *Aging & Mental Health, 8*(4), 330–345. doi:10.1080/13607860410001709683

Crawley, L. M. (2005). Racial, cultural, and ethnic factors influencing end-of-life care. *Journal of Palliative Medicine, 8*(Suppl. 1), S58–S69. doi:10.1089/jpm.2005.8.s-58

Crowley, S. T., Chertow, G. M., Vitale, J., O'Connor, T., Zhang, J., Schein, R. M., … Palevsky, P. M. (2008). Lessons for successful study enrollment from the Veterans Affairs/National Institutes of Health Acute Renal Failure Trial Network Study. *Clinical Journal of the American Society of Nephrology, 3*(4), 955–961. doi:10.2215/CJN.05621207

Curran, G. M., Bauer, M., Mittman, B., Pyne, J. M., & Stetler, C. (2012). Effectiveness-implementation hybrid designs: Combining elements of clinical effectiveness and implementation research to enhance public health impact. *Medical Care, 50*(3), 217–226. doi:10.1097/MLR.0b013e3182408812

De Backer, D., & Schortgen, F. (2014). Physicians declining patient enrollment in clinical trials: What are the implications? *Intensive Care Medicine, 40*(1), 117–119. doi:10.1007/s00134-013-3151-1

de Cosío, F. G., Díaz-Apodaca, B. A., Ruiz-Holguín, R., Lara, A., & Castillo-Salgado, C. (2010). United States-Mexico Border Diabetes Prevalence Survey: Lessons learned from implementation of the project. Revista Panamericana de Salud Pública, 28(3), 151–158. PMID:20963261

DeMarco, R., & Tufts, K. A. (2014). The mechanics of writing policy brief. *Nursing Outlook, 62*, 219–224. doi:10.1016/j.outlook.2014.04.002

Denford, S., Abraham, C., Campbell, R., Busse, H. (2017). A comprehensive review of reviews of school-based interventions to improve sexual-health. *Health Psychology Review, 11*(1), 33–52.

Eaves, Y. D. (1999). Family recruitment issues and strategies: Caregiving in rural African Americans. *Nursing Research, 48*(3), 183–187. doi:10.1097/00006199-199905000-00008

el-Askari, G., Freestone, J., Irizarry, C., Kraut, K. L., Mashiyama, S. T., Morgan, M. A., & Walton, S. (1998). The Healthy Neighborhoods Project: A local health department's role in catalyzing community development. *Health Education & Behavior, 25*(2), 146–159. doi:10.1177/109019819802500204

Erwin, P. C., Greene, S. B., Mays, G. P., Ricketts, T. C., & Davis, M. V. (2011). The association of changes in local health department resources with changes in state-level health outcomes. *American Journal of Public Health, 101*(4), 609–615. doi:10.2105/AJPH.2009.177451

Evans, I., Thornton, H., & Chalmers, I. (2010). *Testing treatments: Better research for better healthcare.* London, UK: Printer & Martin. Retrieved from http://www.testingtreatments.org/

Fine, P. G., & Davis, M. (2006). Hospice: Comprehensive care at the end of life. *Anesthesiology Clinics, 24*(1), 181–204. doi:10.1016/j.atc.2005.12.004

François, B., Clavel, M., Vignon, P., & Laterre, P. F. (2016). Perspective on optimizing clinical trials in critical care: How to puzzle out recurrent failures. *Journal of Intensive Care, 4*, 67. doi:10.1186/s40560-016-0191-y

Gagnon, P., Charbonneau, C., Allard, P., Soulard, C., Dumont, S., & Fillion, L. (2002). Delirium in advanced cancer: A psychoeducational intervention for family caregivers. *Journal of Palliative Care, 18*(4), 253–261.

Gallagher-Thompson, D., Haley, W., Guy, D., Rupert, M., Argüelles, T., Zeiss, L. M., … Ory, M. (2003). Tailoring psychological interventions for ethnically diverse dementia caregivers. *Clinical Psychology: Science and Practice, 10*(4), 423–438. doi:/10.1093/clipsy.bpg042

Gallagher-Thompson, D., Singer, L. S., Depp, C., Mausbach, B. T., Cardenas, V., & Coon, D. W. (2004). Effective recruitment strategies for Latino and Caucasian dementia family caregivers in intervention research. *American Journal of Geriatric Psychiatry, 12*(5), 484–490. doi:10.1176/appi.ajgp.12.5.484

Gance-Cleveland, B., Aldrich, H., Dandreaux, D., Otzel, K. B., & Schmiege, S. (2015). A virtual childhood obesity collaborative: Satisfaction with online continuing education. *Journal of Pediatric Health Care, 29*(5), 413–423. doi:10.1016/j.pedhc.2015.01.006

Gance-Cleveland, B., Aldrich, H., Schmiege, S., & Tyler, K. (2016). Virtual obesity collaborative with and without decision-support technology. *International Journal for Quality in Health Care, 28*(3), 316–323. doi:10.1093/intqhc/mzw029

Gance-Cleveland, B., Dandreaux, D., Aldrich, H., & Kamal, R. (2015). Challenges conducting multicenter translational research: Promoting adherence to childhood obesity guidelines. *IRB: Ethics & Human Research, 37*(1), 6–11.

Garcia, A. B., Cassiani, S. H., & Reveiz, L. (2015). A systematic review of nursing research priorities on health system and services in the Americas. *Revista Panamericana de Salud Publica, 37*(3), 162–171. PMID25988253

Geletta, S., & Sparks, P. J. (2013). Administrator turnover and quality of care in nursing homes. *Annals of Long-Term Care: Clinical Care and Aging, 21*(4), 27–30. Retrieved from http://www.managedhealthcareconnect.com/article/administrator-turnover-and-quality-care-nursing-homes

Given, B. A., Keilman, L. J., Collins, C., & Given, C. W. (1990). Strategies to minimize attrition in longitudinal studies. *Nursing Research, 39*(3), 184–186. doi:10.1097/00006199-199005000-00018

Glickman, S. W., Anstrom, K. J., Lin, L., Chandra, A., Laskowitz, D. T., Woods, C. W., … Cairns, C. B. (2008). Challenges in enrollment of minority, pediatric, and geriatric patients in emergency and acute care clinical research. *Annals of Emergency Medicine, 51*(6), 775–780. e3. doi:10.1016/j.annemergmed.2007.11.002

Grap, M. J., & Munro, C. L. (2003). Subject recruitment in critical care nursing research: A complex task in a complex environment. *Heart & Lung, 32*(3), 162–168. doi:10.1016/S0147-9563(03)00031-1

Grimes, R. M., Courtney, C. C., & Vindekilde, J. (2001). A collaborative program between a school of public health and a local health department to increase HIV testing of pregnant women. *Public Health Reports, 116*(6), 585–589. doi:10.1016/S0033-3549(04)50091-2

Hancock, C., Kingo, L., & Raynaud, O. (2011). The private sector, international development and NCDs. *Global Health, 7,* 1–13. doi:10.1186/1744-8603-7-23

Hanney, S., Greenhalgh, T., Blatch-Jones, A., Glover, M., & Raftery, J. (2017). The impact on healthcare, policy and practice from 36 multi-project research programmes: Findings from two reviews. *Health Research Policy Systems, 15*(1), 26. doi:10.1186/s12961-017-0191-y

Hartog, C. S., Aneman, A., & Ricou, B. (2015). Increasing participation in critical care studies: The need to understand surrogate decision-makers for critically ill patients. *Intensive Care Medicine, 41*(2), 345–347. doi:10.1007/s00134-014-3617-9

Hebert, R. S., Prigerson, H. G., Schulz, R., & Arnold, R. M. (2006). Preparing caregivers for the death of a loved one: A theoretical framework and suggestions for future research. *Journal of Palliative Medicine, 9*(5), 1164–1171. doi:10.1089/jpm.2006.9.1164

Hebert, R. S., & Schulz, R. (2006). Caregiving at the end of life. *Journal of Palliative Medicine, 9*(5), 1174–1187. doi:10.1089/jpm.2006.9.1174

Hotez, P. J., Bottazzi, M. E., Franco-Paredes, C., Ault, S. K., & Periago, M. R. (2008). The neglected tropical diseases of Latin America and the Caribbean: A review of disease burden and distribution and a roadmap for control and elimination. *PLoS Neglected Tropical Diseases, 2*(9), e300. doi:10.1371/journal.pntd.0000300

Hudson, P. L., Zordan, R., & Trauer, T. (2011). Research priorities associated with family caregivers in palliative care: International perspectives. *Journal of Palliative Medicine, 14*(4), 397–401. doi:10.1089/jpm.2010.0345

Hughes, P., Hancock, C., & Cooper, K. (2012). Non-communicable diseases: Calling healthcare educators to action. *Nurse Education Today, 32,* 757–759. doi:10.1016/j.nedt.2012.05.013

International Council of Nurses. (2010). Delivering quality, serving communities: Nurses leading chronic care. Retrieved from http://www.icn.ch/publications/2010-delivering-quality-serving-communities-nurses-leading-chronic-care/

Jenkins, C., Smythe, A., Galant-Miecznikowska, M., Bentham, P., & Oyebode, J. (2016). Overcoming challenges of conducting research in nursing homes. *Nursing Older People, 28*(5), 16. doi:10.7748/nop.28.5.16.s24

Jha, P. (2009). Avoidable global cancer deaths and total deaths from smoking. *Nature Reviews Cancer, 9*(9), 655–664. doi:10.1038/nrc2703

Kavanaugh, K., Moro, T. T., Savage, T., & Mehendale, R. (2006). Enacting a theory of caring to recruit and retain vulnerable participants for sensitive research. *Research in Nursing & Health, 29*(3), 244–252. doi:10.1002/nur.20134

Kazdin, A. E. (2003). *Research design in clinical psychology* (4th ed.). Boston, MA: Allyn & Bacon.

King, D. A., & Quill, T. (2006). Working with families in palliative care: One size does not fit all. *Journal of Palliative Medicine, 9*(3), 704–715. doi:10.1089/jpm.2006.9.704

Klingler, C., Silva, D. S., Schuermann, C., Reis, A. A., Saxena, A., & Strech, D. (2017). Ethical issues in public health surveillance: A systematic qualitative review. *BMC Public Health, 17*(1), 295. doi:10.1186/s12889-017-4200-4

The Lancet. (2014). Research: increasing value, reducing waste. Retrieved from http://www.thelancet.com/series/research

Landry, L., Lee, R., & Greenwald, J. (2009). The San Francisco collaborative: An evaluation of a partnership between three schools of nursing and a public health department. *Public Health Nursing, 26*(6), 568–573. doi:10.1111/j.1525-1446.2009.00816.x

Lindström, K. (2010). *A program for caregivers of hospice patients* (Dissertation, Arizona State University, Phoenix, AZ).

Lindstrom, K. B., & Melnyk, B. M. (2009). Interventions for family caregivers of loved ones on hospice: A literature review with recommendations for clinical practice and future research. *Journal of Hospice & Palliative Nursing, 11*(3), 167–178. doi:10.1097/NJH.0b013e3181a1acb9

Lingler, J. H., Martire, L. M., Hunsaker, A. E., Greene, M. G., Dew, M. A., & Schulz, R. (2009). Feasibility of a patient-driven approach to recruiting older adults, caregivers, and clinicians for provider-patient communication research. *Journal of the American Academy of Nurse Practitioners, 21*(7), 377–383. doi:10.1111/j.1745-7599.2009.00427.x

Lobb, R., & Colditz, G. A. (2013). Implementation science and its application to population health. *Annual Review of Public Health, 34,* 235–251. doi:10.1146/annurev-publhealth-031912-114444

Maas, M. L., Kelley, L. S., Park, M., & Specht, J. P. (2002). Issues in conducting research in nursing homes. *Western Journal of Nursing Research, 24*(4), 373–389. doi:10.1177/01945902024004006

Mann, R. P., Mushtaq, F., White, A. D., Mata-Cervantes, G., Pike, T., Coker, D., … Mon-Williams, M. (2016). The problem with big data: Operating on smaller datasets to bridge the implementation gap. *Frontiers in Public Health, 4*, 248. doi:10.3389/fpubh.2016.00248

McBain, K. L., Payne, E. T., Sharma, R., Frndova, H., Abend, N. S., Sánchez, S. M., … Hahn, C. D. (2016). Strategies to maximize enrollment in a prospective study of comatose children in the PICU. *Pediatric Critical Care Medicine, 17*(3), 246–250. doi:10.1097/PCC.0000000000000642

McMillan, S. C., & Weitzner, M. A. (2003). Methodologic issues in collecting data from debilitated patients with cancer near the end of life. *Oncology Nursing Forum, 30*(1), 123–129. doi:10.1188/03.ONF.123-129

McNeely, E. A., & Clements, S. D. (1994). Recruitment and retention of the older adult into research studies. *Journal of Neuroscience Nursing, 26*(1), 57–61. doi:10.1097/01376517-199402000-00011

Mentes, J. C., & Tripp-Reimer, T. (2002). Barriers and facilitators in nursing home intervention research. *Western Journal of Nursing Research, 24*(8), 918–936. doi:10.1177/019394502237702

Minkler, M., & Wallerstein, N. (Eds.). (2008). *Community-based participatory research for health: From process to outcomes* (2nd ed.). San Francisco, CA: Jossey-Bass.

Miranda, J. J., Bernabé-Ortiz, A., Diez-Canseco, F., Málaga, G., Cárdenas, M. K., Carrillo-Larco, R. M., … Gilman, R. H. (2016). Towards sustainable partnerships in global health: The case of the CRONICAS Centre of Excellence in Chronic Diseases in Peru. *Global Health, 12*(1), 29. doi:10.1186/s12992-016-0170-z. Retrieved from https://www.ncbi.nlm.nih.gov/pubmed/27255370

Miranda, J. J., Bernabe-Ortiz, A., Smeeth, L., Gilman, R. H., Checkley, W., & CRONICAS Cohort Study Group. (2012). Addressing geographical variation in the progression of non-communicable diseases in Peru: The CRONICAS cohort study protocol. *British Medical Journal Open, 2*(1), e000610. doi:10.1136/bmjopen-2011-000610

Moore, M. L.(1997). Recruitment and retention: Nursing research among low-income pregnant women. *Applied Nursing Research, 10*(3), 152–158. doi:10.1016/S0897-1897(97)80248-0

Moreno-John, G., Gachie, A., Fleming, C. M., Nápoles-Springer, A., Mutran, E., Manson, S. M., & Pérez-Stable, E. J. (2004). Ethnic minority older adults participating in clinical research: Developing trust. *Journal of Aging and Health, 16*(Suppl. 5), 93S–123S. doi:10.1177/0898264304268151

Murphy, M. R., Escamilla, M. I., Blackwell, P. H., Lucke, K. T., Miner-Williams, D., Shaw, V., & Lewis, S. L. (2007). Assessment of caregivers' willingness to participate in an intervention research study. *Research in Nursing & Health, 30*(3), 347–355. doi:10.1002/nur.20186

Nabel, E. G., Stevens, S., & Smith, R. (2009). Combating chronic disease in developing countries. *Lancet, 373*(9680), 2004–2006. doi:10.1016/S0140-6736(09)61074-6

Naranjo, L. E., & Dirksen, S. R. (1998). The recruitment and participation of Hispanic women in nursing research: A learning process. *Public Health Nursing, 15*(1), 25–29. doi:10.1111/j.1525-1446.1998.tb00317.x

Natale, J. E., Lebet, R., Joseph, J. G., Ulysse, C., Ascenzi, J., Wypij, D., … Randomized Evaluation of Sedation Titration for Respiratory Failure (RESTORE) Study Investigators. (2017). Racial and ethnic disparities in parental refusal of consent in a large, multisite pediatric critical care clinical trial. *Journal of Pediatrics, 184*, 204–208. e1. doi:10.1016/j.jpeds.2017.02.006

National Association of County and City Health Officials. (2005). *Operational definition of a functional local health department.* Washington, DC: Author.

National Hospice and Palliative Care Organization. (2010). NHPCO facts and figures: Hospice care in America. Retrieved from http://www.nhpco.org

National Institute of Nursing Research. (2011). *NINR strategic plan 2006-2010: Bringing science to life.* Bethesda, MD: National Institutes of Health, U.S. Department of Health and Human Services.

Neiman, T. J., & Kovach, C. R. (2016). Research needs and challenges regarding palliation for individuals in long-term care settings. *Research in Gerontological Nursing, 9*(1), 2–5. doi:/10.3928/19404921-20151211-01

Nichols, L. O., Malone, C., Tarlow, B., & Loewenstein, D. (2000). The pragmatics of implementing intervention studies in the community. In R. Schulz (Ed.), *Handbook on dementia caregiving: Evidence-based interventions for family caregivers* (pp. 127–150). New York, NY: Springer Publishing.

Nichols, L. O., Martindale-Adams, J., Burns, R., Coon, D., Ory, M., Mahoney, D., … Winter, L. (2004). Social marketing as a framework for recruitment: Illustrations from the REACH study. *Journal of Aging and Health, 16*(Suppl. 5), 157S–176S. doi:10.1177/0898264304269727

Northouse, L. L., Rosset, T., Phillips, L., Mood, D., Schafenacker, A., & Kershaw, T. (2006). Research with families facing cancer: The challenges of accrual and retention. *Research in Nursing & Health, 29*(3), 199–211. doi:10.1002/nur.20128

O'Connor Duffany, K., Finegood, D. T., Matthews, D., McKee, M., Venkat Narayan, K. M., Puska, P., … Yach, D. (2011). Community Interventions for Health (CIH): A novel approach to tackling the worldwide epidemic of chronic diseases. *CVD Prevention and Control, 6*(2), 47–56. doi:10.1016/j.cvdpc.2011.02.005

Oliver, D. B., & Tureman, S. (Eds.). (1988). *The human factor in nursing home care.* New York, NY: Haworth Press.

Pan American Health Organization/World Health Organization. (2009). *Policy on research for health.* CD49/10, 61st session of the regional committee. Washington, DC. Author. Retrieved from http://www.paho.org/hq/dmdocuments/2009/CD49-10-e.pdf

Pan American Health Organization/World Health Organization. (2014). *Camino a la Salud. (Su corazón, su vida.) Manual para promotoras y promotores.* Washington, DC: Author. Retrieved from http://iris.paho.org/xmlui/handle/123456789/4313

Pan American Health Organization/World Health Organization. (2016). PAHO/WHO Regional research agenda related to Zika virus infection. Development of a research agenda for characterizing the Zika outbreak and its public health implications in the Americas. Retrieved from http://iris.paho.org/xmlui/handle/123456789/28285

Patrick, J. H., Pruchno, R. A., & Rose, M. S. (1998). Recruiting research participants: A comparison of the costs and effectiveness of five recruitment strategies. *Gerontologist, 38*(3), 295–302. doi:10.1093/geront/38.3.295

Pattison, N., Arulkumaran, N., Humphreys, S., & Walsh, T. (2017). Exploring obstacles to critical care trials in the UK: A qualitative investigation. *Journal of the Intensive Care Society, 18*(1), 36–46. doi:10.1177/1751143716663749

Perry, H., Crigler, L., Lewin, S., Glenton, C., LeBan, K., & Hodgins, S. (2017). A new resource for developing and strengthening large-scale community health worker programs. *Human Resources for Health, 15*(1), 13. doi:10.1186/s12960-016-0178-8

Pessin, H., Galietta, M., Nelson, C. J., Brescia, R., Rosenfeld, B., & Breitbart, W. (2008). Burden and benefit of psychosocial research at the end of life. *Journal of Palliative Medicine, 11*(4), 627–632. doi:10.1089/jpm.2007.9923

Phillips, L. R., & Van Ort, S. (1995). Issues in conducting intervention research in long-term care settings. *Nursing Outlook, 43*(6), 249–253. doi:10.1016/S0029-6554(95)80089-1

Proctor, E. K. (2004). Leverage points for the implementation of evidence-based practice. *Brief Treatment and Crisis Intervention, 4*(3), 227–242. doi:10.1093/brief-treatment/mhh020

Proctor, E. K., & Rosen, A. (2008). From knowledge production to implementation: Research challenges and imperatives. *Research on Social Work Practice, 18*(4), 285–291. doi:10.1177/1049731507302263

Proctor, E., Silmere, H., Raghavan, R., Hovmand, P., & Aarons, G. (2011) Outcomes for implementation research: Conceptual distinctions, measurement challenges, and research agenda. *Administration and Policy in Mental Health and Mental Health Services Research, 38*(2), 65–76.

Randolph, A. G. (2009). The unique challenges of enrolling patients into multiple clinical trials. *Critical Care Medicine, 37*(Suppl. 1), S107–S111. doi:10.1097/CCM.0b013e3181921c9d

REWARD-EQUATOR Conference, Edinburgh, UK.. (2015, September 28-30). Retrieved from http://www.equator-network.org/2015/08/16/research-waste-equator-conference-2015/

Rodríguez-Feria, P., & Cuervo, L. G. (2017). Progress in trial registration in Latin America and the Caribbean, 2007-2013. *Revista Panamericana de Salud Publica, 41,* e31, 1–9. Retrieved from http://iris.paho.org/xmlui/bitstream/handle/123456789/33963/v41a312017.pdf?sequence=1&isAllowed=y

Roman, A. V., Perez, W., & Smith R. (2015). A scorecard for tracking actions to reduce the burden of non-communicable diseases. *Lancet, 386,* 1131–1132. doi:10.1016/S0140-6736(15)00197-X

Rubinstein, A., Colantonio, L., Bardach, A., Caporale, J., Martí, S. G., Kopitowski, K., … Pichón-Rivière, A. (2010). Estimation of the burden of cardiovascular disease attributable to modifiable risk factors and cost-effectiveness analysis of preventative interventions to reduce this burden in Argentina. *BMC Public Health, 10,* 627. doi:10.1186/1471-2458-10-627

Sackett, D. L., Rosenberg, W. M. C., Gray, J. A. M., Haynes, R. B., & Richardson, W. S. (1996). Evidence based medicine: what it is and what it isn't. *British Medical Journal, 312*(7023), 71-72. PMID8555924 PMCID2349778

Salerno, J., Knoppers, B. M., Lee, L. M., Hlaing, W. M., & Goodman, K. W. (2017). Ethics, big data and computing in epidemiology and public health. *Annals of Epidemiology, 27,* 297–301. doi:10.1016/j.annepidem.2017.05.002

School-Based Health Alliance: Redefining health for kids and teens. (2014). 2013-14 Digital Census Report. Retrieved from https://censusreport.sbh4all.org

Shafey, O., Eriksen, M., Ross, H., & Mackay, J. (2009). *The tobacco atlas* (3rd ed.). Atlanta, GA: American Cancer Society.

Sherman, D. W., McSherry, C. B., Parkas, V., Ye, X. Y., Calabrese, M., & Gatto, M. (2005). Recruitment and retention in a longitudinal palliative care study. *Applied Nursing Research, 18*(3), 167–177. doi:10.1016/j.apnr.2005.04.003

Simmons, M. M., Gabrielian, S., Byrne, T., McCullough, M. B., Smith, J. L., Taylor, T J., O'Toole, T. P., … Smelson, D. A. (2017). A hybrid III stepped wedge cluster randomized trial testing an implementation strategy to facilitate the use of an evidence-based practice in VA homeless primary care treatment programs. *Implementation Science, 12,* 46. doi:10.1186/s13012-017-0563-2

Smith, K. N., Gunzenhauser, J. D., & Fielding, J. E. (2010). Reinvigorating performance evaluation: First steps in a local health department. *Public Health Nursing, 27*(5), 425–432. doi:10.1111/j.1525-1446.2010.00875.x

Snyder, M., Tseng, Y. H., Brandt, C., Croghan, C., Hanson, S., Constantine, R., & Kirby, L. (2001). Challenges of implementing intervention research in persons with dementia: Example of a glider swing intervention. *American Journal of Alzheimer's Disease and Other Dementias, 16*(1), 51–56. doi:10.1177/153331750101600106

Sole, M. L., Middleton, A., Deaton, L., Bennett, M., Talbert, S., & Penoyer, D. (2017). Enrollment challenges in critical care nursing research. *American Journal of Critical Care, 26*(5), 395–400. doi:10.4037/ajcc2017511

Sörensen, S., Pinquart, M., & Duberstein, P. (2002). How effective are interventions with caregivers? An updated meta-analysis. *Gerontologist, 42*(3), 356–372. doi:10.1093/geront/42.3.356

Stranges, S., Tigbe, W., Gómez-Olivé, F. X., Thorogood, M., & Kandala, N. B. (2012). Sleep problems: An emerging global epidemic? Findings from the INDEPTH WHO-SAGE study among more than 40,000 older adults from 8 countries across Africa and Asia. *Sleep, 35*(8), 1173–1181. doi:10.5665/sleep.2012

Tarlow, B. A., & Mahoney, D. F. (2000). The cost of recruiting Alzheimer's disease caregivers for research. *Journal of Aging and Health, 12*(4), 490–510. doi:10.1177/089826430001200403

Tattersall, A., & Grant, M. S. (2016). Big data: What it is and why it matters. *Health Information and Libraries Journal 33*(2), 89-91. doi: 10.1111/hir.12147

Tellis-Nayak, M. (2010). *Improving communication: Mentoring and coaching.* Paper presented at the Oklahoma Foundation for Health Care Quality, Tulsa, OK.

Turnock, B. J., Handler, A., Hall, W., Potsic, S., Nalluri, R., & Vaughn, E. H. (1994). Local health department effectiveness in addressing the core functions of public health. *Public Health Reports, 109*(5), 653–658.

VanDevanter, N., Shinn, M., Niang, K. T., Bleakley, A., Perl, S., & Cohen, N. (2003). The role of social and behavioral science in public health practice: A study of the New York City Department of Health. *Journal of Urban Health, 80*(4), 625–634. doi:10.1093/jurban/jtg069

Vedanthan, R., Bernabe-Ortiz, A., Herasme, O. I., Joshi, R., Lopez-Jaramillo, P., Thrift, A. G., … Fuster, V. (2017). Innovative approaches to hypertension control in low- and middle-income countries. *Cardiology Clinics, 35,* 99–115. doi:10.1016/j.ccl.2016.08.010

Villanueva, E. C., Abreu, D. R., Cuervo, L. G., Becerra-Posada, F., Reveiz, L., & Ijsselmuiden, C. (2012). HRWeb Americas: A tool to facilitate better research governance in Latin America and the Caribbean. *Cadernos se Saúde Pública, 28*(10), 2003–2008. doi:10.1590/s0102-311x2012001000018

Wardbegnoche, W., Gance-Cleveland, B., Simpson, P., Parker, J., Jo, C., Dean, J., & Thompson, J. (2009). Effectiveness of a school-based obesity prevention program. *International Journal of Health Promotion and Education, 47*(2), 51–56. doi:10.1080/14635240.2009.10708159

Watts, A. G., Miniota, J., Joseph, H. A., Brady, O. J., Kraemer, M. U. G., Grills, A. W., … Cetron, M. (2017). Elevation as a proxy for mosquito-borne Zika virus transmission in the Americas. *PLOS ONE, 12*(5), e0178211. doi:10.1371/journal.pone.0178211

Welch, V., Jull, J., Petkovic, J., Armstrong, R., Boyer, Y., Cuervo, L. G., … Tugwell, P. (2015a). Protocol for the development of a CONSORT-equity guideline to improve reporting of health equity in randomized trials. *Implementation Science, 10,* 1–11. doi:10.1186/s13012-015-0332-z

Welch, V., Petticrew, M., Petkovic, J., Moher, D., Waters, E., White, H., … PRISMA-Equity Bellagio group. (2015b). Extending the PRISMA statement to equity-focused systematic reviews (PRISMA-E 2012): Explanation and elaboration. *International Journal for Equity in Health, 14,* 1–23. doi:10.1186/s12939-015-0219-2

Weng, C., & Kahn, M. G. (2016). Clinical research informatics for big data and precision medicine. *Yearbook of Medical Informatics, 10*(1), 211–218. doi:10.15265/IY-2016-019

Whalen, G. F., Kutner, J., Byock, I., Gerard, D., Stovall, E., Sieverding, P., … Krouse, R. S. (2007). Implementing palliative care studies. *Journal of Pain and Symptom Management, 34*(Suppl. 1), S40–S48. doi:10.1016/j.jpainsymman.2007.04.010

Whitehead, M. (1992). The concepts and principles of equity and health. *International Journal of Health Services, 22*(3), 429–445. doi:10.2190/986L-LHQ6-2VTE-YRRN

Wiegand, D. L., Norton, S. A., & Baggs, J. G. (2008). Challenges in conducting end-of-life research in critical care. *AACN Advanced Critical Care, 19*(2), 170–177. doi:10.1097/01.AACN.0000318120.67061.82

Williams, A. (2007). Recruitment challenges for end-of-life research. *Journal of Hospice & Palliative Nursing, 9*(2), 79–85. doi:10.1097/01.NJH.0000263529.99552.91

Williams, C. J., Shuster, J. L., Clay, O. J., & Burgio, K. L. (2006). Interest in research participation among hospice patients, caregivers, and ambulatory senior citizens: Practical barriers or ethical constraints? *Journal of Palliative Medicine, 9*(4), 968–974. doi:10.1089/jpm.2006.9.968

Wong, F., Stevens, D., O'Connor-Duffany, K., Siegel, K., & Gao, Y. (2011). Community Health Environment Scan Survey (CHESS): A novel tool that captures the impact of the built environment on lifestyle factors. *Global Health Action, 4,* 5276. doi:10.3402/gha.v4i0.5276

World Economic Forum. (2012). Big data, big impact: New possibilities for international development. Retrieved from http://www3.weforum.org/docs/WEF_TC_MFS_BigDataBigImpact_Briefing_2012.pdf

World Health Organization. (2002). Pain relief and palliative care. In *National Cancer Control Programmes: Policies and managerial guidelines* (2nd ed., pp. 83–91). Geneva, Switzerland: Author. Retrieved from http://www.who.int/cancer/media/en/408.pdf

World Health Organization. (2015). NCD global monitoring framework. Retrieved from http://www.who.int/nmh/global_monitoring_framework/en/

World Health Organization. (2016). EVIPNet in action: 10 years, 10 stories. Retrieved from http://apps.who.int/iris/handle/10665/250581

World Health Organization. (2017). Major research funders and international NGOs to implement WHO standards on reporting clinical trial results. Retrieved from http://www.who.int/en/news-room/detail/18-05-2017-major-research-funders-and-international-ngos-to-implement-who-standards-on-reporting-clinical-trial-results

World Health Organization, 63rd World Health Assembly.. (2010). *WHO strategy on research for health; WHO's roles and responsibilities on health research: Document WHA63.22 and Resolution.* Geneva, Switzerland. Retrieved from http://apps.who.int/gb/e/e_wha63.html

Wyber, R., Vaillancourt, S., Perry, W., Mannava, P., Folaranmi, T., & Celi, L. A. (2015). Big data in global health: Improving health in low- and middle-income countries. *Bulletin of the World Health Organization, 93*(3), 203–208. doi:10.2471/BLT.14.139022

Yach, D., Hawkes, C., Gould, C. L., & Hofman, K. J. (2004). The global burden of chronic diseases: Overcoming impediments to prevention and control. *Journal of the American Medical Association, 291*(21), 2616–2622. doi:10.1001/jama.291.21.2616

Zahner, S. J. (2005). Local public health system partnerships. *Public Health Reports, 120*(1), 76–83. doi:10.1177/003335490512000113

19

Data Management

Sharon M. Lawlor & Kevin E. Kip

This chapter describes the major decisions and approaches to developing an effective and efficient data management system for intervention studies. Although occasionally viewed as somewhat of an afterthought or tangential component of an intervention study, in fact, nothing could be further from the truth (Krishnankutty, Bellary, Kumar, & Moodahadu, 2012). Indeed, no matter how intriguing the study hypotheses, how well the study is designed, and the collective expertise of the study investigators, the data are only as good as the manner in which they are collected and managed. In other words, data management is truly a "rate-limiting" step in conducting a valid and scientifically productive intervention study. Of note, this chapter focuses on a "single-site" intervention study, that is, when all data to be collected are from a single location and investigative group. Data management for multicenter studies is considerably more complex and requires standardization and greater monitoring across participating sites, and a key decision is whether a centralized versus decentralized approach will be used. The reader is referred to additional references for a more complete description of data management within a multicenter setting (Gerritsen, Sartorius, vd Veen, & Meester, 1993; Gluud & Sørensen, 1995).

DATA COLLECTION AND DESIGN OF FORMS

The individual data collection forms (questionnaires and instruments), known as **"case report forms"** (CRFs), are the fundamental mechanism for collection of data. This occurs irrespective of whether the data are to be collected using hard copy forms or electronically, such as through a data entry website or computer-assisted mechanism. Regardless of the method of capture, data elements should be logically organized on paper forms first, according to what data will be collected, who will provide the information, and how the information will be obtained. At the broadest level, selection of CRFs includes whether only established (i.e., reliable and valid) instruments will be used, whether self-developed instruments will be used, or a combination of the two will be used (the most common approach). Regardless, the most basic principles of selection/development of CRFs include the following: (a) collect only those data that are truly necessary to meet the study aims and hypotheses to minimize participant (and data management) burden; (b) make sure the CRFs fully match the study protocol; (c) minimize text write-in responses; (d) embed instructions and definitions into the forms where appropriate and only as necessary according to who will be completing the form (trained study personnel vs. participant); (e) use "skip patterns" when a response to one question eliminates the need to answer subsequent questions—for example, if a participant reports *"No"* to a question on current use of prescription medications, "skip" subsequent questions related to use of beta-blockers, statins, antidepressants, and so forth (Exhibit 19.1); (f) balance print and white space to make the forms clean and clear for the data collector; (g) select variables that have common, established definitions, such as categories used by the U.S. Census Bureau to define race and ethnicity; and (h) ensure that all data forms have a corresponding manual of operation (MOP) that has a complete set of instructions for completing the form and study definitions for every data element on the form.

Self-developed CRFs often include information about participant demographics (DG; e.g., age), lifestyle characteristics (e.g., smoking history), and health history (e.g., presence of diabetes). In addition, many times information about the fidelity of the intervention(s) under study is collected via self-developed forms. An example of a self-developed form is provided in Exhibit 19.2.

No matter what data are to be collected on self-developed CRFs, the most basic design will minimize errors and variability. To this end, the following basic principles should be adhered to:

1. For **continuous variables**, such as height and systolic blood pressure:
   - Explicitly state the unit of measurement on the CRF (e.g., cm, mmHg) and a conversion factor when appropriate (e.g., 1 inch = 2.54 cm).
   - Capture the data in the "raw" scale. For example, collect date of birth rather than age, when possible. The raw data can always be used in calculations or collapsed later for analytic purposes, as needed.
   - Include precision on the CRF. For example, capture hemoglobin as: _____ g/dL.
2. For **categorical variables**, such as self-rating of quality of life or use of medications:
   - Explicitly state on the CRF whether to "select one" response or "select all that apply."
   - Include codes for response choices that are "check one."
   - If the response choices do not represent all possible responses, an "Other" category may be required. Otherwise a "None" category should be provided to encourage a response in every instance.
   - Use code lists when possible so that response sets can easily be expanded over the course of a study.
   - A time reference is typically required for health history variables, such as current condition within the past month, past year, or at any time.

EXHIBIT 19.1 Example of Skip Pattern

---

3. Are you currently taking one or more prescription medications?   ☐ Yes   ☐ No
   If Yes, check all that apply
   a) ☐ Beta blocker
   b) ☐ Statin
   c) ☐ Anti-depressant
   d) ☐ _____
4. Are you currently taking any herbs, "natural" or herbal medications?   ☐ Yes   ☐ No

---

EXHIBIT 19.2 Example of Self-Developed Case Report Form

Title of Intervention Study

Baseline Evaluation

Participant ID: __ __ __ __ __ __ __ __   Date of evaluation: _____/_____/_____
                                                                            mm/dd/yyyy

Instructions: This questionnaire asks about you and your behaviors. Please read each question carefully and then answer each question as completely and honestly as possible. This information is only for study purposes and will remain strictly confidential.

SECTION I: DEMOGRAPHICS

1. Sex at birth: 1 ☐ Male   2 ☐ Female

2. Date of birth *(mm/dd/yyyy):* ___/___/____

3. Do you consider yourself to be Hispanic or Latino? ☐ Yes   ☐ No   ☐ Prefer not to answer

4. What race are you *(check all that apply)*?

   ☐ White or Caucasian   ☐ American Indian or Alaska Native
   ☐ Black or African American   ☐ Native Hawaiian or Other Pacific Islander
   ☐ Asian   ☐ Other _____
   ☐ Prefer not to answer

5. What is your current marital status?

   1. ☐ Never married
   2. ☐ Married or Living in a marriage-like relationship
   3. ☐ Widowed
   4. ☐ Divorced or Separated ☐ Prefer not to answer

6. Which of these categories best represent your total annual household income?

   1. ☐ Less than $25,000
   2. ☐ $25,000–$49,999
   3. ☐ $50,000–$74,999
   4. ☐ $75,000–$99,999
   5. ☐ $100,000–$199,999
   6. ☐ More than $200,000   ☐ Prefer not to answer

SECTION II: HEALTH BEHAVIOR

1. Have you ever used, or do you currently use, a tobacco product (cigarette, cigar, smokeless tobacco)?

   1. ☐ Currently use a tobacco product
   2. ☐ Formerly used a tobacco product
          What year did you stop using the tobacco product *(yyyy):* _____
   3. ☐ Never used a tobacco product

Thank you for your participation.

A special note is directed to the collection of race/ethnicity data (categorical variables), which are often erroneously viewed as synonymous and incorrectly captured. According to the U.S. Census Bureau, the five categories for race include "White," "Black or African American," "American Indian or Alaska Native," "Asian," and "Native Hawaiian or Other Pacific Islander"; and respondents should be instructed to select "one or more races" to which they self-identify. Respondents should be directed for the separate question of ethnicity to indicate whether they consider themselves to be "Hispanic or Latino."

Explicit attention should be directed to the target audience who will complete the forms for all variables on self-developed CRFs, whether it will be study participants or research staff, such as through the conduct of interviews. This includes education, age, culture, and language of the target audience. When in doubt, construct questions and responses using a reading grade level somewhat below the educational level of the target audience. Moreover, "pilot testing" of all forms (self-developed or otherwise) by persons similar to those of the target audience is a critical yet often overlooked step with the potential to identify flaws in the CRFs and minimize data collection errors and incomplete data. Additional details on general guidelines for design of self-developed CRFs in clinical trials have been published (Knatterud, Forman, & Canner, 1983; Pocock, 1983; Wright & Haybittle, 1979).

Established CRFs are frequently used to measure lifestyle characteristics (e.g., dietary patterns), psychosocial status (e.g., depressive symptoms), and general health status (e.g., Charlson Comorbidity Index; Charlson, Szatrowski, Peterson, & Gold, 1994). The primary criterion for selection of such instruments is documented evidence of reliability and validity, preferably in populations similar to persons to be enrolled in the intervention study. Other decisions and guidelines for selection of established CRFs include the following:

- When "short" and "long" forms of an instrument exist (e.g., brief symptom inventory; 18-item vs. 53-item versions; Derogatis, 2000; Derogatis & Melisaratos, 1983), select the short form so long as it is believed to be sensitive to measure the construct or outcome of interest in the intervention study population.
- Determine whether a global (multipurpose) scale, such as the Short-Form Health Survey (SF-36; Ware & Gandek, 1994), is preferred versus domain-specific instruments such as the Center for Epidemiologic Studies Depression Scale (CES-D) used to measure depressive symptomatology (Radloff, 1977). Be wary of overlap in measurement of the same constructs—again, make judicious use of the selection of CRFs.
- Determine whether each instrument to be used in the intervention study has copyright restrictions and a purchase price for use. Of note, some instruments that have undergone revisions have earlier versions that are free for public use. Regardless, make sure to acquire the scoring information for each instrument (e.g., some questions are often reverse scored depending on their wording), and do not modify items because this will no longer ensure acceptable reliability and validity.

As a final and critical step in the design of data collection forms, make sure that every form and every page of each form has an appropriate header and footer. The header should include the study name and form name, and provide space to record the identification (ID) number of the study participant and any other data fields that are considered "key" fields to uniquely identify a record in the study database. Typically, the date of a visit (assessment) or the time points are considered "key" fields. For example, commonly used time points in clinical intervention studies include pretreatment, screening, baseline, treatment, follow-up, and evaluation or summary points (Trocky & Brandt, 2009). An example of a form header is shown in Exhibit 19.3.

The footer should include the date and form version as well as page numbers and any copyright information. Also, consider a short name for each data form and include that short name in the footer. For example, the Laboratory Evaluation (LE) form could be referred to as the LE form. An example of a form footer is provided in Exhibit 19.4.

Also, to maximize tracking of data processes with paper-based collection, consider a "bookkeeping" section on the first or last page of a CRF to track the data collection and entry process, that is, data collector ID and the date the data are collected, entered into the data system, and so forth.

EXHIBIT 19.3 Example of Form Header

Title of Intervention Study

Laboratory Evaluation

Participant ID: _ _ _ _ _ _ _ _ _ _ _   **Visit:** ☐ Screening   ☐ Baseline

Date of sample: _____/_____/_____   ☐ 1-month   ☐ 3-month

　　　　　　　　mm/dd/yyyy   ☐ Study closeout

EXHIBIT 19.4 Example of a Form Footer

June 30, 2017, version 1.0　　　　　　　　LE　　　　　　　　Page 1 of 2

LE, laboratory evaluation.

DATABASE DESIGN AND STRUCTURE

In conjunction with identification of all the data to be collected in the intervention study, it is particularly important to identify and design an appropriate data management system to enter and manage the study data in a secure fashion. This will not only optimize the quality of the study data but also influence the time efficiency involved in data entry, data queries, routine report generation, statistical analyses, and manuscript preparation. There are several related considerations when selecting or designing and developing a data management system that will meet the needs of a study: (a) distributed versus centralized data entry; (b) mode of data collection/entry, that is, whether the data will be entered via key entry (includes web-based entry), optical character recognition (scan/fax), telephone keypad or voice recognition, touchscreen or pen based, or a combination of these; (c) use of commercially available or custom-designed software for the front end (data entry) and back end (database management), balancing the potential limitations of commercially available software with the cost and resources required to design and develop custom software; (d) the database (i.e., Access, Structured Query Language [SQL]); and (e) data security. These considerations can likely be distilled down to the following suggestions for the purposes of a single-center intervention trial with a relatively small number of data forms and limited research personnel and resources: (a) consider Internet-based or other commercially available software including scan software—all of which allow for fairly easy development of data forms and provide a vehicle for data entry; (b) develop a database management system using Access, Statistical Package for the Social Sciences (SPSS), Statistical Analysis Software (SAS), or some other commercially available software that makes database development relatively easy and provides the basic features needed to maintain data integrity; and (c) keep the structure of the database tables simple.

Data Entry and Management System

If the data are to be entered via a web-based system, many universities maintain licenses for online data entry/survey systems such as Qualtrics Survey Software (Qualtrics.com), Survey Monkey® (Survey Monkey.com), and Checkbox (Checkbox Survey, Inc.). These online survey systems require only a modest level of training by the user and offer basic quality control features when designing data entry systems such as embedding range checks for data values (e.g., age in years to range from 0 to 120) and drop-down lists of categorical variables, such as types of medications being taken. In addition, these systems can typically generate descriptive data reports and export the data in multiple formats such as Microsoft Excel and SPSS. Moreover, these systems permit a range of electronic data entry modalities such as smartphones and portable media players. Another popular system being widely used across universities is the Research Electronic Data Capture (REDCap) system (Harris et al., 2009). On the contrary, if sophisticated quality control and report generation features are needed from the data entry or database management system, services of a web or systems programmer will likely be required.

If a commercial software package is to be used, often the study data are collected on hard copy CRFs and manually entered into the database. As a general rule, the software package to be used should have sufficient quality control features (e.g., ability to specify entry of only certain values or text), permit descriptive labeling and formatting of all study variables, and ideally be relational in nature—in other words, the user can specify the relationships between different variables and tables in the database (these features apply to web-based systems as well). An example of relational capacity is for the variable "sex" when entered as "female" to be the only response that permits subsequent entry of a question (variable) related to the use of hormone replacement therapy. Although Microsoft Excel is commonly used for data entry, it should be noted that this package is not a true database management system. Assuming sufficient expertise, the principal investigator (PI) of the intervention study should consider development of a more flexible and robust data entry system using REDCap, Microsoft (MS) Access, SPSS, or the SAS system.

There are several optical scanning systems available nowadays in which data captured on hard copy forms can be directly scanned or faxed into a database. A popular system in use nowadays is the Teleform system (Teleform, n.d.). Although intuitively attractive, these systems require considerable thought in the development of the CRFs to ensure that the data that are scanned are accurately recorded. At the broadest level, text responses should be limited with this type of system, and the CRFs should use sufficiently large fonts and spacing between variables. This is because "coordinates" for each variable are defined on a specific location of the CRF. If the data coordinates are too small or too close to other variables, information may be misread, especially if data collectors are not "neat" when recording data. Multipage forms can be challenging and the data recorded for the "key" fields in the header of each page must be legible in order for the pages to be properly linked. The quality of the printed or faxed document must be good, without any skewing or shrinking/stretching. Providing blank data forms as PDFs eliminates some of the potential variability with printers. Per the above discussion, optical character recognition (OCR) software can be used to develop an efficient and reliable entry system, but proper pilot testing is required. Also, even though the data are electronically scanned into a database, it is good practice to set up the system so that every data field requires "verification." A trained staff person should visually verify from the hard copy forms that the data have been accurately captured by the OCR software. An example of a data form developed using Teleform system is provided in Exhibit 19.5.

Finally, there are other variations (methods) in which data can be captured electronically, particularly with respect to self-report information by the study participant. These include but are not limited to computer-assisted personal interviewing (CAPI), computer-assisted self-interviewing (CASI), and computer-assisted telephone interviewing (CATI). The same guidelines described earlier apply for the development of CRFs as the blueprint by which the self-report data will be collected for these computer-based data entry mechanisms. Typically, for commercial-based systems, the data collected using these computer-assisted programs can be exported into common data formats such as MS Excel, SPSS, and SAS.

EXHIBIT 19.5 Example of a Teleform Data Form

Title of Intervention Trial
Baseline/Hospitalization Form   Form # ⬚⬚⬚⬚ **Participant ID** ⬚⬚⬚⬚⬚⬚⬚⬚

Date of admission: ⬚⬚ / ⬚⬚ / ⬚⬚⬚⬚ *(mm/dd/yyyy)*

I. PARTICIPANT INFORMATION

Date of birth: ⬚⬚ / ⬚⬚ / ⬚⬚⬚⬚ *(mm/dd/yyyy)* Height: ⬚⬚⬚ · ⬚ | height in cm = height in inches × 2.54 |

Sex: ☐ Male ☐ Female   Weight: ⬚⬚⬚ · ⬚ | weight in kg = weight in lbs × 0.45 |

Is participant Hispanic? ☐ No ☐ Yes

Structure of Data Files

When setting up the database, particularly with respect to data entry by use of a commercial software package, it is critical to identify the most efficient structure for the data. Two important design considerations are (a) use of single versus multiple database tables and (b) "row" versus "column" data entry for variables that are repeatedly measured.

As a general rule, one or more different database tables should be developed for information that is collected on different schedules. Oftentimes, database tables reflect the same logical organization of data as on the CRFs with one data table per form. For example, in intervention studies, demographic data and presenting health history information are often collected at study entry only. If so, all of these variables can be captured within a single database table. On the other hand, behavioral (e.g., diet and physical activity) and outcome (e.g., blood pressure, cholesterol) variables are often collected repeatedly throughout the study. In this instance, it is usually best to capture each domain or category of repeatedly collected variables in a separate table. For example, if depressive symptoms (e.g., measured by the CES-D) and quality of life (e.g., measured by the SF-36) measures are administered at study entry and quarterly throughout 1-year follow-up, separate database tables should be set up for the CES-D and the SF-36.

When variables are collected repeatedly throughout the study, the structure of "row" versus "column" entry needs to be defined. Although not apparent to many researchers, the "row" variable approach is typically preferred in terms of both space efficiency and analytical capacity. To illustrate, assume that scores on the CES-D will be captured at study entry and at months 3, 6, 9, and 12 of follow-up, hence five assessments in total. The two primary ways in which these data can be entered (structured in the database) are one row per study participant or one row for each visit (assessment) per study participant. As noted earlier, the latter is the preferred approach. Referring to the fictitious data of three participants in Table 19.1, it is seen that the "column" approach of one row per study participant results in a data matrix of three rows, six columns, and six variables.

If these same data are entered in the database using the "row" entry approach (Table 19.2), this results in a data matrix of 15 rows, 3 columns, and 3 variables. Without getting into all of the technical details, it is generally more efficient to have fewer variables and more rows of data than the reverse. For example, imagine if 50 data variables were collected at 6 different time intervals. This would result in $50 \times 6 = 300$ columns and 300 different variable names.

When conducting statistical analysis on the basis of the "column" approach, it is often unwieldy to specify which variables at which time points are to be analyzed. Moreover, common statistical methods for longitudinal data analysis, including linear mixed models (Goldstein, 2003; Liang & Zeger, 1986), typically require the data to be structured using the more efficient "row" approach. Of note, simple coding in common statistical packages such as SAS and

TABLE 19.1 Example of "Column" Approach of Data Entry for Repeated Measures

STUDY ID	CES-D BASE	CES-D MONTH 3	CES-D MONTH 6	CES-D MONTH 9	CES-D MONTH 12
1	36	24	22	26	20
2	28	12	12	14	10
3	32	16	14	24	26

CES-D, Center for Epidemiologic Studies Depression Scale.

TABLE 19.2 Example of "Row" Approach of Data Entry for Repeated Measures

STUDY ID	TIME POINT	CES-D
1	Baseline	36
1	Month 3	24
1	Month 6	22
1	Month 9	26
1	Month 12	20
2	Baseline	28
2	Month 3	12
2	Month 6	12
2	Month 9	14
2	Month 12	10
3	Baseline	32
3	Month 3	16
3	Month 6	14
3	Month 9	24
3	Month 12	26

CES-D, Center for Epidemiologic Studies Depression Scale.

SPSS can be used to "transform" the data from the "row" to "column" approach if needed for statistical analyses. In general, the database structure should be set up to assure efficient and accurate data collection and entry processes, knowing that data can be reorganized as necessary for the analyst.

Data Formats and Labeling

In the design of the database, each variable is given a specific name and label. The variable name is typically 20 characters or less, and the label is more descriptive of the full meaning of the variable. Although the naming of the study variables is arbitrary, there are several guidelines that can be considered that can aid in not only easy review and interpretation of the entire database but also subsequent statistical analyses.

In general, the variable name should be descriptive but short, because longer names require more typing when writing programs that use the data. Avoid the use of reserved words such as "date" or "time" and special characters that may not be recognized by statistical software. When multiple CRFs are used in the intervention study, it is often helpful to name the specific variables consistently across forms but denote the form in which the variable originated. For example, from the LE form, selected variables could be named as "INR_LE," "CKMB_LE," and so forth. Similarly, from a physical exam (PE) form, variables could be named as "WGTKG_PE" for weight in kilograms and "HGTCM_PE" for height in centimeters. Alternatively, the form abbreviation can be included as a prefix for each variable, such as "PE_WGTKG" for weight in kilograms and "PE_HGTCM" for height in centimeters. Either way, this method helps the data analyst to readily identify specific variables for analyses.

A second guideline refers to naming of suffixes for variables. Specifically, many times validated survey instruments will be used, such as the 20-item CES-D used to measure depressive symptoms. In this instance, it may be helpful to name the variables with a number suffix such as "CES-D_Q1," "CES-D_Q2," "CES-D_Q3," and so forth. The reason for this is that statistical coding written in software packages such as SAS or SPSS permits the analyst to apply data transformation operations or scoring algorithms to ranges of variables, such as "CES-D_Q1–CES-D_Q20." In this way, the code can be written in an efficient manner for all 20 variables as opposed to specifying coding instructions for each individual variable. The downside to naming variables in this way is that the variable name is no longer descriptive, so this naming convention is best for standardized forms that are not likely to change throughout the course of a study.

In terms of variable labels, if possible, it is best to include interpretation information in the label itself. For example, assume on the DG form there is a variable inquiring on history of diabetes, coded as "1" for "Yes" and "0" for "No." The variable name might be "DIABHX_DG" and variable label might be "History of Diabetes: (1 = yes, 0 = no)." Again, the overall goal in selecting variable names and labels is to minimize error, aid in interpretation, and improve efficiency of data analyses.

Data Entry

Even a well-designed database system will fall significantly short of its capabilities in the absence of accurate data entry. As with selection of the CRFs and design of the database, a number of important considerations affect the accuracy and approach to data entry. Entering data in a timely manner will help to avoid missing data and allow for more efficient resolution of data collection errors.

At the most basic level is the question of which individual(s) will perform the data entry. Options include trained research staff personnel (e.g., research assistant), individual study participants, and multiple members of the research team, such as in the case of "double data entry." If the intervention study data are collected on hard copy CRFs, typically the study research staff will enter the data into the study database. In general, study participants will enter study data when this is advantageous, such as when study participants are sampled across broad geographical areas or portable electronic devices such as tablets or laptop computers are available in a clinic setting and web-based data entry is the most efficient approach to collect participant self-assessment data.

If possible, it is best to require double data entry. In this case, one member of the research team enters the data and then a second independent member enters the data. In general, this should not be done in two separate databases but rather into a single database application that evaluates the first entry versus the second entry for consistency. If there is a discrepancy between the two entries, usually the second data entry person will examine and reconcile which value is correct. The goal of double data entry is to reduce the error rate. Of note, both individuals involved in the double data entry must be sufficiently trained in the research protocol. If only one individual is available for data entry, double data entry can be accomplished by having this person enter the data twice with at least 24 hours between the entry sessions. Although there are no firm guidelines on an "acceptable" error rate for data entry, a general rule of thumb is 0.5% or less (in other words, no more than 1 error per 200 data elements entered).

When a web-based data entry system is used (by either research staff or study participants), the system will typically have a design option whereby all questions must be answered in sequence before proceeding to subsequent questions. This approach is very effective as a means to minimize missing data. However, this practice in the strictest sense must always allow a participant to refuse to answer individual questions. The primary reason to offer a "prefer not to answer" option is that when a participant signs the informed consent form to participate in an intervention study, there is always a statement about the voluntary nature of their participation in the study. The same condition applies to voluntary disclosure of information.

It is always important to be able to distinguish between questions intentionally versus accidentally skipped. For example, if a question of a particularly sensitive nature is not answered, such as sexual history, it is not self-evident as to whether it was intentionally or accidentally skipped by the participant. Thus, a good practice is to include appropriate responses such as "unknown" or "refused/prefer not to answer." Having said this, it is best not to make these choices prominent on the CRF so as to encourage their frequent selection. One option is to include these choices separate from the other responses, and perhaps in a smaller font. Moreover, to minimize missing data, general instructions can be included at the beginning of each form, such as "please try to answer each question as candidly as possible, and your response to each question will be kept confidential and will not affect your care."

Regardless of the type of system used to collect/enter data, an audit trail (preferably in electronic format) of all changes made to the data, and by whom, from the time of entry (e.g., to correct data collection or entry errors) should be maintained. An example of an audit trail is provided in Exhibit 19.6. Common database management systems, such as MS Access, allow the ability to track changes made to the data and produce audit trail results.

EXHIBIT 19.6 Example of Audit Trail

PE: Physical Exam			Audit Trail		
ID	Variable Name	Old Value	New Value	Dcid	Date Changed
1	WGTKG_PE	45	54	JDI	07/01/16
1	BPS_PE	120	110	JDI	07/01/16
4	HGTCM_PE	142.4	152.4	DKM	07/15/16
7	EXAMDATE	07/30/16	07/20/16	JDI	08/01/16

"Automatic" Data Entry

Sometimes, no direct data entry will be required, such as when laboratory results from blood tests are generated in an electronic format, such as a Microsoft Excel spreadsheet. In this case, the key challenge will be to establish a set format for the data that will be maintained throughout the course of the study so that these data can be merged into the main study database. At the most basic level, there will be need of a common, unique study ID number used in both the study database and the electronic data source. A limitation of such "automatic" data is that specific desired formats such as variable names and response categories, labels, units of measurement, and so forth cannot always be specified for study purposes. To illustrate, the data shown in Table 19.3 that are fictitiously extracted directly from laboratory analyses show that for the variable "patient sex," too many possible responses are provided, including both "Female" and "F" for female, "Male" and

TABLE 19.3 Example of Fictitious Laboratory Data Automatically Generated

CLIENT NUMBER	DATE OF VISIT	DATE DRAWN	DATE TESTED	PATIENT SEX	TOTAL CHOL (TC)	DESIRED TC
2501	July 14, 2004	July 14, 2004	August 5, 2004	Female	221	<200 mg/dL
2502	July 20, 2005	July 20, 2005	July 28, 2005	Female	190	<200 mg/dL
2503	August 5, 2003	August 5, 2003	September 10, 2003	Female	215	<200 mg/dL
2504	March 15, 2005	March 15, 2005	April 7, 2005	Female	178	<200 mg/dL
2505	August 7, 2003	August 7, 2003	September 10, 2003	Female	155	<200 mg/dL
2506	April 6, 2005	April 6, 2005	April 7, 2005		178	<200 mg/dL
2507	August 12, 2003	August 12, 2003	September 12, 2003	Male	276	<200 mg/dL
2508	August 2, 2005	August 2, 2005	September 2, 2005	U	189	<200 mg/dL
2509	July 21, 2004	July 21, 2004	August 5, 2004	Male	241	<200 mg/dL
2510	August 16, 2004	August 16, 2004	September 8, 2004	Male	208	<200 mg/dL
2511	August 14, 2003	August 14, 2003	September 10, 2003	F	192	<200 mg/dL
2512	August 11, 2005	August 11, 2005	September 2, 2005	Male	174	<200 mg/dL

(continued)

TABLE 19.3 Example of Fictitious Laboratory Data Automatically Generated *(continued)*

CLIENT NUMBER	DATE OF VISIT	DATE DRAWN	DATE TESTED	PATIENT SEX	TOTAL CHOL (TC)	DESIRED TC
2513	August 19, 2003	August 19, 2003	September 10, 2003	Male	251	<200 mg/dL
2514	August 4, 2005	August 4, 2005	September 2, 2005	Male	254	<200 mg/dL
2515	July 29, 2004	July 29, 2004	August 5, 2004	Male	287	<200 mg/dL
2516	September 2, 2005	September 2, 2005	October 7, 2005	Male	160	<200 mg/dL
2517	October 20, 2004	October 20, 2004	November 15, 2004	M	159	<200 mg/dL
2518	August 20, 2003	August 20, 2003	September 10, 2003		161	<200 mg/dL
2519	October 20, 2004	October 20, 2004	November 15, 2004	Female	237	<200 mg/dL
2520	September 2, 2005	September 2, 2005	October 11, 2005	Female	185	<200 mg/dL

"M" for male, missing (blank), and "U" (unknown) for sex not reported. If these data cannot be provided in a more consistent format, the data will have to be recoded to make sure that only the three mutually exclusive categories of "female," "male," and "missing" exist in the database.

Finally, as stated earlier, there exist nowadays various optical scanning systems that can "read" data that are captured on hard copy CRFs into a database system. This method of entry is implemented most efficiently when the CRFs are developed using the OCR software. This type of system may be particularly valuable for intervention studies with multiple forms, a large number of variables, and repeated assessments (i.e., a large volume of study data). Of note, each individual page of the CRFs to be scanned must include the study participant ID number. Critical to the success of use of an optical scanning system is ensuring that all scanned data are verified as accurately captured (scanned) as determined through visual review of the hard copy/PDF version of the completed CRF versus the information that resides in the database.

Quality Control and Assurance

Methods and comprehensiveness of quality control and assurance procedures can vary greatly across intervention studies, particularly in the setting of multicenter clinical trials and whether multiple individuals will be involved in the data collection and entry. Standardization of processes is paramount, that is, all persons involved in data collection and entry capture the data in a consistent, rigorous manner. Data collection/entry systems that provide point of entry checks (i.e., range, data type and format, simple logic) are ideal to identify and resolve data inconsistencies and minimize missing data in real time. At the broadest level, it is always good practice to conduct an audit of a random set of data captured and entered into the study database. This can include auditing a random sample of selected charts for accurate extraction onto the CRFs and subsequent audit of data collected on the CRF accurately entered into the database.

Within the setting of a single-site intervention study, quality control and assurance procedures will frequently center on minimizing missing information, examining ambiguity in participant responses, and accurate reporting of data. To be as proactive as possible, all CRFs should be pilot tested prior to implementation. Similarly, once data have been collected for the first few participants in the intervention study, they should be reviewed in a time-sensitive manner to identify deficiencies early in the process. Notable areas of investigation and potential problems include (a) specific variables that tend to have missing responses and (b) unusual patterns and distributions of data responses.

With respect to missing responses, several potential explanations exist. These include selective omission of data by study participants, such as for questions of a sensitive nature, lack of understanding by the participant in the information being requested, and, depending on the amount of data being collected, participant fatigue. When a significant amount of missing data is identified early in the data collection process, careful examination is needed to identify the root causes and corrective actions. One important point related to data entry (or lack thereof) of variables with missing data—in general, when data are missing for a specific variable—is the following: It is best to properly "code" the reason for missing, or, if this is not possible, to simply leave this field empty in the database. For example, as described earlier, a response choice of "unknown" would be a true indicator of missing data (information), whereas a response choice of "prefer not to answer" would represent a valid (nonmissing) response. As a general rule, missing responses, "unknown" responses, and "prefer not to answer" responses should be coded in the database using letters such as "A," "B," and "C" rather than numbers. The principal reason for this is to make sure that the data analyst recognizes the nature of missing information before performing numerical analyses.

Unusual data patterns are too numerous to list in entirety, but, nonetheless, signal potential problems in the data collection process. For example, assume that a study participant is required to complete a large battery of self-report questionnaires. If responses to questionnaires completed first show more variability (e.g., full use of a 1–5 rating scale) compared with responses to questionnaires completed later (e.g., consistent selection of only the number 3 response), this may be an indication of participant fatigue and haphazard reporting of information. As a second example, if "bimodal" distributions for a continuous variable are seen, this may signal inconsistent interpretation by study participants or data collection personnel. To illustrate, if total cholesterol level is the variable of interest, groups of values ranging from 4.0 to 8.0 and 150 to 300 would indicate data being captured inconsistently in units of mmol/L and mg/dL, respectively. If unusual patterns of data appear to be evident, the best solution is to go back to the source documentation, if possible, to examine accuracy of the information. In the hypothetical example about potential "participant fatigue," there is no obvious solution (i.e., whether to include the potential "problematic" data). One compromise is a "sensitivity" analysis whereby statistical analyses are conducted both with and without the potentially problematic data.

Once all data have been collected, they should be "cleaned" and saved as a "locked" database. The "cleaning" process should be comprehensive and rigorous, but at the most basic level, it involves careful review of the frequencies and ranges of all variables to look for missing, outlying, and potential erroneous values. In the ideal world, all potential inaccuracies and missing data should be rigorously investigated and resolved. However, this may entail considerable effort in reviewing individual medical charts and other source documentation. Therefore, there are general guidelines for prioritization. In particular, in intervention studies, there is normally a primary outcome and one or more secondary outcome variables specified. It is paramount that these variables be accurately collected and entered into the database. At the other extreme, there are usually covariates that are of lesser importance analytically, such as the participant's age at the time of high school graduation. Although every data element should be cleaned, maximum time should be allocated to the primary and secondary outcome variables.

Finally, comprehensive, user-friendly documentation of the study and database is critically important. Data collected from intervention studies tend to be very valuable and unique. Although not always envisioned at the onset, these data may ultimately be made available to other investigators (e.g., faculty and doctoral students). Of note, this practice is permissible when the original informed consent form signed by participants stated that other researchers may make use of the data and will make every effort to maintain strict confidentiality. Given the potential for sharing of data, try to be as complete and diligent as possible in developing the documentation for the data forms, study procedures, and database. Consider existing variable naming and coding conventions when data being collected are common within or across areas of study. For example, demographic information is collected across many fields of study and individual variables (e.g., date of birth, sex, race) can be annotated consistently across studies. This will help to minimize error and maximize efficiency in the use of these data by study personnel and other investigators. Oftentimes, the data are made available as a "limited data set" that include a subset of the main study variables, particularly for intervention studies that are complex and have a very large number of variables.

A data collection timeline to list the data forms, when they are completed and by whom they are completed, is often helpful when there are several data collection forms or research personnel involved with a study. An example of a data collection timeline is provided in Table 19.4.

TABLE 19.4 Example of Data Collection Timeline

	SCREEN	BASELINE	TREATMENT WEEK 4	TREATMENT WEEK 12	TREATMENT WEEK 24	TREATMENT WEEK 48
SE: screening evaluation	RC					
BC: baseline evaluation		RC				
PE: physical exam		PI		PI		PI
SF: SF-36		PT				PT
CD: CES-D		PT		PT	PT	PT
LE: laboratory evaluation		RC	RC	RC	RC	RC

CES-D, Center for Epidemiologic Studies Depression Scale; PI, physician investigator; PT, participant; RC, research coordinator; SF-36, Short-Form Health Survey.

An MOP should be developed to document study-specific definitions and instructions for data collection. An example of an MOP for the PE form is provided in Exhibit 19.7.

An example of documentation (in SAS format) for data collected from a "PE" CRF is provided in Exhibit 19.8.

Form level codebooks help to ensure proper use of data. An example of a form codebook for the PE form in seen in Exhibit 19.9.

Data sharing and data reuse principles and policies have been evolving and there has been increased attention from study sponsors and scientific journals to establish and enforce timelines for sharing clinical trial data. The PI will need to be knowledgeable of the

---

EXHIBIT 19.7   Example of Manual of Operation

Title of Intervention Study

Physical Exam MOP

General Instructions

The physical exam form is completed at the time of the baseline assessment and all subsequent protocol visits.

This form captures information obtained from a combination of sources —participant interview, medical record review, and a physical exam. When information in the medical record conflicts with information provided by the participant, the medical record is normally considered to be the accurate source, although there may be instances when the information provided by the participant is more up to date or accurate. In this instance, the information provided by the participant may be used.

Research personnel are responsible for obtaining the information captured on this form.

Specific Instructions

Participant ID:	Record the participant ID number in the top right corner of each page.
Date of evaluation:	Record the date (month/day/year) that corresponds to the assessment visit.
Protocol time point:	Record the protocol time point that corresponds to the assessment visit.

Section I: Physical Exam

Height:	Record the participant's height in inches at the time of the physical exam. Ask the participant to remove shoes before obtaining the measurement. If height was not measured at the time of the exam, then check "Not done." If for any reason (e.g., wheelchair-bound, equipment failure) a standing measurement is not obtained, record "Not done."
Weight:	Record the participant's weight in pounds at the time of the physical exam. If weight was not measured at the time of the exam, then check "Not done."
Blood pressure:	Record the participant's systolic and diastolic blood pressure in mmHg. Blood pressure should be obtained after the participant has been seated with both feet flat on the floor for at least 5 minutes. If blood pressure was not measured, then check "Not done."

MOP, manual of operation.

EXHIBIT 19.8 Example of Data Set Documentation

Form 5	Physical Exam
Observations	
Baseline	1,998
6 months	315
1 year	1,686
2 year	1,583
3 year	1,548
Baseline data set	
Name	Form5_PE_Base
Observations	1,998
Variables	23
Visits data set	
Name	Form5_PE_Visits
Observations	7,130
Variables	23
All data set	
Name	Form5_PE_All
Observations	2,000 (including 2 without baseline data)
Variables	106

Alphabetical List of Variables and Attributes

Variable	Type	Length Format	Informant Label
IDNUM	Num 8	BEST14. 14.	Participant ID
BMI_PE	Num 8		Body mass index
BP_CLASS_PE	Num 8	BPCLASS.	BP classification
BPD_PE	Num 8	BEST20. 20.	Diastolic BP (mmHg)
BPS_PE	Num 8	BEST20. 20.	Systolic BP (mmHg)
EXAMDATE_PE	Num 8	DATE9.	Date of exam
HGTCM_PE	Num 8	BEST14. 14.	Height (cm)
WGTKG_PE	Num 8	BEST14. 14.	Weight (kg)
HIPCM_PE	Num 8	BEST14. 14.	Hip circumference (cm)
ILIAC_PE	Num 8	BEST14. 14.	Skin fold: iliac crest (cm)
PECTORAL_PE	Num 8	BEST14. 14.	Skin fold: pectoral (cm)
REST_PULSE_PE	Num 8	BEST14. 14.	Resting pulse (minutes)

The complete listing of all variables would follow those listed above.

EXHIBIT 19.9 Example of Form Level Codebook

Title of Intervention Study

Physical Exam

Participant ID: ID
Exam Date: EXAMDATE
Protocol Time point: TMPT

SECTION I: PHYSICAL EXAM

1. Height (cm): **HGTCM_PE**   ☐ Not done   **Note:** 1 inch = 2.54 cm

2. Weight (kg): **WGTKG_PE**   ☐ Not done   **Note:** 1 lb = 0.45 kg

3. Blood pressure (mmHg): _____ / _____   ☐ Not done **BPS_PE/BPD_PE**

---

data-sharing guidelines and requirements of the study sponsor prior to study start. Many intervention studies are funded by federal organizations, such as the National Institutes of Health (NIH), and these organizations have established policies for data sharing (e.g., NIH Data Sharing Policy and Implementation Guidance, grants.nih.gov/grants/policy/data_ sharing/data_sharing_guidance.htm) as well as guidelines for dissemination and reporting of information (grants.nih.gov/grants/guide/notice-files/NOT-OD-16-149.html). The investigator must also be aware of data-sharing requirements from individual journals when preparing and submitting a manuscript.

Data Privacy, Protection, and Security

In today's research environment, and for both federally funded and industry-funded intervention studies, there exists a premium on data privacy, protection, and security. Study protocols and informed consent forms used in intervention studies routinely include specific language for data privacy, protection, and security. Relevant examples include the following:

- "The original signed consent form will be retained in the study participant's file in a locked filing cabinet in the office of the principal investigator (PI) and stored for a period of 5 years."
- "All paper study records will be stored in a locked filing cabinet in the office of the PI, and all electronic study files will be stored on a password-protected computer on a server that is backed up nightly. Access to study files will be limited exclusively to designated members of the research staff."
- "To protect confidentiality, each study participant will be designated with a study-specific identification number that does not contain personal identifying information (e.g., 10001)."

Full compliance with the Health Insurance Portability and Accountability Act (HIPAA) first enacted by the U.S. Congress in 1996 is of utmost importance. This includes the "Privacy Rule" that regulates the use and disclosure of protected health information (PHI; i.e., healthcare information that can be linked to an individual; U.S. Government, 2010) and the "Security Rule" that deals specifically with electronic protected health information (EPHI). This includes (a) physical safeguards (i.e., controlling inappropriate physical access to protected data), (b) technical safeguards (i.e., controlling inappropriate access to computer systems and PHI transmitted electronically over open networks), and (c) administrative safeguards (i.e., organizational commitment to data protection, privacy, and security such as by ongoing training programs on the handling of PHI). Compliance of study personnel with good clinical practice (GCP) training is also necessary for NIH-funded trials (grants.nih.gov/grants/guide/notice-files/NOT-OD-16-148.html). The following general data management and handling guidelines should be rigorously followed for the conduct of a given intervention study:

■ Limit the amount of personal identifying information collected on study participants to only data that are truly essential. For example, collection of Social Security number or medical record number is almost never required in intervention studies.

■ Assign each study participant a unique deidentified (i.e., fictitious) study ID. Maintain a master listing that links participant identifying information to the deidentified IDs in a secure manner (e.g., locked cabinet or password-protected file), separate from participant's study chart, and limit access to this listing to only essential study personnel.

■ Maintain this information in a "double-locked" manner, such as a locked office and locked filing cabinet within the office, for data collected on hard copy CRFs.

■ Permit access by authorized personnel only by use of designated usernames and passwords, and update (change) such information at various intervals throughout the study for data collected and maintained electronically. In addition, back up study data on a frequent basis (e.g., daily) on a secure site, such as restricted access network.

■ Limit the number of research staff members who will have access to study data (hard copy or electronic) and make sure that all such persons have been trained in data privacy, protection, and security.

■ Never leave hard copy CRF data unattended, such as on one's desk, and, similarly, do not leave electronically accessed data unattended, such as walking away from one's computer.

SUMMARY

Development of an effective and efficient data management system is an integral part of conducting a valid and productive intervention study. The same fervor in which scientific hypotheses and areas of inquiries are to be pursued in the intervention study should be applied to data management for the study. This includes involvement from the preplanning phase to study completion. Failure to recognize the critical importance of effective data management will undermine the efforts of even the most committed and well-meaning study investigators.

Key Points From This Chapter

■ Data management, which includes collection, entry, and management of study data, is truly a "rate-limiting" step in conducting a valid intervention study. In short, no amount of ingenuity on the part of the study investigators will rescue an intervention study with poorly collected data.

■ The hard copy CRF is the blueprint for all data collection and management irrespective of whether the data are ultimately collected on paper forms or electronically, such as through a data entry website or computer-assisted mechanism. Exquisite attention to detail is required in developing the CRFs to minimize errors and maximize study efficiency.

- Appropriate design and structure of the study database is paramount. Ideally, the database should be "relational" (i.e., user can specify the relationships between different variables and tables in the database) and possess important quality control features, such as range checks for data values, and the capacity to audit entry of all data collected and modified (e.g., through double data entry).

- Selection of study variables should strive for the minimum amount of data collection required, minimize ambiguity in the data collection process, and include reliable and valid questions. Although not always self-evident, every piece of data to be collected comes with a "price" in terms of effort required for collection, entry, cleaning, and analysis.

- Quality control activities are an integral part of the entire data management process. This includes initial design of CRFs and the study database, pilot testing of forms and systems, random audits of data collected, and thorough cleaning of all data.

REFERENCES

Charlson, M., Szatrowski, T. P., Peterson, J., & Gold, J. (1994). Validation of a combined comorbidity index. *Journal of Clinical Epidemiology, 47*(11), 1245–1251. doi:10.1016/0895-4356(94)90129-5

Checkbox Survey. (n.d.). Checkbox Survey Solutions. Retrieved from http://www.checkbox.com

Derogatis, L. R. (2000). *The Brief Symptom Inventory-18 (BSI-18): Administration, scoring and procedures manual.* Minneapolis, MN: National Computer Systems.

Derogatis, L. R., & Melisaratos, N. (1983). The brief symptom inventory: An introductory report. *Psychological Medicine, 13*(3), 595–605. doi:10.1017/S0033291700048017

Gerritsen, M. G., Sartorius, O. E., vd Veen, F. M., & Meester, G. T. (1993). Data management in multi-center clinical trials and the role of a nation-wide computer network: A 5 year evaluation. *Proceedings of the Annual Symposium on Computer Application in Medical Care,* 659–662.

Gluud, C., & Sørensen, T. I. (1995). New developments in the conduct and management of multi-center trials: An international review of clinical trial units. *Fundamental & Clinical Pharmacology, 9*(3), 284–289. doi:10.1111/j.1472-8206.1995.tb00297.x

Goldstein, H. (2003). *Multilevel statistical models.* New York, NY: Wiley.

Harris, P. A., Taylor, R., Thielke, R., Payne, J., Gonzalez, N., & Conde, J. G. (2009). Research electronic data capture (REDCap): A metadata-driven methodology and workflow process for providing translational research informatics support. *Journal of Biomedical Informatics, 42*(2), 377–381. doi:10.1016/j.jbi.2008.08.010

Knatterud, G. I., Forman, S. A., & Canner, P. L. (1983). The coronary drug project: Design of data forms. *Controlled Clinical Trials, 4*(4), 429–440. doi:10.1016/0197-2456(83)90027-2

Krishnankutty, B., Bellary, S., Kumar, N., & Moodahadu, L. S. (2012). Data management in clinical research: An overview. *Indian Journal of Pharmacology, 44*(2), 168–172. doi:10.4103/0253-7613.93842

Liang, K.-Y., & Zeger, S. L. (1986). Longitudinal data analysis using generalized linear models. *Biometrika, 73*(1), 13–22. doi:10.1093/biomet/73.1.35

Pocock, S. J. (1983). *Clinical trials: A practical approach.* Chichester, UK: Wiley.

Radloff, L. S. (1977). The CES-D Scale: A self-report depression scale for research in the general population. *Applied Psychological Measurement, 1,* 385–401. doi:10.1177/014662167700100306

Survey Monkey. (n.d.). Survey Monkey: Free online survey software and questionnaire tool. Retrieved from http://www.surveymonkey.com

Teleform. (n.d.). Cardiff Teleform. Retrieved from http://www.cardiff.com/products/teleform

Trocky, N., & Brandt, C. (2009). Process of data management. In S. C. Gad (Ed.), *Clinical trials handbook* (pp. 185–202). Hoboken, NJ: Wiley.

U.S. Government, 45 C.F.R. § 164.501 (2010).

Ware, J. E., & Gandek, B. (1994). The SF-36 health survey: Development and use in mental health research and the IQOLA Project. *International Journal of Mental Health, 23*(2), 49–73. doi:10.1080/00207411.1994.11449283

Wright, P., & Haybittle, J. (1979). Design of forms for clinical trials (3). *British Medical Journal, 2*(6191), 650–651. doi:10.1136/bmj.2.6191.650

Analyzing Intervention Studies

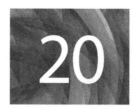

20

Analyzing Intervention Studies

Laura A. Szalacha

> You cannot fix by analysis what you have bungled
> by design. —*Light, Singer, and Willett (1990)*

For those who analyze quantitative data regularly, finally being able to begin the data analyses addressing the research hypotheses and their interpretation is often the "reward" for the past diligent work of properly designing a study with a detailed analytic plan and maintaining good data management practices from the enrollment of the first participant to the end of data collection. Data analysis is sometimes misunderstood as a simple, straightforward application of the analytic plan. It must be noted, however, that even a well-conceived plan requires considerable time, thought, and effort. Poorly executed analyses can introduce bias, which can then result in inaccurate conclusions, and ultimately undermine the intervention entirely (Friedman, Furberg, DeMets, Reboussin, & Granger, 2015).

There exists a plethora of excellent statistical textbooks that provide clear, didactic descriptions of various types of data analysis. As it is well beyond the scope of this chapter to teach how to conduct analytic techniques, you are encouraged to read those texts as you implement the steps of analysis noted herein.

Broadly speaking, there are a minimum of six progressive steps in the analysis of the data from an intervention study:

1. **Evaluate and enhance the quality of your data.** This will involve cleaning the data, assessing the nature of the missing data, and imputing it, if necessary, examining potential outliers and variable distributions indicating the need for transformations.
2. **Assess the psychometric properties** of the scales used, that is, their validity and reliability with your sample.
3. **Assess the potential for bias** by examining study attrition to establish baseline equivalence of the control and intervention groups.

4. **Estimate the univariate descriptive statistics and test bivariate relationships and differences.**
5. **Examine the effects of the intervention** as well as the effects of covariates, mediators, and moderators in the course of the many models you fit with these data.
6. **Conduct** any planned **subgroup analyses.**

After discussing these six steps, this chapter addresses some of the recent developments in the statistical analysis of clustered data and change over time relevant to intervention studies.

The standard analytic approach is to begin with an "eyeball analysis" (Mosteller & Tukey, 1977), that is, plotting out the distributions of all of the variables, using stem-and-leaf displays, box plots, and scatterplots for examination. One then computes descriptive analyses and conducts an exploration of bivariate differences to gain a "feel" for the data. In this exploratory data analysis, there is the opportunity, for example, to consider whether the original scale of measurement for a variable is satisfactory or note potential outliers (Hoaglin, Mosteller, & Tukey, 2000). Subsequently, one tests the specific hypotheses from the study aims, from patterns suggested by the descriptive analyses and examinations of the residuals, and alternate hypotheses from studies reported in the literature. Before data analysis begins in earnest, however, a considerable amount of cleaning, coding, and constructing must be conducted.

EVALUATE AND ENHANCE DATA QUALITY

Data Cleaning

In spite of the numerous advances in data collection procedures, such as Computer-Assisted Survey Information Collection (CASIC) and electronic health record reviews, errors still occur. The first step in the analysis of data is to identify and, if present, correct these errors. Perhaps because it is assumed that these corrections are minor, currently, there exists sparse guidance as to how to set up and conduct efficient and ethical data cleaning. Van den Broeck, Argeseanu Cunningham, Eeckels, and Herbst (2005) propose three phases of data cleaning: screening, diagnosis, and treatment, which ideally occurs throughout the data collection, analysis, and presentation processes.

Screening refers to distinguishing four basic problems: (a) lack or excess of data; (b) outliers, including inconsistencies; (c) unusual patterns in distributions; and (d) unexpected analysis results. This screening can be accomplished with simple descriptive tools (Exhibit 20.1). One can use standard statistical packages to examine normal ranges, distribution shapes, and strength of relationships (Bauer & Johnson, 2000). During the diagnosis phase, one clarifies the true nature of the worrisome data points, patterns, and statistics. "Possible diagnoses for each data point are as follows: erroneous, true extreme, true normal (i.e., the prior expectation was incorrect), or idiopathic (i.e., no explanation found, but still suspect)" (Van den Broeck et al., 2005, p. e267). Some pairs (or more) of related data items are logically or biologically impossible. For example, males cannot have had a pregnancy. Finally, treatment refers to the decisions regarding problematic data points. The three possibilities are to correct, delete, or leave the item unchanged. Impossible values are appropriately corrected or deleted. There is debate as to whether true extreme values should be excluded or remain in the analysis with appropriate sensitivity analyses conducted to ascertain their effect on the outcome (Gardner & Altman, 1994). Regardless, data management must be transparent and responsible researchers must provide the proper documentation of all procedures, including data cleaning (Society for Clinical Data Management, 2005).

EXHIBIT 20.1 Screening Methods

- Checking of questionnaires using fixed algorithms
- Validated data entry and double data entry
- Browsing of data tables after sorting
- Printouts of variables not passing range checks and of records not passing consistency checks
- Graphical exploration of distributions: box plots, histograms, and scatter plots
- Plots of repeated measurements on the same individual, for example, growth curves
- Frequency distributions and crosstabulations
- Summary statistics
- Statistical outlier detection

Source: Adapted from Van den Broeck, J., Argeseanu Cunningham, S., Eeckels, R., & Herbst, K. (2005). Data cleaning: Detecting, diagnosing, and editing data abnormalities. *PLoS Medicine, 2*(10), e267. doi:10.1371/journal.pmed.0020267

Missing Data

As described in the previous chapter, missing observations in an intervention study are, at best, a nuisance and, at worst, a source of the loss of a notable number of subjects' data with the accompanying decrease in precision, loss of statistical power to detect significant differences, complications in data handling and analysis, and the potential introduction of serious bias in estimating both the intervention effects and the within-group differences (Bell & Fairclough, 2013). Little and Rubin (2002) delineated three classes of missing data on the basis of their potential to influence the results of an analysis: (a) missing completely at random (MCAR), the probability of being missing is completely unrelated to all observed and unobserved patient characteristics; (b) missing at random (MAR), often called "ignorable," does not assume that patients with missing values are similar to those with complete data but rather assumes that observed values can be used to "explain" which values are missing and help predict what the missing values would most likely be; and (c) missing not at random (MNAR) or "nonignorable" missing data that occurs when missing values are dependent on unobserved or unknown factors. Formal tests of MCAR versus MAR can be conducted (Little, 1988), but there is no test to distinguish MAR data from MNAR.

There was a time when researchers had to choose among a series of less than ideal solutions with regard to missing data. They could (a) only use complete cases, (b) use the Last-Observation-Carried-Forward (LOCF) method, (c) substitute with the mean from the group, or (d) use multiple regression to estimate the missing values. All of these methods resulted in (a) a severe loss in sample size (and the concomitant loss of statistical power); (b) a biased estimate of the treatment effect; or (c) given that the variance in the sample is artificially reduced, underestimation of standard errors and increased type I error rates (Bell & Fairclough, 2013; Verbeke & Molenberghs, 2000). Fortunately, there are two approaches to attending to MAR data that can produce unbiased estimates with no loss of statistical power: multiple imputation (MI) and maximum likelihood (ML) estimation.

Multiple Imputation

MI is the process of replacing missing data by estimating a distribution of probable values to allow statistical analysis that includes all participants. It is a simulation-based approach that takes into account the uncertainty in the imputed values (Rubin, 2004) and does not suffer from the variance underestimation of simple imputation (Schafer, 1997; 1999).

In MI, each missing data point is replaced by $m > 1$ simulated values (usually five times is sufficient; [Allison, 2003; Li, Stuart, & Allison, 2015]). This produces multiple data sets with identical values for all of the nonmissing values and slightly different values for the imputed values in each data set. Each data set is analyzed separately and the results are subsequently combined. Because of the variation in the imputed values, there should also be variation in the parameter estimates, leading to accurate estimates of standard errors and, therefore, p values that formally incorporate missing data uncertainty. MI is available in SAS, S-Plus, R, SPSS, STATA, and dedicated software such as SOLAS 4.0.

Maximum Likelihood

ML estimation does not impute any data, but rather analyzes each participant's available data to compute ML estimates: the value of the parameter that is most likely to have resulted in the observed data. This likelihood is computed separately for those cases with complete data on some variables and for those with complete data on all variables. These two likelihoods are then maximized together to produce the estimates. Like MI, this method gives unbiased parameter estimates and standard errors that fully account for the fact that some of the data are missing (Allison, 2009). One advantage is that it does not require the careful selection of variables used to impute values that MI requires. On the other hand, it is limited to linear models.

The overarching assumption for both MI and ML is that the data are MAR. Both methods can be extended to data that are MNAR, but the extensions are much more difficult to implement and highly vulnerable to misspecification (Allison, 2003). If the choice is to use MI or ML with MNAR, be certain to conduct a sensitivity analysis (e.g., pattern mixture, selection, and shared parameter models) exploring the consequences of different modeling assumptions as well (Bell & Fairclough, 2013; Little & Rubin, 2002).

PSYCHOMETRICS

In the data reduction phase, one computes many of the variables needed for analysis by constructing scales, indices, and derived variables. Intervention studies will have included a number of scales that have been earlier assessed as reliable and valid with different populations (see Chapter 10). Although some of the classics are the Center for Epidemiologic Studies Depression Scale (CES-D; Radloff, 1977) and General Perceived Self-Efficacy Scale (Schwarzer, 1997), there is considerable enthusiasm for the Patient-Reported Outcomes Measurement Information System (PROMIS) measures.

A National Institutes of Health (NIH)–funded initiative, the **PROMIS** provides access to numerous reliable and valid measures of health status assessing physical, mental, and social well-being for adults and children (Cella et al., 2007).

It is important, nonetheless, to assess the psychometric properties of all of the scales in each study with its specific population. Strictly speaking, one is actually validating the use of the scales with a particular population, rather than the scales themselves.

Scales: A scale is composed of a number of items measuring the same construct. The purpose of a scale is to obtain a more reliable and valid measure of the construct than is possible from any single item. The scale score is summed or averaged across all of the items, after attending to reverse coded items (e.g., "I feel happy" in a depression scale). Established scales will have coding instructions.

Reliability or internal consistency is the ability of an item and of a scale to consistently measure an attribute (DeVon et al., 2007). Scale reliability (internal consistency) is typically assessed by using Cronbach's **alpha coefficient**. Estimating Cronbach's alpha involves examining the relationships between individual items (interitem correlation or agreement), between each item and the remaining items (item–remainder correlation), and between each item and the total scale (item–scale correlation). Cronbach's alpha indicates how well all of the items in a single scale are correlated by estimating the proportion of the total variation of the scale scores that is not attributable to random error. When a reliability coefficient equals 0, the scores reflect nothing but measurement error. Typically, values of 0.70 or greater are acceptable for scales used to analyze associations (Cronbach, 1951). If the scale is used as a clinical instrument for individual patients, its alpha should be at least 0.90 (Nunnally & Bernstein, 1994).

Validity, in a data analytic context, is the degree to which the results of measurement correspond to the true state of the phenomenon being measured. Strictly speaking, validity is not the property of a measure, but an indication of the extent to which an assessment measures a particular construct in a particular context. Scale validity is typically assessed by estimating correlations with measures of other constructs in the study to (a) explicate the theoretical relations among relevant variables (convergent) and (b) examine the degree to which the measure of the construct is not correlated with measures of constructs that it should not (discriminant; see Exhibit 20.2).

Indices: An index is composed of the sum of a group of items, most often binary, to measure a construct, such as a measure of sexual risk behaviors (number of partners, types of partners, use of condoms, use of drugs and alcohol) or lifetime adverse events (divorce, moving, death of a parent). Many times these include lists of check-off items, such as in barriers to breast cancer screening. A summed list of all of the barriers to breast screening covers many different aspects or dimensions, such as not having bus fare or childcare or feeling that medical tests are embarrassing. As each of the items measures a different aspect or dimension, internal consistency measures such as Cronbach's alpha are inappropriate.

Derived variables refer to those that are constructed from a number of different items. For example, the construct of body mass index (BMI) is computed by a combination of age, height, weight, and biological sex (Ogden et al., 2002).

Data Transformations

Many statistical tests have assumptions regarding the normal distribution of variables; many statistical models assume linearity. We use power transformations to meet these assumptions. A transformation is the replacement of a variable by a mathematical function of that variable: for example, replacing a variable x by the square root of x or the logarithm of x.

Various mathematical transformations, up and down "Tukey's ladder" (e.g., logarithms, square root), can be used to "normalize" the outcome variables for appropriate use with such tests. In addition, with severely skewed data, one might establish a cutoff point to recode a continuous variable into a more appropriate binary variable.

EXHIBIT 20.2 Helpful Data Management Hints

Always:
- ✔ Create new variables, rather than recoding the original ones.
- ✔ Inspect individual items before relying on the computed scales, indices, and derived variables.
- ✔ Verify the accuracy of recoding and derived variables by examining contingency tables between the original and derived variables.
- ✔ Examine the scales, indices, and derived variables for floor and ceiling effects, and nonlinearity.

ASSESS POTENTIAL FOR BIAS: ATTRITION

Attrition, the loss of participants from the control or intervention group, is a significant threat to the internal, external, and statistical validity of intervention studies (Marcellus, 2004).

Attrition can occur for the sample as a whole and can be different for the intervention and control groups. Both instances can affect the equivalence of the groups, thus creating potential for bias. There are a number of reasons why participants drop out of intervention studies. Among the most common are greater or milder disease activity, less response to treatment (van den Akker et al., 2007), the presence of mental illness, emotional disturbance, or behavioral concerns (Cotter, Burke, Loeber & Mutchka, 2005; Dierker, Nargiso, Wiseman, & Hoff, 2001). In addition, differential attrition may occur because those participants in a minimal contact control group may become disinterested or participants in intensive intervention group may find the study protocol too burdensome. Analyzing dropout rates and when they occur may give important information about the participant characteristics and intervention characteristics that affect the overall uptake.

Intention-to-Treat

An intention-to-treat (ITT) analysis is a specific data analytic strategy requiring that the outcome data from all of the subjects who were enrolled and randomized to the intervention or attention control groups should be accounted for in the primary analysis (Sackett & Gent, 1979), in the original groups to which they were randomized, regardless of whether they completed the study. The idea of ignoring noncompliance and protocol deviations, even withdrawal, gave rise to the popular phrase, "As randomized, so analyzed." This is a powerful paradigm, as observed differences or associations between groups and differences in relevant outcomes can then be given a causal interpretation (Molenberghs, 2005).

ITT holds that, although not all subjects will have fully complied with the treatment protocol, if the subjects were randomized adequately, noncompliant subjects will be balanced across all the treatment groups (Wang & Bakhai, 2006). The two most important advantages of an ITT analysis are that it preserves the strengths of randomization that was undergone to minimize bias in the first place and it adheres to the a priori power estimates. In its truest form, an ITT analysis can be met only if there are no missing data on the outcome, if missing values are appropriately imputed, fit with ML estimation, or if one fits a pattern mixture, selection, or shared random effects model.

Per-Protocol Analysis

After conducting ITT analyses, a researcher may choose to conduct further analyses of the data with a per-protocol (PP) analysis (also known as an "efficacy analysis"). By focusing analyses only on the fully compliant subjects, you can determine the maximal efficacy of a treatment. Note, however, that a PP analysis could well be biased because those excluded subjects may differ from the analyzed subjects in both measured and unmeasured characteristics. These may be factors that influence the outcome, such as demographics, prognostic factors, and other characteristics that might influence participation or withdrawal from a study (Sedgwick, 2011). Because the subset was not identified prior to randomization, "it cannot be claimed that the properties of randomization apply to this subset, or that the subset provides an unbiased assessment of treatment effects" (Lachin, 2000, p. 169). This bias is the bias in a statistical significance test, that is, the inflation of the type I error beyond the standard 0.05 level.

In summary, an ITT analysis gives a pragmatic estimate of the effect of an intervention in real-world circumstances rather than just the specific efficacy of the intervention itself, as rendered by the PP analysis (Sommer & Zeger, 1991). Ultimately, the ITT analysis provides the most realistic and unbiased assessment of clinical effectiveness.

Establish Baseline Equivalence

Randomization is the preferred approach for equalizing conditions and differences of potentially confounding factors across the different arms of an intervention (Melnyk & Fineout-Overholt, 2005). A crucial step of intervention data analysis is to demonstrate that the intervention and control groups were not significantly different at baseline on key demographic characteristics or other covariates known to be related to the study processes or outcomes. Typically, these include sociodemographic characteristics such as age, biological sex, race/ethnicity, income, health insurance, and education. This may also include predictors strongly related to the study outcomes, such as severity of illness, and the outcome itself. The baseline descriptors are summarized as means and standard deviations or frequencies and percentages depending on the levels of measurement. The analyses are generally bivariate tests of difference (i.e., independent t-tests, F-tests, and contingency table analyses). These analyses are useful not only in assessing comparability but also in describing the sample.

In spite of the best efforts to randomize individuals into the intervention and control groups so that the groups are equivalent, on average, on both observed and unobserved characteristics, systematic differences may still be present. If so, the data analyses must control for these characteristics in all subsequent analyses to ensure that any marginal differences do not bias the impact estimates at follow-up. It is important not to place too much emphasis on any significant differences at baseline, because the cause of differences is either flawed randomization or chance (Assmann, Pocock, Enos, & Kasten, 2000). A nonsignificant imbalance of a strong predictor of the outcome will have more effect on the outcome than a significant imbalance on a variable unrelated to the outcome.

ESTIMATE UNIVARIATE DESCRIPTIVE STATISTICS AND BIVARIATE RELATIONSHIPS AND DIFFERENCES

The substantive analyses begin with the descriptive analyses: measures of frequency (e.g., incidence, prevalence, count) and extent (e.g., means, standard deviations), association, difference, and independence (e.g., correlations, t-tests, F-tests, and contingency table analyses). These serve to describe the sample and to explore responses to the intervention as they may vary by demographic characteristics. Thus, these measures are first estimated for the entire sample and then, if applicable, for subgroups.

Differentiating Efficacy and Effectiveness

There is an often missed, but important distinction between an intervention's efficacy and its effectiveness. Efficacy or explanatory studies determine whether an intervention produces the expected result under *ideal* circumstances. Effectiveness or pragmatic studies measure the degree of beneficial effect under *"real-world"* clinical settings (Godwin et al., 2003). As efficacy research determines the benefit of an intervention to a specific group, it is necessary but not sufficient in establishing effectiveness of interventions (Whittemore & Grey, 2002). Effectiveness research is the critical next step to determine the robustness of the intervention under actual practice conditions (Newman & Tejeda, 1996).

Effect Size

A key question needed to interpret the results of a clinical trial is whether the measured effect size (ES) is clinically important. In other words, knowing the magnitude of an effect enables one to ascertain the practical significance of statistical significance. There are a number of types of ESs. Perhaps the most commonly used is **Cohen's d**, which measures the standardized ES of the difference between two means and is used with t-tests. (Hedge's G

corrects for small sample sizes; Glass's Δ corrects for unequal variances.) It is calculated by subtracting the mean of the control group from the mean of the experimental group and dividing the resultant by the pooled standard deviation. Small, medium, and large effects are designated as 0.2, 0.5, and 0.8, respectively (Cohen, 1988). There are also the **eta-squared** (η^2) and **partial eta-squared** (η_{p}^{2}) that measure the standardized ES of the shared variance between a continuous outcome and categorical predictor(s) and is used with analyses of variance (ANOVAs) and GLMs. **Phi (φ) and Cramer's phi (φ_c)** or V measures the standardized ES of association for the chi-square test. There are various online calculators for these ES measures and they can also be calculated by statistical packages (i.e., SAS, SPSS, and STATA). Moreover, it is possible to convert many ESs to Cohen's d. Other commonly used and easily understood ESs include the following:

Relative risk reduction (RRR): It measures how much the risk is reduced in the intervention group compared with in a control group. For example, if 50% of the control group relapsed and began smoking again and only 25% of the intervention group relapsed, the intervention could be said to be a RRR of 50%.

Absolute risk reduction (ARR): It measures the absolute difference in outcome rates between the intervention and control groups. For example, the ARR for smoking relapse would be 25% or for every 100 participants enrolled in the smoking intervention group, approximately 25 relapses would be avoided.

Number needed to treat (NNT): It measures the number of patients who would need to be in the smoking intervention group to prevent one additional smoking relapse. In this example, NNT = 1/.25 = 4. Thus, for every four participants enrolled in the smoking intervention group, one case of smoking relapse could be prevented.

When interpreting the magnitudes of ESs, "one size" does not fit all. One needs to make a value judgment about the ES (Mordock, 2000). How does the magnitude of the effect fit in the contexts of other interventions? There can be substantial practical and clinical value even in small ESs. According to Litschge, Vaughn, and McCrea (2010), this is especially so, "if a treatment is relatively inexpensive, is easy to execute, is politically feasible, and can be employed on a large scale, thereby affecting large numbers of individuals" (p. 22).

CONTROL AND EXAMINE EFFECTS OF OTHER RELEVANT FACTORS

Covariates

Beyond the effect of the intervention itself, there are three reasons to include a number of covariates in the final model(s). First, several demographic characteristics are standard in examining interventions, such as biological sex, race/ethnicity, age, education, income, relationship status, sexual identification, and so on. Second, there are alternative hypotheses to be tested. Third, to compare and contrast the findings of this intervention with many of the other studies in the same area, one needs to be able to control for those variables controlled for in those other studies as well. Science, in general, is built on replication and intervention science is no different.

Mediators

In intervention studies, the objectives include determining not only whether an intervention is effective but also how or through which mechanism(s) it works. Mediators identify the essential processes that must occur for a predictor to have an effect on an outcome (Shadish, Cook, & Campbell, 2002). The causal steps proposed by Judd and Kenny (1981) and Baron and Kenny (1986) have been challenged on the bases of statistical power and accurate Type I error rates (MacKinnon, Lockwood, Hoffmann, West, & Sheets, 2002). The best balance of Type I error and statistical power among tests of mediation is to test the joint significance of the two effects (predictor to mediator and mediator to outcome) comprising the intervening variable effect.

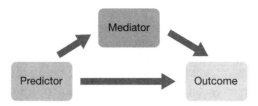

Moderators or Interaction Effects

A moderator is an independent variable that affects the strength and/or direction of the association between a predictor and an outcome. When responses to an intervention vary depending on the level of an individual characteristic, such as biological sex, race/ethnicity, illness- or disease-related factors, the intervention and the individual characteristic "interact." Moderators identify on whom and under which circumstances treatments have different effects.

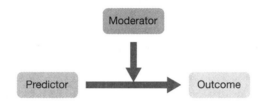

Categorical moderators can be analyzed using standard analysis of covariance procedures, followed by analyses using simple contrasts. Continuous moderators can be tested using regression procedures (Aiken & West, 1991).

An important consideration in interpreting interactions is whether the theorized moderator is the true moderator or some other variable with which the theorized moderator is correlated. Kenny explains the possibilities when examining an interaction with biological sex. The true moderator could be masculinity–femininity, gender role expectations, or even body type. "Unless the moderator is a manipulated variable, you cannot know whether it is a 'true' moderator or just a 'proxy' moderator" (D. A. Kenny, www.davidakenny.net/cm/moderation.htm).

Many statistical interactions can be missed because they can occur even in the absence of any main effects of the independent predictors (Aiken &West, 1991). This is crucial because an interaction could explain why there were no significant group effects or an intervention results in a small overall effect. Moreover, there are more than just two-way interactions. There are three- and four-way interactions. It is incumbent on the data analyst to test all those interactions hypothesized by underpinning theory as well as those suggested by the data analysis (Dawson & Richter, 2006).

SUBGROUP ANALYSES

As noted by Friedman et al. (2015), one of the most frequently asked questions of an intervention is the following: "Among which group of participants is the intervention most beneficial or harmful?" (p. 371). Subgroup analyses, that is, any evaluation of treatment effects for a specific end point in subgroups of participants defined by baseline character-istics, must be conducted to refine the primary hypothesis and to specify for whom the intervention is best. This technique involves extracting the data of a subset of the sample (on the basis of an individual characteristic) and analyzing them separately for interven-tion effect. Such subgroup analyses, however, can also lead to overstated and misleading results (Lagakos, 2006; Rothwell, 2005).

The most appropriate subgroup analyses are those for which there is a clear a priori reason to anticipate differential intervention effects, most often specified in the specific aims of the study. The proper statistical method for assessing differential intervention effects, as mentioned earlier, is a statistical test for interaction. Nevertheless, it is possible that one will find unexpected intervention effects that may prompt conducting relevant subgroup analy-ses. In addition, in the case of multisite interventions, one might expect to examine the results by site in addition to overall, even if just as a data quality and consistency check (Assmann et al., 2000).

One cannot, however, engage in a "fishing expedition," searching for any and all signifi-cant effects. There can be many statistical difficulties with subgroup analyses. First, if not a part of the planned analyses, there may be too few subjects in the subgroups to be able to give a good estimate of the treatment effect. Second, as the number of subgroups increases, the potential for significant findings increases simply by chance because of multiple compari-sons. Stewart and Parmar (1996) explain, "If 10 subgroup analyses are carried out, there is a 40% chance of finding at least one significant false-positive effect (5% significance level)" (p. 271). Finally, even the selection of subgroups post hoc can be biased by the treatment effect itself. In summary, although subgroup analyses should be interpreted cautiously, when properly planned, reported, and interpreted, they can be an important component of inter-vention analyses.

Although it is impossible to adequately present how to fit the many possible models appropriate for analyzing intervention data in one chapter, it is critical to be aware of the developments in multilevel modeling as pertains to intervention research. There are excel-lent texts explaining both the theoretical and statistical underpinnings of multilevel model-ing as well as delineating how to conduct such analyses (e.g., Fitzmaurice, Davidian, Verbeke, & Molenberghs, 2009; Hedeker & Gibbons, 2006; Singer & Willett, 2003).

Clustered Data

There are many intervention study venues in nursing that give rise to clustered data such as when groups are assigned to interventions or when naturally occurring groups in the popu-lation are sampled (Fitzmaurice, 2005). In the first case, in a cluster-randomized intervention study, sites, such as medical clinics or churches, rather than individuals, are randomized to arms of an intervention. Data on the outcomes are collected on all of the individuals, such as patients, healthcare providers, or church attendees, participating within each group. In the second case, clustered data can arise from random sampling of naturally occurring groups, such as patients in hospital units in hospitals, as naturally occurring clusters that might be the primary sampling units in a study. Finally, clustered data are also present in longitudinal interventions. In this case, the cluster is composed of the repeated measurements obtained from each individual at different time points or under different conditions.

The statistical consequences of clustering are, first, that the observations within a group, or within an individual, are more strongly correlated than they are across groups or indi-viduals and, second, the variances are different in different clusters. These correlations and heteroscedasticity violate two crucial assumptions fundamental to many standard statistical techniques: independence and homoscedasticity. When clustering is not addressed in data analysis, the result may be incorrect estimates of precision (e.g., estimated standard errors that are too small, confidence intervals that are too narrow, p values that are too small, or specious inflation of R^2 values; Singer, 1987) and, thus, unavoidable bias in the estimated intervention effects.

Multilevel Models

The modeling approach for the analysis of data organized in hierarchical structures, or, more generally, in multilevel structures, has developed and been applied across a number of disciplines. This has resulted in a variety of names for similar statistical analyses, including "multilevel models" (Snijders & Bosker, 1999), "hierarchical linear models" (Raudenbush & Bryk, 2002), "mixed-effects models" (Laird & Ware, 1982; Pinheiro & Bates, 2000), "random regression models" (Gibbons & Hedeker, 1997), and more.

Multilevel models combine data at different levels in a single model, without aggregation or disaggregation. For a cluster-randomized intervention study, one can model patients (Level 1) in General Practitioners (Level 2), as in the study by Mortsiefer et al. (2008) to optimize the treatment of patients with hypertension. For a random sampling of naturally occurring groups, one can model patients (Level 1) in hospitals (Level 2) as in Cho, Ketefian, Barkauskas, and Smith's (2003) study of the effects of nurse staffing, patient and hospital characteristics on patient adverse events, and medical costs. Finally, for longitudinal interventions, one can model repeated measures (Level 1) over time on several individuals (Level 2), as in the longitudinal study of physical fitness by Haisma et al. (2007) in people with spinal cord injury. Indeed, linear multilevel models have become the standard method of analyzing longitudinal data with continuous outcomes as they allow for the modeling of both average (fixed) effects and individual (random) effects and permit different covariance structures (Peduzzi, Henderson, Hartigan, & Lavori, 2002).

Generalized linear models are routinely used to analyze non-normal response outcomes, that is, dichotomous, ordered categorical, and count data. These have been extended for mixed effects models and are a common choice for analysis of multilevel dichotomous data (Hedeker, 2005, 2008) as well as multilevel longitudinal repeated discrete data. An example of this is the Marion et al. (2008) longitudinal study of the efficacy of the Well Woman Program that modeled the presence of STIs at four points across 15 months using a multilevel random effects model that incorporated time-varying covariates (Guo & Zhao, 2000).

This chapter has touched upon the major steps in analyzing data, with special attention focused on the appropriateness of various types of multilevel analyses for analyzing intervention data. Well-conceived and well-executed analysis is a crucial step in the study and later implementation of interventions.

Key Points From This Chapter

- Neglect exploratory data analysis at your own peril. Getting to know the data well will put you in good stead for later analyses and may even suggest new hypotheses.
- Although it can be tedious, it is imperative to be precise and thorough in data cleaning, assessing the nature of your missing data, coding, and constructing variables.
- An ITT analysis preserves the strengths of randomization that enables the most realistic and unbiased assessment of intervention effectiveness.
- Although subgroup analyses should be interpreted cautiously, when properly planned, reported, and interpreted, they can be an important component of intervention analyses.
- The many types of multilevel analyses hold the most promise for the most accurate intervention analyses.

REFERENCES

Aiken, L. S., & West, S. G. (1991). *Multiple regression: Testing and interpreting interactions*. Newbury Park, CA: Sage.

Allison, P. D. (2003). Missing data techniques for structural equation models. *Journal of Abnormal Psychology, 112*, 545–557. doi:10.1037/0021-843X.112.4.545

Allison, P. D. (2009). Missing data. In R. E. Millsap & A. Maydeu-Olivares (Eds.),*The SAGE handbook of quantitative methods in psychology* (pp. 72–89). Thousand Oaks, CA: Sage Publications.

Assmann, S. F., Pocock, S. J., Enos, L. E., & Kasten, L. (2000). Subgroup analysis and other (mis)uses of baseline data in clinical trials. *Lancet, 355*(9209), 1064–1069. doi:10.1016/S0140-6736(00)02039-0

Baron, R. M., & Kenny, D. A. (1986). The moderator-mediator variable distinction in social psychological research: Conceptual, strategic, and statistical considerations. *Journal of Personality and Social Psychology, 51*(6), 1173–1182. doi:10.1037//0022-3514.51.6.1173

Bauer, U. E., & Johnson, T. M. (2000). Editing Data: What Difference Do Consistency Checks Make? *American Journal of Epidemiology, 151*(9), 921–925. doi:10.1093/oxfordjournals.aje.a010296

Bell, M., & Fairclough, D. (2013). Practical and statistical issues in missing data for longitudinal patient-reported outcomes. *Statistical Methods in Medical Research, 23*(5), 440–159. doi:10.1177/0962280213476378

Cella, D., Yount, S., Rothrock, N., Gershon, R., Cook, K., Reeve, B., … Rose, M. (2007). The patient-reported outcomes measurement information system (PROMIS): Progress of an NIH roadmap cooperative group during its first two years. *Medical Care, 45*(5 Suppl. 1), S3–S11. doi:10.1097/01.mlr.0000258615.42478.55

Cho, S. H., Ketefian, S., Barkauskas, V. H., & Smith, D. G. (2003). The effects of nurse staffing on adverse events, morbidity, mortality, and medical costs. *Nursing Research, 52*(2), 71–79. doi:10.1097/00006199-200303000-00003

Cohen, J. (1988). *Statistical power analysis for the behavioral sciences* (2nd ed.). Hillsdale, NJ: Lawrence Erlbaum.

Cotter, R.B., Burke, J.D., Loeber, R., & Mutchka, J. (2005). Predictors of contact difficulty and refusal in a longitudinal study. *Criminal Behaviour and Mental Health, 15*(2), 126–137. doi.org/10.1002/cbm.46

Cronbach, L. J. (1951). Coefficient alpha and the internal structure of tests. *Psychometrika, 16*(3), 297–334. doi:10.1007/BF02310555

Dawson, J. F., & Richter, A. W. (2006). Probing three-way interactions in moderated multiple regression: Development and application of a slope difference test. *Journal of Applied Psychology, 91*, 917–926. doi:10.1037/0021-9010.91.4.917

DeVon, H. A., Block, M. E., Moyle-Wright, P., Ernst, D. M., Hayden, S. J., Lazzara, D. J., … Kostas-Polston, E. (2007). A psychometric toolbox for testing validity and reliability. *Journal of Nursing Scholarship, 39*(2), 155–164. doi:10.1111/j.1547-5069.2007.00161.x

Dierker, L., Nargiso, J., Wiseman, R., & Hoff, D. (2001). Factors predicting attrition within a community initiated system of care. *Journal of Child and Family Studies, 10*, 367–385. https://doi.org/10.1023/A:1012581027044

Fitzmaurice, G. (2005). Clustered data. In B. S. Everitt & D. C. Howell (Eds.), *Encyclopedia of statistics in behavioral science* (p. 315). Hoboken, NJ: John Wiley & Sons.

Fitzmaurice, G., Davidian, M., Verbeke, G., & Molenberghs, G. (Eds.). (2009). *Longitudinal data analysis*. Boca Raton, FL: Chapman & Hall.

Friedman, L. M., Furberg, C. D., DeMets, D. L., Reboussin, D. M., & Granger, C. B. (2015). *Fundamentals of clinical trials*. New York, NY: Springer.

Gardner, M. J., & Altman, D. G. (1994). *Statistics with confidence*. London, UK: BMJ.

Gibbons, R., & Hedeker, D. (1997). Random effects probit and logistic regression models for three-level data. *Biometrics, 53*(4), 1527–1537. doi:10.2307/2533520

Godwin, M., Ruhland, L., Casson, I., MacDonald, S., Delva, D., Birtwhistle, R., … Seguin R. (2003). Pragmatic controlled clinical trials in primary care: The struggle between external and internal validity. *BMC Medical Research Methodology, 3*, 28. doi:10.1186/1471-2288-3-28

Guo, G., & Zhao, H. (2000). Multilevel modeling for binary data. *Annual Review of Sociology, 26*, 441–462. doi:10.1146/annurev.soc.26.1.441

Haisma, J., Bussmann, J., Stam, H., Sluis, T., Bergen, M., Post, M., . . . Woude, L. V. (2007). Physical fitness in people with a spinal cord injury: The association with complications and duration of rehabilitation. *Clinical Rehabilitation, 21*(10), 932–940. doi:10.1177/0269215507079134

Hedeker, D. (2005). Generalized linear mixed models. In B. Everitt & D. Howell (Eds.), *Encyclopedia of statistics in behavioral science*. New York, NY: Wiley.

Hedeker, D. (2008). Multilevel models for ordinal and nominal variables. In J. de Leeuw & E. Meijer (Eds.), *Handbook of multilevel analysis*. New York, NY: Springer Publishing.

Hedeker, D., & Gibbons, R. D. (2006). *Longitudinal data analysis*. Hoboken, NJ: Wiley.

Hoaglin, D. C., Mosteller, F., & Tukey, J. (2000). *Understanding robust and exploratory data analysis*. Wiley Classics Library. New York, NY: Wiley.

Judd, C. M., & Kenny, D. A. (1981). Process analysis: Estimating mediation in treatment evaluations. *Evaluation Review, 5*(5), 602–619. doi:10.1177/0193841X8100500502

Lachin, J. M. (2000) Statistical conderations of the intent-to-treat principle. *Controlled Clinical Trials, 21*(3), 167–189.

Lagakos, S. W. (2006). The challenge of subgroup analyses: Reporting without distorting. *New England Journal of Medicine, 354*, 1667–1669. doi:10.1056/NEJMp068070

Laird, N. M., & Ware, J. H. (1982). Random-effects models for longitudinal data. *Biometrics, 38*(4), 963. doi:10.2307/2529876

Li, P., Stuart, E., & Allison, D. (2015). Multiple imputation: A flexible tool for handling missing data. *Journal of the American Medical Association, 314*, 1966–1967. doi:10.1001/jama.2015.15281

Litschge, C. M., Vaughn, M. G., & McCrea, C. (2009). The Empirical Status of Treatments for Children and Youth With Conduct Problems: *Research on Social Work Practice, 20*(1), 21–35. doi:10.1177/1049731508331247

Little, R. J. (1988). A Test of Missing Completely at Random for Multivariate Data with Missing Values. *Journal of the American Statistical Association, 83*(404), 1198. doi:10.2307/2290157

Little, R. J. A., & Rubin, D. B. (2002). *Statistical analysis with missing data* (2nd ed.). New York, NY: John Wiley.

MacKinnon, D. P., Lockwood, C. M., Hoffmann, J. M., West, S. G., & Sheets, V. (2002). A comparison of methods to test mediation and other intervening variable effects. *Psychological Methods, 7*(1), 83–104. doi:10.1037//1082-989x.7.1.83

Marcellus, L. (2004). Are we missing anything? Pursuing research on attrition. *Canadian Journal of Nursing Research, 36*, 82–98. PMID: 15551664

Melnyk, B. M., & Fineout-Overholt, E. (2005). *Evidence-based practice in nursing and healthcare: A guide to best practice*. Philadelphia, PA: Lippincott, Williams & Wilkins.

Molenberghs, G. (2005). Intention-to-Treat. In B. S. Everitt & D. C. Howell (Eds.), *Encyclopedia of statistics in behavioral science* (pp. 928–929). Chichester, UK: John Wiley & Sons.

Mordock, J. B. (2000). Outcome assessment: Suggestions for agency practice. *Child Welfare League of America, 79*(6), 689–710.

Mortsiefer, A., Meysen, T., Schumacher, M., Lintges, C., Stamer, M., Schmacke, N., … Schmitten, J. I. (2008). CRISTOPH: A cluster-randomised intervention study to optimise the treatment of patients with hypertension in general practice. *BMC Family Practice, 9*(1). doi:10.1186/1471-2296-9-33

Mosteller, F., & Tukey, J. W. (1977). *Data analysis and regression*. Reading, MA: Addison-Wesley.

Newman, F. L., & Tejeda, M. J. (1996). The need for research that is designed to support decisions in the delivery of mental health services. *American Psychologist, 51*(10), 1040–1049. doi:10.1037//0003-066x.51.10.1040

Nunnally, J. C., & Bernstein, I. H. (1994). *Psychometric theory*. New York, NY: McGraw-Hill.

Ogden, C. L., Kuczmarski, R. J., Flegal, K. M., Mei, Z., Guo, S., Wei, R., … Johnson, C. L. (2002). Centers for Disease Control and Prevention 2000 growth charts for the United States: Improvements to the 1977 National Center for Health Statistics version. *Pediatrics, 109*(1), 45–60. doi:10.1542/peds.109.1.45

Peduzzi, P., Henderson, W., Hartigan, P., & Lavori, P. (2002). Analysis of randomized controlled trials. *Epidemiologic Review, 24*, 26–38. doi:10.1093/epirev/24.1.26

Pinheiro, J. C., & Bates, D. M. (2000). *Mixed effects models in S and S-Plus*. New York, NY: Springer-Verlag.

Radloff, L. S. (1977). The CES-D scale: *Applied Psychological Measurement, 1*(3), 385–401. doi:10.1177/014662167700100306

Raudenbush, S. W., & Bryk, A. S. (2002). *Hierarchical linear models: Applications and data analysis methods* (2nd ed.). Thousand Oaks, CA: Sage.

Rothwell, P. M. (2005). Subgroup analysis in randomised controlled trials: Importance, indications, and interpretation. *The Lancet, 365*(9454), 176–186. doi:10.1016/s0140-6736(05)17709-5

Rubin, D. B. (2004). *Multiple imputation for nonresponse in surveys*. New York, NY: Wiley-Interscience.

Sackett, D. L., & Gent, M. (1979). Controversy in counting and attributing events in clinical trials. *New England Journal of Medicine, 301*(26), 1410–1412. doi:10.1056/nejm197912273012602

Schafer, J. L. (1997). *Analysis of incomplete multivariate data*. London, UK: Chapman & Hall.

Schafer, J. L. (1999). Multiple imputation: A primer. *Statistical Methods in Medical Research, 8*, 3–15. doi:10.1177/096228029900800102

Schwarzer, R. (1997). General perceived self-efficacy in 14 cultures. *Internet Preprint*. Retrieved from http://web.fu-berlin.de/gesund/skalen/Language_Selection/Turkish/Teacher_Self-Efficacy/teacher_self-efficacy.htm

Sedgwick, P. (2011). Analysis by intention to treat. *British Medical Journal, 342*, d2212. doi:10.1136/bmj.d2212

Shadish, W. R., Cook, T. D., & Campbell, D. T. (2002). *Experimental and quasi-experimental design for generalized causal inference*. Boston, MA: Houghton Mifflin.

Singer, J. D. (1987). An Intraclass Correlation model for analyzing multilevel data. *The Journal of Experimental Education, 55*(4), 219–228. doi:10.1080/00220973.1987.10806457

Singer, J. D., & Willett, J. B. (2003). *Applied longitudinal data analysis: Methods for studying change and event occurrence*. New York, NY: Oxford University Press.

Snijders, T., & Bosker, R. (1999). *Multilevel analysis: An introduction to basic and advanced multilevel modeling*. London, UK: Sage.

Society for Clinical Data Management. (2005). *Good clinical data management practices, Version 4.0*. Milwaukee, WI: Author. Retrieved from http://www.bvv.sld.cu/docs/libros/__a_119376865712.pdf

Sommer, A., & Zeger, S. L. (1991). On estimating efficacy from clinical trials. *Statistics in Medicine, 10*, 45–52. doi:10.1002/sim.4780100110

Stewart, L. A., & Parmar, M. K. B. (1996). Bias in the analysis and reporting of randomized controlled trials. *International Journal of Technical Assessment in Health Care, 12*, 264–275. doi:10.1017/S0266462300009612

Van den Broeck, J., Argeseanu Cunningham, S., Eeckels, R., & Herbst, K. (2005). Data cleaning: Detecting, diagnosing, and editing data abnormalities . *PLoS Medicine, 2*(10), e267. doi:10.1371/journal.pmed.0020267

Verbeke, G., & Molenberghs, G. (2000). *Linear mixed models for longitudinal data*. Springer Series in Statistics. New York, NY: Springer-Verlag.

Wang, D., & Bakhai, A. (2006) *Clinical Trials: A practical guide to design, analysis, and reporting*. Chicago, IL: Remedica.

Whittemore, R., & Grey, M. (2002). The systematic development of nursing interventions. *Journal of Nursing Scholarship, 34*(2), 115–120. doi:10.1111/j.1547-5069.2002.00115.x

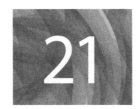

Cost-Effectiveness Analyses for Intervention Studies

Kimberly Arcoleo & Kevin Frick

> The great successful men of the world have used their imagination. They think ahead and create their mental picture in all its details, filling in here, adding a little there, altering this a bit and that a bit, but steadily building—steadily building. —*Robert Collier*

The rapid proliferation of new products, technologies, and interventions in healthcare has led to increasing emphasis on cost-effectiveness analyses (CEAs) to inform policy decisions on the allocation of scarce and potentially diminishing resources. The Centers for Medicare and Medicaid Services estimate that healthcare expenditures are expected to increase, on average, 5.6% annually from 2016 to 2025. Expenditures for 2017 are estimated to be $3,539 billion (18.3% of the gross domestic product [GDP] and projects these figures to increase to $5,549 billion [19.9% of GDP]) by 2025 (Centers for Medicare and Medicaid Services, 2017). In 2016, the Panel on Cost-Effectiveness in Health and Medicine updated and published a set of recommendations for conducting **CEAs** to overcome previous limitations on lack of standardization in methodology and reporting, which hindered appropriate allocation of these resources, and to provide a state of the science review (Sanders et al., 2016). This report provides recommendations for assumptions and methodological practices in CEA that will facilitate broad comparisons across interventions that are studied using randomized controlled trial (RCT) approaches or other types of study designs including modeling exercises. Two significant new recommendations were added. First, the panel suggested that all studies conduct two reference case studies: one from the healthcare system perspective and the other from the societal perspective to more accurately capture the diversity in preferences. Second, as part of the societal case analysis, an "impact inventory" that incorporates all health and nonhealth effects from the intervention should be included providing a more comprehensive assessment of consequences of the intervention (Sanders et al., 2016). There also have been a number of other sets of recommendations since 1996 in the United States and around the world. These recommendations for methods and reporting sometimes focus primarily on the science of comparing a new intervention with the current standard, generalizing results from one setting to another, providing criteria for submitting information for formulary or coverage consideration, or determining thresholds for cost-effective interventions (Chiou et al., 2003; Claxton et al., 2015; Evers, Goossens, deVet, van Tulder, & Ament, 2005; Husereau et al., 2013; Neumann, Cohen, & Weinstein, 2014; Ungar & Santos, 2003).

In this chapter, we discuss the principles of CEA, CEA methodologies, the elements in framing your study, how to design your study to capture relevant cost and outcome data, and organizing your results for publication or presentation.

So what is CEA in healthcare? "Cost effectiveness analysis (CEA) is a method used to evaluate the outcomes and costs of interventions designed to improve health" (Gold, Siegel, Russell, & Weinstein, 1996). Interventions may take many forms: screening tests, primary prevention efforts, biomedical treatment, or social/behavioral intervention programs. Various health outcomes can be evaluated, but the focus is usually on easily quantifiable and critically important outcomes, such as deaths averted, cases of illness avoided, or reduced length of stay for hospitalizations. The goal is to determine whether the improved outcomes of more expensive care are worth the extra costs. Sometimes it is possible to achieve greater effectiveness at lower cost. The results from CEAs are typically reported as the **incremental cost-effectiveness ratio (ICER)**. The numerator represents the incremental cost of intervention B over intervention A. The denominator of the ICER denotes the incremental gain in health status from intervention A to intervention B. Another common reporting method for reporting results is the **quality-adjusted life year (QALY)**, which is described in more detail in the following text.

COST-EFFECTIVENESS ANALYSIS METHODOLOGIES

There are five basic types of economic evaluation methodologies:

1. **Cost-minimization analysis (CMA):** CMA is useful when the outcomes of interest are basically equivalent, and you need to be interested only in comparing costs. For example, in treating hypertension, there are several angiotensin-converting enzyme (ACE) inhibitors currently available that have demonstrated efficacy in reducing mortality. One may choose to carry out a CMA to determine which ones are clinically equivalent (including effectiveness with respect to the primary outcome of interest and side effects) to minimize costs. A published CMA compared two surveillance methods commonly used in intensive care units (ICUs) for screening patients prior to admission for methicillin-resistant *Staphylococcus aureus* (MRSA) infections (Whittington et al., 2017). The two methods are universal preemptive isolation of all patients and targeted isolation of only MRSA-positive patients; the goal was to determine which method minimized inappropriate and overall costs. There are four MRSA-screening tests available and hospitals can choose which to administer. Each screening test was assessed separately for the two surveillance methods. Results of the CMA revealed that for universal preemptive isolation, the total costs were minimized when a polymerase chain reaction screening test, where results are typically returned in 24 hours or less, was used ($82.51/patient). Conventional cultures usually take several days to process resulting in longer periods of isolation and cost $207.60 more per patient for this surveillance method (Whittington et al., 2017). The preferred screening test for the targeted isolation surveillance method was the chromogenic agar 24-hour test that cost $8.54/patient compared with $22.41 more per patient when polymerase chain reaction was used (Whittington et al., 2017).

2. **Cost-consequence analysis (CCA):** The CCA method places the burden of assigning the relative importance of the consequences assessed in relation to their associated costs on the decision maker. Costs and consequences are not aggregated, and the decision maker must make the value judgment trade-offs to integrate all costs and consequences in rendering a final decision (Gold et al., 1996). A CCA was conducted to determine the clinical consequences and costs associated with implementing the Low Risk Ankle Rule for pediatric patients in emergency departments (EDs; Boutis et al., 2015). Of the children presenting to EDs with an ankle injury, 85% to 95% undergo x-ray procedures, yet only 12% of these children actually have a fracture; thus, there are high rates of unnecessary x-rays leading to increased radiation exposure for children and increased costs. There are two validated clinical decision-making tools but only one, the Low Risk Ankle Rule, has high sensitivity and relatively high specificity and thus could potentially dramatically decrease the use of x-rays in these children. This study was conducted in six EDs, three implementing the intervention ($n = 1,055$) and three matched EDs continuing standard practice ($n = 1,096$). EDs that implemented the Low Risk Ankle Rule saved $36.93 per patient compared with standard practice EDs ($p = .02$) and this was attributed to a 23% reduction in ankle x-rays (Boutis et al., 2015). Importantly, the frequency of missed fractures or follow-up use of healthcare resources was not different between groups leading the authors to conclude that widespread implementation of the Low Risk Ankle Rule could result in substantial reductions in children's radiation exposure and healthcare expenses (Boutis et al., 2015).

3. **Cost–benefit analysis (CBA):** CBA values all consequences in monetary units; thus, multiple effects that may not be common to both alternatives can be investigated (Drummond, Sculpher, Torrance, O'Brien, & Stoddart, 2007). A direct comparison of incremental costs and incremental consequences (expressed in the same monetary units as costs) is made, and the preferred strategy is the one demonstrating an incremental net benefit. Both interventions may yield a net benefit compared with no intervention or the status quo, but in this case, we are interested in comparing net benefits between two interventions. There are typically two methods for assigning monetary value to health consequences: willingness to pay and human capital. Willingness to pay can be assessed through validated surveys or by examining trade-off decisions between health and money that individuals make. Human capital values health on the basis of the productive value of people in the economy (Gold et al., 1996). A major criticism of this method is the difficulty and potential subjectivity in assigning monetary values to various nonmonetary outcomes such as lives lost, illness averted, or leisure activities missed. Also, the human capital approach tends to assign a higher value to certain portions of the population, which is sometimes questioned from an ethical viewpoint. It is up to the analyst to assign these values, which may vary widely from study to study. A recent CBA examined the costs and benefits of home-based asthma interventions from the payer perspective (Gomez, Reddy, Dixon, Wilson, & Jacobs, 2017).

    The perspective is an important aspect of every cost-related analysis. Perspective determines what costs and what effects should be considered.

    Home-based asthma interventions have demonstrated efficacy in reducing asthma symptoms, trigger exposure, ED visits and hospitalizations, and missed work and school days, and increasing use of the asthma action plan and controller medications (Krieger, Takaro, Song, Beaudet, & Edwards, 2009), but have not been widely disseminated. This may be because of the fact that many of the economic analyses of asthma interventions are conducted from the societal perspective and rarely the payer perspective. The objective of this study was to evaluate the costs and benefits of the New York State (NYS) Healthy Neighborhoods Program (HNP) from the payer perspective. The NYS HNP conducts home assessments and identifies health and safety hazards and provides information and resources to mitigate those risks. The HNP serves approximately 7,000 households and 2,400 adults and children with asthma across 10 to 15 counties (Gomez et al., 2017). Individuals were classified into an "asthma event" group (individuals with poorly controlled asthma, i.e., one or more clinic, ED, urgent care, or hospital visits because of an exacerbation or an exacerbation in the last 3 months) and an "active asthma" group (individuals in the asthma event group plus those who did not have any medical encounters but were using quick relief and controller medications). The calculation of the average cost of an HNP visit included salary and benefits of the home visitors, travel time, home visit duration, programmatic administrative costs, asthma-specific products, and products provided at all home visits. Benefits measured included the number of healthcare visits (clinic, urgent care, ED, and hospitalizations) for an asthma exacerbation, number of times quick relief medication was used in the past week, and use of daily controller medication in the past week. The results of the CBA revealed that for the asthma event group, $1,083 in medical visits and prescriptions filled per in-home asthma visit was saved. The average cost of the in-home asthma visit was $302. This yielded a net benefit of $781 per asthma visit and benefit:program cost ratio of 3.58. A total of $613 per person was saved per asthma visit and the benefit:program cost ratio was 2.03 and generated a net benefit of $311 for the active asthma group (Gomez et al., 2017). The authors concluded that low-intensity, home environmental asthma interventions produce more modest benefits than higher intensity interventions, but that they are more feasible to scale up while generating substantial cost savings and benefits.

4. **Cost-effectiveness analysis (CEA):** CEA is typically conducted when the aggregated costs of alternative strategies are associated with a single, common consequence (e.g., deaths averted), and the magnitude of the difference between these strategies is examined. The outcomes are measured in natural units such as life years gained, cases averted, or hospital admissions. The results are usually expressed as the ICER and calculated as follows:

$$\text{ICER} = \frac{\text{Cost of strategy A} - \text{Cost of strategy B}}{\text{Effectiveness of strategy A} - \text{Effectiveness of strategy B}}$$

Grabner et al. (2017) carried out a CEA comparing low-density lipoprotein (LDL) levels obtained from nuclear magnetic resonance spectroscopy LDL particle number (LDL-P) with LDL cholesterol (LDL-C) quantified by the standard lipid panel to investigate the economic consequences of treating high-risk patients accordingly to achieve the desired targets on the basis of LDL-P (<1,000 nmol/L) and LDL-C (<100 mg/dL), respectively (Grabner et al., 2017). The number of cardiovascular events was specified as the clinical outcome. Compared with the LDL-C group, the LDL-P group underwent more aggressive treatment to lower lipid levels and had fewer cardiovascular disease (CVD) events during the 36-month follow-up. Although the LDL-P group had greater pharmacy costs, overall medical costs were lower over time. The ICERs varied over time with the intensive intervention actually costing the health plan at 12 months ($23,131 per CVD event avoided), becoming cost equivalent at 24 months ($3,439) and yielding a cost savings (–$4,555) at 36 months. These results suggest that interventions to lower LDL levels using LDL-P thresholds are cost-effective when implemented long-term (Grabner et al., 2017). The 36-month results suggest that the LDL-P dominates LDL-C, as it is more effective and less expensive. If a policy maker had only the 12-month or the 24-month data, a decision on "how much is it worth spending to avert a CVD event?" would need to be made. There are no clear guidelines for each disease condition, so a large element of discretion remains.

5. **Cost-utility analysis (CUA):** CUA is a special type of CEA that includes a quality-of-life measure in the analysis. *Utility* refers to the preference an individual has for a

set of health states and is typically measured on a scale from 0 (death) to 1 (best possible health state). In some cases, it is possible to obtain a negative utility score because an individual may actually prefer death over life in a given health state. Results are usually expressed as QALYs, a metric that combines quality and quantity of life. Other proposed outcome measures are the "healthy years equivalent" (HYE; Mehrez & Gafni, 1993), the "disability-adjusted life year" (DALY; Tan-Torres et al., 2003), and the *saved young life equivalent* (Nord, 1992). The appeal of CUA is that it allows for health-related quality-of-life (HRQOL) adjustments to either a single outcome or a specified set of outcomes, thus weighing more important outcomes and providing a weight for the time in a health state so that survival can be compared with improved quality of life (QoL). The QALY is calculated as the summation of $T \times U$, where T *is the time in health state* and U *the utility of health state*. Discounting (which we discuss later in this chapter) is incorporated to account for the assumption that an individual prefers to sacrifice a portion of the benefits if he or she can accrue them now instead of sometime in the future and also delay costs into the future. In addition, unlike CEA where only a single outcome is assessed, different interventions or programs can be compared using a CUA and resource allocation priorities established more broadly. Results are usually expressed as extra cost/QALY gained. A CUA was recently conducted by Drabo, Hay, Vardavas, Wagner, and Sood (2016) to investigate the cost-effectiveness (using QALYs) of various HIV-prevention strategies for men having sex with men from a societal perspective and lifetime analytical horizon (Drabo et al., 2016). Pre-exposure prophylaxis (PrEP) and test-and-treat (expanded testing and immediate treatment) were demonstrated to provide the greatest decreases in the incidence of HIV and to be highly cost-effective ($27,863/QALY and $19,302/QALY, respectively) compared with standard care (testing and treatment only when CD4 ≤500 cells/μL) and at a willingness-to-pay threshold of $150,000/QALY gained. These analyses also demonstrated that the effectiveness of PrEP is sensitive to the initial HIV prevalence rate, initiation and adherence rates to the medications, probability of HIV transmission, and rates of multiple sexual partners (Drabo et al., 2016). The $150,000/QALY saved threshold is actually high compared with what is commonly used in the United States. The advantage of having a single measure (like QALYs) is that decision makers need to make only one decision on how much it is worth spending to improve health rather than having to decide how much a CVD event averted is worth with a separate figure for all other health conditions. Although only a single threshold is needed, there is no standard in the United States. The $50,000/QALY gained is the most common figure, but it has been used since the 1980s and many authors use $100,000/QALY gained.

Because CUA may involve multiple outcomes derived from different programs, the Public Health Service Panel on Cost-Effectiveness in Health and Medicine (Gold et al., 1996) proposed recommendations for a reference case (a standard set of methodological principles used to capture cost, QOL, and life expectancy). One purpose of the reference case analysis is to compare the health intervention of interest with current practice, best available alternative, or a viable low-cost alternative. In addition, another goal of the reference case analysis is to achieve high-quality, standardized use of science and presentation for ease of study comparability (Gold et al., 1996). The reference case is typically on the basis of the societal perspective. In 2016, the Second Panel on Cost-Effectiveness in Health and Medicine has recommended the addition of a second reference case from the healthcare section perspective because of the differences in preferences and values, interventions, and authority of the decision makers (Sanders et al., 2016).

Table 21.1 summarizes the types of economic methods and the measurement and valuation of the costs and consequences (Drummond et al., 2007).

TABLE 21.1 Measurement and Valuation of Costs and Consequences in Economic Evaluation

EVALUATION METHOD	MEASUREMENT/ VALUATION OF COSTS	IDENTIFICATION OF CONSEQUENCES	MEASUREMENT/ VALUATION OF CONSEQUENCES
CMA	Monetary units	Assumed or shown to be the same	Not necessary because of equivalence
CCA	Monetary units	Multiple effects common to both alternatives	Natural units (e.g., life years gained, cases of disease averted)
CBA	Monetary units	Single or multiple effects, not necessarily common to both alternatives	Monetary units
CEA	Monetary units	Single effect, common to both alternatives but achieved to different degrees	Natural units (e.g., life years gained, cases of disease averted)
CUA	Monetary units	Single or multiple effects, not necessarily common to both alternatives	Healthy years (typically measured as quality-adjusted life years)

CBA, cost–benefit analysis; CCA, cost-consequence analysis; CEA, cost-effectiveness analysis; CMA, cost-minimization analysis; CUA, cost-utility analysis.

Source: Adapted from Drummond, M. F., Sculpher, M. J., Torrance, G. W., O'Brien, B. J., & Stoddart, G. L. (2007). *Methods for the economic evaluation of health care programmes* (3rd ed.). New York, NY. Oxford University Press.

FRAMING THE COST-EFFECTIVENESS ANALYSIS STUDY

The type of economic evaluation you choose will depend on the outcomes to be addressed, the audience/decision maker you are trying to reach, perspective of the analysis, boundaries of the study, interventions or programs to be analyzed, target population, and analytic horizon. Prior to selecting your method, you need to "frame" your study. Framing your study involves careful consideration of decisions to be made regarding the description and design of your study. Understanding how your study results will contribute to the decision-making process is essential because it will guide your selection of the audience and perspective for the study. These key decisions will then inform the remaining design elements such as interventions/programs to be studied, relevant outcomes, intervention time frame, analytical method, types of data to be collected, and analytic horizon. We next discuss these key elements of the study frame in more detail.

Audience for the Study

You want to carefully consider who your target audience is for your study. Normally, the target audience will be those who have decision-making responsibility. Examples of these groups are hospital administrators, managed care organizations, policy makers, and individual healthcare providers. There may also be a secondary audience that is interested in the results but does not hold any decision-making authority. This group may include patients, researchers, and advocacy groups. Sometimes particular decision makers will have specific requirements for how studies are to be conducted and reported (Drummond et al., 2007; Gold et al., 1996).

Perspective of the Analysis

The choice of perspective is important because it guides the types of costs and effects included and their valuation. Typically, studies that address broad allocation of resources adopt the societal perspective. The societal perspective includes all costs and all health effects, regardless of who bears the costs and who obtains the effects. The Second Panel on Cost-Effectiveness in Health and Medicine recommends that a second reference case analysis be included from the healthcare sector perspective (Sanders et al., 2016). If all analysts include all costs and all effects in the reference case analysis, it will help to make studies more comparable. Other perspectives include the patient, caregiver, or insurers.

Boundaries of the Study

The boundaries, or scope, of the study must also be defined. In almost any intervention study, there will be other outcome effects from your program or intervention that are not the primary focus. Some examples might be QOL changes for caregivers, infant health outcomes on the basis of interventions with mothers when pregnant, or impact on children's academic success. As the researcher/analyst, you need to balance incorporating all relevant outcomes with the feasibility of being able to capture all of the data required.

Program or Intervention to Be Analyzed

It is critical that, in framing your study, you precisely define what programs or interventions will be analyzed. Your audience should be able to determine the comparability of your economic evaluation results to other analyses. Describe whether the comparator for the reference case will be standard of care, best available alternative, or a "do nothing" alternative. Include details on frequency and duration of the overall program or intervention and each session, setting where it will take place (e.g., clinic, home, school, and workplace), the target population, and outcomes to be assessed.

Target Population

Choosing the appropriate target population for your study is essential because it can influence your choice of programs/interventions, your economic evaluation, and interpretation of the results. In some circumstances, you may choose to divide the target population into effectiveness, cost, or preference subgroups (Drummond et al., 2007; Gold et al., 1996). The effectiveness subgroups are groups that, on the basis of previous empirical data, would be expected to obtain differing levels of health outcomes from the program or intervention. For example, in a contralateral prophylactic mastectomy study, subgroup analyses were conducted on the basis of presence or absence of the *BRCA* gene because these women have demonstrated a higher risk for developing breast cancer, and age because older women have less risk of future cancer (Zendejas et al., 2011). Cost subgroups might be considered if it is expected that there will be different resource consumption or cost savings between groups because of the program or intervention (Drummond et al., 2007; Gold et al., 1996). The Creating Opportunities for Parent Empowerment (COPE) program for parents of premature infants has been shown to be a cost-effective intervention for reducing depression and anxiety in mothers of preterm infants and length of stay for the babies (Melnyk & Feinstein, 2009). Subgroup analyses also were conducted for babies who weighed less than 1,500 g at birth because these babies typically incur longer lengths of stay and require more medical intervention. Another subgroup that might be considered would be a preference subgroup. Differences in preferences for a given health outcome will lead to differing cost/QALY estimates between groups. Your analysis may reveal that the program or intervention is more cost-effective with a particular preference group. A good example of this is hormone replacement therapy (HRT) for menopausal women. HRT can lower the risk of heart disease and osteoporosis and decrease or eliminate hot flashes, sleep problems, and night sweats but may increase the risk of uterine and breast cancer. One preference group may be more risk-averse to the QOL outcomes from suffering heart disease or osteoporosis, whereas another may fear the risk of cancer more (Gold et al., 1996). A key when analyzing preference subgroups is to determine whether data are available to characterize preferences by subgroup. Because preferences from the societal perspective are usually recommended and are often produced by standard algorithms that score available instruments, a data source would need to be found that provides information about preferences for the subgroups.

Analytic Horizon

The analytic horizon is not the same as your intervention time frame. You want your analytic horizon to extend far enough into the future to capture the major health and economic outcomes. In some cases, this will be until death or even future generations. Because funding for carrying out your study may not cover this period, data modeling techniques must be used. The *keepin' it REAL* substance use prevention intervention has demonstrated efficacy when delivered to middle-school students (Hecht et al., 2003; Marsiglia, Kulis, Booth, Nuño-Gutierrez, & Robbins, 2015). In the original study, the time frame for assessing intervention effects was 14 months postintervention. If we were to carry out an economic evaluation of this program, we may be interested in examining substance use patterns through completion of high school. It may not be possible to secure funding to follow the participants for another 4 to 5 years, so we could use modeled data to carry out the economic evaluation. This is an accepted methodological approach, although the ability to attribute long-run outcomes to short-run interventions is always a matter of concern.

DESIGNING THE STUDY

The conceptual model for your study also will guide your economic evaluation of the study. Your intervention will be designed to have an impact on a single outcome or set of health outcomes. Participants' movements through various health states over the course of the intervention trigger changes in associated costs as well, so it is important at the outset to consider what might be those costs.

Types of Study Designs

Ideally, you would plan to collect your cost and outcome data simultaneously in a single prospective RCT. An advantage of this design is that costs associated with changes in health status are captured at the time they occur, not retrospectively. However, there are a few disadvantages to this design. Many times, piggybacking the economic evaluation onto the RCT is not a feasible option because of financial and research design constraints. Costs may be inflated because of protocol-required visits or tests that may not occur in the real-world setting, and there may be low external validity because of eligibility criteria.

Another option is to design an RCT specifically for the economic evaluation, not to establish efficacy of an intervention. Participants are randomly assigned to the intervention or comparator groups with few additional constraints. With this design, you are investigating the impact of the intervention in a real-world setting, not in a highly controlled clinical environment. External validity will be higher with this design than with the piggybacked design because it more closely approximates what would happen in the general healthcare setting. Several disadvantages include cost—this design is more costly than the piggyback RCT because the entire cost-effectiveness RCT must be funded. These RCTs tend to require more participants and are of longer duration. Because there are no stringent ineligibility/eligibility criteria and few protocol constraints, these types of studies may suffer from participant crossover, bias because of lack of blinding, and introduction of other confounding variables (Drummond et al., 2007; Gold et al., 1996).

A third option is a secondary or retrospective analysis using existing data. These data may be obtained from RCTs, administrative databases, medical records, meta-analyses, or observational studies. These types of designs typically require obtaining data from multiple sources collected at varying points in time. The advantages of this design are that it is relatively inexpensive and can be completed quickly because the data are readily available. Disadvantages are that you need large and comprehensive datasets of the intervention and comparator conditions to control for confounding and selection bias. In addition, these datasets may not contain all of the outcomes or cost data for which you are interested. For example, insurance claims data will provide information about service utilization but nothing about patient survival.

As mentioned earlier, in some cases it may be necessary to use modeling designs to capture all of the outcome effects attributable to your intervention. There are two types of modeling designs: clinical decision-analytic models and epidemiologically based models. Clinical decision-analytic models are typically used when you are carrying out an economic evaluation of programs/interventions targeting current disease/health status. Epidemiologically based models are used when you are interested in examining the probability of future disease/health outcomes. Many prevention interventions would fall into this category. Figure 21.1 illustrates a simple decision tree for two interventions and the associated probabilities for each possible health outcome.

These designs rely on data published earlier, expert clinical opinion, and/or clinical data collected earlier. Similar to the retrospective design, the advantages of modeling designs are the low cost and rapid availability of the data. Disadvantages may include inaccurate estimates and complexity and difficulty of validating the models.

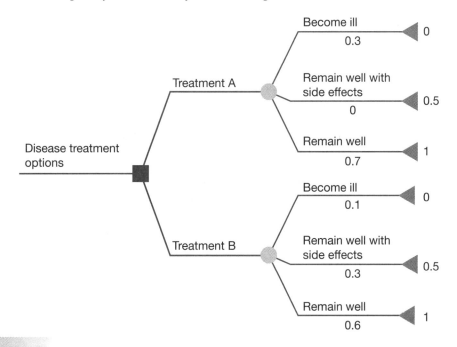

FIGURE 21.1 Decision-analytic model for evaluating two disease-treatment options.

The last design option is a combination design, which may include elements of two or more of the aforementioned designs. You may integrate data obtained from your primary intervention study with similar data published by other researchers and then incorporate modeling techniques to arrive at the final decision.

Data to Be Collected

Once you have determined the type of design you wish to use, you need to consider the relevant cost and other data that you want to include in the economic evaluation, in addition to the clinical outcome data you will collect. These may include healthcare costs associated with the study's outcome events, such as cost to deliver the intervention, hospitalization costs, healthcare provider's fees, outpatient services, pharmaceuticals, and so forth. You also need to consider appropriate nonhealthcare costs such as transportation, child care, loss of productivity, patient time, and caregiver time. If you are conducting a CUA, you will also want to obtain a measure of HRQOL. There are several validated instruments for assessing HRQOL: the Medical Outcomes Survey (MOS) 36-item short-form health survey (SF-36; Ware & Sherbourne, 1992), EQ-5D (EuroQol Group, 1990), and the Health Utilities Index (HUI) Mark 3 (Furlong, Feeny, Torrance, & Barr, 2001).

Discounting and Inflation

When you are prepared to perform the analysis, you will often find that you are using data that were reported or gathered several years earlier. Decision makers (and other audiences who read the peer-reviewed articles that you write) are not interested in knowing how much the intervention and its associated impact cost several years ago. The audience for which you are writing will be interested in the costs at the time they read the article. Thus, reviewers and decision makers will expect that you adjust the costs for inflation. Inflation is common in our day-to-day lives. An audience does not want to know how much an intervention vehicle or fuel cost at the time of intervention but at the time of making a new decision. Even if the analytic horizon is many years into the future, the inflation adjustment is only to the year of publication. We are not in a position to speculate on future inflation.

Discounting is a separate process that places a relative valuation on outcomes and costs in the future compared with those that occur immediately. The relative valuation is on the basis of a discount rate. It is similar to the idea of compound interest. Next year's costs and outcomes are valued a little less. The year after is valued the same amount less than next year as next year to this year. This means that costs and health outcomes in the distant future are valued much less. The key is that discounting provides a structured way of performing this weighing process and the weight on future outcomes can be varied from saying that all outcomes are worth the same, no matter when they occur, to a much lower valuation. After costs and outcomes have been discounted, we refer to the result as the present value.

ORGANIZING RESULTS FOR PUBLICATION AND PRESENTATION

You have carried out your study and analyzed the results, and now it is time to prepare for dissemination of your findings. Just as the reference case analyses have been established to create standardized methodologies for capturing costs, QOL, and life expectancy, there have been various reporting formats proposed for standard reporting of economic evaluations. Although the objectives of these different formats may differ, there are a set of elements common to all that should be included. The Second Panel on Cost-Effectiveness in Health and Medicine has developed a checklist to standardize reporting of economic evaluations (Sanders et al., 2016). The major elements of the checklist are as follows:

- Introduction;
- Study Design and Scope (objectives, audience, analysis type, target population, interventions, boundaries, time horizon, perspective, reference cases, analytical plan);
- Methods and Data (trial- or model-based analysis, outcomes, data sources and preference weights, methods for estimating costs, effects and preference weights, data quality, costing year, inflation and discounting methods, and currency type)
- Impact Inventory
- Results (model validation, reference cases, sensitivity analysis, estimates and graphs of uncertainty, results graphs, aggregate results, and secondary analyses)
- Disclosures
- Discussion (summary of reference case results and sensitivity analyses, comparison to similar economic evaluations, ethical implications, limitations, relevance to policy; Sanders et al., 2016)

If you prepare your document addressing the items mentioned earlier, it will go a long way toward standardizing economic evaluation reports and facilitate interpretation of results across studies. The word or page limitations of some journals may preclude being able to provide all of the aforementioned information, but you may be able to include a technical appendix. If this is not permissible, you may be able to provide the technical document on the Internet through the journal or your institution.

> Nothing can stop the man with the right mental attitude from achieving his goal; nothing on earth can help the man with the wrong mental attitude. —*Thomas Jefferson*

Key Points From This Chapter

- There is increasing emphasis on CEAs to inform policy decisions on allocation of diminishing resources.
- Appropriate selection of CEA methodology is on the basis of the study's objectives.
- Pay close attention to the essential elements for framing and designing a high-quality, scientifically rigorous economic evaluation.
- Adjustments for inflation and discounting should be carried out when using retrospective data (inflation) or assessing valuation of costs and outcomes in the future (discounting).
- The Reporting Checklist for Cost-Effectiveness Analyses guides the publication and interpretation of economic evaluation results.

REFERENCES

Boutis, K., von Keyserlingk, C., Willan, A., Narayanan, U. G., Brison, R., Grootendorst, P., … Goeree, R. (2015). Cost consequence analysis of implementing the low risk ankle rule in emergency departments. *Annals of Emergency Medicine, 66*(5), 455–463. e4. doi:10.1016/j.annemergmed.2015.05.027

Centers for Medicare and Medicaid Services. (2017). National health expenditure data. Retrieved from https://www.cms.gov/Research-Statistics-Data-and-Systems/Statistics-Trends-and-Reports/NationalHealthExpendData/NationalHealthAccountsProjected.html

Chiou, C. F., Hay, J. W., Wallace, J. F., Bloom, B. S., Neumann, P. J., Sullivan, S. D., … Ofman, J. J. (2003). Development and validation of a grading system for the quality of cost-effectiveness studies. *Medical Care, 41*(1), 32–44. doi:10.1097/01.MLR.0000039824.73620.E5

Claxton, K., Martin, S., Soares, M., Rice, N., Spackman, E., Hinde, S., … Sculpher, M. (2015). Methods for the estimation of the NICE cost effectiveness threshold. *Health Technology Assessment, 19*(14), 1–503, v–vi. doi:10.3310/hta19140

Drabo, E. F., Hay, J. W., Vardavas, R., Wagner, Z. R., & Sood, N. (2016). A cost-effectiveness analysis of preexposure prophylaxis for the prevention of HIV among Los Angeles county men who have sex with men. *Clinical Infectious Diseases: An Official Publication of the Infectious Diseases Society of America, 63*(11), 1495–1504. doi:10.1093/cid/ciw578

Drummond, M. F., Sculpher, M. J., Torrance, G. W., O'Brien, B. J., & Stoddart, G. L. (2007). *Methods for the economic evaluation of health care programmes* (3rd ed.). New York, NY: Oxford University Press.

EuroQol Group. (1990). EuroQol: A new facility for the measurement of health-related quality of life. *Health Policy, 16,* 199–208. doi:10.1016/0168-8510(90)90421-9

Evers, S., Goossens, M., deVet, H., van Tulder, M., & Ament, A. (2005). Criteria list for assessment of methodological quality of economic evaluations: Consensus on health economic criteria. *International Journal of Technology Assessment in Health Care, 21*(2), 240–245. doi:10.1017/S0266462305050324

Furlong, W. J., Feeny, D. H., Torrance, G. W., & Barr, R. D. (2001). The health utilities index (HUI) system for assessing health-related quality of life in clinical studies. *Annals of Medicine, 33*(5), 375–384. doi:10.3109/07853890109002092

Gold, M. R., Siegel, J. E., Russell, L. B., & Weinstein, M. C. (Eds.). (1996). *Cost-effectiveness and health and medicine.* New York, NY: Oxford University Press.

Gomez, M., Reddy, A. L., Dixon, S. L., Wilson, J., & Jacobs, D. E. (2017). A cost-benefit analysis of a state-funded healthy homes program for residents with asthma: Findings from the New York state healthy neighborhoods program. *Journal of Public Health Management and Practice: JPHMP, 23*(2), 229–238. doi:10.1097/PHH.0000000000000528

Grabner, M., Winegar, D. A., Punekar, R. S., Quimbo, R. A., Cziraky, M. J., & Cromwell, W. C. (2017). Cost effectiveness of achieving targets of low-density lipoprotein particle number versus low-density lipoprotein cholesterol level. *American Journal of Cardiology, 119*(3), 404–409. doi:10.1016/j.amjcard.2016.10.028

Hecht, M. L., Marsiglia, F. F., Elek, E., Wagstaff, D. A., Kulis, S., Dustman, P., & Miller-Day, M. (2003). Culturally grounded substance use prevention: An evaluation of the keepin' it R.E.A.L. curriculum. *Prevention Science, 4*(4), 233–248. doi:10.1023/A:1026016131401

Husereau, D., Drummond, M., Petrou, S., Carswell, C., Moher, D., Greenberg, D., … Loder, E. (2013). Consolidated health economic evaluation reporting standards (CHEERS) statement. *Cost Effectiveness and Resource Allocation, 11*(1), 6. doi:10.1186/1478-7547-11-6

Krieger, J., Takaro, T. K., Song, L., Beaudet, N., & Edwards, K. (2009). A randomized controlled trial of asthma self-management support comparing clinic-based nurses and in-home community health workers: The Seattle–King county healthy homes II project. *Archives of Pediatrics & Adolescent Medicine, 163*(2), 141–149. doi:10.1001/archpediatrics.2008.532

Marsiglia, F. F., Kulis, S. S., Booth, J. M., Nuño-Gutierrez, B. L., & Robbins, D. E. (2015). Long-term effects of the keepin' it REAL model program in Mexico: Substance use trajectories of Guadalajara middle school students. *Journal of Primary Prevention, 36*(2), 93–104. doi:10.1007/s10935-014-0380-1

Mehrez, A., & Gafni, A. (1993). Healthy-years equivalent versus quality-adjusted life years: In the pursuit of progress. *Medical Decision Making, 13,* 287–292. doi:10.1177/0272989x9301300404

Melnyk, B. M., & Feinstein, N. F. (2009). Reducing hospital expenditures with the COPE (creating opportunities for parent empowerment) program for parents and premature infants: An analysis of direct healthcare neonatal intensive care unit costs and savings. *Nursing Administration Quarterly, 33*(1), 32–37. doi:10.1097/01.NAQ.0000343346.47795.13

Neumann, P. J., Cohen, J. T., & Weinstein, M. C. (2014). Updating cost-effectiveness: The curious resilience of the $50,000-per-QALY threshold. *New England Journal of Medicine, 371*(9), 796–797. doi:10.1056/NEJMp1405158

Nord, E. (1992). An alternative to QALYs: The saved young life equivalent (SAVE). *BMJ (British Medical Journal), 305*(6858), 875–877. doi:10.1136/bmj.305.6858.875

Sanders, G. D., Neumann, P. J., Basu, A., Brock, D. W., Feeny, D., Krahn, M., … Ganiats, T. G. (2016). Recommendations for conduct, methodological practices, and reporting of cost-effectiveness analyses second panel on cost-effectiveness in health and medicine. *Journal of the American Medical Association, 316*(10), 1093–1103. doi:10.1001/jama.2016.12195

Tan-Torres, E. T., Baltussen, R., Adam, T., Hutubessy, R., Acharya, A., Evans, D. B., & Murray, C. J. L. (2003). *Making choices in health: WHO guide to cost-effectiveness analysis.* Geneva, Switzerland: World Health Organization.

Ungar, W. J., & Santos, M. T. (2003). The pediatric quality appraisal questionnaire: An instrument for evaluation of the pediatric health economics literature. *Value Health, 6*(5), 584–594. doi:10.1046/j.1524-4733.2003.65253.x

Ware, J. E., Jr., & Sherbourne, C. D. (1992). The MOS 36-item short-form health survey (SF-36): I. conceptual framework and item selection. *Medical Care, 30*, 473–483. doi:10.1097/00005650-199206000-00002

Whittington, M. D., Curtis, D. J., Atherly, A. J., Bradley, C. J., Lindrooth, R. C., & Campbell, J. D. (2017). Screening test recommendations for methicillin-resistant staphylococcus aureus surveillance practices: A cost-minimization analysis. *American Journal of Infection Control, 45*(7), 704–708. doi:10.1016/j.ajic.2016.12.014

Zendejas, B., Moriarty, J. P., O'Byrne, J., Degnim, A. C., Farley, D. R., & Boughey, J. C. (2011). Cost-effectiveness of contralateral prophylactic mastectomy versus routine surveillance in patients with unilateral breast cancer. *Journal of Clinical Oncology, 29*(22), 2993–3000. doi:10.1200/JCO.2011.35.6956

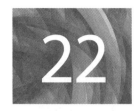

22

Explaining Intervention Effects

Kimberly Arcoleo

> Belief in oneself is one of the most important bricks in building any
> successful venture. —*Lydia M. Child*

Because of the escalating cost of providing healthcare and diminishing financial resources in the United States, many researchers have shifted their focus to developing and testing preventive interventions. The goal of preventive intervention research is to intervene early to improve social, physical, and mental health (Society for Prevention Research, 2017). Preventive intervention programs and strategies are designed to change the intended outcome by targeting risk and protective factors that are hypothesized to be causally related to the outcome (MacKinnon, Fairchild, & Fritz, 2007) and identifying how interventions work and who can benefit most (Fairchild & MacKinnon, 2014). Through empirically derived data, we want to identify potentially modifiable risk factors that *increase* the probability of negative outcomes and protective factors that *decrease* this probability. It is important to not only assess efficacy and cost-effectiveness but also understand the mechanism through which an intervention influences health outcomes to make decisions about resource allocations. All of this information is critical in determining the core components responsible for health outcomes that are essential in disseminating the intervention on a broader scale.

Because we are interested in the investigation of causal pathways from independent variable(s) (IVs) to outcome(s), the required analytical methods are more complex. The focus of this chapter is to define mediation and moderation in intervention research and present various analytical methods to be considered when designing the intervention study. Incorporation of mediating and moderating variables in the analytical model provides valuable information about how, why, when, and for whom the intervention works. So how does one decide what mediating and moderating variables to include? The theoretical framework for the intervention will guide the selection of some of these variables. One may also want to review the empirical evidence for additional variables that have been identified for similar research hypotheses and/or interventions. Mediating and moderating variables can be continuous or categorical and the choice of analytical method may depend on variable type.

MEDIATION

Mediation is a process through which an IV (exogenous) causes variation in another variable (mediator), which then causes variation in a dependent variable (DV; endogenous; Fairchild & MacKinnon, 2014; MacKinnon & Fairchild, 2009). **Mediating variables** explain how or why the outcome occurs, clarifying the underlying mechanism for change. Mediating variables are amenable to change and, thus, are targets of the intervention. Figure 22.1 illustrates a simple mediation model.

In this model, the IV precedes and is a cause of the mediator. The mediator precedes and is a cause of the DV. Traditionally, the conditions for carrying out mediation analyses were the following:

- Significant association between the independent and dependent variables.
- Significant association between the independent variable and the mediator.
- Significant association between the mediator and dependent variable.
- Association between the independent and dependent variables is significantly attenuated after controlling for the mediator (Baron & Kenny, 1986).

Full mediation is present when the relationship between the IV and the DV is reduced to zero after controlling for the mediator. Partial mediation results when the relationship between the IV and the DV is attenuated but not reduced to zero. The drawback of these conditions is that many intervention study designs include multiple mediators. How can additional mediators be tested if the initial mediator completely attenuates the IV–DV relationship?

Recent research into mediation analyses has led to a relaxation of some of these conditions and a shift in emphasis to examining the magnitude and significance of the indirect effects of mediating and suppressor variables (Fairchild & MacKinnon, 2014; Hayes, 2009; MacKinnon et al., 2007; MacKinnon & Pirlott, 2015). Sample size must also be considered when interpreting the results of mediation analyses. Determining whether partial or full mediation is present relies on the p value for the direct effect that is influenced by sample size. The smaller the sample, the more likely mediation will be designated as full because it is easier to achieve a nonsignificant direct effect (Baron & Kenny, 1986). Holding all other factors constant, if the sample size increases, so does the likelihood of statistically significant total effects (Fritz, Cox, & MacKinnon, 2015; Rucker, Preacher, Tormala, & Petty, 2011). Evidence is being generated demonstrating that significant indirect effects may occur in the absence of significant direct or total effects (Fairchild & MacKinnon, 2014; Fritz et al., 2015; Rucker et al., 2011). This may be, in part, because of suppressor variables. A suppressor variable is defined as "a variable that increases the predictive validity of another variable (or a set of variables) by its inclusion in a regression

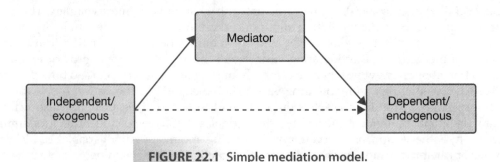

FIGURE 22.1 Simple mediation model.

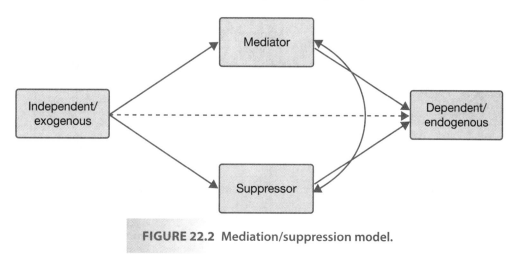

FIGURE 22.2 Mediation/suppression model.

equation" (MacKinnon, Krull, & Lockwood, 2000). When suppression is present, the sign for the indirect effect is *opposite* that for the total effect, and omitting the suppressor variable may result in a small or nonsignificant total effect. Figure 22.2 illustrates a model with mediator and suppressor variables.

If the suppressor variable is omitted, the effect of the IV on the DV is weakened, which can lead to nonsignificant direct and total effects. The following example demonstrates this phenomenon. Knowlden (2014) conducted a study examining the impact of environment, emotional coping, expectations, self-control, and self-efficacy on physical activity and screen time behaviors in children. A secondary objective of this study was to investigate the effects of suppressor variables identified earlier in pediatric obesity-prevention intervention research that can help inform design strategies for these interventions (Knowlden, 2014). Mapping the variables of interest from this study to Figure 22.2, environment, expectations, self-control, and self-efficacy were the IVs, emotional coping was the mediator, and child physical activity behavior was the DV. The correlation matrix, impact of emotional coping on the standardized beta weights of the IVs, multicollinearity, and the beta weight for emotional coping were examined to determine whether emotional coping, in fact, was a suppressor variable. The results revealed that emotional coping was not correlated with child physical activity behavior ($r = 0.09$) but was significantly, positively correlated with environment ($r = 0.48$) and self-efficacy ($r = 0.60$). Removing emotional coping from the structural equation model resulted in a decrease in the R value from 0.22 to 0.14 and self-efficacy was no longer a statistically significant IV ($\beta = 0.09$, $p = .31$). The beta weight for environment also decreased (from 0.47 to 0.32) but remained statistically significant ($p = .001$). There was no evidence of multicollinearity. Although there was positive correlation between emotional coping and child physical activity behavior (0.09; not statistically significant), in the regression model, emotional coping had a negative beta weight suggesting its role as a negative suppressor (Knowlden, 2014). The results of these analyses now provide the researchers with important information, not only about the mechanism of action but also regarding future study designs and analytical models.

Longitudinal mediation may also need to be considered if the goal of the intervention is to change mediating and/or outcome variables from their baseline values and examine these changes over time. It is a mistake to simply include the baseline variable in a standard regression model as a covariate because this does not account for the dependency of the variable measured at (time) T2 on its measurement at T1. Figure 22.3 illustrates a simple longitudinal mediation model. The mediator and outcome variables are measured at baseline prior to the

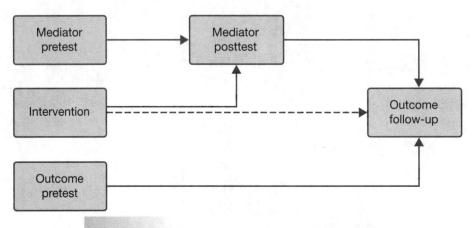

FIGURE 22.3 Simple longitudinal mediation model.

start of the intervention. The mediator is then measured postintervention, and the outcome variable is assessed at some specified time after the postintervention mediator measurement. This method allows the examination of whether the effect of the mediator is stable over time. Longitudinal models also inform causal ordering of mediating variables in the model.

There are three major types of longitudinal mediation models: (a) autoregressive (or cross-lagged panel) model, (b) latent growth model (LGM), and (c) latent difference score model (MacKinnon & Fairchild, 2009; MacKinnon & Pirlott, 2015). The autoregressive model incorporates the dependency between the adjacent mediators as part of the estimation of the longitudinal relationships. The covariances among the variables at T1 and the covariances among the residual variances of the independent, mediating, and DVs at later time periods are specified as well. Figure 22.4 shows a model with four measurement periods and specifies the covariance between the variables over time. One of the restrictions of this model is that variables are influenced only by adjacent variables. As can be seen, mediator T3 is affected only by IV T2, and not IV T3. The only exception to this is that the DV is affected by IV at T2.

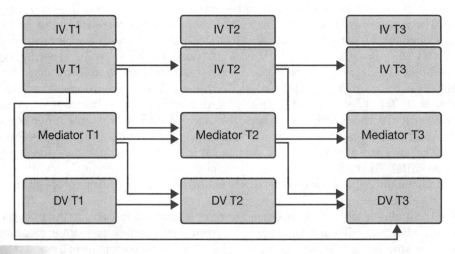

FIGURE 22.4 Autoregressive mediation model.

DV, dependent variable; IV, independent variable.

A major drawback of this model is that it does not explicitly incorporate the effect of time. The variables are ordered so that it is implied that X_2 is measured after X_1 but the actual length of time between these measurements is not specified. Selection of the study duration and lag (length of interval between measurements) is critical. You want to make sure that the study lasts long enough to observe mediation and that you have selected the appropriate developmental intervals to measure the variables. Remember, you will be able to interpret the results from only one interval to the next. This model is most appropriate when you are interested in examining interindividual change and should be used only when it is anticipated that intraindividual change remains fairly stable over time.

When you are interested in evaluating the interindividual and intraindividual changes over time, you may choose to use a LGM. The LGM investigates whether the growth in the IV affects the growth of the mediator, which affects the growth of the DV. One limitation of this model is that the mediation relationship is correlational (MacKinnon et al., 2007; MacKinnon & Pirlott, 2015). The slope of the IV is correlated with the slope of the mediator, and the slope of the mediator is correlated with the slope of the DV. Thus, change in the mediator is associated with a change in the DV *at the same time*, not that a change in the mediator is related to a later change in the DV. With these types of models, measurement invariance is critical because change in measurement over time confounds how we interpret the observed changes in outcomes over time.

We have discussed what mediating and suppressor variables are and walked through an example highlighting the importance of their inclusion in the analyses. We now define and discuss moderation and moderated mediation.

MODERATION

A **moderating variable** is one that affects the strength and/or direction of the relationship between an IV and the DV. Moderating variables help to understand under what conditions the IV influences the DV, for whom the intervention works, and under what conditions the intervention works. In essence, we are seeking information about external validity because we are examining how universal the effect of the intervention was. In an example, which is explored in detail later in this chapter, it was demonstrated in a study of a nurse home visiting intervention that a reduction in physical aggression at the age of 2 years led to an increase in verbal ability at the age of 6 years among females but not among males (Sidora-Arcoleo et al., 2010). Thus, sex was a moderator of the influence of physical aggression on verbal ability.

The choice of moderators should be guided by the theory underlying the intervention, empirical evidence, and/or clinical expertise. Ideally, you want to measure the moderator before measuring the IV. In some cases, the moderator may be a variable that does not change, such as ethnicity, and then the timing of measurement is not as critical. Moderating variables do not need to be correlated with the IVs and, in fact, if they are correlated and the relationship is too strong, there may be problems with estimation (Kenny, 2015). Typically, the effects of moderation are assessed through the interaction of the IV and moderator variable on the DV. A simple regression equation is presented here:

$$Y = i + b_1X + b_2M + b_3XM + e$$

where Y = dependent variable; i = intercept; X = independent variable; b_1 = path coefficient for X; M = moderator; b_2 = path coefficient for M; XM = interaction of X and M; b_3 = path coefficient for XM; and e = error term.

Level of Measurement

Moderators may be continuous or categorical. If the moderator is a continuous variable, then we are examining how the relationship between the IV and the DV differs across different values of the moderator. If the moderator is categorical, then we are assessing how the relationship between IV and DV differs by level of the moderator (Aiken & West, 1991; Fairchild & MacKinnon, 2014; Kenny, 2015). How we interpret the results will depend on the level of measurement of the IV (continuous or categorical). There are four possible combinations: (a) both moderating variable and IVs are categorical, (b) categorical moderator and continuous IV, (c) continuous moderator and categorical IV, and (d) both moderating variable and IV are continuous.

Categorical Moderator and Independent Variables

In the simplest case, each variable will have two levels. Using the previous example, physical aggression may have been coded as a dichotomous variable indicating the presence or absence of physically aggressive behavior. If we were interested in examining physical aggression by males and females, we need to dummy code each of the variables using codes of 0 and 1. Thus, sex would be coded 0 = male and 1 = female, and physical aggression would be coded 0 = absent and 1 = present. Path coefficient a represents the effect of X (physical aggression) when M is 0 (sex = male). Path coefficient b is the effect of M (sex) when X is 0 (physical aggression = absent). Path coefficient c denotes how much the effect of X (physical aggression) changes as M (sex) goes from 0 (male) to 1 (female). When c is positive, the effect of X (physical aggression) on Y (verbal ability) increases as M (sex) goes from 0 (male) to 1 (female). If c is negative, the effect of X on Y decreases as M goes from 0 to 1. If X and M have more than two levels, then it will be necessary to use multiple dummy variables (the number of levels minus 1) and create a set of interaction variables (Kenny, 2015).

Categorical Moderator and Continuous Independent Variable

Continuing with the physical aggression example, in this scenario M (sex) is categorical, X (physical aggression) is a continuous variable, and Y is verbal ability (continuous variable). The assumptions are that the effect of X on Y is linear, and moderation is linear. As M increases (moves from male to female), the linear relationship between X (physical aggression) and Y (verbal ability) increases or decreases (Kenny, 2015). In this example, as M moved from male to female, the relationship between physical aggression and verbal ability decreased and was not statistically significant for females.

Continuous Moderator and Categorical Independent Variable

Here, we might be interested in how maternal depression (M) moderates the effect of the nurse home-visiting intervention (X) on children's physical aggression (Y). One cautionary note: Make sure that 0 is a meaningful value for the moderator variable because the moderator needs to be centered prior to analysis. In this example, a depression score of 0 is valid. There are situations, however, where there is a moderator that was derived from a standardized scale, and the lowest possible score is non-0. It will be necessary to center this variable prior to analysis. There may be interest in examining the effects of X at various levels of M to interpret the results. The specification of these levels should be on the basis of some conceptual rationale. Depression may be classified as exceeding clinical cutoff, borderline, or within normal range. It is also appropriate to use values that are 1 standard deviation (SD) above and 1 SD below the mean.

Continuous Moderator and Independent Variables

As demonstrated earlier, the assumption is made that change is linear. The effect of X (physical aggression) on Y (verbal ability) changes by a constant amount as M (maternal depression) increases or decreases by a fixed amount (Kenny, 2015). If 0 is not a meaningful value for X and M, the variables need to be centered prior to analysis. Another assumption is that X and M are measured without error, a questionable assumption. It has also been demonstrated that power for tests of moderation when the moderator and IV are continuous is typically low, particularly when interaction effects are specified (Judd, Yzerbyt, & Muller, 2014; McClelland & Judd, 1993).

In many intervention studies, there may be multiple moderators in the model. In these cases, the effect of the moderator (M1) on the relationship between the IV and the DV is influenced by the level of another moderator (M2). The regression equation for this model is as follows:

$$Y = i + b_1X + b_2M1 + b_3M2 + b_4XM1 + b_5XM2 + b_6M1M2 + b_7XM1M2 + e$$

We now explore an example of a multiple moderator model. Researchers were interested in testing an adaptive weight loss intervention for obesity targeting African American adolescents (Naar-King et al., 2016). Adolescents aged 12 to 16 years ($n = 181$) who were obese were first randomized (along with their caregivers) to either a 3-month home-based or office-based motivational interviewing plus skills-building intervention. Nonresponders during the first phase were subsequently randomized to the home-based intervention or to receive contingency management. The primary outcome variable was percent overweight and potential moderators of intervention effects were adolescent depression and executive functioning (Naar-King et al., 2016). The primary aims of the study were to examine changes in percent overweight before and after the 3-month intervention to determine whether home-based versus office-based intervention yielded better results. The second aim was to investigate whether contingency management resulted in greater weight loss than continued skills training for adolescents who were nonresponders in phase 1. Weight loss over time was examined for all participants. Moderation was explored by determining whether baseline adolescent depression and executive functioning had differential effects on changes in percentage overweight at each of the posttest periods (3 and 7 months postintervention). Separate models were specified for each moderator. Adolescents with lower executive functioning at baseline in the home-based intervention group did not demonstrate greater reductions in percentage overweight at month 3 [$t = (313.84) = -0.51$, $p = .61$)] or month 7 [$t = (313.90) = -0.18$, $p = .86$)] compared with the office-based group. A similar finding was observed for the moderating effect on weight loss between contingency management and continued skills building in phase 2. Figure 22.5 illustrates that adolescents with greater executive functioning at baseline exhibited greater reductions in percentage overweight at month 7, irrespective of intervention group. The higher executive-functioning group decreased their percentage overweight by 4.39% (95% confidence interval [CI]: 2.53, 6.24) versus 1.51% (95% CI: −0.35 to 3.38) for the lower executive-functioning group (Naar-King et al., 2016).

The same analytical models were run substituting adolescent depression for executive functioning as a moderator. Adolescents with higher levels of depression assigned to the home-based intervention group did not demonstrate greater reductions in percentage overweight compared with their office-based intervention counterparts at month 3 [$t = (313.89) = 0.80$, $p = .94$)] or month 7 [$t = (313.96) = 0.97$, $p = .92$)]. No moderating effect of adolescent depression was observed between contingency management and continued skills building in phase 2. At the end of month 3, there was a marginal moderating effect for adolescent depression on weight loss, irrespective of intervention group [$t(313.89) = 1.73$, $p = .085$], which was attenuated at month 7 [$t(313.96) = 0.65$, $p = .514$]. Adolescents with lower depression scores decreased their percentage overweight by 2.55% (95% CI: 0.70, 4.40) versus 0.27% (95% CI: −1.55 to 2.10) for those with higher depression scores. Interestingly, the findings were reversed from month 3 to 7. Adolescents with *higher* depression scores at baseline had greater reductions in percentage

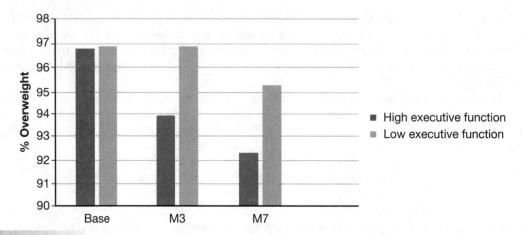

FIGURE 22.5 Moderating effects of executive functioning on longitudinal changes in percentage overweight.

overweight (2.51% [95% CI: 0.66, 4.35]) compared with those with lower depression scores (0.04% [95% CI: F02D1.77 to 1.85]; Naar-King et al., 2016).

This example has provided insight for the researchers as they think about redesigning their intervention. They now have information regarding for whom the intervention might be most effective and under what conditions the intervention might be most effective, and identified mechanisms and processes that might make the intervention differentially effective.

MODERATED MEDIATION

In many intervention studies, we may also want to carry out subgroup analyses to investigate whether the pathways by which the intervention-influenced outcomes differ by these subgroups. This is known as **moderated mediation**. Perrino and colleagues conducted a study synthesizing the results using integrated data analysis from three longitudinal, randomized clinical trials of the Familias Unidas intervention, a family prevention intervention targeting internalizing behaviors in Latino adolescents. The goals of this study were to investigate the mediators and moderators of the intervention on internalizing symptoms (anxiety and depression) to address the questions of how the Familias Unidas intervention works and whether there are differential effects by adolescent subgroups (Perrino et al., 2014). The proposed moderators were internalizing and externalizing symptoms and family communication. The Familias Unidas intervention was theorized to result in greater reductions of internalizing symptoms among adolescents with: (a) higher internalizing symptoms at baseline compared with adolescents with lower symptoms (H1a); (b) higher externalizing symptoms at baseline versus lower symptom levels (H1b); and (c) lower levels of family communication at baseline as opposed to those with higher family communication (H1c). It was hypothesized that improving family communication would mediate the impact of the intervention on adolescents' internalizing symptoms and that this effect would be stronger for adolescents with low levels of family communication at baseline (H2). Linear LGMs were specified for examining each hypothesis and allowing for examining changes over time. Covariates for each model were age, sex, baseline externalizing symptoms and parent–child communication, and the latent intercept for internalizing symptoms. Interactions for each of these variables with intervention were specified. Separate models for each hypothesis assessing moderation were run that tested internalizing symptoms, family communication, and externalizing symptoms (all measured at baseline) as moderators of treatment effects. Figure 22.6 illustrates the results of the moderator analyses for baseline family communication and internalizing symptoms. The results support the hypothesis that baseline internalizing symptoms are a significant moderator of the relationship between the Familias Unidas intervention and trajectory of internalizing symptoms ($b = 0.74$, $SE = 0.32$, $p = .02$). Externalizing symptoms were not a significant moderator of treatment effect on internalizing symptoms ($b = 0.04$, $SE = 0.03$, $p = .22$). Hypothesis 1c was also supported. The effects of Familias Unidas intervention on internalizing symptoms were greater for those adolescents with reported lower levels of baseline family communication ($b = -0.05$, $SE = 0.03$ $p = .03$).

Moderated mediation (H2) was modeled by specifying postintervention family communication as a mediator of the relationship between intervention condition and trajectory of internalizing symptoms. Baseline family communication was specified as a moderator between intervention and postintervention family communication and the internalizing trajectory.

The moderated mediation model included a baseline family communication by intervention interaction term as a predictor of postintervention family communication (mediator) and the trajectory of internalizing symptoms (outcome). Figure 22.7 depicts the basic model.

Figure 22.8 demonstrates that baseline family communication significantly moderated the effect of the Familias Unidas intervention on postintervention family communication ($b = 0.25$, $SE = 0.07$, $p < .001$), reflecting increased communication in the intervention group versus control for those who had low levels of communication at baseline. Postintervention family communication was also significantly associated with the slope of internalizing symptom trajectory ($b = -0.06$, $SE = 0.02$, $p = .002$), indicating that better communication yielded

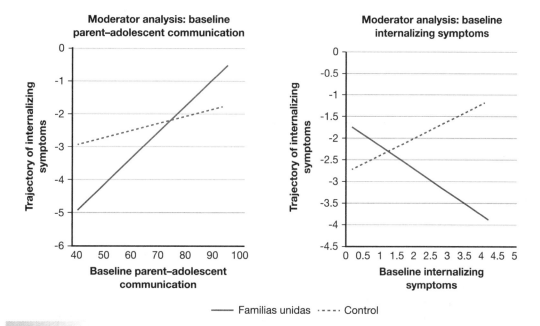

FIGURE 22.6 Moderation effects of baseline family communication and internalizing symptoms on postintervention internalizing symptoms.

Source: Adapted from Perrino, T., Pantin, H., Prado, G., Huang, S., Brincks, A., Howe, G., Brown, C. H. (2014). Preventing internalizing symptoms among Hispanic adolescents: A synthesis across familias unidas trials. *Prevention Science, 15*(6), 917–928.

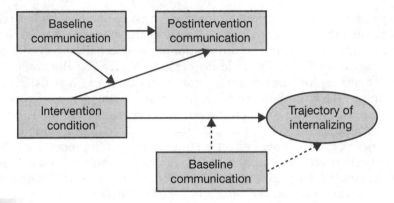

FIGURE 22.7 Basic moderated mediation model.

Source: Adapted from Perrino, T., Pantin, H., Prado, G., Huang, S., Brincks, A., Howe, G., Brown, C. H. (2014). Preventing internalizing symptoms among Hispanic adolescents: A synthesis across familias unidas trials. *Prevention Science, 15*(6), 917–928.

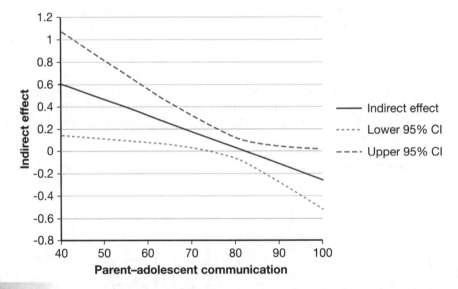

FIGURE 22.8 Moderated mediation results for different levels of family communication.

CI, confidence interval.
Source: Adapted from Perrino, T., Pantin, H., Prado, G., Huang, S., Brincks, A., Howe, G., Brown, C. H. (2014). Preventing internalizing symptoms among Hispanic adolescents: A synthesis across familias unidas trials. *Prevention Science, 15*(6), 917–928.

a greater reduction in symptoms. There was a significant indirect effect of the average level of baseline family communication ($b = 0.13$, $SE = 0.06$, $p = .02$). Full mediation was observed because the direct effect of the interaction term on internalizing trajectories became nonsignificant in the presence of the indirect effect (Figure 22.8).

The examples presented earlier have illustrated how multiple mediator models help identify the most effective potential targets for intervention. Moderator models help identify the subgroups for which the intervention was most effective. Mediation, moderation, and moderated mediation models provide critical information for redesigning interventions prior to large-scale effectiveness trials and dissemination. We now move to a discussion of analytical methods for assessing mediation, moderation, and longitudinal moderated mediational models.

ANALYTICAL METHODS FOR EXAMINING MEDIATION, MODERATION, AND LONGITUDINAL MODERATED MEDIATION

A shift is occurring in analytical methodologies in intervention research away from correlational analyses and simple linear regression analyses between predictors and outcomes. Because greater emphasis is placed on understanding the processes and mechanisms by which interventions work and for whom they are most effective, more complex analytical methods are being used because of an increase in moderated mediational models. Traditionally, when researchers have been interested in combining mediation and moderation in their analyses, they have used approaches that were fraught with methodological issues. One method is to analyze mediation and moderation separately but the results are interpreted together (piecemeal approach). There are several limitations to this approach. Which of the paths relating the IV, mediator, and DV varying as a function of levels of the moderator cannot be determined. Use of the causal steps method to assess mediation may hide a mediated effect through the requirement that a significant relationship exists between the IV and the DV (discussed earlier; Edwards & Lambert, 2007; Fairchild & MacKinnon, 2014). A second method is to split the sample into subgroups representing various values of the moderator and then assess mediation within each subgroup (subgroup approach). The mediation analyses are typically carried out using the causal steps approach. Subgroups are created on the basis of naturally occurring conditions (e.g., sex, intervention group), or continuous variables are collapsed into two or more categories (Edwards & Lambert, 2007; Fairchild & MacKinnon, 2014). Creating categorical variables from continuous variables has been criticized because useful information is discarded, frequently biased parameter estimates are obtained, and there is a decrease in statistical power (MacCallum, Zhang, Preacher, & Rucker, 2002; Maxwell, 2004; McClelland, Lynch, Irwin, Spiller, & Fitzsimons, 2015). The subgroup approach does not yield statistical tests of the differences in mediation across the levels of the moderator. Mediation is implied when it is present for one group but not the other, but this does not actually tell whether mediation differed between the groups (Edwards & Lambert, 2007; Fairchild & MacKinnon, 2014). Mediation is generally assessed with the causal steps procedure in the subgroup approach. Another approach is known as the "moderated causal steps approach." Moderation and mediation are combined by adding product terms to the causal steps regression equations. In addition to the limitations of the causal steps procedure described earlier, there are several other drawbacks to this method. In many circumstances, moderation is examined only for a subset of the paths between the IV and the DV, there is no information on how the mediator affects the form of the interaction between the IV and the moderator, and rarely are the coefficients relating IVs, moderator, and DV at the specific levels of the moderator reported (Edwards & Lambert, 2007; Fairchild & MacKinnon, 2014).

Many researchers are turning to structural equation modeling (SEM) techniques to address the limitations of the various analytical approaches described earlier. SEM is a collection of statistical techniques that allow for not only directly observed variables but also latent variables (defined later). We focus on an introduction to SEM and provide an illustrative example of moderated mediation.

Structural Equation Modeling

SEM evolved from and is an extension of general linear modeling techniques. It is a technique that allows for the examination of observed and latent variables through path analysis and factor analysis. In contrast to inferring indirect pathways from a series of sequential regression analyses, SEM provides direct estimation of direct and indirect effects of the exogenous (independent) variables on the endogenous (dependent) variables. When all of the variables in the model are observed, then a path analysis is conducted. Latent variables are not directly observed but are inferred through a mathematical model from several observed variables (Duncan,

Duncan, & Strycker, 2013). Observed variables that are used in creating the latent construct are referred to as "indicators." For example, in follow-up analyses on the differential effect of a nurse home-visiting intervention on physically aggressive behavior in children (Sidora-Arcoleo et al., 2010), we were interested in examining children's academic success at the end of sixth grade. A latent variable representing this construct was created from the observed indicators for grade point average for math and reading, standardized test scores, and scores from a test of sustained attention. The capacity to include observed and latent variables in the analytical model differentiates SEM from analysis of variance (ANOVA) and multiple regression where only observed variables can be analyzed. Another distinguishing feature of SEM is that error variance is modeled, and the degree to which this error variance influences results can be interpreted.

The researcher must have a priori hypotheses regarding the causal relationships among the variables in the model on the basis of theory and/or empirical evidence. SEM seeks to understand the patterns of covariance among the set of observed and/or latent variables and to explain as much of the variance as possible in the specified causal model (Duncan et al., 2013; Kline, 2011). Means can also be estimated in SEM. The advantage of SEM over ANOVA is that means for latent variables can be estimated in addition to observed variables. One cautionary note—SEM is a large-sample technique. So what is a large enough sample size to generate reliable estimates? The answer depends on several factors: complexity of the model, the type of estimation algorithm used, and the distributional properties of the outcome variables. Maximum likelihood is the most common estimation algorithm used in SEM. Kline (2015) states that there is no set minimum number because there are several important factors to consider. First, more model parameters or model complexity will require larger samples to maintain precision. Second, models where all DVs are continuous, normally distributed, effects are linear, and no interaction terms are included will allow for smaller sample sizes. Third, larger sample sizes will be required if there are a lot of missing data or reliability coefficients for measures are low. Fourth, different types of SEM models (e.g., factor analysis) may require larger sample sizes (Kline, 2015). Jackson (2003) proposes that a rule of thumb on the basis of empirical support is a ratio of the number of cases to the number of model parameters. An ideal sample size:parameters ratio is 20:1. Thus, if the model has 15 parameters, then an ideal sample size would be 20 × 15, or $N = 300$. As the ratio decreases below 10:1, the reliability of the results also decreases (Jackson, 2003). Many times a "typical" sample size of 200 is recommended, as this corresponds to the median sample size across studies published using SEM methodologies (Kline, 2015). Because of the lack of a gold-standard minimum sample size, Wolf and colleagues conducted a series of Monte Carlo simulations across different SEM models to evaluate sample size requirements (Wolf, Harrington, Clark, & Miller, 2013). Various model parameters were manipulated to observe how these changes impacted required sample sizes on the basis of parameter estimate bias and solution propriety. A wide range (30–460) of sample sizes resulted (Wolf et al., 2013).

The core of the SEM analysis will provide estimates of how well the data fit the hypothesized model and identify the statistically significant path coefficients for the latent and observed variables. There are numerous goodness-of-fit indicators and the choice will depend on the type of outcome variables (continuous or categorical). Many of the statistical software packages for SEM will generate several of these. The most commonly reported are the Tucker–Lewis index (TLI), comparative fit index (CFI), root mean square error of approximation (RMSEA), and standard root mean square residual (SRMR). Cutoff values have been established for these indicators, and if the majority provide support for a good fit, it is reasonable to assume that the data fit the model well. The following are the suggested cutoff values: RMSEA < .06, TLI > .95, CFI > .95, and SRMR < .08 (Kline, 2015). Interpretation and reporting of the path coefficients is similar to that of linear regression models. The output will provide unstandardized and standardized estimates, p values, and 95% CIs.

We now go through an illustrative example. The nurse–family partnership (NFP) is an intensive nurse home-visiting intervention targeting first-time, low-income mothers.

A secondary analysis was conducted to explore whether there were differential effects of the NFP on verbal ability and the development of physically aggressive behavior in children from 2 to 12 years of age (Sidora-Arcoleo et al., 2010). The theoretical framework used for the analyses is known as the language–aggression hypothesis (Boone & Montare, 1976). It is posited that language is inversely related to physical aggression. Low levels of language proficiency are associated with high levels of aggressive behavior. The research questions addressed were the following:

- Was the NFP effective in reducing physically aggressive behaviors through the age of 12 years?
- Did the intervention effects on the development of physical aggression over time differ by sex?
- Did maternal psychological resources (IQ, mental health, mastery, self-efficacy, and coping) mediate the relationship between the intervention and physical aggression?
- Were the effects of the intervention on physical aggression mediated by children's verbal ability?

Four models were examined: (a) intervention main effects, (b) intervention × child's sex, (c) intervention × maternal psychological resources, and (d) intervention × sex × maternal psychological resources. Two covariates (negative parenting beliefs and household poverty) were included in the model because there were baseline differences between intervention groups. Figure 22.9 presents the simplified hypothesized moderated mediational model.

Examination of the goodness-of-fit statistics revealed that both the CFI and the TLI exceeded .90 and RMSEA was .06. Nurse-visited children demonstrated lower levels of physical aggression at the age of 2 years than the control-group children, but these effects were attenuated at the ages of 6 and 12 years. Adding a child's sex to the model as a moderator showed that there was no significant interaction of intervention and sex on verbal ability and a trend toward statistical significance on physical aggression ($t = 1.95$, $p < .10$). Further probing of the interaction revealed that nurse home visitation significantly protected against aggression at the age of 2 years in girls ($t = -3.43$, $p < .01$) but not in boys ($t = -0.23$, nonsignificant). This effect was not evident at 6 and 12 years of age. The next model added maternal psychological resources and the interaction of intervention and psychological

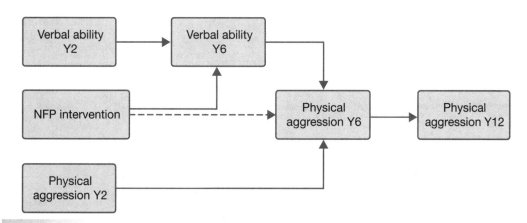

FIGURE 22.9 NFP language–aggression mediational model.

NFP, nurse–family partnership.
Source: Adapted from Sidora-Arcoleo, K., Anson, E., Lorber, M., Cole, R., Olds, D., & Kitzman, H. (2010). Differential effects of a nurse home visiting intervention on physically aggressive behavior in children. *Journal Pediatric Nursing, 25*(1), 35–45.

resources. No statistically significant interactions were found for verbal ability at 2 and 6 years of age or physical aggression at the age of 2 years. The intervention × maternal psychological resources interaction on physical aggression, however, was significant ($t = -2.49$, $p < .05$) and was sustained through the age of 12 years ($t = -2.35$, $p < .05$). Further examination of the interaction revealed that among the high-psychological-resource mothers, the nurse-visited children had significantly lower physical aggression scores than their comparison-group counterparts at 6 and 12 years ($t = -1.79$, $p < .10$; and $t = -2.50$, $p < .05$). There were no intervention effects on children's physical aggression among the low-psychological-resource mothers. The last model included all two-way and three-way interactions of intervention, sex, and maternal psychological resources. There were no statistically significant three-way interactions in predicting verbal ability or physical aggression. Mediation was evaluated only where there was a measure of child's verbal ability assessed at the same time as or before physical aggression to ensure that there was not violation of the temporal precedence criterion. This analysis was further limited to females—the subgroup for whom the intervention effects on physical aggression were concentrated. The mediation analysis revealed that our original hypothesis that the intervention would work through improvements in children's verbal ability to reduce physical aggression was not supported because the intervention had no direct effect on verbal ability at the age of 2 years. In fact, the results suggested an alternate direction of mediation. There was a significant intervention effect on physical aggression at the age of 2 years, and a marginal effect on verbal ability at the age of 6 years among the females. It was plausible, given these results, that the improvements in verbal ability at the age of 6 years among the nurse-visited children were mediated by reductions in physical aggression at the age of 2 years. This alternate model and support for the model that was demonstrated were tested. The path from intervention to aggression at the age of 2 years was significant ($t = -3.149$, $p < .01$); the path from aggression to verbal ability at the age of 6 years was marginally significant ($t = -1.826$, $p < .10$); the 95% CI for the unstandardized indirect effect estimate did not include 0 (95% CI = 0.001 to –0.786); and the direct effect from intervention to verbal ability at the age of 6 years dropped to a nonsignificant level after controlling for physical aggression at the age of 2 years (Figure 22.10).

These secondary SEM analyses yielded several important findings regarding the NFP intervention. It was revealed that there were significant moderation effects on the basis of child's sex and mother's psychological resources. The NFP's effects were concentrated among females and children of high-psychological-resource mothers. The lack of intervention effects for boys suggests that there may be a different set of etiological factors important in predicting physically aggressive behavior among this group. These findings were also

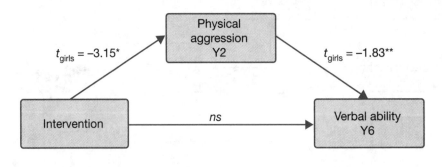

$^*p < .01$; $^{**}p < .10$

FIGURE 22.10 Alternate hypothesis mediational model.

Source: Adapted from Sidora-Arcoleo, K., Anson, E., Lorber, M., Cole, R., Olds, D., & Kitzman, H. (2010). Differential effects of a nurse home visiting intervention on physically aggressive behavior in children. *Journal Pediatric Nursing, 25*(1), 35–45.

consistent with positive outcomes reported earlier among the high-psychological-resource mothers (Kitzman et al., 1997, 2000; Olds et al., 2002; Olds, Kitzman, et al., 2004; Olds, Robinson, et al., 2004). We theorize that through improvements in parenting behaviors, these mothers were better able to provide competent care and promote optimal child development.

The goal of this chapter was to provide you with an introduction to how powerful mediation, moderation, and moderated mediation methodologies can be in your intervention studies. The results of these analyses will guide the development and refinement of your intervention. We know that a "one-size-fits-all" approach is neither effective nor efficient. Use of these techniques, particularly SEM, will allow you to identify those risk factors and predictors most amenable to change through your intervention and for whom your intervention is going to have the greatest effect. So grab your statistical toolkit and tinker with expanding your current analytical framework to more complex models.

Key Points From This Chapter

- It is important to understand the mechanisms through which an intervention influences health outcomes and who benefits most from the intervention to make decisions about resource allocations.
- The selection of mediators and moderators should be on the basis of the theoretical framework and/or empirical evidence.
- Suppressor variables are many times overlooked but may play a significant role when nonsignificant direct and total effects are observed.
- SEM techniques are quite powerful and will provide valuable information on modifiable mediating factors, potential moderators that influence for whom the intervention is most effective, and outcomes required for large-scale dissemination.

REFERENCES

Aiken, L. S., & West, S. G. (1991). *Multiple regression: Testing and interpreting interactions.* Thousand Oaks, CA: Sage.

Baron, R. M., & Kenny, D. A. (1986). The moderator-mediator variable distinction in social psychological research: Conceptual, strategic, and statistical considerations. *Journal of Personality and Social Psychology, 51*(6), 1173–1182. doi:10.1037/0022-3514.51.6.1173

Boone, S. L., & Montare, A. (1976). Test of the language-aggression hypothesis. *Psychological Reports, 39,* 851–857. doi:10.2466/pr0.1976.39.3.851

Duncan, T. E., Duncan, S. C., & Strycker, L. A. (2013). *An introduction to latent variable growth curve modeling: Concepts, issues, and application.* New York, NY: Routledge Academic.

Edwards, J. R., & Lambert, L. S. (2007). Methods for integrating moderation and mediation: A general analytical framework using moderated path analysis. *Psychological Methods, 12*(1), 1–22. doi:10.1037/1082-989X.12.1.1

Fairchild, A. J., & MacKinnon, D. P. (2014). Using mediation and moderation analyses to enhance prevention research In Z. Sloboda & H. Petras (eds.), *Defining Prevention Science* (pp. 537–555). New York, NY: Springer.

Fritz, M. S., Cox, M. G., & MacKinnon, D. P. (2015). Increasing statistical power in mediation models without increasing sample size. *Evaluation & the Health Professions, 38*(3), 343–366. doi:10.1177/0163278713514250

Hayes, A. F. (2009). Beyond Baron and Kenny: Statistical mediation analysis in the new millennium. *Communication Monographs, 76,* 408–420. doi:10.1080/03637750903310360

Jackson, D. L. (2003). Revisiting sample size and number of parameter estimates: Some support for the N:Q hypothesis. *Structural Equation Modeling, 10,* 128–141. doi:10.1207/S15328007SEM1001_6

Judd, C. M., Yzerbyt, V. Y., & Muller, D. (2014). Mediation and moderation. *Handbook of Research Methods in Social and Personality Psychology, 2,* 653–676. doi:10.1017/CBO9780511996481.030

Kenny, D. A. (2015). Moderator variables: Introduction. Retrieved from http://davidakenny.net/cm/ moderation.htm#GO

Kitzman, H., Olds, D. L., Henderson, C. R., Jr, Hanks, C., Cole, R., Tatelbaum, R., ... Barnard, K. (1997). Effect of prenatal and infancy home visitation by nurses on pregnancy outcomes, childhood injuries, and repeated childbearing: A randomized controlled trial. *Journal of the American Medical Association, 278*, 644–652. doi:10.1001/jama.1997.03550080054039

Kitzman, H., Olds, D. L., Sidora, K., Henderson, C. R., Jr, Hanks, C., Cole, R., ... Glazner, J. (2000). Enduring effects of nurse home visitation on maternal life course: A 3-year follow-up of a randomized trial. *Journal of the American Medical Association, 283*, 1983–1989. doi:10.1001/jama.283.15.1983

Kline, R. B. (2011). *Principles and practice of structural equation modeling* (3rd ed.). New York, NY: Guilford Press.

Kline, R. B. (2015). *Principles and practice of structural equation modeling*. New York, NY: Guilford Press.

Knowlden, A. P. (2014). Role of suppressor variables in primary prevention obesity research: Examples from two predictive models. *International Scholarly Research Notices Obesity, 2014*, 567523, 1–9. doi:10.1155/2014/567523

MacCallum, R. C., Zhang, S., Preacher, K. J., & Rucker, D. D. (2002). On the practice of dichotomization of quantitative variables. *Psychological Methods, 7*(1), 19–40. doi:10.1037//1082-989X.7.1.19

MacKinnon, D. P., & Fairchild, A. J. (2009). Current directions in mediation analysis. *Current Directions in Psychological Science, 18*(1), 16–20. doi:10.1111/j.1467-8721.2009.01598.x

MacKinnon, D. P., Fairchild, A. J., & Fritz, M. S. (2007). Mediation analysis. *Annual Review of Psychology, 58*, 593–614. doi:10.1146/annurev.psych.58.110405.085542

MacKinnon, D. P., Krull, J. L., & Lockwood, C. M. (2000). Equivalence of the mediation, confounding and suppression effect. *Prevention Science, 1*, 173–181. doi:10.1023/A:1026595011371

MacKinnon, D. P., & Pirlott, A. G. (2015). Statistical approaches for enhancing causal interpretation of the M to Y relation in mediation analysis. *Personality and Social Psychology Review, 19*(1), 30–43. doi:10.1177/1088868314542878

Maxwell, S. E. (2004). The persistence of underpowered studies in psychological research: Causes, consequences, and remedies. *Psychological Methods, 9*, 147–163. doi:10.1037/1082-989X.9.2.147

McClelland, G. H., & Judd, C. M. (1993). Statistical difficulties of detecting interactions and moderator effects. *Psychological Bulletin, 114*, 376–390. doi:10.1037/0033-2909.114.2.376

McClelland, G. H., Lynch, J. G., Jr, Irwin, J. R., Spiller, S. A., & Fitzsimons, G. J. (2015). Median splits, type II errors, and false positive consumer psychology: Don't fight the power. *Journal of Consumer Psychology, 25*(4), 679–689. doi:10.1016/j.jcps.2015.05.006

Naar-King, S., Ellis, D. A., Idalski Carcone, A., Templin, T., Jacques-Tiura, A. J., Brogan Hartlieb, K., ... Jen, K. L. (2016). Sequential multiple assignment randomized trial (SMART) to construct weight loss interventions for African American adolescents. *Journal of Clinical Child & Adolescent Psychology, 45*(4), 428–441. doi:10.1080/15374416.2014.971459

Olds, D. L., Kitzman, H., Cole, R., Robinson, J., Sidora, K., Luckey, D. W., ... Holmberg, J. (2004). Effects of nurse home visiting on maternal life-course and child development: Age-six follow-up results of a randomized trial. *Pediatrics, 114*, 1550–1559. doi:10.1542/peds.2004-0962

Olds, D. L., Robinson, J., O'Brien, R., Luckey, D. W., Pettitt, L. M., Henderson, C. R., Jr, ... Talmi, A. (2002). Home visiting by paraprofessionals and by nurses: A randomized, controlled trial. *Pediatrics, 110*, 486–496. doi:10.1542/peds.110.3.486

Olds, D. L., Robinson, J., Pettitt, L., Luckey, D. W., Holmberg, J., Ng, R. K., ... Henderson, C. R., Jr,. (2004). Effects of home visits by paraprofessionals and by nurses: Age 4 follow-up results of a randomized trial. *Pediatrics, 114*, 1560–1568. doi:10.1542/peds.2004-0961

Perrino, T., Pantin, H., Prado, G., Huang, S., Brincks, A., Howe, G., ... Brown, C. H. (2014). Preventing internalizing symptoms among Hispanic adolescents: A synthesis across Familias Unidas trials. *Prevention Science, 15*(6), 917–928. doi:10.1007/s11121-013-0448-9

Rucker, D. D., Preacher, K. J., Tormala, Z. L., & Petty, R. E. (2011). Mediation analysis in social psychology: Current practices and new recommendations. *Social and Personality Psychology Compass, 5*(6), 359–371. doi:10.1111/j.1751-9004.2011.00355.x

Sidora-Arcoleo, K., Anson, E., Lorber, M., Cole, R., Olds, D., & Kitzman, H. (2010). Differential effects of a nurse home visiting intervention on physically aggressive behavior in children. *Journal of Pediatric Nursing, 25*(1), 35–45. doi:10.1016/j.pedn.2008.07.011

Society for Prevention Research. (2017). Society for Prevention Research mission statement and strategic plan. Retrieved from http://www.preventionresearch.org/about-spr/mission-statement

Wolf, E. J., Harrington, K. M., Clark, S. L., & Miller, M. W. (2013). Sample size requirements for structural equation models an evaluation of power, bias, and solution propriety. *Educational and Psychological Measurement, 73*(6), 913–934. doi:10.1177/0013164413495237

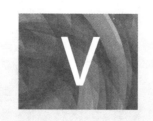

Writing Successful Grants
and Progress Reports

23

Writing Grants That Fund!

Bernadette Mazurek Melnyk & Dianne Morrison-Beedy

> If you never swing, you never hit. Baseball players with the best averages actually miss the ball many more times than they hit it. Keep swinging the bat until you hit the ball and your grant funds, as success is going from one failure to the next with enthusiasm! —*Bern Melnyk*

The world of grant writing is highly competitive. Therefore, it is extremely important that every time you submit a grant application, it is near perfection. Remember, you never get a second chance to make a great first impression (Melnyk & Fineout-Overholt, 2015)!

INCREASING CHANCES OF SUCCESSFUL GRANT FUNDING

Many funding agencies, such as the National Institutes of Health (NIH), the Agency for Healthcare Research and Quality (AHRQ), Patient-Centered Outcomes Research Institute (PCORI), and professional organizations and foundations, list areas of priority for grant applications. Many funders also publish requests for applications that specifically call for grants on certain topics with deadlines for submission. If possible, it is beneficial to direct your application to one of these high-priority areas as the funders allocate substantial dollars to their priorities. However, several funders (e.g., NIH) routinely accept applications in an investigator's area of research that are not specified as high priority; these are typically referred to as "investigator-generated" applications.

It is often helpful to obtain presubmission consultation from the funding agency. Many funding agencies list primary contacts or program officers for grant applications who can advise you on your project idea and help guide you on your competitive grant submission. These program officers are often publicized on the agency's website. If you do request a consultation from the funding agency, it is best to prepare an abstract of the study or project that you would like to propose, which outlines its background/significance, innovation, sample, methods, and analysis with implications for clinical practice and/or future research. Incorporating how your study will extend the science in the area, fill a gap in knowledge, or improve population health outcomes will help spark the interest of the funding agency. It also is very helpful to review grants that have been earlier funded by the agency that you are targeting for your submission. Some funders publish examples of funded grants. If they do not, it is perfectly fine to contact the investigator and ask for a copy of their grant. Applications that are funded by the federal government (e.g., NIH, AHRQ, PCORI) are in the public domain and also can be requested from the agency, although the process for receiving the grants may be much lengthier than calling the investigator personally and asking for a copy of his or her grant.

> Remember to avoid the old and predictable when writing research grants. Be innovative and groundbreaking. —*Bern Melnyk*

It is critical that you never assume the reviewers will know what you mean. Clear explanations and rationales for why you have chosen certain methods, measures, or analyses are important. Be careful not to promise too little or too much; either case is likely to result in a poor grant review. Also, make sure that your grant is aesthetically pleasing without typographical and grammatical errors. If the application has typographical and grammatical errors, the reviewers will doubt your ability to carry out your project meticulously. Take time to thoroughly review the application guidelines as well as the funding agency's established criteria for grant reviews. Most funding agencies publish the criteria that are used in the review of their grants so that you can carefully target these important criteria in your application. Furthermore, it is imperative to follow directions to a "tee." Failure to follow directions could result in the return of your grant application and a missed opportunity for funding.

Before submitting the application, it is helpful for a **mock review** of your application to be conducted. Mock reviews typically mimic formal grant reviews by having three to four seasoned funded researchers critique your application before it is submitted to the funding agency. The reviewers who participate in the mock review should be provided the published review criteria from the funder, if available, so that they can specifically address those criteria in their reviews. Feedback from these reviewers allows you the opportunity to address areas of limitation and strengthen your application before it is submitted. It is best to have experts in the field as well as a researcher who does not conduct work in your area to critique your grant, as the latter can be very helpful in making sure that the content is understandable to those without expertise in the field. If seasoned researchers are not available at your institution, it is advisable to seek outside experts who would be willing to review your grant and provide feedback. Most seasoned researchers are willing to provide a review of your grant for a small honorarium (e.g., $500). Expert consultants also should be used whenever possible to strengthen your application in areas that may be needed to fill in the gaps on your research team. Fees for these consultants should be built into your grant application's budget. Finally, it is highly recommended to have an editor review your grant before submitting it to make sure the content flows and the grammar is correct.

SPECIFIC STEPS IN WRITING A GRANT PROPOSAL

The Abstract

Because the abstract is critical in peaking the interest and excitement of the reviewers, it is important to spend considerable time writing it. Abstracts should be clear, concise, and compelling. Because grant reviewers typically receive multiple applications, you want to "whet

---

EXHIBIT 23.1 An Abstract From Grant #R01 NR012171 Funded by the NIH/NINR (Bernadette Melnyk, Principal Investigator)

The prevention and treatment of obesity and mental health disorders in adolescence are two major public health problems in the United States today. The incidence of adolescents who are overweight or obese has increased dramatically over the past 20 years, with approximately 17.1% of teens now being overweight or obese. Furthermore, approximately 15 million children and adolescents (25%) in the United States have a mental health problem that is interfering with their functioning at home or at school, but less than 25% of those affected receive any treatment for these disorders. The prevalence rates of obesity and mental health problems are even higher in Hispanic teens, with studies suggesting that the two conditions often coexist in many youth. However, despite the rapidly increasing incidence of these two public health problems with their related health disparities and adverse health outcomes, there has been a paucity of theory-based intervention studies conducted with adolescents in high schools to improve their healthy lifestyle behaviors as well as their physical and mental health outcomes. Unfortunately, physical and mental health services continue to be largely separated instead of integrated in the nation's health care system, which often leads to inadequate identification and treatment of these significant adolescent health problems.

Therefore, the goal of the proposed randomized controlled trial is to test the efficacy of the COPE (Creating Opportunities for Personal Empowerment)/Healthy Lifestyles TEEN (Thinking, Emotions, Exercise, and Nutrition) program, an educational and cognitive-behavioral skills building intervention guided by cognitive behavior theory, on the healthy lifestyle behaviors and depressive symptoms of 800 culturally diverse adolescents enrolled in Phoenix, Arizona high schools. The specific aims of the study are to (a) use a randomized controlled trial to test the short-term and more long-term efficacy of the COPE TEEN program on key outcomes, including healthy lifestyles behaviors, depressive symptoms, and body mass index percentage; (b) examine the role of cognitive beliefs and perceived difficulty in leading a healthy lifestyle in mediating the effects of COPE on healthy lifestyle behaviors and depressive symptoms; and (c) explore variables that may moderate the effects of the intervention on healthy lifestyle behaviors and depressive symptoms, including race/ethnicity, gender, socioeconomic status (SES), acculturation, and parental healthy lifestyle beliefs and behaviors. Six prior pilot studies support the need for this full-scale clinical trial and the use of cognitive-behavioral skills building in promoting healthy lifestyles beliefs, behaviors, and optimal mental health in teens.

This study is consistent with the NIH roadmap and goals of improving people's health, and preventing the onset of disease and disability as well as promoting the highest level of health in a vulnerable population.

NIH/NINR, National Institutes of Health/National Institute of Nursing Research.

their appetite" for reading your entire proposal and get them excited about your study. Examples of well-formulated abstracts from grants funded by the NIH/National Institute of Nursing Research (NINR) can be found in Exhibits 23.1 and 23.2.

Introduction and Specific Aims

The significance of the problem should be introduced immediately in the proposal, such as: "Over 500,000 premature infants are born every year in the United States, costing the health-care system approximately $26 billion annually. Prematurely born infants have a host of adverse neurodevelopmental, mental health, and academic outcomes, which call for the urgent testing of interventions to avert these major problems." In the introduction, note how your study is innovative and will extend the science in the area, such as "This study will be the first to test a manualized theory-based intervention for parents of preterm infants that commences very early in the neonatal intensive care unit (NICU) stay, before the development of premature stereotyping by parents. It will extend the science by analyzing the mediating processes through which the intervention will work to affect parent and child outcomes."

EXHIBIT 23.2 An Abstract From Grant #R01 NR008194 Funded by the NIH/NINR
(Dianne Morrison-Beedy, Principal Investigator)

Adolescence is the only age category where the number of females becoming infected with HIV outnumbers the number of males. Despite these data, only *four* randomized controlled trials have evaluated the efficacy of a gender-specific HIV-risk reduction program for adolescent females. The proposed research aims to address this gap in HIV prevention science, and will evaluate the short- and long-term efficacy of an HIV-prevention intervention for adolescent girls. We will recruit 640 adolescent females aged 15–19 years from family planning clinics and randomly assign them to one of two conditions: (a) an HIV-risk reduction intervention based on the Information-Motivation-Behavioral Skills (IMB) model (Fisher & Fisher, 1992) or (b) a structurally equivalent health promotion control group (CTL), both supplemented by booster sessions at 3 and 6 months. At a short-term (3-month) follow-up, we hypothesize that IMB participants will increase HIV-related knowledge, motivation, and behavioral skills and decrease the frequency of risky sexual practices relative to CTL participants. We will reassess all participants at 6 and 12 months to evaluate the long-term efficacy of the interventions. At these long-term follow-ups, we hypothesize that IMB participants will demonstrate higher levels of HIV knowledge, motivation, and behavioral skills; decreased risky sexual practices; and decreased rates of STDs (chlamydia, gonorrhea) relative to the CTL participants. The final aim of the proposed research is to determine whether the constructs in the IMB model (Fisher & Fisher, 1992), can account for variability in HIV-related behavior. We hypothesize that preventive behavior at 6 and 12 months will be a function of a participant's HIV-related information, motivation, and behavioral skills at the 3-month follow-up, and that information and motivation will be partially mediated by behavioral skills to influence the initiation and maintenance of HIV preventive behavior. The long-term intent of the proposed research is to develop a risk-reduction program that can be used by community-based health organizations to reduce the risk of HIV infection among adolescent females.

NIH/NINR, National Institutes of Health/National Institute of Nursing Research; STDs, sexually transmitted diseases.

In the introduction to the application, it is critical to be clear about the goal and specific aims of your study so that the grant reviewers will know exactly what your research will accomplish. For example:

The goal of the proposed randomized controlled trial (RCT) is to test the efficacy of the COPE (Creating Opportunities for Personal Empowerment)/Healthy Lifestyles TEEN (Thinking, Feeling, Emotions, and Exercise) program, an educational and cognitive behavioral skills building intervention guided by cognitive behavioral theory on the healthy lifestyle behaviors and depressive symptoms of 800 culturally diverse adolescents enrolled in Phoenix, Arizona, high schools. The specific aims of the study are to (a) use an RCT to test the short- and more long-term efficacy of the COPE TEEN program on key outcomes, including healthy lifestyle behaviors, depressive symptoms, and body mass index (BMI) percentage; (b) examine the role of cognitive beliefs and perceived difficulty in leading a healthy lifestyle in mediating the effects of COPE on healthy lifestyle behaviors and depressive symptoms; and (c) explore variables that may moderate the effects of the intervention on healthy lifestyle behaviors and depressive symptoms, including race/ethnicity, gender, socioeconomic status (SES), acculturation, and parental healthy lifestyle beliefs and behaviors.

Hypotheses and Research Questions

"Hypotheses" are statements about the predicted relationships between the **independent variables** (i.e., the intervention or treatment) and the **dependent** or **outcome variables**. If preliminary data have been gathered that indicate how the intervention is likely to impact the outcome variables in the study, hypotheses should be included immediately following the goal and aims of the study. Hypotheses should always be clear and testable. An example of a well-written hypothesis from the aforementioned intervention study testing the COPE/Healthy Lifestyles program with teens is the following: "Adolescents who receive the COPE program will report less depressive symptoms than those who receive an attention control program." If pilot data are not available and it is not known how the intervention to be tested might affect the outcome variable(s), it is best to ask research questions than to test hypotheses. For a first-time pilot study testing the COPE program, an appropriate research question is, What is the effect of the COPE program on depressive symptoms in adolescents?

THE RESEARCH STRATEGY

The research strategy of a grant application contains the significance of the project, the background of the problem, the preliminary studies/progress report section, and the research design and methods.

Background and Significance

In the background section, it is important to convince the reviewers that the problem is worthwhile to study (e.g., the findings will improve the health outcomes of a high-risk population). It also is critical to describe how the proposal will extend the science in the area as well as how the project is innovative and breaks new ground (e.g., Does it use new groundbreaking methods? Is the intervention likely to improve the quality of care and outcomes for a particularly vulnerable population?). A comprehensive but concise review of the literature should be included in this section, followed by a critical analysis of the literature that explains the strengths and gaps of prior work in the area. It is very helpful to use a table to present prior relevant research that summarizes the sample, design, measures, outcomes, and strengths as well as limitations of each study (see Table 23.1). Remember, it is not enough to describe or summarize prior studies; they must be synthesized and critically analyzed.

A solid theoretical or conceptual framework should be included to guide your research, with a description of how the framework is guiding your study hypotheses, intervention(s), and the relationship between or among the study's variables. This section also should include clear definitions of the constructs in your study. A model of how the constructs to be studied relate to one another or a model of how you expect the intervention to exert its effects is especially useful, such as the one depicted in Figure 23.1.

Preliminary Studies

If you have conducted prior preliminary work/pilot studies, it is important to describe the findings from that work and explain how they support the proposed research. An error that is sometimes made in grant applications is that investigators "go overboard" in describing their prior studies and leave little room to describe in detail their proposed study's design and methods, so be careful to balance these sections.

Research Design and Methods

When writing the research design and methods section, it is important to provide rationales for your decisions. For example, if you have chosen to conduct a **quasi-experimental** study instead of an RCT, you must provide outstanding rationale for your choice of design. Leave nothing to the reviewers' imaginations so that they know you have very carefully considered your options and chosen the best one.

(text continues on page 406)

TABLE 23.1 Example of a Table Summarizing Studies with Teens in High Schools Targeting Prevention and/or Treatment of Overweight

AUTHOR/LOCATION/ DESIGN/THEORY	PURPOSE/SAMPLE/SETTING	INTERVENTION/OUTCOMES/ FOLLOW-UP	SIGNIFICANT FINDINGS	STRENGTHS/ LIMITATIONS
Killen et al. (1989) Northern California The Stanford Adolescent Heart Health Program Two group RCT Theoretical framework: Social cognitive theory Social inoculation theory	**Purpose:** Create, implement, and test a school-based multiple risk factor reduction program for high school students. **Sample:** 4 high schools N = 1,447 (1,130 in F/U) 10th grade students Age 15 (70%), 14 (14%), 16 (14%) 69% Whites 13.1% Asians 6.4% Latinos 2% African Americans 0.3% American Indians 0.4% Pacific Islanders 8.9% others **Setting:** High school PE classes	**Intervention:** 20 classroom sessions for 50 minutes (33 per week for 7 weeks). Delivered by school staff and research team with local guest instructors. Cardiovascular disease risk factors, physical activity, nutrition, cigarette smoking, stress, goal setting, problem-solving skills, self-managed incentives, and action plan creation for behavioral change. **Control:** Traditional PE class **Outcome measures:** Knowledge: physical activity, nutrition, and smoking, physical activity checklist, nutrition checklist Cigarette smoking/drug use, height, weight, skinfold, HR and BP resting **F/U:** 2 months postintervention	Increased knowledge in physical activity, nutrition, and cigarette smoking Increase in the number of nonexercisers who became exercisers More likely to choose healthy snacks More experimental smokers who quit Decrease in resting HR Beneficial effect on BMI and skinfold	**Strengths:** No significant differences at baseline between groups Theoretical framework Randomization to group Multicomponent intervention Pretesting/posttesting Self-monitoring skills taught **Limitations:** **Follow-up:** Only short-term effects No equal attention comparison group No measurement of mediating and moderating variables to understand the process through which the intervention worked and under what circumstances the intervention best worked.

Fardy et al. (1996)

New York City

Coronary disease risk factor reduction and behavioral modification in minority adolescents: The PATH Program

Two group RCT

Purpose: Evaluate a health promotion program combining circuit training and health lecture for its effect on knowledge, behavior, CVD risk factors, and cardiovascular fitness.

Sample: One inner city public high school, 346 students (80% 9th and 10th grades, 20% 11th and 12th grades)

Treatment group: 181 (91 females, 90 males)

Control group:

165 (109 females, 56 males)

9% Asians

47% African Americans

21% Hispanics

3% Whites

19% others

Setting: High school PE classes

Intervention:

30-minute classes 5 days per week for 11 weeks. 4 weeks of intervention; 7 weeks of testing. Taught by PE teachers.

Each session: circuit training 20 to 25 minutes (resistance and aerobic) and health behavior lecture 5 minutes (exercise, nutrition, smoking cessation, stress management, heart disease, cancer, and motivation).

Control: Volleyball class for 11 weeks

Outcome measures: Height, weight, total cholesterol, percentage body fat (skinfold), resting systolic/diastolic BP

Questionnaires: PA checklist, dietary habits, food frequency, Luckhohn's value orientation schema (health attitude), 3-minute step test, CV health knowledge

F/U: Immediate postintervention

(Both boys and girls) Cardiovascular health knowledge significantly greater

(Girls) Significant improvement in self-report dietary habits

(Girls) Significant decrease in cholesterol

(Girls) Significant improvement in CV fitness

(Boys) Control group activity improved fitness

Strengths:

Placebo attention control group

Randomization to group

Multicomponent intervention

Pretesting/posttesting

Limitations:

Both groups at same school—potential for cross-group contamination

No measurement of mediating and/or moderating variables

(continued)

TABLE 23.1 Example of a Table Summarizing Studies with Teens in High Schools Targeting Prevention and/or Treatment of Overweight *(continued)*

AUTHOR/LOCATION/ DESIGN/THEORY	PURPOSE/SAMPLE/SETTING	INTERVENTION/OUTCOMES/ FOLLOW-UP	SIGNIFICANT FINDINGS	STRENGTHS/ LIMITATIONS
O'Neil and Nicklas (2002) New Orleans, Louisiana Gimme 5: An innovative, school-based nutrition intervention for high school students Two group RCT (matched pair randomization)	**Purpose:** Evaluate a 4-year, school-based intervention designed to increase daily fruit and vegetable consumption by high school students to five or more servings. **Sample:** 12 high schools *N* = 2,213 ninth grade students 56% girls 84% Whites 4% African Americans 12% others **Setting:** Catholic high schools	**Intervention:** 1. School media marketing: Promotes positive attitudes toward fruit and vegetables. 2. Workshops: Five 55-minute workshops on eating habits, eating and athletic performance, evaluating fast food, reading labels, and cooking. 3. Increase availability, variety, and taste of fruits and vegetables in school meals. 4. Parent: Taste-test activities, recipes, and media displays at Parent Teacher Organization meetings. Brochures and newsletters mailed to parents. **Control:** Program not reported, presumably usual school curriculum **Outcome measures:** Knowledge, attitudes, and practices questionnaire Intake of fruits and vegetables **F/U:** 4 years	Knowledge scores were significantly higher in intervention group. Increased awareness in intervention group. Increased consumption of fruits and vegetables in the intervention group.	**Strengths:** Longitudinal study Randomization to group Large sample Parent component Multicomponent intervention Pretesting/posttesting **Limitations:** No equal attention control for comparison group No measurement of mediating and/or moderating variables

				Strengths:
Neumark-Sztainer, Story, Hannan, and Rex (2003) Twin Cities, Minnesota New Moves: A school-based obesity prevention program for adolescent girls Two group RCT (cluster randomized trial)	**Purpose:** Test the feasibility of an innovative school-based program for obesity prevention among adolescent girls. **Sample:** 6 schools N = 201 high school girls 41.9% Whites 28.6% African Americans 21.1% Asian Americans 4.4% Latinos 1% Native Americans 3% others **Setting:** High school PE class	**Intervention:** 1 semester (16 weeks) PA 43 per week (1-day community guest, 1-day strength training, 2-day PE teacher PA); nutrition class every other week; social support class every other week; 8 weekly lunches after the program for maintenance. **Control:** Program not reported, presumably school curriculum **Outcome measures:** BMI, PA stages of change Participation in PA, dietary intake, binge eating, personal factors, Harter's self-perception profile for children, media internalization, self-efficacy to be active, socioenvironmental support **F/U:** 16 weeks and 8 months	Trend in intervention group for increased time in PA, decreased soda pop intake, and increased fruit and vegetable intake. High-program satisfaction among participants: girls, parents, and school staff.	RCT Pretest–posttest Parent component No significant differences at baseline between groups Acceptable attrition Collected information from different sources using quantitative and qualitative methods Theory-based: Social cognitive theory Limitations: Allocation by unit but evaluated by individual No equal attention comparison group No measurement of mediating or moderating variables

(continued)

TABLE 23.1 Example of a Table Summarizing Studies with Teens in High Schools Targeting Prevention and/or Treatment of Overweight *(continued)*

AUTHOR/LOCATION/ DESIGN/THEORY	PURPOSE/SAMPLE/SETTING	INTERVENTION/OUTCOMES/ FOLLOW-UP	SIGNIFICANT FINDINGS	STRENGTHS/ LIMITATIONS
Pate et al. (2005) Promotion of PA among high school girls: an RCT South Carolina Two-group RCT (school unit of randomization) Theory: Social ecological theory, social cognitive theory Model: Coordinated School Health Program Model	**Purpose:** Examine effects of a school-based intervention on PA among high-school girls. Aim was to increase percentage of girls who meet PA guidelines by increasing the intensity and the duration of PA during PE classes and promoting PA participation in other settings. **Sample:** 24 high schools Ninth grade girls in two cohorts 2,744 at baseline 1,604 with complete data (pre and post) 48.7% African Americans 46.7% Whites **Setting:** High school	**Intervention:** Change instructional practices: content/delivery of PE and health education, enhance PA self-efficacy and enjoyment, teach physical and behavioral skills to adopt and maintain an active lifestyle, and adopt moderate to vigorous PA to 0.50% of PE. Change school environment: Role model PA, increased communication about PA, promotion of PA by school nurse, and family and community-based activities. **Control:** Program not reported, presumably school curriculum **Outcome measures:** Height and weight, 3-day physical activity record, amount of vigorous or moderate physical activity **F/U:** Postintervention 9 months	**Findings:** Prevalence of regular vigorous physical activity was greater in the LEAP intervention schools than in the control schools ($p = .05$). 8% greater participation in vigorous physical activity in intervention schools versus control schools.	**Strengths:** Large sample and number of schools in intervention RCT design Diversity of schools participating Measures well validated Theory-based: Social cognitive theory **Limitations:** Self-report measure for physical activity No equal attention comparison group No measurement of mediating or moderating variables

	Purpose: Evaluate an innovative program for inner-city girls that focused on addictive food avoidance, exercise, and self-esteem building.	Intervention: 9-month program; 29 weekly 2-hour sessions. Content focus on:	Findings:	Strengths:
Chehab, Pfeffer, Vargas, Chen, and Irigoyen (2007)		1. Doing something nice for others	Obese and overweight subjects: 1 Pearson's correlation of 0.6 ($p < .10$) between weight loss and extent of program participation	Innovative concepts: food addiction
New York City	**Sample:**	2. Positive affirmations		Positive weight loss
"Energy up": A novel approach to the weight management of inner-city teens	46 girls	3. Avoiding foods containing flour, sugar, and salt		Minority sample
	98% girls of color, predominantly Latina	4. Regular exercise	Obese girls lost an average of 12.9%	**Limitations:**
Nonexperiment one group design		**Outcome measures:** Height and weight		Small sample size
	Setting: All-girls high school	**F/U:** Intervention completion at 9 months		Not equal attention comparison group
				No measurement of mediating or moderating variables
				Sample may have attracted more motivated girls

BP, blood pressure; BMI, body mass index; F/U, follow-up; HR, heart rate; PA, physical activity; PE, physical education; RCT, randomized controlled trial.

Source: From Grant #R01 NR012171, funded by the NIH/National Institute of Nursing Research; PI: Bernadette Melnyk.

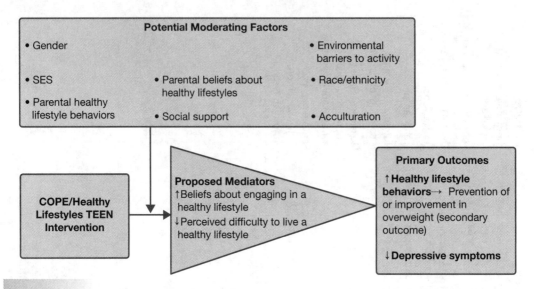

FIGURE 23.1 COPE conceptual model (From Grant #R01 NR012171, funded by the NIH/NINR; PI: Bernadette Melnyk).

COPE, Creating Opportunities for Personal Empowerment; NIH, National Institutes of Health; NINR, National Institute of Nursing Research; PI, principal investigator; SES, socioeconomic status; TEEN, Thinking, Feeling, Emotions, and Exercise.

> Leave nothing to the reviewers' imaginations!
> —*Bern Melnyk & Dianne Morrison-Beedy*

Sample

Describe the sample that you will target in your study and outline your inclusion and exclusion criteria, providing explanations for why you chose to eliminate individuals with certain characteristics. Include a **power analysis** in determining your sample size unless you are conducting a small pilot study the purpose of which is to calculate **effect sizes** to be used in a power analysis for a future large-scale clinical trial (Mays & Melnyk, 2009). Remember, the power to detect statistically significant findings in your study increases when sample size increases.

Describe the sampling design that you will use (e.g., random sampling; convenience sampling) and provide a rationale for your decision. If random sampling is not possible, it is important to address how you will attempt to increase representativeness of your sample (e.g., conducting the study at multiple sites; inclusion of diverse participants). Explain how threats to **external validity** will be minimized (see Chapter 9). In addition, specify exactly how the subjects will be recruited into the study and the feasibility of recruiting your targeted number. Provide letters of support from key administrative personnel at your study sites that support access to the population which you are targeting in your grant application. In the sample section of the grant, describe how you will include subjects of both genders, from diverse cultural groups, and children younger than 21 years. If your study does not include these groups, a strong rationale should be included.

The Intervention(s)

Clearly describe each component of the intervention(s) being proposed in your study. If the experimental intervention is one that has multiple sessions or doses, it is important to list the content of each session of the intervention. Again, leave nothing to the reviewers' imaginations. Reviewers will want the intervention clearly and fully described. In this section, reinforce how the theoretical framework guided the development and content of the intervention. In addition, discuss the reproducibility and feasibility of intervention delivery in real-world practice settings. It also is important to discuss the control group condition in detail. If you will have an **attention control group**, describe exactly what will be included in that intervention in a manner similar to how you described your experimental intervention. Remember, the attention control condition must be credible. For example, if you are targeting obese adults with a multicomponent experimental intervention to enhance their nutritional practices and physical activity, a credible attention control condition would not be teaching the control group about dental hygiene or motor vehicle safety. In this section, it also is important to discuss strategies that will be implemented to ensure cultural sensitivity of the intervention as well as intervention **fidelity**. Fidelity in intervention work means that the intervention was delivered to the participants in the precise manner as it was intended to be delivered. Explaining how fidelity of the intervention will be maintained in the project is a key methodological requirement of an intervention study.

Manipulation checks also are an important aspect to describe in this section of the grant application. They assure that the participants processed the intervention content and/or are adhering to activities prescribed for them. For example, if the intervention was educational in content, a multiple choice test might be given to participants after receiving the educational content to determine whether they truly received and processed the information. If the participants were directed to engage in physical activity, they might be asked to keep a record of the days and times that they actually engaged in physical activity as the manipulation check.

Measures

One of the first pointers in writing your measurement section of the grant application is to ensure that you describe thoroughly all variables that you include in your study and their related measures and, conversely, do not include measures without also addressing why they are being used. Above everything else, remember that all measures are not created equal, so selectivity is key. Presenting a description of all of the measures in a consistent manner is helpful to reviewers. The instrument name, description of the construct it is assessing, number of items, type of answer response format, example of answer options, scoring range, and psychometric properties (i.e., validity and reliability) should all be presented. **Validity** indicates that the instrument is measuring what it is intended to measure. Include face, content, and construct validity of the instrument if known. For **internal consistency reliability** (i.e., the measure is consistently measuring its construct), the value (e.g., Cronbach's alpha) should ideally be 0.80, 0.70 at the very least. Using measures with established validity and reliability is critical for the success of the grant. For intervention studies, the instruments used should also be sensitive to change over time (i.e., those with low test–retest reliabilities so there is opportunity to show a change in outcomes) and culturally sensitive. Interrater reliability for objective measures should be at least 90% and assessed routinely to monitor for observer drift. Justify why you chose a specific measure, especially if there are multiple instruments available that tap the same construct. Include self-report as well as nonbiased observations whenever possible because if the findings from both types of these measures converge, study conclusions will be stronger.

EXHIBIT 23.3 Common Criticisms in the Measurement Section of Proposals

---

- Simply listing the name of a measure without describing it in some detail (e.g., number of items, response options, construct being assessed) is not an effective or convincing presentation.
- Do not report "this measure is valid and reliable" without accompanying details.
- Descriptions should specify the type of psychometric evaluation approach used to establish validity and reliability (e.g., interrater reliability between two trained raters).
- Present pilot data that provide evidence of reliability and validity.
- Measures validated in one culture, race, age, or unique population should not automatically be considered valid for other groups.
- Do not include measures with reliability statistics lower than the standard threshold *without* addressing this concern.
- Do not select a measure on the basis of its name without confirming that the items specifically relate to your study construct.
- Steer clear of selecting so many measures that your list reads like an encyclopedia rather than a well-thought-out choice.

When faced with page limitations, tables are very useful for the measurement section of a grant application. Exhibit 23.3 presents pearls of wisdom for strengthening the measures section of your grant application.

Procedure

The procedure section of a grant application includes the protocol for the study. In this section, it is important to clearly describe each step of the protocol (e.g., exactly how the participants will be recruited, when the interventions will be delivered, the exact timing of when the measures will be collected). Again, it is very helpful to create a table to summarize the protocol. See Table 23.2 for an example of a table that outlines the data collection schedule for a clinical trial. Including a timeline that outlines major study activities is a component of the application that documents for reviewers your grasp of the "big picture" of study implementation as well as need for desired years of funding. Table 23.3 presents an example of a 5-year RCT timeline, which provides a fairly detailed explanation of anticipated components, from logistical start-up to analysis and dissemination.

Data Analysis

In the data analysis section of your grant application, be specific and clear about how you will analyze the data from your study to answer each of the study questions or test each of the hypotheses. It is helpful to repeat the research questions or hypotheses in this section and describe the analysis for each of them. Grant applications are strengthened by having a seasoned statistician as part of your team.

Potential Limitations With Alternative Approaches

At the conclusion of the grant application, it is important to discuss potential limitations with alternative strategies that you would use if these limitations become an issue during the study. This section of the grant demonstrates to reviewers that you have thought carefully about the potential limitations of your study design and methods with strategies for overcoming them. For example, if you know that cross-contamination between intervention groups or attrition may be potential problems in your study, it would be important to acknowledge them and to include your strategies to minimize these issues.

TABLE 23.2 Example of a Data Collection Summary Table

VARIABLE FROM OUR THEORETICAL FRAMEWORK	INSTRUMENT/SOURCE OF DATA	DATA COLLECTION TIMES				MEASURE USED IN STATISTICAL ANALYSIS
		PRE	POST	6 MONTHS	12 MONTHS	
Demographics (potential covariates/moderators)	Demographic questionnaire	X				Item ratings/answers
Acculturation (moderator)	The AHIMSA Scale	X				Total score
Healthy lifestyle behaviors (primary outcome)	Healthy Lifestyle Behaviors Scale and pedometer steps	X	X	X	X	Total score on the Healthy Lifestyle Behaviors Scale and total number of pedometer steps
Depressive symptoms (primary outcome)	Beck Youth Inventory II	X	X	X	X	Total score
Weight (secondary outcome)	BMI%	X	X	X	X	BMI%
Cognitive beliefs about a healthy lifestyle (mediator)	Healthy Lifestyle Beliefs Scale	X	X	X		Total score
Perceived difficulty in leading a healthy lifestyle (mediator)	Perceived difficulty scale	X	X	X		Total score

AHIMSA, Acculturation, Habits, and Interests Multicultural Scale for Adolescents; BMI, body mass index.

Source: From Grant #R01 NR012171, funded by the NIH/National Institute of Nursing Research; PI: Bernadette Melnyk.

TABLE 23.3 Exemplar Time Table From *HIP Teens* Study (Funded by the National Institutes of Health/National Institute of Nursing Research #R01 NR0081994)

MONTHS	RESEARCH ACTIVITIES
1–3	Finalize procedures, establish school liaisons, hire/train staff, CAB/TAB managements
4–6	Focus groups, transcribe/analyze transcripts; pilot measures
7–9	Refine/finalize all study manuals, materials, procedures, and protocols
10–12	Train interventionists/recruiters; ACASI programming
13–33	Start RCT recruitment during month 13; end recruitment in month 33
14–34	Start HIV and CTL sessions in month 14; end in month 34
18–38	Begin 3-month follow-up assessments in month 18; end 3-month follow-ups in month 38; ongoing data management
21–41	Begin 6-month follow-up assessments in month 21; end 3-month follow-ups in month 41; ongoing data management
24, 36, 48	Prepare reports for DSMB, IRBs, and NICHD/NIH; hold annual DSMB meeting
27–47	Begin 12-month follow-up assessments in month 27; end 3-month follow-ups in month 47; ongoing data management
33–53	Begin 18-month follow-up assessments in month 33; end 3-month follow-ups in month 53; ongoing data management
48–54	SEM data analysis on 3-, 6-, and 12-month data; papers/presentations
54–60	Complete 18-month data management, data analyses; NICHD reports; manuscripts

ACASI, audio computer-assisted self-interview; CAB/TAB, Community Advisory Board/Teen Advisory Board; CTL, control group; DSMB, Data and Safety Monitoring Board; IRB, Institutional Review Board; NICHD/NIH, National Institute of Child Health & Human Development/National Institutes of Health; RCT, randomized controlled trial; SEM, structured equation modeling.

Human Subjects and Their Protection

In this section of the grant application, it is important to describe (a) the demographic characteristics of the sample you intend on recruiting, (b) how informed consent will be obtained, (c) the risks and benefits of the research, (d) how confidentiality will be obtained, and (e) knowledge to be gained from the study. Plans for the inclusion of women, minorities, and children must be described, particularly for NIH grants. If one of these groups will not be included, a strong justification must be provided.

Data Safety and Management Plan

A data safety and management plan needs to be included for all clinical trials. This section should include the potential risks of the clinical trial and a plan for the appropriate oversight and monitoring of the conduct of the study to ensure the safety of the participants as well as the validity and integrity of the data. For those intervention studies that are multisite clinical trials with potential risk to participants, a Data and Safety Monitoring Board (DSMB) is required by NIH. The DSMB assesses study safety and recommends early closure if significant risks have

---

EXHIBIT 23.4 Example of Responsibilities of the DSMB Members From *Hip Teens* Study

---

1. Maintain confidentiality of the data and the results of the monitoring.
2. Review the research protocol and plans for data and safety monitoring.
3. Review on a yearly basis and as-needed basis the quality of outcome data at all sites; participant recruitment, randomization, and retention; risk versus benefit ratio for participants, including unanticipated adverse effects; and other factors that may affect outcome.
4. Determine whether the trial should continue as designed, should be changed, or should be terminated on the basis of the data and make recommendations to the NIH, IRBs at each site, and site investigators considering conclusion or continuation of the study.
5. Monitor reports of related studies to determine whether the current study needs to be changed or terminated.
6. Following DSMB meetings, provide appropriate NIH staff and the PIs with written information concerning their findings.
7. Submit summary reports of discussions regarding unexpected adverse effects or unanticipated problems involving risks to participants or others. These reports should include a review of data and outcomes across all sites, summary of the review of these events, and any recommendations for modification of the study protocol.
8. Oversee that reports are relayed to the IRB and to the OHRP.
9. Review proposed modifications to the study prior to their implementation.

DSMB, Data and Safety Monitoring Board; IRB, Institutional Review Board; NIH, National Institutes of Health; OHRP, Office of Human Research Protections; PI, principal investigator.

arisen or if new information indicates that the trial is unlikely to be successfully completed. The DSMB are scientific experts selected by the principal investigator (PI), who review the study on a regular (usually yearly) basis. See Exhibit 23.4 for an example of the responsibilities of a DSMB taken from a study funded by the NIH/NINR.

Budget

Details regarding planning the budget for an intervention study are provided in Chapter 12. If you are writing a grant for the NIH, permission must be obtained to submit an application with yearly direct costs of more than $500,000. Reviewers will look critically at whether you have appropriate personnel and time allotted to those personnel to carry out your study. The PI should be at least 30% effort on the project. Remember, do not overestimate or underestimate your budget and remember to "justify, justify, and justify" each item of your budget with strong rationale.

CRITERIA USED IN REVIEWING GRANTS WITH COMMON FEEDBACK FROM REVIEWERS

Funding agencies typically use similar criteria to evaluate the quality of grant submissions and most publish these criteria so that investigators are aware of how their applications will be evaluated. Therefore, it is important to review and take into consideration those criteria before starting your grant application. The criteria given in the following subsections are used by the NIH in the review of grant applications; however, these criteria are very similar to those used by other federal funding agencies, foundations, and professional organizations.

Impact

The overall impact of the grant, which reflects whether the research is worth conducting, is a major criterion in the review process. Impact is the probability that the study will exert a sustained powerful influence on the field or improve outcomes in the real world. Common feedback from reviewers in the area of impact includes the following:

- The probability of clinicians using and sustaining this intervention in real-world practice settings is unlikely.
- Key outcomes related to this problem are not being measured; as a result, the opportunity for major impact in the field is minimal.
- Efforts to reduce attrition in this high-risk population need more consideration because loss of several subjects from this trial will threaten the internal validity of the study.
- Dose–response to treatment is not being assessed; therefore, it will not be known how much of the intervention is absolutely necessary to produce positive outcomes.
- The power calculation used for this study is on the basis of a moderate **effect size** for the intervention on the study's primary outcome; however, there is no prior evidence in the application to expect a moderate intervention effect.

Significance

Significance of a study addresses whether the research directs an important problem or a critical barrier to progress in the field. Furthermore, it focuses on whether scientific knowledge, technical capability, and/or clinical practice will be advanced if the aims are achieved. Common feedback from reviewers in the area of significance includes the following:

- The argument for why an intervention in this particular population is needed is not strong.
- Examining the process through which the intervention works would increase the significance of the study.
- The conceptual framework as presented underlies the intervention but is not consistent with the overall study.

Investigator and Team

Reviewers look at the research team very critically to determine whether the investigators are appropriately trained and suited to carry out the proposed study. They also determine whether the proposed work is appropriate to the experience level of the PI and other researchers on the team. The publication record of the PI and coinvestigators will be scrutinized, especially noting whether manuscripts were a product of the team's prior grants. Common feedback in this area includes the following:

- The PI is inexperienced and does not have strong coinvestigators.
- The PI has limited publications.
- The team does not have a seasoned statistician.
- The percentage of time devoted to the study by the PI is not sufficient to complete the project.

Innovation

Innovation of the project is heavily evaluated in grant applications. Questions related to innovation include the following: (a) Does the project use novel concepts, approaches, or methods? (b) Are the aims original and innovative? (c) Does the project challenge existing paradigms or develop new methodologies or technologies? Common feedback from reviewers about innovation includes the following:

- The use of an educational booklet to deliver the intervention is not innovative.
- The intervention being proposed has already been tested in several other populations, and the investigator is not really adding anything new to what has already been done.
- It is unclear whether the intervention would be routinely delivered by clinicians as designed.
- The dependent variables being used in the study are not innovative.

Approach

The approach section of a grant deals with the study's methods and whether they are rigorous. Specifically regarding approach, reviewers will assess whether the conceptual framework, design, methods, and analyses are adequately developed, well integrated, and appropriate to the aims of the project. Reviewers also will be looking for whether the application acknowledged potential problem areas and considered alternative strategies. Common feedback on approach includes the following:

- The theory does not drive the intervention proposed or variables selected for the study.
- The study design is weak, which will threaten internal validity.
- Some of the details of the methodology are unclear or questionable.
- Sample size will not be adequate to detect medium intervention effects.
- The investigator did not designate on which outcome variable the power analysis was based.
- The measures are not adequately described.
- The possibility of cross-contamination between study groups is not addressed.
- The data analysis plans need further discussion of statistical analyses to be used to test each hypothesis.
- The number of measures being used creates too much burden for subjects.
- The project is too ambitious for the timetable proposed.

Environment

Reviewers will look carefully at whether the scientific environment in which the work will be conducted contributes to the probability of success. They also will expect to see whether there is evidence of institutional support (e.g., letters from key administrative personnel). In addition, reviewers will assess whether the proposed study takes advantage of unique features of the scientific environment or uses useful collaborative arrangements. Common feedback on environment includes the following:

- The investigator does not capitalize on the extensive resources in the environment.
- The General Clinical Research Center (GCRC) is not being used.
- There is no letter of support from the dean or associate dean for research.

For a summary of tips for writing strong grant applications, please see Exhibit 23.5. Tips for writing applications can be found online at https://grants.nih.gov/grants/how-to-apply-application-guide/format-and-write/write-your-application.htm.

DEADLY SINS AND MAJOR CHARACTERISTICS OF FUNDED GRANT PROPOSALS

There are 10 deadly sins of grant proposals that immediately decrease their probability of funding. These deadly sins are listed in Exhibit 23.6. Conversely, major characteristics of funded grant applications are listed in Exhibit 23.7.

EXHIBIT 23.5   Tips for Increasing Grant Funding Success

- Write a grant that is in the funding agency's priorities.
- Consider obtaining presubmission consultation from the funding agency.
- Review guidelines for the submission of applications as well as the funder's established criteria for the review of grants, which are frequently posted on its website.
- Review funded applications from the agency and use them as a template for success.
- Develop a proposal that is significant, innovative, and groundbreaking.
- Follow directions meticulously.
- Conduct a "mock review" of your proposal prior to submission with seasoned funded investigators.
- Obtain external consultants to strengthen your research team in needed areas.
- Obtain editorial review of your grant prior to submission.
- Remember that you never get a second chance to make a great first impression!

EXHIBIT 23.6   Ten Deadly Sins of Grant Proposals

1. Failure to follow directions to a "tee"
2. Lack of new or original ideas
3. Failure to acknowledge published relevant work
4. Lack of innovation
5. Fatal flaws (e.g., lack of an attention control group; use of instruments that are not valid and reliable)
6. Applications that are incomplete or do not contain enough detail about the methods to be used in the study
7. Over- or underambitiousness
8. Uncritical approach
9. Spelling and grammatical errors
10. Uncertainty about future directions

EXHIBIT 23.7   Major Characteristics of Funded Grant Applications

1. Innovative/creative
2. Clear and well written
3. Potential for significant impact in the field/extension of the science
4. Sophisticated
5. Rigorous in methods
6. A highly qualified team
7. Depth in conceptual issues

STRATEGIES FOR RESUBMITTING NONFUNDED GRANTS

When a grant application that took you weeks to months to write does not fund, it is normal to feel discouraged and question whether you should try to resubmit it. Remember, everyone goes through a period of shock and disbelief when their grant does not score or fund; then, the shock turns to stress and finally fatigue sets in as you wonder whether you can get up enough energy to write a resubmission on top of all of your other responsibilities. After reading the critique or summary statement from the grant review, it is common to feel sad, depressed, anxious, angry, and/or frustrated. Many individuals also commonly question whether the reviewers actually read through their proposal in detail because their comments sometimes reflect missing certain points when they were actually included in the grant. Remember, reviewers are human and often receive several grants to review. The reviewers are typically experts in their fields and try their very best to give each grant the most thoughtful review and consideration. After a period of grieving the summary statement or critique, it is important to get back to your dream and passion of making a difference with your research and revise your application for submission if permitted by the funding agency. Federal agencies, such as the NIH and the AHRQ, currently allow one resubmission of a grant proposal. Most agencies also allow the investigator to provide a one-page introduction to the revised application to explain how they addressed the reviewers' comments and suggestions.

If an introduction to the revised application is permitted by the funding agency, tell the review committee that their critique has assisted you in clarifying and strengthening your application. Respond point by point to the critical issues raised by the review panel. Do agree with as many constructive comments by the reviewers. If you disagree with a comment, do so gently with excellent rationale, such as "We agree that contamination is always a concern in clinical intervention studies and have given it thoughtful consideration. However, we believe that this potential problem can be minimized by taking several precautions, such as placing the intervention materials in similar-colored binders for both experimental groups and randomly assigning subjects by blocks of time instead of by individuals."

In the resubmission, do not completely rewrite the application as if it were new. Some agencies, such as the NIH, require that all changes be made in different or italicized font so that the reviewers will know exactly what content was changed in the application. Unhelpful responses in the resubmission of grants include (a) ignoring the reviewers' criticisms, (b) uncritically changing the research design in an attempt to please the review panel, and (c) denigrating the review panel's criticism.

> Never, never, never, never, never, never, never quit
> (until your study is funded)! —*Winston Churchill*

SUMMARY

In conclusion, writing a grant application is similar to eating a 2-ton chocolate elephant. If you sit down in front of the elephant and look up at the whole animal, it looks way too large to consume. However, if you keep your eyes only on the chunk of chocolate that is right in front of your eyes and consume that piece, then move to the next piece of chocolate and focus only on eating that piece, pretty soon the whole elephant will be eaten as a result of eating it one bite at a time. Remember, success is getting up one more time when you fall. In the world of grant writing, nothing is terminal. Everything is transitional. What looks like the end of the road will turn out to be only a bend in the road. The important thing is for you to stay focused on your dream/vision of making a difference and remain persistent through the character builders (i.e., nonfunded applications). Keep swinging the bat until you hit the ball and your grant funds!

Key Points From This Chapter

■ Consider obtaining presubmission consultation from the funding agency that you are targeting with your grant application.

■ Follow directions to a "tee."

■ Obtain the funding agency's grant review criteria and concentrate on writing your application to address those criteria.

■ Obtain one or two successfully funded grants from the funding agency that you are targeting and review them carefully.

■ Arrange for a "mock" review of your proposal prior to submission.

■ If your grant was not funded and resubmission of your application is allowed, address each comment from the reviewers' summary statement or critique in a positive manner.

■ Remember, with every rejection you get, you are one step closer to a funded grant.

REFERENCES

Chehab, L. G., Pfeffer, B., Vargas, I., Chen, S., & Irigoyen, M. (2007). "Energy up": A novel approach to the weight management of inner-city teens. *Journal of Adolescent Health*, *40*(5), 474–476. doi:10.1016/j.jadohealth.2006.12.009

Fardy, P. S., White, R. E., Haltiwanger-Schmitz, K., Magel, J. R., McDermott, K. J., Clark, L. T., & Hurster, M. M. (1996). Coronary disease risk factor reduction and behavior modification in minority adolescents: The PATH program. *Journal of Adolescent Health*, *18*(4), 247–253. doi:10.1016/1054-139X(95)00283-X

Fisher, J. D., & Fisher, W. A. (1992). Changing AIDS-risk behavior. *Psychological Bulletin*, *111*(3), 455–474. doi:10.1037/0033-2909.111.3.455

Killen, J. D., Robinson, T. N., Telch, M. J., Saylor, K. E., Maron, D. J., Rich, T., & Bryson, S. (1989). The Stanford Adolescent Heart Health Program. *Health Education Quarterly*, *16*(2), 263–283.

Mays, M. Z., & Melnyk, B. M. (2009). A call for the reporting of effect sizes in research reports to enhance critical appraisal and evidence-based practice. *Worldviews on Evidence-Based Nursing*, *6*(3), 125–129. doi:10.1111/j.1741-6787.2009.00166.x

Melnyk, B. M., & Fineout-Overholt, E. (2015). Writing a successful grant proposal to fund research and evidence-based practice implementation projects. In B. M. Melnyk & E. Fineout-Overholt (Eds.), *Evidence-based practice in nursing & healthcare: A guide to best practice* (3rd ed., pp. 490–514). Philadelphia, PA: Wolters Kluwer.

Neumark-Sztainer, D., Story, M., Hannan, P. J., & Rex, J. (2003). New Moves: a school-based obesity prevention program for adolescent girls. *Preventive Medicine*, *37*(1), 41–51. doi:10.1016/S0091-7435(03)00057-4

O'Neil, C. E., & Nicklas, T. A. (2002). Gimme 5: An innovative, school-based nutrition intervention for high school students. *Journal of the American Dietetic Association*, *102*(Suppl. 3), S93–S96. doi:10.1016/S0002-8223(02)90432-3

Pate, R. R., Ward, D. S., Saunders, R. P., Felton, G., Dishman, R. K., & Dowda, M. (2005). Promotion of physical activity among high-school girls: A randomized controlled trial. *American Journal of Public Health*, *95*(9), 1582–1587. doi:10.2105/AJPH.2004.045807

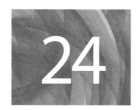

Submitting a Research Grant Application to the National Institutes of Health: Navigating the Application and Peer Review System

Mindy B. Tinkle & Ann Marie McCarthy

> Character consists of what you do on the third and fourth tries. —*John Albert Michener*

If you are committed to a career in research, particularly clinical intervention research related to improving the health of a population, chances are good that you will at some point submit a research grant application to the National Institutes of Health (NIH). The NIH is a major source of funding for relevant clinical research, and the NIH peer review system is widely accepted as one of the premier peer review systems around the world. Although the NIH process will be used as a model, much of what is included in this chapter will also apply to other funding sources.

The mission of the NIH is to "seek fundamental knowledge about the nature and behavior of living systems and the application of that knowledge to enhance health, lengthen life, and reduce the burdens of illness and disability" (NIH, 2015, Mission and Goals section, para. 1). The NIH supports the research of scientists in universities, hospitals, and research institutions in the United States and abroad to accomplish this mission. It sits organizationally in the U.S. Department of Health and Human Services and is one of 11 federal agencies providing health and human services and critical research for all Americans, such as the Centers for Disease Control and Prevention, the Food and Drug Administration, the Agency for Healthcare Research and Quality, and the Indian Health Service.

The NIH is the largest source of funding for biomedical research in the world, with an annual budget in 2016 of $32.3 billion (NIH, 2017). More than 80% of this funding is awarded through approximately 50,000 competitive grants to more than 300,000 researchers at more than 2,500 universities in every state and across the globe (NIH, 2017).

Most of these awarded funds support the direct costs of conducting research or those costs that can be directly attributed to a specific research project, such as scientists' and project staffs' salaries and equipment. About one-quarter of the NIH investment in research reimburses indirect costs or those general expenses that are used collectively for construction, maintenance, and operation of facilities used for research and for supporting administrative expenses, such as financial management, institutional review boards, and environmental health and safety management (U.S. Government Accountability Office, 2007). These indirect reimbursements (often referred to as "F&A," or "facilities and administrative costs") are critical to the development and maintenance of research infrastructure in universities and research organizations across the country. Each institution negotiates with the federal government to set its own indirect cost rate; therefore, it is important to work with your university's Office of Sponsored Projects to be aware of this rate and how it is managed.

The NIH is composed of 27 different institutes and centers, each of which has its own specific research agenda, and all but three are funded by Congress, manage their own budgets, and award grants. Most of the institutes are categorical, or focus on specific disease conditions, such as the National Cancer Institute, or have a body system focus, such as the National Eye Institute or the National Heart, Lung, and Blood Institute. The National Institute of Nursing Research (NINR) and the National Institute for Dental and Craniofacial Research are the only institutes that are discipline focused. Even though there are many categorical institutes, most health conditions are not funded solely at one institute. Although critical care research is funded mostly through the National Heart, Lung, and Blood Institute because of the high incidence of respiratory issues in critical illness, many other institutes also support research in this area. For example, the National Institute of Child Health and Human Development funds critical care research that focuses on the pediatric population, the National Institute on Aging supports research on critical care issues affecting the older adult, and the NINR funds research on issues of decision making in critical care. Each institute or center produces a strategic plan and vision document that identifies the science areas that are considered highest priority in terms of potential impact on the health of the public. Linking your application's research focus to the relevant strategic plan helps to make sure your project is aligned with the institute or center's program priorities.

NIH is composed of both Extramural and Intramural Programs. The Extramural Program provides funding for grants from researchers outside the NIH campus. The Office of Extramural Research (OER) at the NIH provides an invaluable array of tools and guidance for investigators applying for funding. The OER website (grants.nih.gov/grants/oer.htm) contains information about the NIH grant process and policies, types of grant programs, the peer review system, and how to apply. One important tool that can be accessed from the OER website is the NIH RePORTER. This tool allows you to search the database of awarded NIH grants to learn about funded projects in your science area of interest. Another tool on the OER website is the NIH Data Book (report.nih.gov/nihdatabook), which provides basic statistics on extramural grants, success rates for different grant mechanisms, and data about funded investigators. The OER sponsors two interactive NIH Regional Seminars on Program Funding and Grants Administration each year for the extramural community in different areas of the country to learn more about the grant application and peer review process, and highlight current issues of special interest to the NIH. These seminars are specifically geared to investigators new to the NIH, grants administrators, and graduate students.

The NIH also houses a robust Intramural Research Program (IRP), with 1,200 principal investigators (PIs) and more than 4,000 postdoctoral fellows conducting research across the NIH campus and the NIH 240-bed research hospital (NIH, n.d.-c). The IRP accounts for approximately 10% of the NIH annual budget (NIH, 2017). The NINR IRP investigators conduct a focused program of clinical research on symptom science in their laboratories on the NIH campus. In addition, the NINR IRP also supports research-training opportunities at the NIH for nurse scientists across the country, such as the Graduate Partnership Program, the Summer Genetics Institute, and other special-topics summer research-training workshops. Other NIH institutes and centers also offer intramural research-training opportunities, such as the Office of Behavioral and Social Sciences Research's Training Institute on Dissemination and Implementation Research and Mobile Health Summer Training Institute. These intramural training programs are unique and rich opportunities to engage with cutting-edge science, interact with NIH scientists, and learn more about the NIH systems and processes.

NIH FUNDING OPPORTUNITY ANNOUNCEMENTS

The NIH uses the funding opportunity announcement to publicize its intention to award grants, most often as a result of competition for funds through the peer review process. Institutes and centers issue these announcements to stimulate and encourage research in high-priority science areas to advance their respective missions. The NIH requests research through two types of funding opportunity announcements: Program Announcements (PAs) and Requests for Applications (RFAs). A PA typically is an ongoing solicitation, allows for multiple receipt dates, and is usually active for 3 years. RFAs, however, are typically one-time solicitations for grant applications addressing a defined research topic and usually include a set aside of funds for these projects. Both PAs and RFAs specify the participating institutes and centers and describe the scope and objectives of the research of interest, application requirements, and review criteria to be applied. You can search the *NIH Guide to Grants and Contracts* (grants. nih.gov/grants/guide/index.html) for active funding opportunity announcements in your scientific area. In addition, each institute and center generally includes a list of active-funding opportunity announcements they are participating in on their respective websites.

NIH also supports unsolicited research applications that are outside the scope of the targeted announcements but still consistent with the NIH mission and one or more of the institutes or centers. These unsolicited applications are often called "investigator-initiated" submissions. Investigators submitting an unsolicited research grant application specify a "parent announcement" or an NIH-wide funding opportunity announcement specific for the type of grant mechanism in the application.

There are a number of award mechanisms available through the NIH. F and K training awards provide opportunities to both obtain further training and begin a program of research for early investigators. An F32, the Ruth L. Kirschstein National Research Service Award Individual Postdoctoral Fellowship (NIH, n.d.-b), provides mentored, postdoctoral training with strong senior faculty. Research Career Development Awards (NIH, n.d.-c), referred to as "K Awards," are training grants that support junior faculty as well as established investigators interested in enhancing their careers. Similar to the F32, K Awards for junior faculty include mentoring by senior researchers, training as needed, and funding for pilot projects. The most common K Awards for junior faculty are the K01 Mentored Research Scientist Career Development Award, K08 Mentored Clinical Scientist Research Career Development, and K23 Mentored Patient-Oriented Career Development Award. Although K Training Awards provide excellent opportunities, the remainder of this chapter focuses on the R-series research grants.

OVERVIEW OF NIH RESEARCH GRANTS (R-SERIES) MECHANISMS

Some of the most frequently used R-series grant mechanisms at the NIH include the NIH Small Grant Program (R03), the NIH Academic Research Enhancement Award (R15), the Exploratory/ Developmental Research Grant (R21), and the NIH Research Project Grant Program (R01). Each of these mechanisms has a distinct focus, has different features and requirements, and provides varying levels of funding (see Table 24.1). (Technically, the specific research program, e.g., the NIH Small Grant Program, is called a "grant mechanism," whereas the specific number, e.g., R03 or R01, is called an "activity code"; however, the two terms are often used interchangeably, and for the purposes of this chapter, the term "grant mechanism" is used for both.) It is important to note that not all NIH institutes and centers accept applications for all types of grant mechanisms, or they may apply specialized eligibility criteria. You will want to determine which institute and center participates and any specifics regarding eligibility. Talking with an Institute/Center Program Officer, the Office of Sponsored Projects, and senior colleagues at your institution and closely reviewing the relevant NIH funding opportunity announcements are all helpful in determining which grant program you should target.

The R01 is the traditional and historically oldest grant mechanism used by the NIH to support health-related research. The R01 program supports discrete and specified research projects to be conducted by PIs who are focused in the investigators' scientific area of interest and competencies (NIH, 2016d). R01 funding (or its equivalent) is the type of NIH grant often considered a critical factor in performance assessments for promotion and tenure. Almost all of the NIH institutes and centers fund R01 grants.

In February 2007, the NIH began allowing for research grant submissions, including the R01, from more than one PI on a single project, which is the multiple PI option (NIH, 2006). This option was extended to encourage interdisciplinary, translational, and other team approaches to research. This change signals a dramatic culture shift that appreciates the growing importance of teamwork in science that spans university boundaries (Jones, Wuchty, & Uzzi, 2008). Institutions are increasingly developing formal policies for sharing F&A costs received from grant funding and realigning tenure and promotion criteria with the team science model as ways to reduce barriers to interdisciplinary research (Inside Higher Ed, 2011; Kulage, Larson, & Begg, 2011; Mazumdar et al., 2015).

The NIH also has instituted new policies and initiatives to encourage and assist new investigators or those who have not successfully competed for R01-level grants in obtaining research funding and at an earlier age. After the doubling of the NIH budget between 1998 and 2003, the number and percentage of new investigators who were R01 recipients declined. In addition, the average age of investigators at the time of the first R01 award has been steadily increasing since 1980. Spiegel (2010) projected that if trends continue, the average age of a new R01 investigator would increase from the current age of about 42 to almost 60 by 2020. A similar trend can be seen by looking beyond R01s to all NIH R-series grants. The proportion of research grant funding awarded to investigators younger than 36 years has declined from 5.6% in 1980 to 1.2% in 2012 (Daniels & Rothman, 2014).

The NIH has implemented several strategies to address these concerns about age at first award, including the identification of new investigators and early-stage investigators (ESIs). New investigators are those who have not earlier competed successfully as a PI for a substantial NIH research award. ESIs are new investigators who are within 10 years of completing their terminal research degree or medical residency at the time of application for R01 grants. The goal at the NIH is for at least half of the new-investigator R01 applications being reviewed be from researchers in the early stage of their careers or ESIs (NIH, 2016b). The applications from ESIs and all new investigators receive special considerations both during peer review and at the time of funding.

TABLE 24.1 Frequently Used NIH R-Series Grant Mechanisms	
CODE	DESCRIPTION
R01	NIH Research Project Grant Program (R01) ■ Used to support a discrete, specified, circumscribed research project ■ NIH's most commonly used grant program ■ No specific dollar limit unless specified in the FOA ■ Advance permission required for $500,000 or more (direct costs) in any year ■ Generally awarded for 3 to 5 years ■ Utilized by all ICs ■ See parent FOA: PA-16-160
R03	NIH Small Grant Program (R03): ■ Provides limited funding for a short period of time to support a variety of types of projects, including the following: pilot or feasibility studies, collection of preliminary data, secondary analysis of existing data, small, self-contained research projects, development of new research technology, etc. ■ Limited to 2 years of funding ■ Direct costs generally up to $50,000 per year ■ Not renewable ■ Utilized by more than half of the NIH ICs ■ See parent FOA: PA-16-162
R15	NIH AREA ■ Supports small research projects in the biomedical and behavioral sciences conducted by undergraduate and/or graduate students and faculty in institutions of higher education that have not been major recipients of NIH research grant funds ■ Eligibility limited (see https://grants.nih.gov//grants/funding/area.htm) ■ Direct cost limited to $300,000 over the entire project period ■ Project period limited to up to 3 years ■ All NIH ICs utilize except Fogarty International Center and National Center for Advancing Translational Sciences ■ See parent FOA: PA-16-200
R21	NIH Exploratory/Developmental Research Grant Award (R21) ■ Encourages new, exploratory, and developmental research projects by providing support for the early stages of project development. Sometimes used for pilot and feasibility studies ■ Limited to up to 2 years of funding ■ Combined budget for direct costs for the 2-year project period usually may not exceed $275,000 ■ No preliminary data are generally required ■ Most ICs utilize ■ See parent FOA: PA-16-161

AREA, Academic Research Enhancement Award; FOA, Funding Opportunity Announcement; ICs, institutes and centers; NIH, National Institutes of Health; PA, Program Announcement.

Source: National Institutes of Health. (2016g). Types of grant programs. Retrieved from https://grants.nih.gov/grants/funding/funding_program.htm#RSeries

Another initiative to address these troubling trends about age is the Early Career Review Program through the NIH's Center for Scientific Review (CSR, n.d.-b). Building on the findings from Ginther et al. (2011) that service on an NIH peer review study section was related to successful grant applications, this program targets early-career scientists with the goal of developing researchers as more competitive applicants earlier in their careers. The CSR

Program seeks to recruit junior faculty without prior CSR review experience to participate in peer review committees and learn how applications are evaluated and rated.

Racial and ethnic disparities in funding rates of investigator-initiated R01 applications have also been identified as a tenacious concern. Studies demonstrate that scientists from racial minority groups, particularly African American scientists, are less likely to receive funding from the NIH. In the landmark study conducted by Ginther et al. (2011), the gap in funding success rates among African American scientists amounted to 13% points compared with that among White scientists, even after controlling for educational background, country of origin, training, previous research awards, publication record, and employer characteristics. Oh et al. (2015) found that these award disparities for R01 or equivalent grants persist. The NIH leadership is actively working to understand and eliminate discrepancies for minority investigators. For example, CSR is experimenting with strategies to maximize fairness and eradicate unconscious bias in peer review (CSR, 2014; NIH, 2014). The NIH is also increasing investment in the diversity pipeline by supporting the National Research Mentoring Network (2017), a $19 million initiative at Boston College to improve the mentorship of scientists from underrepresented groups.

TIPS TO CONSIDER IN PLANNING YOUR NIH RESEARCH GRANT APPLICATION

The first step when planning to submit an application for an NIH research grant is to work with your sponsoring institution. Within your department, the chair or associate dean for research is a good starting point. Advice on the process for developing a grant and the content of your proposal should be discussed. Some departments provide reviews to colleagues, including mock review sessions. Secretarial help may be available to facilitate targeted aspects of the process, such as obtaining biosketches and letters of support and uploading components of the grant to the NIH system. Guidance on developing your budget can be critical. Your institution also will likely have a central office that must approve the budget and the grant and officially submit the proposal to NIH. It is important to remember that NIH grants are awarded to an institution, not to the individual, although the PI is responsible for carrying out the proposed research.

The NIH OER website offers an excellent description of tips and strategies to follow for planning (grants.nih.gov/grants/planning_application.htm) and writing (grants.nih.gov/grants/writing_application.htm) your application. It is always advisable to discuss your application with the relevant program officer at the institute or center you are targeting. These NIH staff are available to discuss strategies for the preparation of your application and also to consider the fit of your proposed study with the scientific priorities of the specific institute or center. You may also want to review the institute or center's website for information on grants and funding. For example, the NINR has a frequently-asked-questions document focused on preparation for a grant application that is a must-read for new investigators (NINR, 2016).

In addition to these helpful strategies, you will want to carefully review the peer review criteria that are used to evaluate and score your application during the review process (see Table 24.2). In addition to the five core review criteria that are used to score an application, there are additional criteria that reviewers consider and that you will want to carefully address, such as protection of human subjects. Overall, the NIH is focused on funding science that not only is slightly incremental but also has the potential to make significant advances in the science field involved. Starting with an important problem and making a sound case for how your study will build scientific knowledge and potentially improve health are key factors in crafting a competitive application.

TABLE 24.2 NIH Core Peer Review Criteria for R-Series Grants

CRITERION	DEFINITION
Significance	Does the project address an important problem or a critical barrier to progress in the field? If the aims of the project are achieved, how will scientific knowledge, technical capability, and/or clinical practice be improved? How will successful completion of the aims change the concepts, methods, technologies, treatments, services, or preventative interventions that drive this field?
Investigator(s)	Are the PDs/PIs, collaborators, and other researchers well suited to the project? If ESIs or new investigators, or in the early stages of independent careers, do they have appropriate experience and training? If established, have they demonstrated an ongoing record of accomplishments that have advanced their field(s)? If the project is collaborative or multi-PD/PI, do the investigators have complementary and integrated expertise; are their leadership approach, governance, and organizational structure appropriate for the project?
Innovation	Does the application challenge and seek to shift current research or clinical practice paradigms by utilizing novel theoretical concepts, approaches or methodologies, instrumentation, or interventions? Are the concepts, approaches or methodologies, instrumentation, or interventions novel to one field of research or novel in a broad sense? Is a refinement, improvement, or new application of theoretical concepts, approaches or methodologies, instrumentation, or interventions proposed?
Approach	Are the overall strategy, methodology, and analyses well reasoned and appropriate to accomplish the specific aims of the project? Are potential problems, alternative strategies, and benchmarks for success presented? If the project is in the early stages of development, will the strategy establish feasibility and will particularly risky aspects be managed? If the project involves clinical research, are the plans for (a) protection of human subjects from research risks and (b) inclusion of minorities and members of both sexes/genders, as well as the inclusion of children, justified in terms of the scientific goals and research strategy proposed?
Environment	Will the scientific environment in which the work will be done contribute to the probability of success? Are the institutional support, equipment, and other physical resources available to the investigators adequate for the project proposed? Will the project benefit from unique features of the scientific environment, subject populations, or collaborative arrangements?

ESI, early-stage investigator; NIH, National Institutes of Health; PD, project director; PI, principal investigator.

Source: National Institutes of Health. (2016a). Definitions of criteria and considerations for research project grant (RPG/X01/R01/R03/R21/R33/R34) critiques. *Scored Review Criteria.* Retrieved from https://grants.nih.gov/grants/peer/critiques/rpg_D.htm#rpg_01

Demonstrating the qualifications and suitability of the PI(s) and research team to conduct the proposed research is another key element in building a successful application. If you are submitting a major research grant application as a PI, you will want to portray the fit of your project with your research trajectory and demonstrate your scientific expertise and competency to successfully lead the project. There are many opportunities in the grant application to document your expertise and that of your team members. For example, the quality and clarity of the specific aims, research strategy, and analysis plan indicate the expertise of the PI. The NIH biosketch, completed by all senior/key personnel, provides evidence of each team member's prior research experience under the researcher's Contribution to Science section, which includes statements on research expertise along with relevant publications. The Personal Statement on each biosketch should include a description of that investigator's research expertise and a statement of that investigator's role and contribution to the proposed research. Other sections of the application, such as the Resources section, Budget Justification, and Letters of Support, can also provide documentation of PI and team expertise.

You will also want to demonstrate evidence in the application that the research team you have assembled provides adequate expertise in the major substantive and methodological areas needed to conduct the research. For example, if you do not have a statistician on your team with expertise relevant to your quantitative study or do not have a health economist on your team and you are proposing a cost-effectiveness analysis, your application will probably not fare well. Documenting that the research team has worked together in the past, through either completed studies or joint publications, will also strengthen your application. If you are using the multiple PI model, you will need to include a leadership plan in your application that provides a sound rationale for the choice of this approach and outlines how the investigators will share the authority and responsibility for leading and directing the project.

If you are submitting an R01 application, you will need to provide pilot data in your application that are foundational for the project you are proposing. These data should be placed in your application wherever it makes best sense for your proposal. Preliminary data are often woven into the Significance or Innovation sections and/or as part of the Approach. If you qualify as a new investigator and as an ESI (applicable only to R01 submissions), you do need to include pilot data as well, but the emphasis in peer review will be more on your experience and training and less on your ongoing record of accomplishments. The smaller R-series grant mechanisms, such as the R03 and R21, do not require pilot data, but if you have done some preliminary work, you should include your data.

It is critical to carefully address all of the required components of the proposed R mechanism. Researchers tend to focus their attention on the description of the research to be conducted, the Specific Aims, Research Strategy, and Approach, which are the heart of the application. However, there are other components that must be included, and attention to these sections is often neglected. These sections include the Abstract, Narrative, Facilities and Other Resources, Equipment, Biosketches, Budget and Personnel Justification, Human Subjects, and Letters of Collaborators and Support.

It is also important to be aware of changes made by the NIH to the application format and review process. For example, in 2017, what is allowed in the Appendix of an R-series grant has changed. In the past, applicants would include relevant articles, protocols, instruments, and other materials. The new policy (NIH, 2016c) states that the only materials allowed in appendices are blank informed consent/assent forms and blank proposed instruments. Clinical trial application appendices may also include clinical trial protocols and the investigator's brochure from an investigational new drug application. In 2016, the NIH added the requirement that applications address the reproducibility of research findings through increased scientific rigor and transparency (NIH, 2016h). Scientific rigor ensures robust and unbiased experimental design, methodology, analysis, interpretation, and reporting of results. One aspect of this expectation is that sex and other biological variables are factored into the design and analyses of the proposed project.

Being able to view a funded R-series NIH application may also be helpful. The NINR (2016) has instructions for how you may be able to use the Freedom of Information Act to access a funded NIH project, or a colleague may be willing to share his or her funded application with you. The National Institute of Allergy and Infectious Diseases (NIAID, 2017), with the permission of the PIs, has published on their website a set of successful R-series grant applications and their corresponding summary statements (www.niaid.nih.gov/grants-contracts/sample-applications). These successful examples may be useful to you as you begin to plan and write your application.

PEER REVIEW OF YOUR APPLICATION

The peer review system at the NIH is designed to provide a process for the evaluation of grant submissions that is fair, timely, accurate, and free of bias (NIH, 2018). This process is carried out in two levels (see Figure 24.1). The first level of review is conducted by a Scientific Review Group, commonly called a "study section," where the application receives an independent outside review for scientific and technical merit. The second level of review takes place at the relevant institute or center of National Advisory Council or Board, where funding recommendations for applications reviewed in study sections are made to the NIH staff in relation to program priorities and relevance. The institute or center director makes the final decision on funding, considering programmatic priorities and the input from the council and staff.

Where Your Application Is Reviewed

Most of the investigator-initiated research grant applications received by the NIH are peer reviewed in the NIH CSR. The NIH reviews approximately 88,000 applications each year (NIH, 2013b), and of that number, the CSR reviews 75% of the research grant submissions (CSR, n.d.-a). About one-fourth of the applications are reviewed outside the CSR, primarily in one of the NIH institutes or centers. The review offices in the NIH institutes and centers generally review applications submitted in response to the RFAs. The CSR operates somewhat like a peer review service center for all of the institutes and centers at the NIH, although it is an independent center with its own scientific staff and leadership. The CSR has a website for

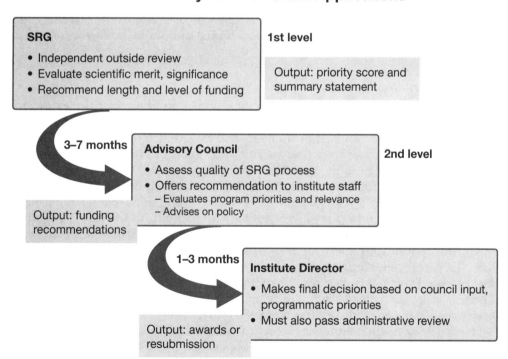

Review System for Grant Applications

FIGURE 24.1 Review system for grant applications.

SRG, Scientific Review Group.

Reprinted with permission from Paul Sheehy, National Institutes of Health.

applicants, which is an excellent resource to learn more about the specific steps involved in peer review (public.csr.nih.gov/ApplicantResources/Pages/default.aspx).

One important piece of homework you will want to do in thinking ahead about the peer review of your application is to search out the CSR study section(s) you feel is most appropriate to review your application and identify the institute or center most suited to fund your application. This information should be specified in the cover letter that accompanies your grant application. CSR staff review these cover letters, and investigator requests for study section assignment are generally honored. CSR study sections are clustered together in integrated review groups (IRGs) around a common scientific area. A list of IRGs is available on the CSR website that links to descriptions of each IRG and the specific study sections within that particular scientific cluster (public.csr.nih.gov/ StudySections/IntegratedReviewGroups/Pages/default.aspx). You will want to look closely at these descriptions and identify the IRG and study section you think is best suited to review your application.

This website also lists the membership roster and CSR scientific review officer for each study section. You will probably recognize the names of some of the study section members as imminent researchers in your field, and some of their backgrounds and publications should be relevant to your proposed work. If not, then you probably want to keep looking for a better fit. Talking to an institute or center program officer and colleagues in your scientific field for advice about identifying the most appropriate study section is an important strategy. In addition, you may also contact the scientific review officer at the CSR associated with the study section you may be targeting to talk further about the fit of your proposed research with this study section. The NIH RePORTER database of funded grants is another source for identifying study sections that reviewed successful applications in your scientific field. The CSR website provides a comprehensive list of other items to consider, including what to put in your cover letter, as well as a suggested cover letter format (https://grants. nih.gov/grants/how-to-apply-application-guide/format-and-write/write-your-application. htm#coverletters).

Review Meeting Overview

Once your application has been assigned to a study section, the scientific review officer will analyze it, review the cover letter, decide which reviewers from among the members of the study section can best evaluate it, and assign it to three or more reviewers. The scientific review officer may also recruit additional or "temporary" reviewers to augment the study section with specific scientific expertise that may be needed for the applications submitted for that particular review round. Regular or "chartered" study sections meet three times a year, generally in February, June, and October, in face-to-face meetings. Before the meeting, reviewers prepare and submit to the CSR a preliminary critique of your application and assign preliminary scores reflecting their evaluation of the scientific merit of your application.

The NIH peer review scoring system uses a 9-point scale using whole numbers only, without decimals (see Exhibit 24.1). A score of 1 indicates an exceptionally strong application without weaknesses, whereas a score of 9 indicates an application with major weaknesses that severely limit the scientific impact and very few strengths (NIH, 2013a). Each assigned reviewer uses this 9-point scale to assign preliminary scores to each of the 5 individual review criteria and to assign an overall impact/priority score to the application. The overall impact/priority score reflects the reviewer's overall evaluation of the application in terms of the likelihood for the proposed project to exert a sustained, powerful influence on the research field(s) involved.

Before the meeting and after receiving the reviewers' preliminary critiques and overall impact/priority scores for each of their assigned applications, the scientific review officer uses the preliminary impact scores to determine the order of review of applications for the meeting

EXHIBIT 24.1 Scoring Guidance for Research Applications

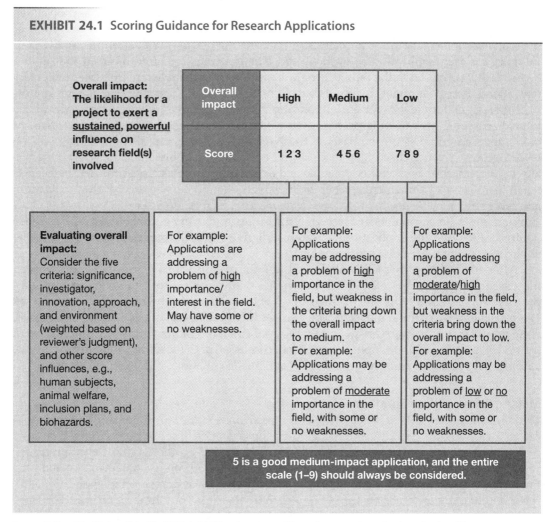

Overall impact:
The likelihood for a project to exert a <u>sustained</u>, <u>powerful</u> influence on research field(s) involved

Overall impact	High	Medium	Low
Score	1 2 3	4 5 6	7 8 9

Evaluating overall impact:
Consider the five criteria: significance, investigator, innovation, approach, and environment (weighted based on reviewer's judgment), and other score influences, e.g., human subjects, animal welfare, inclusion plans, and biohazards.

For example: Applications are addressing a problem of <u>high</u> importance/interest in the field. May have some or no weaknesses.

For example: Applications may be addressing a problem of <u>high</u> importance in the field, but weakness in the criteria bring down the overall impact to medium.
For example: Applications may be addressing a problem of <u>moderate</u> importance in the field, with some or no weaknesses.

For example: Applications may be addressing a problem of <u>moderate/high</u> importance in the field, but weakness in the criteria bring down the overall impact to low.
For example: Applications may be addressing a problem of <u>low</u> or <u>no</u> importance in the field, with some or no weaknesses.

5 is a good medium-impact application, and the entire scale (1–9) should always be considered.

Source: National Institutes of Health. (2013a). Additional scoring guidance for research applications. Retrieved from https://grants.nih.gov/grants/peer/guidelines_general/scoring_guidance_research.pdf

with the best-scoring applications discussed first. Applications from new investigators are clustered together for review to improve consistency. Generally, if a grant mechanism (e.g., R01s) has 10 or more applications being reviewed, only applications that fall in the top 50% of the preliminary impact scores are discussed and scored at the meeting, whereas applications that fall in the lower half are not discussed. For example, in a study section meeting that reviews 100 applications, all of them are reviewed, but only about 50 of them will actually be discussed and assigned an impact/priority score at the meeting. If your application is not discussed at a review meeting, you will receive your reviewers' critiques and will have the opportunity to resubmit a revised and improved application, considering this valuable feedback. The NIH allows for one resubmission of an unfunded application that must be submitted within 37 months of the original, new application. If the resubmission is unsuccessful, the NIH now permits you to submit your same idea as a new application (NIH, 2016f).

Study section meetings are generally composed of about 20 to 35 reviewers and are held over 1 to 2 days, depending on the number of applications to be reviewed. Each meeting is led by a scientific review officer, who is an extramural staff scientist and the designated federal official responsible for ensuring that each application receives a fair and objective initial peer review and that all relevant federal laws and policies are followed. The chair of the study section is a nonfederal scientist who leads the discussion of scientific and technical merit for each application being reviewed. The meetings are announced in the Federal Register and are closed to the public. Program officers from the relevant institutes or centers may attend these peer review meetings but are not involved in the evaluation of applications.

The assigned reviewers for each application (generally three reviewers per application) to be discussed at the meeting present their preliminary priority scores and a summary of their prepared critiques on the basis of the NIH review criteria to all the members of the review group. An open discussion moderated by the study section chair follows, and, generally, each application is discussed for an average of 10 to 15 minutes. Less time may be needed when there is broad agreement among the reviewers about the evaluation of the application, and more time may be needed if the assessments are discrepant. After discussion, the chair summarizes the major points addressed in the group, and every eligible reviewer (i.e., those not in conflict with the application) privately assigns an overall impact/priority score to the application using the 9-point scoring scale.

After the meeting, the CSR tabulates the final overall impact/priority score for each discussed application by calculating the average score from all of the reviewers' impact/priority scores, multiplying the average by 10 and rounding to the nearest whole number. The possible range of final impact/priority scores is from 10 (high impact) to 90 (low impact). Final impact/priority scores are generally released to investigators within 3 business days of the review meeting. If your application was not discussed at the meeting, you will not receive a numerical impact/priority score and will have the designation "ND" for not discussed.

Making Sense of Your Summary Statement

The scientific review officer is responsible for preparing a summary statement for each application reviewed by the study section, including those not discussed at the meeting. Examples of summary statements from successful R01s are provided on the NIAID website (https://www.niaid.nih.gov/grants-contracts/sample-applications). Summary statements include the final impact/priority score, the critiques from the reviewers assigned to the application, and the individual review criterion scores from each reviewer. If your application was discussed at the review meeting, a resume and summary of the discussion prepared by the scientific review officer are also included. A percentile may also be reported on the summary statement for a subset of applications. A percentile reflects the percentage of applications that received a better overall impact/priority score from the study section during the past three study section meetings or past year (NIH, 2016e). For example, if an application receives an impact/priority score of 20 and a percentile of 7, this indicates that only 7% of applications reviewed in this study section over the past three meetings had an impact/priority score better than 20. Percentile rankings and overall impact scores are among the most important factors used to help in determining funding decisions. Other factors that relate to the second level of review also enter into funding decisions, such as the institute and center program priorities, the balance of short-term and longer duration grants being supported, and the new-investigator and/or ESI status of R01 applications (NIH, n.d.-a).

Summary statements are generally released to new-investigator R01 applicants within 10 days of the review meeting to facilitate the resubmission of the application for the next review round. Other applicants generally receive their summary statements within 30 days of the review meeting. If you have questions about your summary statement, your program officer from the institute or center listed on the first page of your summary statement is your contact. In many cases, the program officer assigned to your application will have attended the review meeting, will have listened to the discussion, and may be able to guide you about your next steps.

Receiving a summary statement that includes critique of your work can sometimes be difficult. You will want to read it carefully and analytically, and talk with your colleagues and mentors to get more feedback. The resume and summary of discussion in your summary statement may look somewhat different from the individual reviewer critiques because this summary is a synthesis of what was actually discussed at the review meeting. The individual critiques include the assigned reviewers' statements of strengths and weaknesses for each criterion (e.g., significance, investigators) and criterion scores from 1 to 9. If your application was not discussed at the review meeting, your summary statement will not include a resume but will include the assigned reviewers' statements of strengths and weaknesses for each criterion and the criterion scores.

If your application did not get discussed, or the impact score is not competitive, ask yourself and seek input from colleagues about whether the weaknesses identified in your summary statement are fixable (see Exhibit 24.2). If there is a fatal flaw, take some time to decide the best route to approach your next submission. Most often, the weaknesses can be corrected, so focus on fixing the weaknesses and submitting a revised application (see Exhibit 24.3). Most investigators must submit multiple applications before they achieve funding success for their work, so persistence and practice can make a difference. An application that is not funded in the first review has a better chance of being funded on resubmission. In 2015, the NIH reported that the success rate for R01 applications was 13.1%, but the success rate for resubmission applications was 33.5% (NIH, n.d.-a). Most investigators report that the critiques received from the NIH peer reviews have helped them improve their applications and their overall science.

EXHIBIT 24.2 Common Reasons for NIH Applications Scoring Poorly in Peer Review

---

- The work is not important and will have little scientific impact.
- The significance of the work is not convincing.
- The work has already been done.
- The key areas of needed scientific expertise are not present in the project team.
- The conceptual model for the project is poorly integrated throughout the application.
- The proposed methods are not sound.
- The links between the aims, conceptual framework, measures, and analysis are not clear.
- Critical components of the project are underdeveloped, such as proposed intervention or data management and analysis plan.
- The application is poorly written, not well organized, and difficult to follow.

NIH, National Institutes of Health.

EXHIBIT 24.3 Tips on Resubmission of Applications to the NIH

- Funding on the first attempt is difficult, so be persistent.
- Determine whether people with the right expertise reviewed your application.
- Decide if you want to resubmit to the same or a different study section.
- Throw out the weak parts of your application and capitalize on your strengths.
- Respond point by point to reviewers' comments and suggestions, even if you disagree.
- If you disagree, explain why and provide additional information.
- Be respectful of the reviewers' evaluations, and never, never be hostile.

NIH, National Institutes of Health.

Key Points From This Chapter

- The NIH is a major source of funding for clinical research, and its peer review system is considered one of the best in the world.
- When submitting a grant to the NIH, demonstrate your scientific expertise to successfully lead the project and show the expertise of your research team.
- Start with a really important problem and make a sound case for how your study will build scientific knowledge and potentially improve health.
- Work with experienced researchers and your institution for advice and guidance.
- Identify the CSR study section that you feel is most appropriate to review your application.
- The NIH peer review system is a 9-point scoring system.
- Only applications that fall in the top 50% of the preliminary impact scores are discussed and scored at the review meeting.
- Receiving a summary statement that includes critique of your work can sometimes be difficult. Discuss it with your colleagues and mentors to get more feedback.
- Most problems identified in a summary statement can be resolved, so be persistent. Fix the problems and resubmit.

REFERENCES

Center for Scientific Review. (2014). Peer review notes Sep 2014. Retrieved from https://public.csr.nih.gov/aboutcsr/NewsAndPublications/PeerReviewNotes/Pages/Peer-Review-Notes-Sep-2014Part5.aspx

Center for Scientific Review. (n.d.-a). About CSR. Retrieved from https://public.csr.nih.gov/aboutcsr/Pages/default.aspx

Center for Scientific Review. (n.d.-b). Early Career Reviewer (ECR) Program. Retrieved from https://public.csr.nih.gov/ReviewerResources/BecomeAReviewer/ECR/Pages/default.aspx

Daniels, R. J., & Rothman, P. (2014, March 4). How to reverse the graying of scientific research. *Wall Street Journal*. Retrieved from https://www.wsj.com/articles/SB10001424052702304026804579411293375850348

Ginther, D. K., Schaffer, W. T., Schnell, J., Masimore, B., Liu, F., Haak, L. L., & Kington, R. (2011). Race, ethnicity, and NIH research awards. *Science, 333*(6045), 1015–1019. doi:10.1126/science.1196783

Inside Higher Ed. (2011). Tenure across borders. Retrieved from http://www.insidehighered.com/news/2011/07/22/usc_rewards_collaborative_and_interdisciplinary_work_among_faculty

Jones, B. F., Wuchty, S., & Uzzi, B. (2008). Multi-university research teams: Shifting impact, geography, and stratification in science. *Science, 322*(5905), 1259–1262. doi:10.1126/science.1158357

Kulage, K. M., Larson, E. L., & Begg, M. D. (2011). Sharing facilities and administrative cost recovery to facilitate interdisciplinary research. *Academic Medicine, 86*(3), 394–401. doi:10.1097/ACM.0b013e31820924ea

Mazumdar, M., Messinger, S., Finkelstein, D. M., Goldberg, J. D., Lindsell, C. J., Morton, S. C., … Parker, R. A. (2015). Evaluating academic scientists collaborating in team-based research: A proposed framework. *Academic Medicine, 90*(10), 1302–1308. doi:10.1097/ACM.0000000000000759

National Institute of Allergy and Infectious Diseases. (2017). Sample applications & more. Retrieved from https://www.niaid.nih.gov/grants-contracts/sample-applications

National Institute of Nursing Research. (2016). NINR policy on data and safety monitoring (DSM) of clinical trials – updated September 2014. Retrieved from https://www.ninr.nih.gov/researchandfunding/grant-development-and-management-resources

National Institutes of Health. (2006). Establishment of multiple principal investigator awards for the support of team science projects. Retrieved from http://grants.nih.gov/grants/guide/notice-files/NOT-OD-07-017.html

National Institutes of Health. (2013a). Additional scoring guidance for research applications. Retrieved from https://grants.nih.gov/grants/peer/guidelines_general/scoring_guidance_research.pdf

National Institutes of Health. (2013b). NIH peer review: Grants and cooperative agreements. Retrieved from https://grants.nih.gov/grants/peerreview22713webv2.pdf

National Institutes of Health. (2014). Rock talk. Retrieved from https://nexus.od.nih.gov/all/2014/05/29/new-efforts-to-maximize-fairness-in-nih-peer-review/

National Institutes of Health. (2015). Mission and goals. Retrieved from https://www.nih.gov/about-nih/what-we-do/mission-goals

National Institutes of Health. (2016a). Definitions of criteria and considerations for Research Project Grant (RPG/X01/R01/R03/R21/R33/R34) critiques. *Scored Review Criteria*. Retrieved from https://grants.nih.gov/grants/peer/critiques/rpg_D.htm#rpg_01

National Institutes of Health. (2016b). A history of new and early stage investigator policies and data. Retrieved from https://grants.nih.gov/policy/new_investigators/history.htm

National Institutes of Health. (2016c). New policy eliminates most appendix material for NIH/AHRQ/NIOSH applications submitted for due dates on or after January 25, 2017. Retrieved from https://grants.nih.gov/grants/guide/notice-files/NOT-OD-16-129.html

National Institutes of Health. (2016d). NIH Research Project Grant Program (R01). Retrieved from https://grants.nih.gov/grants/funding/r01.htm

National Institutes of Health. (2016e). Peer review. Retrieved from https://grants.nih.gov/grants/peer-review.htm#Summary

National Institutes of Health. (2016f). Resubmission applications. Retrieved from https://grants.nih.gov/grants/policy/amendedapps.htm

National Institutes of Health. (2016g). Types of grant programs. Retrieved from https://grants.nih.gov/grants/funding/funding_program.htm#RSeries

National Institutes of Health. (2016h). Updated application instructions to enhance rigor and reproducibility. Retrieved from https://www.nih.gov/research-training/rigor-reproducibility/updated-application-instructions-enhance-rigor-reproducibility

National Institutes of Health. (2017). Budget. Retrieved from https://www.nih.gov/about-nih/what-we-do/budget

National Institutes of Health. (2018). Updated application instructions to enhance rigor and reproducibility. Retrieved from https://grants.nih.gov/grants/peer-review.htm

National Institutes of Health. (n.d.-a). Applicant guidance: Next steps "Your application was reviewed; what to do next…." Retrieved from https://grants.nih.gov/grants/next_steps.htm

National Institutes of Health. (n.d.-b). Department of Health and Human Services. Part 1. Overview information. Retrieved from https://grants.nih.gov/grants/guide/pa-files/PA-16-307.html

National Institutes of Health. (n.d.-c). Intramural Research Program. Retrieved from https://irp.nih.gov

National Research Mentoring Network. (2017). Unlocking scientific potential through mentoring. Retrieved from https://nrmnet.net

Oh, S. S., Galanter, J., Thakur, N., Pino-Yanes, M., Barcelo, N. E., White, M. J., … Burchard, E. G. (2015). Diversity in clinical and biomedical research: A promise yet to be fulfilled. *PLOS Medicine*, *12*(12), e1001918. doi:10.1371/journal.pmed.1001918

Spiegel, A. M. (2010). Commentary: New guidelines for NIH peer review: Improving the system or undermining it? *Academic Medicine*, *85*(5), 746–748. doi:10.1097/ACM.0b013e3181d7e130

U.S. Government Accountability Office. (2007). National Institutes of Health extramural research grants: Oversight of cost reimbursements to universities. Retrieved from http://www.gao.gov/products/GAO-07-294R

25

Writing Progress and Final Reports

Margaret Roudebush & Shirley M. Moore

> To get it done, you have to sit down and get started. Tell your story because no one knows it better. —*Dianne Morrison-Beedy*

Progress and final reports are opportunities to indicate to the funder how the aims of the project were achieved, how the money was spent, what was learned from the project, and what the future plans are for continuation of the project or sustainability and dissemination of project results. This chapter provides information about the structure and content of research progress and final reports, general principles and writing tips, and submission procedures. Preparation of both the summary narrative and financial portions of federal and foundation grant reports is included. Examples of progress and final reports are provided. Special attention is given to writing reports of intervention studies. General information regarding progress and final reports is offered first, followed by information specific in writing reports for the National Institutes of Health (NIH).

PROGRESS REPORTS

When you accept the funds, you accept the responsibility to report the progress of the project and how the monies are being spent. Whether the grant is a small, internally funded pilot study, a private foundation project, or a federally funded study, a progress report is written to provide an update on your progress. The progress report should describe how your project is meeting its established goals, activities you have engaged in to date to meet those goals and any that have not been completed on schedule, and other relevant issues you are addressing. Your progress report will be reviewed by your program officer or foundation grants manager. A funding agency budget manager may read it as well.

A progress report should also be viewed as an opportunity to build and maintain a relationship with your funding agency. The progress report is a time to tell your unfolding story of the project and engage your program officer in the importance and quality of your work. Finally, it is important to note that on the basis of the information you provide, your program officer may contact you to ask for clarification or additional information during the course of your grant.

ORGANIZING A SYSTEM FOR WRITING YOUR PROGRESS REPORTS

At the time of receipt of project funding, set up a progress report filing system so that you will have the data you need at your fingertips to write your future progress and final reports. These are files in which you can store ongoing information about the project in an organized fashion to enhance the speed and accuracy of developing your progress reports. For example, an electronic progress report file might include the following subfiles: project milestones, personnel changes, analyses/results, unexpected events, enrollment reports, popular media contacts/reports, and presentations or manuscripts related to the project. Be sure to include a file that contains the guidelines for the preparation of the progress reports. Because no two funders are alike, it is important to know the guidelines for progress reports specific to that funder. There are usually specific guidelines available at the time of the notice of award (NOA), and, in some cases, at the time of the call for applications. It is important to read the grant NOA for information about the requirements for the report. The NOA often includes information about the following:

- Key dates for progress report and final reports
- The information on which you will need to report
- Report format, such as a specific form to use
- The person who will need to sign off on the report
- The department where you will send the report

The progress report for an intervention study may also be enhanced by keeping a set of field notes that will assist report writing, such as characterization of changes in the intervention protocol as the project unfolded, historical events that occurred during the study that might confound the interpretation of results, or personnel changes that affected intervention delivery. A more accurate description of important project changes over time can then be summarized for progress report writing.

THE PROGRESS REPORT SUMMARY NARRATIVE

Although there is no "one-size-fits-all" format, a progress report generally consists of a summary narrative and a financial report. The summary narrative usually contains four key elements:

- Background
- Work Completed
- Preliminary Results
- What's Next

Background
A progress report summary narrative usually starts with a restatement of the specific aims or the purpose of the project. If you are reporting on only a subset of the project aims, the particular subset of aims to be addressed should be clearly stated. Always provide the dates

of the period covered early in the report. Briefly summarize the significance of the project. If applicable, refer to previous progress reports and describe any funding for the project you may have received from other sources.

Work Completed

A major purpose of a project report is to describe what work has been completed during the reporting period. Use the project timeline and/or milestones as a reference point in describing the progress. A set of project tasks is usually associated with a time period or predetermined milestone. A bulleted list of the completed tasks is a succinct way to display a list of tasks completed; however, remember not to make the list too long. Group the tasks so that the list is no longer than six to eight items. In general, it is recommended to write using active verbs and in chronological order, or, if more logical, write in order of subtasks of the larger project. Include also any major project tasks associated with a milestone that have not been completed.

Preliminary Results

If you have preliminary results, provide them in a section that is clearly marked as such. Report both the positive and the negative results. State positive progress first, such as, "The study team has successfully recruited 100 participants who are currently receiving the intervention. Participants have expressed positive feedback." Then state the more problematic details, for example: "We had hoped to recruit 50% of minority subjects, but current participants represent only 20% of minority populations. We have taken steps to increase recruitment for minority subjects by the addition of two new recruitment sites that have a higher minority population than those we are currently using." Do not report a long list of problems, but rather, clearly state the challenge, what you have learned or discovered that may have changed your approach or have given you new insights, and state your strategy for solving the problem.

What's Next

In this section of the summary narrative, describe the work you expect to complete for the next time period. Describe any anticipated changes in the scope or objectives. A progress report should not be the first time a program officer learns about a change in scope or objective. Such changes should be requested in advance, following a discussion with your program officer, and the approval should be obtained in writing. If the changes impact the budget, a budget revision may be needed. This is not the place to write "We really need more staff to complete this project. I now see this project is terribly underfunded, and we will need additional funds to complete the project as originally stated." Rather, a clear statement that you have the problem under control is, "With the addition of a new clinic site to recruit participants, we expect to soon be on track with our proposed timeline." As a general rule, reports need to be concise and cover all reporting requirements of the funder.

TIPS FOR WRITING REPORTS

Exhibit 25.1 provides a list of tips for writing a successful report. Pay special attention to the page limit. Remember, your report is not the only report that is being read by the program official. Keep it brief. Many funders will set a maximum report length in their guidelines, but if they do not, aim for between 5 and 10 printed pages. Break the report up into short paragraphs with subheadings and use short lists and bullet points to assist the reader to pick out what you want to highlight. Make sure all exhibits and graphs are easily readable and carefully labeled; be careful not to overwhelm the reader with too many tables or exhibits. Color can enhance the visual appeal of your report and tables and graphs, but keep in mind that not all reviewers will print the report on a color printer. Make sure the image is

---

EXHIBIT 25.1 Tips for Writing a Successful Report

---

1. Follow the funder's guidelines for the elements to include in the report.
2. Use subheadings and indents to make your report ideas easy to find and follow.
3. Use bullet points for important details that you wish to highlight.
4. Use tables and graphs (but do not overwhelm with too many tables).
5. Make sure the font size is legible.
6. Use color to enhance the visual appeal of your report and tables and graphs.
7. Include stories and testimonials.
8. Use pictures.
9. Make sure reports are concise and cover all requirements.
10. Meet the reporting deadlines.

Source: Adapted from Satterfield, B. (2007). An introduction to grant reports: Tips and tools for preparing reports for your funders. Retrieved from http://www.cityvision.edu/wiki/introduction-grant-reports-tips-and-tools-preparing-reports-your-funders

also visually appealing if it were printed in black and white. Emotional impact can be incorporated in a progress report by the use of short stories, testimonials, and pictures. Finally, every effort should be made to meet the funder's deadline for when progress reports should be submitted. If you cannot meet the deadline for some reason and your report will be late, be sure to contact the funder. Most funders have an understanding attitude regarding grant reports that will be submitted late, as long as you give advance notice. This should not be a habit, however, as continual lateness in reporting may raise concerns by the funder about your grant management skills and may reduce your chances for future funding.

THE FINANCIAL REPORT

A detailed financial report is usually required with all progress reports. This typically involves both principal investigator (PI) and institutional sign-off. The financial report should include the details of how the monies were spent and should match your proposal and proposed timeline. Explanations should be provided, if needed, of why your spending does not match the proposal. Unexpended funds should be explained, with plans provided if those funds are to be used in the future as planned, or are to be shifted to a new purpose. As with a change in scope or aims, any changes in budgets are to be discussed in advance with a program officer, and permission for such changes should be obtained in writing. An example of a financial report for a progress report is provided in Exhibit 25.2.

BIBLIOGRAPHY, APPENDICES, AND ATTACHMENTS

A bibliography is often a required part of a progress report. Closely follow the bibliography formatting requirements of the funding agency. The bibliography provides a record of the publicly available products produced during your project. It is a complete listing of the following materials from your project:

■ Publications, such as books, book chapters, journal articles, reports, or websites
■ Proceedings and materials from national/regional events such as conferences and workshops
■ Published presentations and testimony

EXHIBIT 25.2 Sample Financial Report for Progress Reporting

FINANCIAL REPORT
The Robert Wood Johnson Foundation
P.O. Box 2316
Princeton, NJ 08543-2316
Phone: (609) 452-8701 Fax: (609) 627-6416

65114 Developing and conducting psychometric testing on a tool to measure systems thinking	**Project Director: Mary A. Smith**	**216**-###-####
CQI Improving the Science of Continuous Quality Improvement Program and Evaluation	**Financial Officer: Janet A. Jones**	**216**-###-####

Case Western Reserve University, Frances Payne Bolton School of Nursing

Budget Period: 10/01/2013 to 12/31/2015		**Grants Administrative Assistant:**
Project Period: 10/01/2013 to 12/31/2015		**Team Coordinator:** **Program Officer:** **Communications Associate:**
Budget for Period: 10/01/2013 to 12/31/2015	**Reporting Periods:** Final	**Communications Officer:** **Grants Administrative Senior Officer:**

EXPENDITURES

Item	Approved Budget Amount	10/2013 to 12/2015
Personel		
Project Director/Principal Investigator	25,152	25,773
Program Staff	39,219	41,995
Subtotal	**64,371**	**67,768**
Fringe Benefits	11,575	8,616
Personnel TOTAL	**75,946**	**76,384**
Other Direct Costs		
Office Operations	2,573	3,693
Communications/Marketing	400	248
Travel	5,916	3,694
Surveys	60	61
Equipment	1,460	1,821
Other Direct Costs	375	819
Other Direct Costs TOTAL	**10,784**	**10,336**
Purchased services		
Consultants	2,500	2,500
Purchased Services TOTAL	**2,500**	**2,500**
Indirect Costs	10,708	10,706
Indirect Costs TOTAL	**10,708**	**10,706**
Grant Total	**99,938**	**99,926**

Authorized Signature _____ Date: _____

Appendices and attachments may or may not be permitted with the progress report. Watch for specific guidelines regarding appendices and attachments. If appendices are permitted, there are sometimes specific tables or categories of information that are requested to be put in the appendices or attachments; there may be a specific form to be completed. Often, appendices and attachments are not permitted or are restricted in number. Unless otherwise specified, a general rule is not to include more than four to six appendices. When preparing the report, note also whether a cover letter is permitted and how the front page should be formatted, such as the display of organizational and project information.

FINAL REPORTS

A final report is written to provide a summary of the outcomes of a funded project. Similar to a progress report, a final report usually includes a summary narrative, a financial report, and a bibliography, and may include appendices as well. A final report specifies how the money was spent and the results for the entire project. The NOA for a project may contain the date and time when the final report is due. If not, it is usually provided by at least the beginning of the last year of the project. Refer to the report template required for use by the funding agency for the exact components to be included in the final report. The writing tips described in Exhibit 25.1 also apply to the writing of final reports.

Exhibit 25.3 provides a sample outline of a final report using the guidelines of a private foundation (Cleveland Foundation, n.d.). Describe the project aims, how you measured them, and the extent to which they were met. If there were additional accomplishments or results, describe them as well. Use evidence to describe the extent to which your project achieved its aims. Tables are useful for displaying results, but use tables sparingly. Use a bulleted format for major findings of your research, with one bullet for each key finding.

Your goal when writing a final report is to clearly describe the overall impact of the project. The report should describe what was found or produced, and how the information/product was or will be disseminated. A dissemination summary or bibliography is usually provided with the final narrative report. This dissemination summary is a record of certain kinds of products available to the public (e.g., books, journal articles, reports, brochures, websites), national/regional events (e.g., conferences and workshops), as well as published presentations and testimonies your project produced (Robert Wood Johnson Foundation, 2016).

EXHIBIT 25.3 Sample Outline of a Final Report for a Foundation Grant

1. Summary of original expected outcomes for project and planned activities to achieve them
   a) Project goal and objectives
   b) Activities to achieve objectives
2. Principal accomplishments of the project
3. Difficulties that have been encountered
4. Most challenging or surprising aspects of this project
5. Advice to others planning a similar project
   a) Strengths
   b) Limitations of the project
6. Postgrant plans

Source: Adapted from Cleveland Foundation. (n.d.). Grantee toolkit, online grant reporting instructions. Retrieved from https://www.clevelandfoundation.org/grants/grantee-toolkit/

Sustainability is an important issue to address in a final report for community intervention projects. Include a plan for how you will ensure ongoing benefits once the funding runs out for community-based projects. Include what portions of the project will continue, or how the impact of the project will remain. If you plan to assess the effects of your project over a longer period in the future, include those plans. If known, include who program officials can contact in the future to receive follow-up information on the project.

An abstract summarizing the project is often requested as part of a final report. Final abstracts are usually one to two pages in length and include the aims of the project, the results or findings of the project, and the significance of the results. Sometimes, special challenges and new insights gained from the project are included as well. An example of an abstract for a final report is included in Exhibit 25.4.

Finally, remember that a final report is often used by a funding agency to assess the extent to which it is meeting its strategic goals. Look at the strategic goals of the funding initiative of your project and include in your summary report how your project results support the achievement of those goals.

PREPARING NIH PROGRESS, INTERIM, AND FINAL REPORTS

Research Performance Progress Report (RPPR) System

Although there are several federal grant-funding agencies, including the Agency for Healthcare Research and Quality (AHRQ), the Centers for Disease Control and Prevention (CDC), and the Department of Defense (DOD), in this chapter, we focus on the reporting requirements of research funded by the NIH. All NIH noncompeting (Type 5) grant progress reports are submitted online using the RPPR system. The Public Health Service (PHS) 2590 form earlier used for NIH progress reports has been phased out and is no longer accepted except for very select programs (e.g., Type 4 noncompeting awards). NIH progress reports are generally required on an annual basis, 45 to 60 days before the end of the grant period, depending on the award. The PI or the "grantee" is responsible for submitting the report on time (NIH, 2017). Failure to submit the report on time could delay funding for the upcoming year or even delay funds altogether. One of the useful aspects of an NIH progress report is that the timing and requirements of the report are known even before you receive funding. Detailed guidelines are described online in the *NIH and Other PHS Agency RPPR Instruction Guide* (2017).

The RPPR requires no forms to download, and grantees access it through their NIH Electronic Research Administration (eRA) Commons status page. The eRA Commons is the web-based NIH interface for accessing and sharing grant information between NIH administrative staff and grantees. All PIs are required to register in eRA Commons at the time of the grant submission and to use the eRA Commons to exchange information throughout the life cycle of the grant. With the RPPR integrated with the eRA Commons system, much of the grantee's information, including name, grant number, project title, and period, prepopulates in the RPPR.

NIH, in the interest of saving time for all parties involved, created the Streamlined Noncompeting Award Process (SNAP) for progress reports of noncompeting awards. The SNAP provides a streamlined approach in that the direct costs for the entire project period are determined at the time of the initial award, and, thus, annual negotiations for funding are eliminated. The majority of NIH "R" series grants (i.e., R01 and R21) are SNAP awards. The RPPR deadline for a SNAP-issued award is 45 days before the next budget start date. Non-SNAP award (e.g., T32 and P30) RPPRs have a deadline of 60 days before the next budget period. The NIH NOA will state the award SNAP status. Be sure to check the grant status in eRA Commons for your exact progress report due date.

EXHIBIT 25.4 Sample Abstract for Final Report

TEAMS AND SYSTEMS: EFFECTIVENESS OF AN INTERDISCIPLINARY
TRAINING PROGRAM ON TEAMWORK SKILLS

Shirley M. Moore, Mark S. Richard, Laura Cummings, Jacqueline Niesen,

David Roberts, Diana Smetana, Ethel Smith, Steve Zepp,

Case Western Reserve University, and MetroHealth Medical Center, Cleveland, Ohio

BACKGROUND

Professional training programs in medicine, nursing, and pharmacy rarely systematically impart the skills necessary to function as part of an interdisciplinary team to provide team care. In addition, there are few prospective studies of the effectiveness of interdisciplinary team training programs that use comparative designs with control groups. The purpose of this study was to determine the effectiveness of the *Catalyst for Kids* model on participants' attitudes and knowledge of teamwork. For 3 years, the *Catalyst for Kids* CITE project has been preparing health professions trainees to function in interdisciplinary teams in pediatric primary care units. Trainees are taught collaborative teamwork skills and continuous quality improvement techniques to deliver and improve the care they give to pediatric patients and their families. This project has been part of a national team training project sponsored by Partnerships for Quality Education, an initiative of the Robert Wood Johnson Foundation.

METHODS

The study sample consisted of 30 health professions trainees (19 pediatric residents, 10 advanced practice nursing students, one pharmacy resident) assigned to 10 primary care pediatric clinics of a public urban teaching hospital for their clinical training. Using convenience assignment, trainees in the afternoon clinics comprised the *Catalyst for Kids* intervention group ($n = 17$) and those in the morning clinics comprised the control group ($n = 13$). Subjects did not self-select into the study groups. The *Catalyst for Kids* program (intervention) consisted of three half-day training workshops, during which the skills of teamwork and continuous quality improvement of care were taught, and an 8-month field experience during which the trainees provided team care and designed and implemented improvement projects for the clinic. A two-group, pretest–posttest design was used to measure the impact of the training program on four dimensions of teamwork: attitudes toward teamwork, knowledge of teamwork skills, appropriate use of authority in teams, and interdisciplinary collaboration. ANCOVA was used to test for group differences at completion of the program, controlling for pretest scores on standardized instruments.

RESULTS

There were no differences between the study groups at baseline. Significant differences from pretraining to posttraining were found between experimental and control groups on measures of team skills ($F = 7.5$; $df = 1$; $p = .01$) and use of authority in teamwork ($F = 6.6$; $df = 1$; $p = .01$); thus, participants increased their knowledge of team skills and had greater understanding of the appropriate use of authority in teamwork. No differences were found on measures of attitudes toward teamwork or interdisciplinary collaboration. No differences were found by gender or discipline.

CONCLUSIONS AND IMPLICATIONS

These findings suggest that the *Catalyst for Kids* model is an effective training program to enhance participants' knowledge of teamwork skills and use of authority in teamwork. Importantly, we have shown that the skills of interdisciplinary collaborative teamwork and quality improvement can be taught as part of already existing residency and clinical practice training experiences of health professionals. We currently are collecting data on the impact of this training model on patient outcomes.

ANCOVA, analysis of covariance; CITE, Collaborative Interdisciplinary Team Education.

EXHIBIT 25.5 RPPR PDF Formatting Requirements

- Use font size of 11 point or larger.
- Use a typeface of Arial, Helvetica, Palatino Linotype, or Georgia typeface.
- Symbol fonts at size 11 may be used to insert Greek letters or special characters.
- Use English only and avoid jargon.
- Abbreviations need to be spelled out the first time used, followed by the abbreviation in parentheses.
- Figures, charts, tables, and footnotes may be smaller in size, but must be legible.
- Before uploading, convert file to PDF.

RPPR, Research Performance Progress Report.

The annual NIH progress report in RPPR consists of nine separate screens, A to I, and can be worked on in any sequence, saved, and returned to at a later time before the final submission. The grantee or grantee designator clicks through the screens, answering check boxes, inserting text in text boxes, and uploading PDF files to complete the RPPR. Exhibit 25.5 describes the NIH general requirements for the RPPR PDF file uploads.

The RPPR is organized into the following sections: Section A—Cover Page; Section B—Accomplishments; Section C—Products; Section D—Participants; Section E—Impact; Section F—Changes; Section G—Special Reporting Requirements; Section H—Budget for Non-SNAP Awards Only; and Section I—Outcomes, which applies to Final and Interim reports only. Greater detail on each of these report requirements follows.

RPPR Section A—Cover Page
This section requires basic organizational and project information.

RPPR Section B—Accomplishments
The Accomplishments section is considered essential to the overall evaluation of the project. The specific aims/goals of the project are inserted, and any changes in the specific aims are noted. A discussion of what was accomplished under these goals should include (a) major activities, (b) study results, (c) significance, and (d) key outcomes or other achievements. The NIH notes that the emphasis in this section should move from reporting activities to reporting accomplishments as the study progresses. The narrative is saved as a PDF and uploaded in the RPPR. The NIH recommends the accomplishment narrative should be concise and brief, approximately two pages, not including exhibits or tables. This page limit can be challenging when reporting on an intervention study. An example of an NIH RPPR accomplishment narrative can be found in Exhibit 25.6. The use of tables with dates of the project period and milestones on steps toward achieving the aims of the grant is one way to display results efficiently. Use exhibits and tables to focus on data and results. State progress on major outcomes first, and then acknowledge any major challenges and/or changes to your approach.

One of the advantages of the RPPR system is that it allows for easy reporting of a competitive revision/administrative supplement associated with the parent award. Under Section B.3, a table is provided and serves as the framework for the supplement progress report where details on aims and accomplishments are entered.

Section B.4 requests information on training and professional development if it is part of the research of the project; otherwise, select "Nothing to Report." A description on the use of Individual Development Plans (IDPs) must be included for projects that have graduate students and/or postdoctoral fellows working on the study.

EXHIBIT 25.6 RPPR Accomplishment Narrative—Section B2

MAJOR ACTIVITIES

During the early months of Year 2, June to October 2016, significant effort was given to the conclusion of Phase 1, development and design of our "INVOLVE" prototype, through an iterative, user-centered process and generated qualitative data that were used to enhance the usability and efficacy of the intervention. The INVOLVE program consists of exposures to an avatar-based decision support technology that is administered via tablet computer and allows SDMs opportunities to practice their communication and decision-making skills through interactions with avatars that portray a decision coach and various healthcare providers. The Ottawa Decision Framework has guided the development of the interventions, design, and variable selection. This model postulated that if SDMs are exposed to an effective decision support strategy, they will have improvements in the decision-making readiness and decision-making quality, which will, in turn, reduce their decision regret, anxiety, and depression.

In October 2016, we finalized beta-testing of the INVOLVE prototype and concluded collection of qualitative data. Phase 1 successfully concluded with a deployable version of the INVOLVE intervention that will address the needs of SDMs faced with end-of-life care decisions that commonly occur in the ICU. This will be the first study to test interventions tailored to the unique needs of the SDMs of CCI patients delivered using an interactive avatar-based format. The intervention is a promising innovation that offers SDMs an "on-demand" experiential resource to address their decisional needs. This is a format that is easily delivered, well accepted, and well suited for this vulnerable and difficult-to-reach cohort of decision makers. If the interventions are efficacious, we will not only improve decision-making readiness and quality but improve SDM and patient outcomes as well.

Phase 2, clinical evaluation of decision support, began late October 2016. Since the beginning of Phase 2, we have successfully recruited 40 (as of 4/1/17) SDMs that aligns with our project monthly recruitment rate of eight to 10 subjects per month. This phase of our project consists of a three-arm, unblinded, clinical trial using pretests and posttests to evaluate the efficacy of two electronic decision-support interventions, INVOLVE and IS, compared with each other and with UC among 270 SDMs of cognitively impaired CCI patients. This design allows us to prospectively compare the efficacy of our experiential avatar-based decision support tool (INVOLVE) with both an IS condition and UC. Our second condition, IS, exposes SDMs to the educational resources of INVOLVE without the experiential components. Subjects assigned to an experimental condition (INVOLVE or IS) will receive two doses of the intervention, at enrollment and 1 day later. After the second dose, these subjects will have access to their assigned condition for subsequent self-administered doses, which will be electronically captured until the patient's ICU discharge or death. Each dose of this condition is expected to last no longer than 15 to 20 minutes. Data will be collected at (T1) baseline (Day 3 or 4 of the patient's ICU stay), and then on Days 1, 3, 7, and 90 postbaseline. In an effort to achieve balance among study groups, we will continue to use covariate adaptive randomization (minimization) rather than traditional randomization method (simple or blocked randomization). The allocation schedule is concealed and specified by the Q-Minim program.

In March 2017, we convened a data- and safety-monitoring board meeting, and established decision points for the assessment of subject safety and adherence to the study protocol as well as explored differential rate of consent among racial/ethnic minorities. During this meeting, the committee recommended notifying those participants with elevated Hospital Anxiety and Depression Scale (HADS) scores at the time of the interview instead of mailing a letter several days later. The Data and Safety Monitoring Board (DSMB) will reconvene in August 2017.

SPECIFIC OBJECTIVES

The aim of Phase 1 was to engage SDMs with prior experience in making healthcare decisions for a cognitively impaired CCI patient. These SDMs assisted us in refining the prototype avatar-based decision support intervention (INVOLVE). To address Aim 1, a series of several focus groups were conducted to identify key features of the INVOLVE intervention and its educational content. Because of the availability of subjects, we had to conduct more than four focus group discussions to achieve the minimum target sample size of 20 subjects.

(continued)

EXHIBIT 25.6 RPPR Accomplishment Narrative—Section B2 *(continued)*

STUDY RESULTS

On the basis of our preliminary analysis of the transcripts from the focus groups, we have been able to refine content, graphics, animations, and audio for the INVOLVE to enhance the usability of this intervention for SDMs. With that, we have been able to acquire sufficient data to address Specific Aim 1.

Aim 1: Identify the essential elements of the graphical user interface and educational content needed to revise the INVOLVE prototype for a set of common end-of-life decisions that occur in the ICU.

The aims of Phase 2 will be comparing INVOLVE with IS and UC to evaluate group differences for their effect on the primary outcomes: decision-making readiness and quality.

Aim 2: Evaluate whether there are differences in the decision-making readiness and decision-making quality between subjects exposed to INVOLVE, IS, or UC on Days 1, 3, and 7 postbaseline while accounting for covariates (prior SDM experience, SDM knowledge of the patient's preferences, and SDM's religious beliefs).

Aim 3: Determine whether there are differences in the postdecision outcomes of SDMs and their CCI patients by study condition while accounting for covariates at 90 days postbaseline.

SIGNIFICANCE

The importance of finding strategies to improve the quality of decision making for end-of-life care in the ICU has been well recognized. From a public health perspective, these technology-based interventions may offer sustainable solutions that can be easily adapted to varied populations to improve the health outcomes of SDMs and their loved ones who are cognitively impaired.

KEY OUTCOMES

This project is on target to meet all of the stated objectives. The investigators have successfully completed Phase 1 aim and plan to publish these findings in the coming months. Because of the early stages of subject recruitment, we do not have any preliminary results to report regarding Phase 2. Subject recruitment rates have been consistent with projected estimates and, at this time, there are no foreseen recruitment challenges that may hamper subject accrual.

CCI, chronically critically ill; DSMB, Data and Safety Monitoring Board; HADS, Hospital Anxiety and Depression Scale; INVOLVE, Interactive Virtual Decision Support for End-of-Life and Palliative Care; IS, informational support; RPPR, Research Performance Progress Report; SDMs, surrogate decision makers; UC, usual care.

Section B.5 asks, "How have results been disseminated to the communities of interest?" A response is required if this activity is part of the study protocol; otherwise, "Nothing to Report" is appropriate. Scientific publications and the sharing of research resources are reported in the section RPPR Section C—Products. Section B concludes with a text box for the grantee to briefly describe plans for the next reporting period. See Exhibit 25.7 for a list of all the components of the Accomplishments section. Be sure to discuss your methods and approach to ensure robust and unbiased results (NIH, 2016b).

RPPR Section C—Products

NIH progress reports include a list of published manuscripts that are the result of the currently funded grant that have not been reported earlier. Publications such as these are required to be listed in RPPR Section C along with other products such as websites, technology, inventions, or sharable resources. If the grantee has publications to report, selecting "yes" and checking the box "Associate with this RPPR" allows the grantee to

---

EXHIBIT 25.7 Components of the RPPR Section B—Accomplishments

B.1 Specific Aims/Goals: If aims of the project have changed or been modified, provide an explanation for the revised aims. This does not substitute for prior approval to change specific aims (text box).

B.2 Accomplishments: Briefly describe the major activities and the results of the study completed during the report time period. Address any major challenges that were encountered. Emphasize the significance of the findings and potential impact. Discuss efforts taken to *ensure robust and unbiased results*. This should not exceed two pages (PDF upload).

B.3 Competitive Revisions/Administrative Supplements: Goals and accomplishments of the supplement are reported here (yes/no—if yes, text box table).

B.4 Training and Professional Development Opportunities: These are described if they are part of the research study, or describe use of the institution's IDP if graduate students or postdocs are working on the study (PDF upload).

B.5 Dissemination of Results: Results are given to communities that are part of the study protocol. Routine dissemination such as press releases or websites is not required. Scientific publications go under Section C—Products (PDF upload).

B.6 Plans: Discuss what will be done in the next reporting period to further your specific aims. Include any changes or modifications that may have been made to the original plan. Discuss approach to *ensure scientific rigor and robust and unbiased results* (text box).

IDP, Individual Development Plan; RPPR, Research Performance Progress Report.

---

easily link publications from the grantee's My NCBI account with the RPPR. See the *NIH RPPR Instruction Guide* (2017) for details on My NCBI. Please note: Any NIH-funded study must include the PubMed Central ID number (PMCID). This PMCID number is not to be confused with the PMID number. Additional information on the NIH Public Access Policy and obtaining the PMCID is available at the NIH website including an online tutorial and step-by-step instructions (NIH, 2014).

A Note on Published Manuscripts

Intervention researchers are often challenged regarding the need to publish data from their study while it is still in progress. Often, there is a "blinding" of the outcome data until completion of the study. However, manuscripts that could be produced during the course of an intervention study might address topics such as the success of a new recruitment strategy, baseline data that provide new insights into a population, or the design and findings of the study process evaluation.

RPPR Section D—Participants

Each person who has worked on the project for at least 1 calendar month (8.3% effort for 12 months or 11% effort for 9 months) is entered into the participant table regardless of the source of support (e.g., in-kind effort, training effort). The eRA Commons ID is required for the project director (PD)/PI, students, and postdoctoral fellows, and, when entered, will self-populate several of the informational fields. The PI must be included regardless of effort. For example, a PI with 5% in-kind effort is entered in at 1.0 calendar month. All effort is entered as a rounded whole number. The system will not accept a decimal. Participation on a diversity supplement or other type of administrative supplement can also be indicated in this section, and if an individual has a primary affiliation with a foreign organization.

All personnel updates or changes are indicated in Section D.2 through a series of five questions:

- **Will there be, in the next budget period, a significant change in the level of effort for key personnel on the NOA from what was approved for this project?** A "significant change" is considered to be a 25% or greater reduction in time devoted to the project. If "yes," please explain; otherwise, select "no."
- **Are there or will there be new key personnel?** If "yes," upload an NIH Biosketches and Other Support form for each new key person in a single PDF file. The NIH Other Support form includes information on all active grants, and does not need to include pending grants.
- **Has there been a change in the "other support" of key personnel since the last reporting period?** For each key person on a grant, any changes in grant effort, the termination of a grant active earlier, or activation of a previous pending or new grant must be reported. Select "yes," and submit the NIH Other Support form indicating what has changed from the previous submission. If there is no change in "other support," the grantee selects "no" (see Exhibit 25.8 for a sample completed NIH Other Support form).
- **Are there or will there be new significant contributors?** If "yes," upload biosketches for all new significant contributors.
- **Will there be a change in the Multiple Principal Investigator (MPI) Leadership Plan for the next budget period?**
  Although a change in the MPI Leadership Plan does not require NIH prior approval, the revised plan must be entered into the RPPR.

RPPR Section E—Impact
This title is somewhat misleading as the section is not applicable for most NIH awards. The Impact section refers to awards that form infrastructure and also collects data on certain subawards to foreign entities. See *NIH RPPR Instruction Guide* for more details (2017).

RPPR Section F—Changes
In this section, the grantee describes any significant challenges and how these challenges were resolved. Significant changes to human subjects, vertebrate animals, biohazards, and/or select agents are also addressed here. If your project has experienced significant changes, these should be discussed with your program officer before submitting the RPPR.

RPPR Section G—Special Reporting Requirements
The Special Reporting Requirements section includes human subjects, inclusion enrollment data, clinical trials, foreign involvement, and certain budget issues. Check your NOA for any agency-specific award terms and conditions. The progress report guides the grantee through a series of questions related to each of these issues. Projects involving human subjects (Section G.4.b) provides a link to the "planned" and the "cumulative" enrollment tables. The cumulative enrollment, not to be confused with the planned enrollment table that is completed at the time of a grant application, is usually required as part of an NIH progress report. The *NIH RPPR Instruction Guide* emphasizes saving your work often and before selecting the enrollment link so as not to lose data already entered on your screen (2017). This report is discussed here in some detail because it often causes confusion and results in reporting error.

The cumulative enrollment report is a cumulative summary of the race and ethnicity of all participants in the study by gender, including individuals who entered, but then dropped from the study. The enrollment number cannot decrease from the previous progress report.

EXHIBIT 25.8   NIH Other Support

OMB No. 0925-0002 (Rev. 11/16 Approved Through 10/31/2018)

PHS 2590/RPPR OTHER SUPPORT FORMAT PAGE

Samples

NEW SENIOR/KEY PERSONNEL (D.2.b)

BENNETT, P.
ACTIVE

Investigator Award (Bennett)	9/1/2015 to 8/31/2010	6.0 calendar
Howard Hughes Medical Institute	$581,317	
Gene Cloning and Targeting for Neurological Disease Genes		

This award supports the PI's program to map and clone the gene(s) implicated in the development of Alzheimer's disease and to target expression of the cloned gene(s) to relevant cells.

5 R01 HG 000000-07 (Daumier)	3/1/2009 to 2/28/2018	3.6 calendar
NIH/NHGRI	$196,639	
Identification of the Risk Factor Genes for Alzheimer's Disease		

The major goals of this project are to identify new Alzheimer's disease genes and predict Alzheimer's disease.

(THIS AWARD)		
2 R01 HL 000000-14 (Anderson)	3/1/2002 to 2/28/2017	1.2 calendar
NIH/NHLBI	$186.529	
Chloride and Sodium Transport in Airway Epithelial Cells		

OVERLAP: No overlap

RICHARDS, L.
No Other Support

CHANGES IN OTHER SUPPORT (D.2.c)

ANDERSON, R.R.
ACTIVE

(THIS AWARD)		
2R01 HL 000000-14 (Anderson)	3/1/2002 to 2/28/2017	3.6 Calendar
NIH/NHLBI	$186,529	
Chloride and Sodium Transport in Airway Epithelial Cells		

The major goals of this project are to define the biochemistry of chloride and sodium transport in airway epithelial cells and clone the gene(s) involved in transport.

5 R01 HL 00000-04 (Baker)	4/1/2012 to 3/31/2016	1.2 calendar
NIH/NHLBI	$122,717	
Ion Transport in Lungs		

The major goal of this project is to study chloride and sodium transport in normal and diseased lungs.

R000 (Anderson)	9/1/2001 to 8/31/2016	1.2 calendar
Cystic Fibrosis Foundation	$43,123	
Gene Transfer of CFTR to the Airway Epithelium		

(continued)

EXHIBIT 25.8 NIH Other Support *(continued)*

The major goals of this project are to identify and isolate airway epithelium progenitor cells and express human CFTR in airway epithelium cells.

(NEW)
R01 DK000000-01 (Zimmerman)   9/1/2015 to 8/31/2019   1.2 calendar
NIH/NIDDK $187,265
Cystic Fibrosis–Related Diabetes and Lung Function

The major goals of this project are to determine how CFRD contributes to lung function decline.

OVERLAP: No overlap

INACTIVE

DCB 950000 (Anderson)   12/1/2008 to 11/30/2011   2.4 calendar
National Science Foundation $82,163
Liposome Membrane Composition and Function

The major goals of this project are to define biochemical properties of liposome membrane components and maximize liposome uptake into cells.

HERNANDEZ, M.
ACTIVE
5 R01 CA 00000-08 (Hernandez)   4/1/2007 to 3/31/2017   3.6 academic
NIH/NCI $110,532   3.0 summer
Gene Therapy for Small Cell Lung Carcinoma

The major goals of this project are to use viral strategies to express the normal *p53* gene in human SCLC cell lines and to study the effect on growth and invasiveness of the lines.

(NEW)
5 P01 CA 00000-02 (Chen)   7/1/2011 to 6/30/2016   1.8 academic
NIH/NCI $104,428 (sub only)
Mutations in p53 in Progression of Small Cell Lung Carcinoma

The major goals of this subproject are to define the *p53* mutations in SCLC and their contribution to tumor progression and metastasis.

BE 00000 (Hernandez)   9/1/1999 to 8/31/2016   1.8 academic
American Cancer Society $86.732
p53 Mutations in Breast Cancer

The major goals of this project are to define the spectrum of *p53* mutations in human breast cancer samples and correlate the results with clinical outcome.

(THIS AWARD)
2 R01 HL 000000-13 (Anderson)   3/1/2002 to 2/28/2017   0.6 calendar
NIH/NHLBI $186,529
Chloride and Sodium Transport in Airway Epithelial Cells

OVERLAP: There was scientific overlap between aim 2 of 5 R01 CA 00000-08 and aim 4 of project 2 in 5 P01 CA 00000-02. In conjunction with agency staff, it was decided to remove aim 4 of project 2 from the P01 and adjust the budget and PI level of effort accordingly.

CFRD, cystic fibrosis-related diabetes; NCI, National Cancer Institute; NHGRI, National Human Genome Research Institute; NHLBI, National Heart, Lung, and Blood Institute; NIH, National Institutes of Health; PI, principal investigator; RPPR, Research Performance Progress Report; SCLC, small cell lung cancer.

Studies may have more than one enrollment table. The table consists of collecting data on gender (male, female, or unknown), ethnicity (Hispanic and Latino, not Hispanic or Latino, and unknown), and race (seven categories) of the study participants. These categories cannot be changed or combined in any way. If unknown sex/gender, ethnicity, or race is noted, the PI should provide an explanation in the comment section at the top of the table, such as "Several subject participants chose not to complete the ethnicity category." Multiple studies under one grant require a separate enrollment report for each study or protocol, both a planned and a cumulative table. Also, separate enrollment reports may be completed for different populations of study participants. For example, a project examining the effects of a healthy diet in school-aged children and their mothers requires a separate enrollment report for the children and the mother participants. Exhibit 25.9 shows a sample cumulative enrollment report. If the study has a year with no enrollment, it is important to note this in the comment section at the top of the table (click on edit Inclusion Data); otherwise, an error message will occur. Keeping accurate records on an ongoing basis throughout the study makes completing the inclusion enrollment report a relatively easy task. Significant challenges or concerns with the enrollment should be addressed in Section F.3.a along with changes or concerns in the planned enrollment. Once again, prior communication with your program officer on significant changes with planned or inclusion enrollment or any other significant change is essential for a successful project report.

Other items to note in this section include Section G.4.c, which requires the grantee to register a clinical trial at ClinicalTrials.gov and record the clinical trial number there. The NIH's definition of a clinical trial is not dependent on the sample size; an NIH clinical trial is a research study where one or more human subjects are randomly assigned to a biomedical or behavioral intervention. Section G.5 addresses human subjects educational requirements for new personnel. In addition to human subjects training, the NIH requires good clinical

EXHIBIT 25.9 Sample Cumulative Enrollment Report

| Racial Categories | Ethnic Categories | | | | | | | | | Total |
| | Hispanic or Latino | | | Not Hispanic or Latino | | | Unknown/Not Reported Ethnicity | | | |
	Female	Male	Unknown/ Not Reported	Female	Male	Unknown/ Not Reported	Female	Male	Unknown/ Not Reported	
American Indian/ Alaska Native	1	0	0	3	0	0	0	0	0	4
Asian	0	0	0	0	0	0	0	0	0	0
Native Hawaiian or other Pacific Islander	2	0	0	0	0	0	0	0	0	2
Black or African American	417	130	0	2	5	0	0	0	0	554
White	30	10	0	16	6	0	0	0	0	62
More than one race	13	2	0	0	1	0	0	0	0	16
Unknown or not reported	2	2	0	62	16	0	0	0	0	82
Total	465	144	0	83	28	0	0	0	0	720

practice (GCP) training for all clinical trial research investigators and staff as of January 2017; see NIH NOT-OD-16-148 (2016a). Although there is no requirement to include it on the RPPR as of this writing, your program office might appreciate seeing that all your research personnel completed the good clinical practice (GCP) training, listing each person's name and a one-sentence description of the training.

Section G.10 asks, "**Is it anticipated that an estimated unobligated balance (including prior year carryover) will be greater than 25% of the current year's total budget?**" If "yes," state the approximate percentage of carryover and explain the reason for this unobligated balance and how it will be spent if carried into the next budget year. If not, state "no."

RPPR Section H—Budget

The Budget section in the RPPR applies to non-SNAP awards only. Select the SF424 Research and Related budget from the drop-down menu and complete the budget for the next budget period. The budget is typically similar to what was originally submitted in the grant application, taking into account any personnel or project changes and any carryover funds. Attach a detailed budget justification describing any line items that have significantly changed from the earlier awarded budget (greater than 25%).

RPPR Section I—Outcomes (Applicable for Final and Interim Reports)

The Outcomes section is required for the Final or the Interim RPPR. This section contains a concise summary of the cumulative outcomes or findings of the project. The outcomes will be made available to the general public and should be written in laymen's terms. Proprietary or confidential information should not be included. The NIH recommends the Outcomes section should not be more than half a page.

NIH Final and Interim Reports and RPPR

The RPPR system is used for NIH annual, final, and interim reports. The Final RPPR replaced the Final Progress Report (FPR) and the NIH no longer accepts the FPR. If a competing renewal application is submitted before the 120-day deadline, an interim report is due instead of the final. Both the Final RPPR and the Interim RPPR are due 120 days after the grant end date and are accessed through the grant closeout documents in eRA Commons. Should the renewal application receive funding, the Interim RPPR serves as the annual RPPR for the last previous competitive segment of the grant. If the application is not funded, the Interim RPPR becomes the Final RPPR (see Exhibit 25.10). With the addition to project outcomes, the data fields for the Final and Interim RPPR are the same as for the annual RPPR, except for the budget and plans for next year, which are not required.

The RPPR Submission

The RPPR system allows for error checking any time before the RPPR submission and displays a detailed error or warning message. All errors must be corrected before a RPPR can be submitted. The RPPR contains several different sections, various types of data fields, and a few new terms and acronyms, but do not let it scare you. The RPPR is user-friendly and walks you through the necessary information for the NIH progress report. By using the same system for progress, interim, and final reports, the grantee becomes very familiar with the process of the RPPR. The RPPR also allows for collecting data on complicated grant structures, including multicomponent awards and administrative supplements. Remember to save your work frequently, and as you move from section to section. Once completed, the RPPR is routed to the institution's business signing official for submission to the NIH, unless the institution has delegated this signing authority to the individual PI. Exhibit 25.11 provides tips for the RPPR.

EXHIBIT 25.10 Final or Interim RPPR Workflow Process

Competing Renewal Application Status	Action	
Not submitting a Competing Renewal application	Submit a Final RPPR no later than 120 days from the project period end date	
Submitting a Competing Renewal application	Submit an Interim RPPR no later than 120 days from the project period end date	
	Funded	**Not Funded**
	The Interim RPPR is accepted as the annual RPPR	The Interim RPPR is accepted as the Final RPPR

RPPR, Research Performance Progress Report.

EXHIBIT 25.11 Tips for the NIH RPPR

- Text boxes are limited to 8,000 characters, about three pages.
- The NIH encourages concise responses and states a recommended length for some questions.
- Headers and footers including pagination are not recommended on documents that are uploaded.
- Save all PDF attachments with descriptive file names of 50 characters or less. Use only standard characters.
- PDF files that are larger than 6 MB are not accepted by the system.

NIH, National Institutes of Health; RPPR, Research Performance Progress Report.

NIH Close-Out Documents

The NIH grant close-out process requires two additional documents in addition to the Final RPPR: the Federal Financial Report (FFR) and the Final Invention Statement (FIS). The close-out document links are accessed and viewed through the PI's eRA Commons grant status page, and all are due 120 days after the grant ending date. The FFR is completed by your institution and typically requires the PI to sign off before the institution submits to the NIH. The Final Invention link gives easy access to the FIS and Certificate. During the grant period, any inventions conceived or used during the course of the grant work must be documented here. If there were no inventions, the PI selects "no." Once completed, the FIS is routed to the institutional signing official for signature and submission to NIH.

Progress Report Additional Materials (PRAM)

It is not unusual for the NIH grants management officer to request additional information to clarify or further evaluate the progress of the study. The response to this additional information is submitted through PRAM, the link in the PI's eRA Commons grant status page. The PRAM is also used for noncompliant publications, and the PI will receive an automatic email notification requesting publications be brought into NIH public access compliance. A My NCBI PDF report to document compliance or a justification of why a publication cannot be brought into compliance can be uploaded in the PRAM link in eRA Commons in response to the email. It is important to respond to all requests in a timely manner or funding of the award could be delayed or reduced. The NIH requires all official correspondence with your NIH program officer or grants manager to go through your institutional signing official. Once the PI submits PRAM, it will route through your signing official for submission to the NIH.

If there are any questions regarding what to include or not include in your progress report, contact your NIH program officer. Finally, do not wait until progress report time to inform your program officer about a major hurdle or significant change in your project. Contact them immediately. Your program officer wants you to succeed just as much as you do.

Carryover Request. NIH awards that are not subject to SNAP often require prior approval from the NIH grants management officer to carry over unobligated funds into the next budget period. If a carryover request is anticipated for the next funding period, state so in the progress report. The exact amount will not be known until the annual FFR is completed, but a best estimate should be included. Explain any unobligated balance greater than 25% of the current year budget, including previous carryover, and how it will be spent in the next funding period. Once the FFR is complete (usually by your institution's grant accounting office), the exact carryover amount should be written, in Item 12 Remarks of the FFR, and submitted to the NIH (see Exhibit 25.12 for a sample financial report).

EXHIBIT 25.12 Financial Status Report

Financial Status Report	Final		
1. Federal Agency and Organizational Element to Which Report is Submitted	**2. Federal Grant or Other Identifying Number**		
NATIONAL INSTITUTE OF NURSING RESEARCH	5P30NR000000-3		
3. Recipient Organization (Name and complete address, including ZIP code) CASE WESTERN RESERVE UNIVERSITY 10900 EUCLID AVE CLEVELAND OH 441067015	**4. Employer Identification Number** 10000000000		
	5. Recipient Account Number RES504260 CON105962		
	6. Final Report ☒ Yes ☐ No		**7. Basis** ☒ Cash ☐ Accrual
8. Funding/Grant Period		**9. Period Covered by This Report**	
From 09/29/2012 **To** 06/30/2017		**From** 07/01/20014 **To** 06/30/2015	

(continued)

EXHIBIT 25.12 Financial Status Report *(continued)*

10. Transactions:	Previously Reported	This Period	Cumulative
a. Total outlays	663,416.88	450,292.01	1,113,708.89
b. Refunds, rebates, etc.	0.00	0.00	0.00
c. Program income used in accordance with the deduction alternative	0.00	0.00	0.00
d. Net outlays (line a, less the sum of the lines b and c)	663,416.88	450,292.01	1,113,708.89
Recipient's share of net outlay, consisting of:			
e. Third party (in-kind) contributions	0.00	0.00	0.00
f. Other Federal awards authorized to be used to match this award	0.00	0.00	0.00
g. Program income used in accordance with the matching or cost sharing alternative	0.00	0.00	0.00
h. All other recipient outlays not shown on lines e, f, or g	0.00	0.00	0.00
i. Total recipient share of net outlays (sum of lines e, f, g, and h)	0.00	0.00	0.00
j. Federal share of net outlays (line d less line i)	663,416.88	450,292.01	1,113,708.89
k. Total unliquidated obligations			0.00
l. Recipient's share of unliquidated obligations			0.00
m. Federal share of unliquidated obligations			0.00
n. Total Federal share (sum of lines j and m)			1,113,708.89

(continued)

EXHIBIT 25.12 Financial Status Report *(continued)*

o. Total Federal funds authorized for this funding period			1,149,937.00
p. Unobligated balance of Federal funds (line o minus line n)			36,228.11
Program income, consisting of:			
q. Disbursed program income shown on lines c and/or above			0.00
r. Disbursed program income using addition alternative			0.00
s. Undisbursed program income			0.00
t. Total program income realized (sum of lines q, r, and s)			0.00

11. Indirect expense	a. Type of rate	Provisional ☐ Predetermined ☐ Final ☒ Fixed ☐		
	b. Rate	c. Base	d. Total Amount	e. Total Amount Federal Share 151,979.51
	54.50	278,861.49	151,979.51	
Total	54.50	278,861.49	151,979.51	

12. Remarks	Carryover of the unobligated balance requires prior approval. The unobligated balance includes EAB travel balance in the amount of 2,854.00 and pilot projects balance in the amount of 28,812.00.	**Carryover Request** $28,812
13. Authorized official	**Name** Robin Tiller **Title** Associate Director, OSPA	**Telephone (Area code, number, and extension)** 216-368-4516	**Date Report Submitted** 09/23/2015
14. Approved by	**Name** Jean Mason		**Date Report Accepted** 09/29/2015

EAB, external advisory board; OSPA, Office of Sponsored Projects Administration.

EXHIBIT 25.13 Sample Carryover Request Letter

Date
Name
Grants Management Specialist
Address
E-mail

Re: Carryover Request for NIH Grant#

Dear Grants Management Specialist:

I am writing to formally request approval for carryover of an unobligated balance from Year 3 of $18,649 directs + $10,163 indirects = $28,812 total.

The unobligated balance is caused by a delay in start-up and hiring personnel for pilot study #2. Pilot study #2 is now up and running, and we anticipate meeting the project timeline for Year 4. The carryover is critical for the successful completion of the project.

The unobligated balance will be used for funding the necessary personnel and other costs to carry out the three pilot interventions as noted in the specific aims of the project.

Attached please find a detailed budget and budget justification.

Thank you in advance for your consideration of this request. If you have any questions, please do not hesitate to contact me.

Sincerely,
Principal Investigator

EAB, external advisory board; NIH, National Institutes of Health; OSPA, Office of Sponsored Projects Administration.

At this time, a written request must be submitted to your NIH program officer or grants management specialist requesting a carryover of unobligated funds as outlined in your NOA. This request should state the amount of the unobligated funds, direct and indirect, the reason for the balance, a detailed justification of the need for the carryover, and how the funds will be spent in the upcoming grant period. Your NIH NOA will provide details on to whom to send the request. Your NIH program officer may be able to offer guidelines for the requirements specific to that agency. The letter is submitted to the NIH through your institution's signing official (see Exhibit 25.13 for a sample carryover request letter).

Once a file is uploaded and submitted to the NIH, there is no option to reupload a revised report. If a revision is necessary, you must contact your NIH program officer or grants manager and submit the revised report directly to your NIH program officer through your institutional signing official.

SUMMARY

Writing progress and final reports for intervention research studies involves careful planning from the onset of the project. Developing a system early in the project for keeping the information you will need for the reports is a wise investment of time. Pay close attention to the funding agency's guidelines so that you are able to adequately address the content, structure, and submission of the reports. Use your study aims as the focus around which to build your report and write in a clear, concise manner to tell the story of your project. Remember also that your program officer is usually happy to answer any questions you may have about preparing the report. This is an opportunity to build a good relationship with your program officer and gain his or her investment in your work.

Writing reports are important phases in the life course of a research project. As a researcher, use report writing as an opportunity for reflection on how things are progressing according to your plan, and what you are discovering. This is your opportunity to present your good work, ask for help if needed, and show how you are responsibly using the funds that were given to you.

Key Points From This Chapter

- By accepting funding for your research, as PI, you also accept responsibility for reporting how you are meeting your study goals and how you have spent the funding agency's money.
- Progress reports provide the opportunity to showcase your work, but be sure to follow the funding agency's guidelines (usually reported on the NOA).
- Avoid "surprising" your program officer by discussing changes in budgetary allowances or unexpected challenges prior to submitting your report.
- For an NIH award, an unobligated balance of more than 25% requires thorough explanation; a written request for carryover of these monies must be submitted with detailed justification and future plans.
- NIH progress, interim, and final reports are submitted through the RPPR system in eRA Commons.
- Focus your final report on the study aims and significant findings, both positive and negative, that you have identified, including all dissemination activities.

REFERENCES

Cleveland Foundation. (n.d.). Grantee toolkit, online grant reporting instructions. Retrieved from https://www.clevelandfoundation.org/grants/grantee-toolkit/

National Institutes of Health. (2014). NIH Public Access Policy: When and how to comply. Retrieved from http://publicaccess.nih.gov

National Institutes of Health. (2016a). Policy on good clinical practice training for NIH awardees involved in NIH-funded clinical trials. Retrieved from https://grants.nih.gov/grants/guide/notice-files/NOT-OD-16-148.html

National Institutes of Health. (2016b). Rigor and reproducibility. Retrieved from https://grants.nih.gov/reproducibility/index.htm

National Institutes of Health. (2017). NIH and Other PHS Agency Research Performance Progress Report (RPPR) Instruction Guide, March 2, 2017. Retrieved from https://grants.nih.gov/grants/rppr/rppr_instruction_guide.pdf

Robert Wood Johnson Foundation. (2016). Grantee reporting instructions. Retrieved from http://www.rwjf.org/en/how-we-work/grants/grantee-resources/reporting-and-accounting-information/instructions.html

Satterfield, B. (2007). An introduction to grant reports: Tips and tools for preparing reports for your funders. Retrieved from http://www.cityvision.edu/wiki/introduction-grant-reports-tips-and-tools-preparing-reports-your-funders

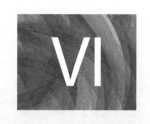

Moving Intervention Findings Into the Real World

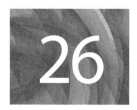

26

Disseminating Findings of Intervention Studies

Marion E. Broome

> Knowing how hard it is to collect a fact, you understand why most people want to have some fun analyzing it. —*Jesse L. Greenstein*

The systematic accumulation of scientific data into a body of knowledge that can support the translation of research to practice mandates that researchers disseminate their findings in the literature. The dissemination of findings from intervention studies is a primary responsibility of every researcher and scientific team. So much time, effort, and energy goes into developing an intervention, finding funding to test the effectiveness of the intervention, and then dealing with the practical and logistical implementation of the study that thinking about dissemination is not something most investigators give attention to at the beginning of their study. Yet, thinking about the "cycle of dissemination" early on is very important. Dissemination of information related to an intervention can be done at many stages throughout the study, although when to provide which information about the outcome will vary depending on the stage of implementation.

The purpose of this chapter is to

1. Describe the process, procedures, and mechanics of publishing the results of an intervention study;
2. Describe the essential components of appropriate reporting for an intervention study;
3. Identify challenges that can arise when deciding authorship on manuscripts from an intervention study;
4. Discuss alternate dissemination venues beyond scientific journals, including posters, presentations, and social media, as well as feedback about study results to the participants;
5. Describe how to write an abstract and points about presenting one's work in poster and podium venues at conferences.

HOW AND WHEN TO WRITE

Developing a manuscript is hard work and other tasks can easily take priority. Many researchers put this off, waiting for "the right time." Barriers to writing are numerous (see Table 26.1). If you are having difficulty getting started, ask yourself the questions in Table 26.1, identify your barriers, and then carefully plan your approach to decrease the barriers. There are many excellent resources you should access prior to writing and it is worth the time to access some of these resources (LeBrun, 2011; Oermann & Hays, 2015; Silvia, 2007).

Most experienced authors will acknowledge that it is never easy to find the time and motivation to develop a manuscript. One must make time and schedule that time as

TABLE 26.1 Strategies for Removing Barriers to Writing

BARRIER	SUGGESTED STRATEGIES FOR REDUCING BARRIER
I have too many interruptions when I work on a manuscript.	■ Find a quiet place to work: at home; in the library. ■ Turn email and cell phone ringer off.
I have no time in my schedule to write.	■ Schedule 2–6 hours as if you had class or any other appointment on a weekly or, at the very least, biweekly basis. Do not accept any other appointments during this time.
I need peace and quiet to get my ideas organized.	■ Discuss your goals with your chairperson or dean.
I don't feel like I will be rewarded for publishing.	■ Ask about expectations for scholarship to support application for promotion. ■ Think about whether external rewards alone are satisfactory to you given effort publishing research requires. Think about what you will learn when writing.
I want my ideas to be perfectly developed before I share them.	■ There are no perfect ideas. ■ Give yourself a specific amount of time and drafts to write one section of the manuscript and then give to a colleague to read and critique. ■ Write in teams. Ask others on the team to read what you write.
I have difficulty with expressing myself in writing.	■ Writing takes practice, critique, and rewrites. It is a skill, not an intrinsic ability. But you have to be open to accepting feedback.
Once I write something, I don't want to read or rewrite it.	■ Put a time limit on how long you write a section and the number of times you will reread before passing on to another colleague to read.
I wonder how people will respond to my ideas.	■ People are much more generous and helpful to us than we are to ourselves when it comes to writing.
I'm not sure I have anything important to say.	■ Given your research experience, it is likely you have quite a bit to say that others don't know. ■ Ask your colleague who reviews your drafts to concentrate on how you develop your argument for the need for the intervention study.

consistently as one does any other appointment. Everyone differs in their approach to developing a manuscript, but there are several commonalities across all approaches. Common approaches include using a method to organize one's thoughts, such as an outline of the content of the manuscript; using a model from the literature that is a well-written article (in terms of subheadings, style, approach to synthesis); and taking time to draft one's thoughts on paper. Most authors find it takes a block of time (i.e., 3–4 hours) to develop various drafts of a manuscript section. However, the smaller sections (e.g., introduction; description of the sample and sampling plan) can be done in a shorter period (2 hours) and then one can come back to the manuscript over several sittings and expand the draft each time.

What Findings to Publish?

Most intervention studies are very complex and include numerous comparison groups, measures, and data points across the study, such as baseline and follow-up. Hence, there are often multiple papers containing information that will be of interest to different audiences: other researchers, clinicians, and/or students in the field. Authors often ask "how many" papers can be published from one intervention study without being considered "salami publishing" (Baggs, 2008). There is no simple answer to this question, except "it depends." Various factors must be considered, such as the following:

- Are the baseline findings for the experimental and comparison groups important as a stand-alone description of the variables studied?
- Have new methods (assays, questionnaires, surveys) been used to study the phenomenon in this study? Do you have psychometric data for these methods that document the reliability and validity of the measure? Did you adapt any measure to your population that readers could find useful?
- Were both quantitative and qualitative data collected to address different dimensions of the phenomenon? Are there subgroups within the study (e.g., preschool vs. adolescent; ethnic groups) who responded differently to the intervention?

A team has to think carefully about how many different ways to report its findings. Salami publications are a concern and authors need to give this serious consideration (Baggs, 2008; Henly, 2014). "Salami publishing" refers to a practice of publishing multiple manuscripts from the same study that "slice" the study findings into such discrete slices that the context of the study is lost. Transparency about what papers are reported from one study is an important ethical responsibility of the lead investigator of the study. That person needs to track all the potential presentations and publications—both prior to submission and after publication.

Readers of an article should always be told that the findings in that specific paper are part of a larger investigation and provide enough information about the larger study, including citations, that will provide a context for them to judge the findings reported in that specific paper. However, there are also some conventions followed by most journal editors about how the findings of the effectiveness of an intervention study should be reported and these should be followed (Conn & Groves, 2011). For instance, the publication of findings related to outcomes of the intervention should not be published in several papers if the study participants are followed postintervention at several time points (e.g., 6 months, 1 year). Long-term follow-up should be viewed as just that—behavior and lasting effects can change over time. Publishing different papers for each time point could result in other investigators interpreting the success (or failure) of an intervention if they accessed only one article reporting on one point in time. Also, if three different time points for data collection are reported in three different papers, investigators conducting a meta-analysis would treat those three time points as independent, which could artificially inflate the effect sizes and potentially change the overall findings of the meta-analysis.

Journal Selection

There are currently more than 1,300 journals listed in the Cumulative Index to Nursing and Allied Health Literature (www.ebscohost.com) alone that are available from which to choose once one decides on which aspect of the intervention study to focus in a particular manuscript. The focus is important as it will help narrow the field of journals to consider. For instance, if a researcher has translated a measurement tool for physical activity and piloted it in a smaller sample prior to the intervention obtaining satisfactory reliability and validity estimates, a measurement-focused paper might be of interest to other researchers. The investigator might consider several journals for submission. Research journals such as *Western Journal of Nursing Research, Nursing Research, Research in Nursing and Health, Online Journal of the Southern Nursing Research Society*, and so forth would be interested in this topic. But another option would be the *Journal of Nursing Measurement*. If the intervention research team decides to publish the findings from its study with an emphasis on the policy implication, then journals such as *Nursing Outlook* would be an appropriate venue in which to disseminate.

Given that most intervention research teams are interdisciplinary, it is highly likely that journals outside of the nursing discipline will also be of interest. Most team members will be familiar with the journals in their own discipline and know which are more highly regarded, which reach a particular audience, and which have the highest impact factors (IFs). As mentioned earlier, these discussions should be held early in the life of a study so due consideration can be given to all possibilities for dissemination. Another source that is very useful for authors who want to generate a list of journals that may be options for their manuscripts is the Journal/Author Name Estimator (JANE, 2017). The author places the abstract of his or her manuscript in a box provided on the website (or title or keywords) and a list of potential journals will be provided. This is an interdisciplinary website.

There are no hard and fast rules about which journal is more appropriate to choose for disseminating one's work (see Exhibit 26.1). When considering journal choice, the audience or readers of the journal should be considered. If the methods and primary findings are the focus of the paper, it may be more appropriate to select a journal that reports empirical findings from interventions, but targets those investigators and clinicians who belong to a specific profession. For instance, *Pediatrics* (medicine), *Journal of Pediatric Nursing*, and *Pediatric Psychology* are all well-respected journals from different disciplines that all publish intervention studies. If the primary findings have been published and the focus of the manuscript is on the translation of the intervention, another journal, such as *Clinical*

EXHIBIT 26.1 Criteria for Selecting an Appropriate Journal

1. Editorial purpose: What does the journal editor consider the primary purpose of that journal to be (policy, research findings, new pedagogies, etc.)? This can be found in the author guidelines section of the journal website.
2. Audience: Whom do I want to hear about my research? Who has a "need to know?" Who will be the most likely to use my findings in their work (research, practice)?
3. IF: What is the latest IF? Has this journal had a consistent trend in its IFs?
4. Acceptance rate: What is the overall acceptance rate of the journal? What is the time from submission to first decision by the editor?
5. Has the journal published a similar paper recently? If so, how does my manuscript differ?
6. Length of manuscripts, format, etc.

IF, impact factor.

Nurse Specialist: The Journal for Advanced Practice Nursing or *Cancer Nursing Practice*, may be more appropriate.

At some point during the "life" of a particular intervention study, an investigator should be interested in disseminating the findings to clinicians in practice. In some cases, depending on the focus of the intervention, the choice will be an interdisciplinary journal, health professions journal, or nursing journal. One way to choose could be to embed the description of the specific intervention study within an integrative review or a meta-analysis of all similar studies. Another option is to use a table in which the intervention method and major findings are described but the manuscript focuses on how the findings could be used in practice. This would require particular attention to the readiness of the findings for translation to practice and feasibility for application.

Authors should go to a journal's website and read the "Guidelines for Authors" section (Lewallen & Crane, 2010) when considering to which journal to submit but before the final draft is completed. This will provide information about the editorial purpose of the journal and the required format for the paper, including reference style, the number of pages, suggestions for charts and figures, and so forth.

Every author should be informed about and wary of predatory publishers and journals when selecting a journal in which to disseminate their research. The "Open Access" movement began in mid-2000s (Broome, 2014) which created new journals that did charge a fee but also provided authors with typical services including peer review and editing, while also providing free access to the manuscript for anyone wanting it after being accepted. This free access to the literature was thought to expand the reach of research—especially in poorly resourced countries. In Open Access journals (always online), the author(s) retain the copyright to the paper. Predatory publishers emerged around 2008 and charged authors high fees to publish their manuscripts without providing the usual support and service, including peer review, editing, and so forth. Over the past 10 years, these predatory "journals" have proliferated at an unprecedented rate, with 116 predatory journals documented in 2011 and 882 in 2016 (Beall, 2017). The intent of these publications is to provide authors with a quick and easy route to online publication of their manuscript, often within 24 to 72 hours (Broome, 2017).

These predatory journals are published online only and often have titles that are very close to reputable journals. Their websites list editorial board members—some of whom are well known in the field and who often are not even aware their names are listed. In a recent study of predatory open access nursing journals (Oermann et al., 2016), the authors documented a dramatic increase in predatory journals in the nursing field, with 140 nursing journals identified from 75 publishers, with most having begun publishing in the past 1 to 2 years, charging fees from $75 to $1,500. One of the most important differences (and there are many) between reputable and predatory journals is that no reviewers are invited to evaluate the manuscript for significance of the topic, relevance, rigor, analytic methods, conclusions, depth of discussion, and validity of conclusions on the basis of data/arguments in the paper. In summary—buyer beware. Know that open access journals are not the same thing as predatory journals, although sometimes the differences are difficult to assess. So carefully select the journal in which to publish (Broome, 2017).

Consideration of the Journal's Impact Factor

Clarivate Analytics now provides the rankings of the individual IFs for over 230 journals in nursing. This list is most easily accessed by asking a librarian for it, or by checking the website for a specific journal. The calculation of the IF is on the basis of the number of times that articles appearing in the target journal are cited by authors published in the other journals listed in the citation database. The calculation covers a 2-year period after the target article is published (Polit & Northam, 2011).

There are many factors that influence the calculation of the IF of a journal. These include the number of articles published by a journal, the types of articles published (i.e., review articles are cited more often), how fast changes in the discipline occur, and so forth. In a recent study, the median IF for the 74 journals indexed in 2009 was 0.91, similar to that in other health disciplines (Polit & Northam, 2011). The IF of a journal is published annually and some universities require submission of this information when an individual submits his or her dossier for promotion. IF, when used as a quality assessment, has been very controversial across disciplines; however, there are few other reasonable metrics available. See Polit and Northam (2011) for a more complete and contemporary discussion of IFs, a historical analysis of changes in IF in nursing journals, and the factors that affect the IF of a specific journal.

FORMATTING THE INTERVENTION REPORT

Intervention studies follow the typical format for reporting empirical studies. The major headings include the following:

- Introduction
- Background/Review of Literature/Theoretical Framework
- Purpose and Specific Aims
- Methodology
  1. Design
  2. Sample
  3. Intervention
  4. Measurement
  5. Procedure
  6. Analysis Plan
- Findings
- Discussion
- References
- Tables, Figures and Graphs

The aforementioned outline can be especially useful if a team approaches writing the paper and each person is assigned a section to draft initially. In general, although journals differ in required page length (which are most often found in the "Authors' Guidelines" section), research reports of intervention studies will be 15 to 18 manuscript pages (or 5 to 6 journal pages) including references and tables. Each of the earlier sections is discussed subsequently, including recommendations about the length of each section.

Abstract
The abstract will be read by all journal peer reviewers first as well as many readers when they are deciding which articles in a journal to read. Hence, it is very important as this may be the last thing the reader chooses to look at. If the abstract is vague, not well developed, uninteresting, too full of findings, or incomplete, reviewers and readers will lose interest quickly, affecting the dissemination of the research. The abstract contains a brief description of the problem and purpose of the study, the methods and procedures, major findings, and a discussion about the impact of the study (i.e., the usefulness of the findings in extending what is known and solving problems; LeBrun, 2011). Most journals restrict the number of words in

an abstract and authors should carefully choose their words to be as concise, yet descriptive, as possible.

Introduction (1½ Pages)

The introduction to the paper is one of the most difficult sections to write and yet one of the most important. This section introduces the reader to the topic, provides some description of the scope of the issue, a concise review of what is known about the area, and what gaps there are in the literature. After reading this section, the reader should understand why this study was needed and what potential contribution the study could make.

Purpose and Specific Aims (½ to ¾ Page)

The introduction should lead seamlessly into a statement of the purpose and specific aims of the study. In some journals, authors are also asked to add in this section the hypotheses they tested under each aim. In other journals, the hypotheses can be added to the data analysis plan or findings section.

Background (3 Pages)

This section provides the opportunity for the authors to provide a more in-depth discussion of the study's theoretical framework, previous research studies in the area, a description of common approaches to studying the problem, and so forth. The purpose of including the theoretical framework in this section is to explicitly describe how the intervention attributes are linked with concepts in the theory (Conn & Groves, 2011). If space allows, a graphic depicting these relationships is useful for readers.

Methodology
Design

The design section includes a description of the type of experimental or quasi-experimental design such as "a randomized three-group, repeated measures design" for intervention reports. Statements about institutional review board (IRB) approval and human subject protections (e.g., consent procedures, incentives) can also be placed here.

Sample

Information about the participants in the study should include the inclusion and exclusion criteria, number of participants and their ages, gender and ethnicity, as well as any other relevant demographic information. This is also the section in which one can provide information about the power calculations used to determine how many participants to recruit. Sometimes authors choose to add the power analysis to the data analysis section, which is also acceptable.

Intervention

The intervention should be clearly described in enough detail to provide the reader with a complete understanding of what the participants received, how it was delivered, when it was delivered, what the control group's experience was, and how it differed from that in the intervention group (Conn & Groves, 2011). Successful replication of the intervention in future studies with different populations will require this level of detail. Authors need to provide details about the integrity of the intervention, training procedures for the interveners, as well as procedures that were put in place to prevent "drift" of delivery across interveners or across time for each intervener. Table 26.2 includes the various components of an intervention that should be described (Conn & Groves, 2011).

TABLE 26.2 Essential Intervention Content in Research Reports

INTERVENTION ELEMENT	DESCRIPTION	CONSIDERATIONS
Theory	*Why* was a particular intervention (or set of interventions) chosen and what is the mechanism by which it is thought to function?	Explicitly identify the theory. Link the intervention attributes to theoretical concepts. Describe how the intervention functions to achieve the desired goals.
Intervention recipient	*Who received* the intervention?	Differentiate between the intervention target and recipient. Describe individual or group recipients. Describe their preparation. Indicate treatment preference. Describe incentives, compensation, and/or rewards.
Interventionist	*Who delivered* the intervention to the recipients?	Identify the interventionist and the relationship to the recipient. Identify personal characteristics specific to this project (e.g., ethnicity). Describe their professional qualifications. Identify specific intervention competence (e.g., training).
Intervention content	*What* does the intervention entail?	Provide clear operational definitions. Describe procedures and materials in sufficient detail so they can be replicated. Indicate how interventions were or could be targeted or tailored. Provide information about obtaining further intervention descriptions.
Intervention delivery	*How* was the intervention delivered? *Where* and *when* was the intervention delivered? *How much* of the intervention was delivered?	Describe the delivery mode. Describe the physical and contextual settings. Describe the dosage of the intervention (amount, frequency, and duration), including both intended and administered dosages. Report on the fidelity of the intervention.

Source: Adapted from Conn, V. S., & Groves, P. S. (2011). Protecting the power of interventions through proper reporting. *Nursing Outlook, 59*(6), 318–325. doi:10.1016/j.outlook.2011.06.003

Measurement

In the measurement section, each instrument is described. The name and source of the measure, the number of items, subscales and their labels, and response format (Likert scale: from 1 = *strongly disagree* to 5 = *strongly agree*) are identified. It is very helpful for the readers to understand the potential range of total scores on the measures so that later, when they read the analysis section, they can place the overall scores, mean, and standard deviations in context of what was possible. Previous reliability and validity reports in similar samples, and the current reliability estimates (i.e., Cronbach's alpha, test–retest reliability) should be provided. Any estimates of criterion validity that were computed (i.e., correlations between similar measures of the same construct) should also be included in this section.

Procedure

This section should provide the reader with enough information to replicate the study. Whether the participants were randomized and what specific randomization procedure was used is described here. If the recruitment and randomization procedures were complicated, it may be useful to use an algorithm that graphically depicts how participants "moved through the study" from entry to data collection (Schulz, Altman, & Moher, 2010). Blinding procedures of participants, data collectors, and interveners (if appropriate) should be described. How and when and from whom data were collected are outlined.

Analysis Plan

Information about how the dataset was cleaned and managed is found in this section. The Statistical Package for the Social Sciences (SPSS) or Statistical Analysis Systems (SAS) package (and version) is identified. If a qualitative dataset and analysis software package was used, information should be provided for the qualitative data software. Information related to how the data were managed, including security procedures and "cleaning process" (i.e., eliminating errors and incorrect entries), is described in this section.

Findings

The presentation of the findings can be organized by the hypotheses that were tested, by the research questions, or by variables tested in the study. Depending on the journal, early in the findings section, a description of the sample and subgroups is sometimes included here in the "sample" section. Many editors prefer the sample description be placed in the sample section, both for flow and because it reduces space needs.

If one uses hypotheses to organize the findings section, it will be helpful for readers to describe what data were extracted from what source, and what statistical test was applied to test each hypothesis. The effect size, the actual test value, probability level ($p < .01$), confidence intervals, or odds ratios would follow. The findings section should be very straightforward with little interpretation of the findings in this section.

Discussion

Many new authors restate the findings in the discussion section. Yet, the discussion section is the authors' opportunity to be creative in terms of interpreting what the findings really mean. In addition, this section gives the authors an opportunity to make known the contribution of the study findings to the knowledge base. This is the section of the paper in which the authors' experience with the theory that was tested, the populations of participants, and/or the measurement strategies used and the insights gleaned from the implementation of the study being reported can extend knowledge and inform future research. If the opportunity is not taken, the study will likely just "add to" and not actually transform what is known in the area.

A one- or two-paragraph summary of the findings is to open the discussion section. This summary should focus first on the primary findings that supported the hypotheses, followed by those that were not supported. Then, each primary finding should be interpreted by the authors in the context of what has been reported in the literature before. Many authors struggle with choosing how many and which findings to discuss.

In some ways, this is an arbitrary decision, but each author should give it considerable thought. For instance, choosing to discuss only the positive (i.e., those hypotheses that were supported) findings may leave readers with the impression that those that were not supported should continue to be studied in future research. In fact, no one study would be sufficient to reject a hypothesis supported by theory and earlier believed to be viable. If the findings are not congruent with previous research, the authors should examine their sample, examine the fit of their findings with the theoretical framework, and examine the measures that were used with this sample. The following questions should be asked:

■ What parts of the theoretical model were supported? Which were not? Why? Did the configuration of relationships change?
■ If the sample in the study was different from those investigated earlier, did the measures perform adequately (reliable and valid)? How was the sample different?
■ If parts of the model were not supported, is it possible that some of the relationships need to be reexamined?
■ Were the measures culturally appropriate?

References

There are many opinions about how many references one should include. Again, there is no one single correct answer. Including references that will assist readers to understand the context of previous research in the area, where the findings might fit in the existing body of knowledge, the source for statistics and controversial ideas, and so forth, are some useful guides to what and how many references. As in any research report, it will be essential to reference literature that provides the reader with an understanding of how knowledge in the specific area has evolved, what the commonalities across the literature are, and, most importantly, what the gaps are. Reviewers often expect the most recent research related to the intervention (i.e., past 5 years) be included in the reference list, and do not find references more than a decade earlier useful. The number of references may differ by topic as well, depending on how fast knowledge in the field is changing—the more rapid the pace of knowledge evolution in the field, the more recent the references should be.

Tables, Figures, and Graphs

There are several basic rules for inclusion of figures/graphs and tables. Select the content for any figures and tables carefully. Space in every journal is costly. Some journals restrict the number of tables, whereas other journals that have websites have chosen to place extensive tables and reference lists in the online version rather than restrict the number.

■ Figures are useful if the study design itself is complicated and the reader would benefit from a graphic that depicted the various relationships between the study variables and the intervention itself.
■ Do not put content in tables that is already included in the text.
■ Cite the original source for a table unless the author creates the table with original information specific to the study.
■ If using a table or figure already reported in the literature, you must obtain permission to include the table. Obtaining permission for a table is relatively simple and can be requested from the journal website (e.g., https://www.nursingoutlook.org/content/permission).

COMPLETE REPORTING OF INTERVENTION FINDINGS

Publication Guidelines

Over the past decade, several guidelines have been developed to improve the consistency of information found in research reports, which would enhance the availability of information to meta-analysts, researchers, and clinicians seeking evidence on which to practice. The first of these—Consolidated Standards of Reporting Trials (CONSORT)—was developed to enable more transparent reporting of trials so they could be assessed accurately and findings compared across studies (CONSORT, 2017; Schulz et al., 2010). Over the years, the CONSORT group has refined the standards and a checklist has been developed to facilitate transparent and consistent reporting that provides guidance for all randomized controlled trials (RCTs) that should be published in peer-reviewed journals (see Table 26.3). Adherence to the checklist by authors enhances clarity of presentation, completeness, and inclusion of all relevant information (Smith et al., 2008).

TABLE 26.3 CONSORT 2010 Checklist of Information to Include When Reporting a Randomized Trial Literature Review

SECTION/TOPIC	ITEM NO.	CHECKLIST ITEM
Title and abstract	1a. 1b.	■ Identification as randomized trial in the title ■ Structured summary of trial design, methods, results, and conclusions (for specific guidance, see CONSORT for abstracts)
Introduction		
Background and objectives	2a. 2b.	■ Scientific background explanation of rationale ■ Specific objectives or hypotheses
Methods		
Trial design	3a. 3b.	■ Description of trial design (such as parallel, factorial) including allocation ratio ■ Important chances to methods after trial commencement (such as eligibility criteria) with reasons
Participants	4a. 4b.	■ Eligibility criteria for participants ■ Settings and locations where the data were collected
Interventions	5.	■ The interventions for each group with sufficient details to allow replication, including how and when they were actually administered
Outcomes	6a. 6b.	■ Completely defined as prespecified primary and secondary outcome measures, including how and when they were assessed ■ Any changes to trial outcomes after the trial commenced, with reasons
Sample size	7a. 7b.	■ How sample size was determined ■ When applicable, explanation of any interim analyses and stopping guidelines

(continued)

TABLE 26.3 CONSORT 2010 Checklist of Information to Include When Reporting a Randomized Trial Literature Review *(continued)*

SECTION/TOPIC	ITEM NO.	CHECKLIST ITEM
Randomization		
Sequence generation	8a. 8b.	■ Method used to generate the random allocation sequence ■ Type of randomization; details of any restriction (such as blocking and block size)
Allocation concealment mechanism	9.	■ Mechanism used to implement the random allocation sequence (such as sequentially numbered containers), describing any steps taken to conceal the sequence until interventions were assigned
Implementation	10.	■ Who generated the random allocation sequence, who enrolled participants, and who assigned participants to interventions
Blinding	11a. 11b.	■ If done, who was blinded after assignment to interventions (e.g., participants, care providers, those assessing outcomes) and how ■ If relevant, description of the similarity of interventions
Statistical methods	12a. 12b.	■ Statistical methods used to compare groups for primary and secondary outcomes ■ Methods for additional analyses, such as subgroup analyses and adjusted analyses
Results		
Participant flow (*a diagram is strongly recommended*)	13a. 13b.	■ For each group, the numbers of participants who were randomly assigned, received intended treatment, and were analyzed for the primary outcome ■ For each group, losses and exclusions after randomization, together with reasons
Recruitment	14a. 14b.	■ Dates defining the periods of recruitment and follow-up ■ Why the trial ended or was stopped
Baseline data	15.	■ A table showing baseline demographic and clinical characteristics for each group
Numbers analyzed	16.	■ For each group, number of participants (denominator) included in each analysis and whether the analysis was by original assigned groups
Outcomes and estimation	17a. 17b.	■ For each primary and secondary outcome, results for each group, and the estimated effect size and its precision (such as 95% confidence interval) ■ For binary outcomes, presentation for both absolute and relative effect sizes is recommended
Ancillary analyses	18.	■ Results of any other analyses performed by subgroup analyses and adjusted analyses, distinguishing prespecified from exploratory

(continued)

TABLE 26.3 CONSORT 2010 Checklist of Information to Include When Reporting a Randomized Trial Literature Review *(continued)*

SECTION/TOPIC	ITEM NO.	CHECKLIST ITEM
Harms	19.	■ All important harms or unintended effects in each group (for specific guidance see CONSORT for harms)
Discussion		
Limitations	20.	■ Trial limitations, addressing sources of potential bias, imprecision, and, if relevant, multiplicity of analyses
Generalizability	21.	■ Generalizability (external validity, applicability) of the trial findings
Interpretation	22.	■ Trial limitations, addressing sources of potential bias, imprecision
Other information		
Registration	23.	■ Registration number and name of trial registry
Protocol	24.	■ Where the full trial protocol can be accessed, if available
Funding	25.	■ Sources of funding and other support (such as supply of drugs), role of funders

CONSORT, Consolidated Standards of Reporting Trials.

Source: Adapted from Schulz, K. F., Altman, D. G., & Moher, D., CONSORT Group. (2010). CONSORT 2010 statement: Updated guidelines for reporting parallel group randomised trials. *British Medical Journal, 340,* 698–702.

In 2004, a group of researchers and editors recognized that nonrandomized interventions and evaluation studies with randomization also reported valuable information that should be reported consistently, as the findings from these studies would also be used to make public health and clinical decisions. The Transparent Reporting of Evaluations with Nonrandomized Designs (TREND) statement was developed and includes another 22-item checklist (Des Jarlais, Lyles, & Crepaz, 2004; EQUATOR, 2013). Emphasis is placed on additional areas of a manuscript in the TREND guidelines, such as the theories underlying the intervention and methods used to adjust for threats to validity in nonrandomized designs (see Table 26.4). Subsequently, several additional guidelines have been developed as well for quality improvement studies and qualitative designs. These can also be found on the EQUATOR website.

AUTHORSHIP ISSUES

Most researchers, at some point in their academic careers, experience or observe differences of opinion about who should be an author on a research report, or what the order of authorship should be. These are challenging experiences and everyone has an opinion. Fortunately, there are also well-established and accepted guidelines to which an author may refer when beginning the conversation with the scientific team about who will be included in authoring a paper and what the order of authors might be. These are important

TABLE 26.4 The TREND Checklist (Version 1.0)

PAPER SECTION/ TOPIC	ITEM NO.	DESCRIPTOR
Title and abstract	1	■ Information on how units were allocated to interventions ■ Structured abstract recommended ■ Information on target population or study sample ■ Scientific background and explanation of rationale
Introduction		
Background	2	■ Theories used in designing behavioral interventions
Methods Participants	3	■ Eligibility criteria for participants, including criteria at different levels in recruitment/sampling plan (e.g., cities, clinics, subjects) ■ Method of recruitment (e.g., referral, self-selection), including the sampling method if a systematic sampling plan was implemented ■ Recruitment setting ■ Settings and locations where the data were collected
Interventions	4	■ Details of the interventions intended for each study condition and how and when they were actually administered, specifically including: Content: what was given? Delivery method: how was the content given? Unit of delivery: how were subjects grouped during delivery? Deliverer: who delivered the intervention? Setting: where was the intervention delivered? Exposure quantity and duration: how many sessions, episodes, or events were intended to be delivered? How long were they intended to last? Time span: how long was it intended to take to deliver the intervention to each unit? Activities to increase compliance or adherence (e.g., incentives)
Objectives	5	■ Specific objectives and hypotheses
Outcomes	6	■ Clearly defined primary and secondary outcome measures ■ Methods used to collect data and any methods used to enhance the quality of measurements ■ Information on validated instruments such as psychometric and biometric properties
Sample size	7	■ How sample size was determined and, when applicable, explanation of any interim analyses and stopping rules
Assignment method	8	■ Unit of assignment (the unit being assigned to study condition, e.g., individual, group, community) ■ Method used to assign units to study conditions, including details of any restriction (e.g., blocking, stratification, minimization) ■ Inclusion of aspects employed to help minimize potential bias induced because of non-randomization (e.g., matching)
Blinding (masking)	9	■ Whether or not participants, those administering the interventions, and those assessing the outcomes were blinded to study condition assignment; if so, statement regarding how the blinding *was accomplished* and how it was assessed

(continued)

TABLE 26.4 The TREND Checklist (Version 1.0) *(continued)*

PAPER SECTION/ TOPIC	ITEM NO.	DESCRIPTOR
Unit of analysis	10	■ Description of the smallest unit that is being analyzed to assess intervention effects (e.g., individual, group, or community) ■ If the unit of analysis differs from the unit of assignment, the analytical method used to account for this (e.g., adjusting the standard error estimates by the design effect or using multilevel analysis)
Statistical methods	11	■ Statistical methods used to compare study groups for primary outcome(s), including complex methods for correlated data ■ Statistical methods used for additional analyses, such as subgroup analyses and adjusted analysis ■ Methods for imputing missing data, if used ■ Statistical software or programs used
Results, Participant flow	12	■ Flow of participants through each stage of the study: enrollment, assignment, allocation and intervention exposure, follow-up, analysis (a diagram is strongly recommended) 　■ Enrollment: the numbers of participants screened for eligibility, found to be eligible or not eligible, declined to be enrolled, and enrolled in the study 　■ Assignment: the numbers of participants assigned to a study condition 　■ Allocation and intervention exposure: the number of participants who received each intervention 　■ Follow-up: the number of participants who completed the follow-up or did not complete the follow-up (i.e., lost to follow-up), by study condition 　■ Analysis: the number of participants included in or excluded from the main analysis, by study condition ■ Description of protocol deviations from study as planned, along with reasons
Recruitment	13	■ Dates defining the periods of recruitment and follow-up
Baseline data	14	■ Baseline demographic and clinical characteristics of participants in each study condition ■ Baseline characteristics for each study condition relevant to specific disease prevention research ■ Baseline comparisons of those lost to follow-up and those retained, overall and by study condition ■ Comparison between study population at baseline and target population of interest
Baseline equivalence	15	■ Data on study group equivalence at baseline and statistical methods used to control for baseline differences
Numbers analyzed	16	■ Number of participants (denominator) included in each analysis for each study condition, particularly when the denominators change for different outcomes; statement of results in absolute numbers when feasible ■ Indication of whether the analysis strategy was "intention to treat" or, if not, description of how noncompliers were treated in the analyses

(continued)

PAPER SECTION/ TOPIC	ITEM NO.	DESCRIPTOR
Outcomes and estimation	17	■ For each primary and secondary outcome, a summary of results for each study condition, the estimated effect size, and a confidence interval to indicate the precision ■ Inclusion of null and negative findings ■ Inclusion of results from testing prespecified casual pathways through which the intervention was intended to operate, if any
Ancillary analyses	18	■ Summary of other analyses performed, including subgroup or restricted analyses, indicating which are prespecified or exploratory
Adverse events	19	■ Summary of all important adverse events or unintended effects in each study condition (including summary measures, effect size estimates, and confidence intervals)
Discussion, interpretation	20	■ Interpretation of the results, taking into account study hypotheses, sources of potential bias, imprecision of measures, multiplicative analyses, and other limitations or weaknesses of the study ■ Discussion of results taking into account the mechanism by which the intervention was intended to work (casual pathways) or alternative mechanisms or explanations ■ Discussion of the success of and barriers to implementing the intervention—fidelity of implementation ■ Discussion of research, programmatic, or *policy implications*
Generalizability	21	■ Generalizability (external validity) of the trial findings, taking into account the study population, the characteristics of the intervention, length of follow-up, *incentives, compliance rates, specific sites/ settings involved in the study*, and other contextual issues
Overall evidence	22	■ General interpretation of the results in the context of current evidence and current theory

TABLE 26.4 The TREND Checklist (Version 1.0) *(continued)*

TREND, Transparent Reporting of Evaluations with Nonrandomized Designs.

Source: Adapted from Des Jarlais, D. C., Lyles, C., & Crepaz, N., TREND Group. (2004). Improving the reporting quality of nonrandomized evaluations of behavioral and public health interventions: The TREND statement. *American Journal of Public Health, 94*(3), 361–366. doi:10.2105/AJPH.94.3.361

conversations to have and to document, as authorship of scientific papers in well-respected journals is heavily weighted during decisions for promotion and tenure. The International Committee of Medical Journal Editors (www.icmje.org) worked on a set of principles over a decade ago that most journals now accept as criteria for authorship. These principles basically state that all authors listed on a manuscript should be involved in a substantial way in the conceptualization, and/or implementation, and/or analysis, and writing the report of a study. These guidelines suggest that all authors be involved in at least two of the following steps in a study:

1. The conceptualization of the study
2. The overall design and planning of the study implementation
3. Data collection and analysis
4. Drafting the manuscript providing substantive critique for all aspects of the final manuscript

There are individuals who have participated in the study at one point or the other (i.e., data collection and analysis), but who do not make any substantive contribution to the manuscript. The authors of the study can include these individuals in the "Acknowledgment" section of the paper, along with any description of any funding received for the study.

Conventions for deciding who is the first author differ according to discipline, that is, in some disciplines, the last author is considered the senior author. In nursing, most commonly the first or lead author is the one who takes primary responsibility for coordinating and writing a first draft and provides the overall direction for incorporating all authors' comments and suggestions. However, in most disciplines, the order of authors reflects the quantity and quality of contributions to the project being presented.

Decisions about order of authorship should be documented after a group meeting of all of the potential authors in which the decision is made. It is possible that these decisions will be revisited at a later time (e.g., if an author fails to contribute his or her section of a manuscript). There are some special instances of potential authorship that consistently present challenges and primary investigators need to be aware of the sensitive nature of these relationships (Oberlander & Spencer, 2006). These include student–faculty advisor and employee–supervisor (e.g., chair and faulty member). The need for early and often discussions about who is an author, and in what order, gets a little more challenging in these cases when compared with discussions among peers. This is a case where team discussions and documentation can be exceptionally helpful, as well as consultation by journal editors in the university if these individuals are available to authors. A third party can usually address common misconceptions or assumptions about authorship and can smooth negotiations among those involved.

SUBMISSION AND PEER REVIEW OF THE MANUSCRIPT

Submission and Review

The review process in refereed journals will require 4 to 16 weeks, depending on the journal. Most journals now manage all submissions through a website devoted to the journal and editors assign specific manuscripts to referees on the basis of those reviewers' areas of expertise. Some editors ask prospective authors for names of referees, but most well-respected journals select reviewers either from their own database or by searching the literature and/or publisher website for experts on papers published earlier in the area. In most (if not all) journals, referees are not paid for this service and most referees are very busy individuals. This is important for authors to remember. Editors, the majority of whom have another full-time job, will assign reviewers within 2 weeks of the paper being submitted. Then the editor will invite reviewers and ask for a review to be submitted back to the website in 3 to 4 weeks. Reminders are sent 1 week prior to the deadline. However, there is no penalty for submitting a review late or even not at all, although most editors can "rate" their reviewers' quality of review for future reference. On occasion, editors will request four to five referees to accept the paper to review, and occasionally none will. This can slow down the review process as well. In this author's experience, the more cutting edge the paper, the more interest there will be from reviewers. Once the reviews are returned to the editor by at least two reviewers (preferably three), the editor can make a decision within a few weeks, depending on the complexity of the reviewers' comments.

Almost every journal now requires papers be submitted through the journal's website because all correspondence, processing, and so forth is handled electronically. In many ways, this speeds up the review process and an author should always be able to communicate easily with an editor. In fact, on most web-based systems, the authors themselves can check on the status of the manuscript, that is, whether it has been assigned to reviewers, if it is with the editor after reviews have come in, and so forth.

Every author who has had their work published should submit their name for consideration as a reviewer to at least one journal, as should clinical experts. It should be clear from the above discussion that this is a service to colleagues by experts who give their time and experience to improve the reporting of research published in the literature. It is incumbent on any author to make himself or herself available for the same service to others. Reviews take 3 to 5 hours and most editors will ask an individual to conduct a review only every 3 to 4 months.

Handling Rejection

All successful authors have had at least one (and likely many more) manuscript rejected during their careers. The reasons for rejection vary—sometimes the topic is not a good fit with the journal's editorial purpose, the methods are not considered rigorous by the reviewers, the topic itself is dated, or the writing style is poor. Rejections are very hard to take, no matter how experienced an author is. Authors spend a great deal of time writing a manuscript and it is expected that disappointment will be experienced when one's product is rejected. However, not all is lost—in fact, much is gained. The reviewers' comments are almost always included in a rejection notice and an author should use these reviews to his or her advantage before he or she submits the paper to another journal. Ignoring the reviews and just resubmitting the paper to another journal is shortsighted and will often result in a second rejection. Instead, the author should carefully read the critique, make any warranted changes, and then submit to another journal. Novice authors may want to request assistance with this review and revision process from someone more experienced with the process.

Managing Revisions

A revision request is good news, although authors rarely see this as an exciting development. We all expect to have our paper accepted on the first review! However, a revision request, in this author's (and editor's) experience, always results in a better final product. The wisdom and suggestions of reviewers invariably strengthen the manuscript (Broome, 2017; Thomas, 2011).

Those authors who are most successful at revising a manuscript on the basis of recommendations of reviewers approach this task with some level of objectivity as they read the reviews. It is helpful to begin the process by developing a table that includes all the major points that reviewers made, a summary of what revision was (or is planned to be) made, and in a third column where the revision can be found (see Table 26.5). It is important that each reviewer's request be considered carefully. If a reviewer asks for a revision that is counter to another reviewer, or if the reviewer asks for a revision that the authors do not believe is appropriate, it is usually a good idea to contact the editor to get another opinion. This revision table should be included in a revised submission for the editor and reviewers. Using such a table is extremely useful during the revision process if different members of the team are asked to address certain comments. However, it is the first author's responsibility to pull all the changes together and make sure the manuscript still reads with one "voice." It is especially important to make sure every author is given the opportunity to read the final revised version and indicate his or her acceptance of the final product before resubmitting.

ADDITIONAL DISSEMINATION VENUES

Abstracts

Investigators usually have a list of professional meetings where they want to disseminate the results to facilitate the translation of research findings into practice and promote further research in the area. Some of these are scientific meetings at which research is presented in various areas, usually clustered by topic. In most cases, these meetings cannot accept all the

TABLE 26.5 Revision Response Table		
REVIEWER COMMENTS	**AUTHOR RESPONSE**	**PAGE NO.**
The abstract is not in the format we use for the practice applications section.	We could not find any sample articles from the practice applications section so we referenced the following guidelines: www.pediatricnursing.net/authorguidelines.html. The word count for the abstract is 176.	1
Last section of introduction discusses how research has not been conducted across racial and ethnic lines but is not mentioned as a focus of the current study … needs clarification.	Clarification of the focus of the current study (it is to include children regardless of gender, race, or ethnicity) was added.	3
APA requires spelling out of abbreviations when first mentioned … does this apply to a gene marker	Name of gene marker was spelled out with its abbreviation following in parentheses.	3
Be more specific on what exactly the studies referenced define as "reduced sleep."	Referenced both articles mentioned and included specific number of hours generally considered to be "reduced sleep" for children of this age.	4
Sentence is confusing and close to a run-on … better to break into two sentences	The sentence is separated into two sentences as suggested to enhance clarity.	4
Statement [improperly] assumes that providers are using only their clinical judgment for diagnosis … Providers are using BMI but don't treat once overweight is discovered … two different issues are being addressed here.	We agreed that the two ideas discussed here were not linked together. We deleted the last sentence in this section to avoid raising a new topic for the reader that was not expanded on.	4
Replace "as well as" with "and."	Changed as recommended.	5
Change "report" to "reported."	Changed as recommended.	5
Remove the word "likely."	Changed as recommended.	5
Change the ";" to a ",".	Changed as recommended.	6
Insert a ",".	Changed as recommended.	6
Separate into two sentences.	Separated into two sentences.	6
This last sentence is a bit of a disconnect with the developmental stage of younger children … I don't believe developmentally that this age of a child has the capacity to abstractly think about size as it might affect social interaction … so they would not have any self-esteem related to this concept.	We added a reference to support the developmental capabilities of preschool children. We also included a brief discussion about how society has changed and is reflected in children's exposure to ideas concerning body image in the media at a very young age.	6

(continued)

TABLE 26.5 Revision Response Table *(continued)*

REVIEWER COMMENTS	AUTHOR RESPONSE	PAGE NO.
Research questions should be displayed in a numbered list format … and should be more formally written.	Changed research questions to a numbered list format. We were not clear on what the reviewer meant by "more formally written." However, we did attempt to word them more typically.	7
The design of the study is described to be descriptive … but the research questions also discuss a correlation.	Clarification that the design of the study did involve correlational analysis was added.	7
"They" … clarify who is they.	Changed "they" to "the center directors" to clarify the subject of the sentence.	8
What were the inclusion criteria	Added specific eligibility criteria for inclusion in the study.	8
Need to discuss assent of the child versus consent of the parent and how both were obtained … consent should be blindly distributed and explained by the researcher.	Clarification added about how we addressed both consent of the parents and assent from the children … we made it clear that the consents were distributed by day-care centers and that parents had a phone number at which they could contact the investigators with questions.	8

APA, American Pyschological Association; BMI, body mass index.

submissions they receive. They will request that an abstract of the study findings be submitted for review by several experts in the area. Some abstracts are accepted for oral and some for poster presentation.

Several myths abound about the value of competitive abstracts, of the relative value of poster versus oral presentation, and about how many times one should present the findings of a study. Everyone has an opinion about each of these, so here are a few from this author:

- Question: Is an oral presentation of a study more highly rated than a poster?
  This depends on the university and the criteria it uses for rating individuals for promotion. In terms of rigor of review, the same reviewers rate both formats. Many times, a presentation is provided only a poster slot (and not oral) because the findings are not completed in time for the submission deadline. One relatively new practice at conferences is to group posters on a similar topic and schedule the poster session for a selected time in which each author talks for about 5 minutes about his or her research and then the audience asks all poster presenters questions. The moderator, usually a senior person in the field, manages the discussion. As an investigator, this author actually prefers to disseminate in a poster session. Only interested participants come to view it, usually ask more in-depth and interesting questions, and the connections with these same individuals are much more satisfying.
- How many times, and over what time, can research be presentted before it is published? There is no specific answer to this. My own personal rule about this is no more than three times over a year to 15 months. Given that abstract deadlines are now due

6 to 9 months prior to a reputable conference, and that some conferences require the submission be a first presentation of that research, the answer to this question takes some deliberation and planning. It is possible that one could complete a study in January and the national clinically focused conference is held in October and the regional research conference the next March. In that case, presenting the same intervention research findings twice—for different audiences—should be sufficient, with the assumption that the findings are being drafted in a manuscript for submission in summer of that first year. In that case, if submitted concurrently with the presentations, the manuscript should have been reviewed and most likely be pending request for revision. Given the author now also has the suggestions from conference participants to incorporate into the revision, and the revised manuscript will be even stronger, the paper can be accepted within 12 to 15 months of completion.

ADDITIONAL VENUES FOR DISSEMINATION

In addition to the scholarly article(s) as a mechanism for dissemination of the scientific findings of an intervention study, there are several other dissemination vehicles that intervention researchers should consider.

Participants: The first is how feedback about the results will be provided to participants in the study. One method would be to send each a copy of a study abstract. However informative, most participants in an intervention would likely find it more helpful and interesting to receive a more in-depth, colorful, and descriptive report. This report could include pictures (no real participants should be identified unless permission has been obtained from both the participant and the IRB), bulleted points about what was found, and a section that provides some guidance on how to apply the findings in their lives. PowerPoint presentations, stapled or placed in a folder, are colorful and useful formats to use. Also, references to the scientific reports can be provided for participants in the study who might be interested.

Study facilitators: To provide feedback to the professionals who facilitated access to the population or provided input for the development of the intervention, a poster presentation is usually viewed very positively—especially if it includes a small section in which those who were facilitators are included. These can then be hung in the clinic or inpatient unit where the study took place. A handout can also be produced with the poster on it for distribution. In some facilities, staff rarely have this loop closed and appreciate knowing what happened. As a result, they may be more likely in the future to host the investigator.

Social media: The use of social media (i.e., individual faculty and school websites, Facebook, blogs, twitter) has become increasingly viewed as a useful dissemination vehicle for one's research. These are not to be considered as sole or final venues for reputable research but rather a mechanism in a toolkit that researchers can use to gain a wider audience and uptake (and hopefully translation) of his or her findings. Some studies have demonstrated that use of social media, which pushes findings to users as opposed to requiring the user to seek the information, can increase the dissemination and use of the original article (Allen, Stanton, Di Pietro, & Moseley, 2013; Terras, 2012). Interestingly, in the study by Allen et al., although the number of views and downloads was significantly higher in the week following release when the paper was highlighted in social media, the number of citations a year later was not greater. Terras (2012) also found similar download spikes from open access publications when she blogged about the studies she conducted. The acceptance of these social media cites by promotion committees is becoming better recognized as a metric for extent of reach, but not necessarily impact of one's work. What is clear is that social media has advantages to highlighting one's work if in open access journals, and if in subscription-based journals can also be used after publication to highlight one's research and point other researchers to where one's work is published.

SUMMARY

Dissemination of research occurs throughout a study in various venues. However, the final responsibility of the lead investigator for any intervention study is to publish, in a refereed journal, the final results describing the effectiveness of the intervention. Science is incremental in most cases, so publication in a refereed journal closes the loop on that study and opens the possibility for others to build on that work and extend knowledge further. Consistent and transparent reporting of study findings is enabled if authors refer to standards developed in the health professions. Other options for dissemination include presentations of the findings for professional and lay audiences, a report of the findings for those who participated in the study, and feedback of findings to those who facilitated entry to the "system" in which the study was implemented and provided access to the participants.

Key Points From This Chapter

- Dissemination plans for publications and authorship should be discussed early and revisited often by the research team.
- Choice of journal is dependent on many factors, including goodness of fit with editorial purpose of the journal, target audience, and IF of the journal.
- Authors should use established guidelines—that is, CONSORT and TREND—to guide their inclusion of content in a manuscript reporting an intervention study.
- Intervention reports must include details about theory and method, as well as findings, that will enable replication of the study and comparison with similar interventions.
- Revision requests for submitted manuscripts should be viewed as an opportunity to strengthen one's scholarship on the basis of reviews from experts in the field.

REFERENCES

Allen, H. G., Stanton, T. R., Di Pietro, F., & Moseley, G. L. (2013). Social media release increases dissemination of original articles in the clinical pain sciences. *PLOS ONE, 8*(7), e68914. doi:10.1371/journal.pone.0068914

Baggs, J. G. (2008). Issues and rules for authors concerning authorship versus acknowledgements, dual publication, self plagiarism, and salami publishing. *Research in Nursing & Health, 31*(4), 295–297. doi:10.1002/nur.20280

Beall, J. (2017). Research integrity corner: Special issue on predatory publishing. *Biochemia Medica, 27*(2), 273–278. doi:10.11613/BM.2017.029

Broome, M. E. (2014). Open access publishing: A disruptive innovation. *Nursing Outlook, 62*(2), 69–71. doi:10.1016/j.outlook.2014.02.004

Broome, M. E. (2017). Predatory publishing is everyone's concern. *Nursing Outlook, 65*(6), 667–668. doi:10.1016/j.outlook.2017.10.003

Conn, V. S., & Groves, P. S. (2011). Protecting the power of interventions through proper reporting. *Nursing Outlook, 59*(6), 318–325. doi:10.1016/j.outlook.2011.06.003

CONSORT: Transparent reporting of trials. (2017). Retrieved from http://www.consort-statement.org

Des Jarlais, D. C., Lyles, C., & Crepaz, N., TREND Group. (2004). Improving the reporting quality of nonrandomized evaluations of behavioral and public health interventions: The TREND statement. *American Journal of Public Health, 94*(3), 361–366. doi:10.2105/AJPH.94.3.361

EQUATOR. (2013). Guidelines for reporting health research: How to promote their use in your journal. Retrieved from http://www.equator-network.org

Henly, S. J. (2014). Duplicate publications and salami reports: Corruption of the scientific record. *Nursing Research, 63*(1), 1–2. doi:10.1097/NNR.0000000000000015

JANE. (2017). Journal/Author Name Estimator. Retrieved from http://Jane.biosemantics.org

LeBrun, J. L. (2011). *Scientific writing 2.0: A reader and writer's guide.* Hackensack, NJ: World Scientific.

Lewallen, L. P., & Crane, P. B. (2010). Choosing a publication venue. *Journal of Professional Nursing, 26*(4), 250–254. doi:10.1016/j.profnurs.2009.12.005

Oberlander, S. E., & Spencer, R. J. (2006). Graduate students and the culture of authorship. *Ethics & Behavior, 16*(3), 217–232. doi:10.1207/s15327019eb1603_3

Oermann, M. H., Conklin, J. L., Nicoll, L. H., Chinn, P. L., Ashton, K. S., Edie, A. H., … Budinger, S. C. (2016). Study of predatory open access nursing journals. *Journal of Nursing Scholarship, 48*(6), 624–632. doi:10.1111/jnu

Oermann, M. H., & Hays, J. C. (2015). *Writing for publication in nursing* (3rd ed.). New York, NY: Springer Publishing.

Polit, D. F., & Northam, S. (2011). Impact factors in nursing journals. *Nursing Outlook, 59*(1), 18–28. doi:10.1016/j.outlook.2010.11.001

Schulz, K. F., Altman, D. G., & Moher, D., CONSORT Group. (2010). CONSORT 2010 statement: Updated guidelines for reporting parallel group randomised trials. *British Medical Journal, 340,* 698–702. doi:10.1136/bmj.c332

Silvia, P. J. (2007). *How to write a lot: A practical guide to productive academic writing.* Washington, DC: American Psychological Association.

Smith, B. A., Lee, H. J., Lee, J. H., Choi, M., Jones, D. E., Bausell, R. B., & Broome, M. E. (2008). Quality of reporting randomized controlled trials (RCTs) in the nursing literature: Application of the consolidated standards of reporting trials (CONSORT). *Nursing Outlook, 56*(1), 31–37. doi:10.1016/j.outlook.2007.09.002

Terras, M. M. (2012). The impact of social media on the dissemination of research: The results of an experiment. *Journal of Digital Humanities, 1*(3).

Thomas, S. P. (2011). Conceptual debates and empirical evidence about the peer review process for scholarly journals. *Journal of Professional Nursing, 27*(3), 168–173. doi:10.1016/j.profnurs.2010.09.015

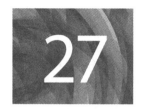

Social Media Use in Intervention Research and Dissemination

Linsey N. Grove & Dianne Morrison-Beedy

> Tweet me, snapchat me, text me, email me…
> just don't forget me. Use this need people have to connect to
> make change in the world. —*Dianne Morrison-Beedy*

Social media has changed how people around the world connect, communicate, and interact with each other. Many different industries have harnessed the power of social media to increase profits, solve complicated problems, and market their goods. There are many uses for social media in healthcare, research, and public health, and as social media changes, innovation and adaptation must follow. Social media use in clinical settings to improve public health, healthcare, and research must be strategic; however, for many professionals, how best to use social media to successfully implement and disseminate research interventions can be confusing or misunderstood (Aase & Timimi, 2013). To understand how social media has been used in research interventions by investigators, it is important to first understand the definition and types of social media.

BACKGROUND AND DEFINITION OF SOCIAL MEDIA

Since its inception, the Internet has strived not only to provide a wealth of information to its users but also to connect people around the globe. Early communication channels included discussion forums and chat rooms. The digital landscape changed dramatically as Internet speeds and data storage increased, allowing for larger, multifunctional platforms for users to interact (Obar & Wildman, 2015). There is no global consensus on this terminology because many social media platforms provide the same communication functionality as traditional media applications. The constantly changing social media landscape also makes defining social media difficult (Aase & Timimi, 2013; Obar, Zube, & Lampe, 2012). Social media platforms come and go from the Internet and mobile world, each providing different communication, content, and user functionality that keep the definition of social media changing (Obar et al., 2012). These social media platforms include Facebook, Twitter, Snapchat, Instagram, Pinterest, blogs, and wikis and many more depending on region and audience (Pew Research Center, 2017). In this chapter, we discuss various social media platforms and their use particularly in health interventions. Understanding the limitations, functionality, and potential pitfalls of using social media in research can help researchers plan effective health interventions in diverse settings.

TYPES OF SOCIAL MEDIA

Table 27.1 presents a snapshot of popular social media platforms. These platforms are ever changing, and by the time this chapter is published, it is likely that there could be new or more popular social media platforms.

BACKGROUND IN LITERATURE

As noted in Aase and Timimi (2013), the healthcare industry has been slow to embrace social media in patient engagement and other interaction opportunities. However, since the Aase & Timimi article was published, multiple research studies have been conducted to evaluate the use of social media in various venues including (a) social support groups for patients, (b) health information dissemination and evaluation, (c) data mining and surveillance, and (d) health behavior and intervention design.

Social Support Groups

For patients and caregivers, social media offers easily accessible global support groups to help cope with diagnoses, caregiver fatigue, peer-to-peer education, and treatment experiences (Alotaibi et al., 2017; Hamm et al., 2013; Koskan et al., 2014; Patel, Chang, Greysen, & Chopra, 2015). A scoping review of social media use in patient and caregiver populations yielded 284 studies that met the review criteria (primary research, focused on patient and caregiver experiences in healthcare, and used social media in the study as a tool). This review found that 77.1% of these studies used social media as a tool to promote self-care among both caregivers and patients, with 72.9% of studies presenting positive conclusions in overall social media use (Hamm et al., 2013). Different diseases can also impact the types and frequency of social media used for social support; a systematic review of social media use in cancer found that different types of cancers yielded differing amounts of use for emotional support, information exchange, and self-disclosure (Koskan et al., 2014). Different social media platforms were more frequently used by users on the basis of cancer type. For instance, breast cancer studies in the review were focused on mostly online forums (as a form of social media) that addressed information dissemination, emotional support, and self-expression (Koskan et al., 2014).

Health Information Dissemination and Evaluation

The Internet not only has provided a way to disseminate information to large audiences but also has allowed different individuals and organizations to disseminate information, whether credible or not. There were numerous studies focusing on how and what information (both created by the study itself or independent content creators) is disseminated

TABLE 27.1 Top Five Most Used Social Media Platforms in the United States

SOCIAL MEDIA PLATFORM	DESCRIPTION	AUDIENCE

Facebook	Online and mobile social media platform with almost 2 billion users worldwide (Statista, 2017). Started in 2004 by Mark Zuckerberg, Facebook was initially created for college students but quickly allowed anyone to access. Users can create "profiles" and connect with "friends" through mutual access to profiles, posts, and photos. Businesses and organizations can also create pages for users to interact with by "follow," "post," or "comment" functions.	All online adults: 79%
		
		Men: 75%
		Women: 88%
		Age (years)
		  18–29: 88%
		  30–49: 84%
		  50–64: 72%
		  ≥65: 62%
		
		Urban: 81%
		Suburban: 77%
		Rural: 81%

Instagram	Instagram allows users to take photos and apply filters through its mobile app. These photos can then be shared with others (either publicly or privately; Instagram, 2018). Started in 2010 Kevin Systrom and Mike Krieger and bought by Facebook in 2012, Instagram has 600 million users globally (Leonard, 2012; Statista, 2017).	All online adults: 32%
		
		Men: 26%
		Women: 38%
		Age (years)
		  18–29: 59%
		  30–49: 33%
		  50–64: 18%
		  ≥65: 8%
		
		Urban: 39%
		Suburban: 28%
		Rural: 31%

LinkedIn	LinkedIn is a professional social media platform for job seekers, recruiters, industry experts, and companies. Users can create professional profiles similar to resumes and network with other users in their field (LinkedIn, 2016b). It was launched in 2003, and now hosts 106 million worldwide users (LinkedIn, 2016a; Statista, 2017).	All online adults: 29%
		
		Men: 31%
		Women: 27%
		Age (years)
		  18–29: 29%
		  30–49: 34%
		  50–64: 28%
		  ≥65: 16%
		
		Urban: 30%
		Suburban: 34%
		Rural: 25%

(continued)

SOCIAL MEDIA PLATFORM	DESCRIPTION	AUDIENCE*
TABLE 27.1 Top Five Most Used Social Media Platforms in the United States *(continued)*		
Pinterest	Pinterest allow users to "pin" graphics to "boards" (Pinterest, 2018). Its 150 million users (Statista, 2017) can create thematic boards and with small images of online content (Madrigal, 2012).	All online adults: 31%
		Men: 17%
		Women: 45%
		Age (years)
		18–29: 36%
		30–49: 34%
		50–64: 28%
		≥65: 16%
		Urban: 30%
		Suburban: 34%
		Rural: 25%
Twitter	Started in 2006, Twitter is a social network of 140 character-limited messages with 317 million users currently (Arrington, 2006; Twitter, 2017a). Posts or "tweets" can contain text, photos, videos, and links to other webpages and can be shared with "followers" or made public (Twitter, 2017a). Hashtags or (#) are used with keywords or terms as a way to categorize tweets via search (e.g., #WorldAIDSDay; Twitter, 2017b).	All online adults: 24%
		Men: 24%
		Women: 25%
		Age (years)
		18–29: 36%
		30–49: 23%
		50–64: 21%
		≥65: 10%
		Urban: 26%
		Suburban: 24%
		Rural: 24%

(Bell, Douglas, & Cutts, 2014; Logsdon et al., 2014; Paige, Stellefson, Chaney, & Alber, 2015; Robillard, Cabral, Hennessey, Kwon, & Illes, 2015) by whom, as well as on evaluating information currently available to different groups for accuracy, credibility, behavioral impact (Boyle, LaBrie, Froidevaux, & Witkovic, 2016; McGregor et al., 2014), and specific messaging (Puljak, 2016). Lin, Zhang, Song, and Omori (2016) evaluated factors that drive personal information disclosure among U.S., South Korean, and Hong Kong teens after seeing and obtaining prescriptions from medical professionals. Lin et al. (2016) found that even with the surge in online information seeking, medical professionals are still regarded as credible stakeholders for patient self-disclosure. They also found that higher trust in social media information sources is positively associated with online self-disclosure of health issues or concerns among U.S. and South Korean teens but not Hong Kong teens (Lin et al., 2016). Some articles looked at specific social media platforms and the types of health information being disseminated. The types of audiences targeted on each of these platforms were also evaluated; this included Facebook (Hales, Davidson, & Turner-McGrievy, 2014; Puljak, 2016), Twitter (Robillard et al., 2015), and Instagram. Paige et al. (2015) analyzed one specific social media platform called Pinterest to see what types of chronic obstructive pulmonary disease (COPD) information were being disseminated to users. Many of the "pins" were related to disease self-management and general information about COPD and included more targeted information to female users (Paige et al., 2015). Other studies looked at which social media platforms had more influence on specific audiences' health behaviors. In particular, these studies examined exposure to alcohol-related posts (Boyle et al., 2016; Westgate & Holliday, 2016) and weight loss (Hales et al., 2014). In the Westgate and Holliday (2016) article, researchers found that adolescents exposed to drinking-related content on Facebook predicted a significant increase in drinking behavior. Hales et al. (2014) found that counselor-generated posts in Facebook groups dedicated to weight loss programs can help program participants lose weight by increasing social media engagement. Social media can also be used as a way to promote professional development in the healthcare field through information dissemination, social network support, and continuing education opportunities (Weaver, Lindsay, & Gitelman, 2012).

Data Mining and Surveillance

Social media has provided an enormous amount of data for researchers, communities, and for-profit industries to analyze. Health data can be collected from, and linked to, different social media and can be used by different audiences (including clinicians, patients, and healthcare administrators) to better understand public health indicators, information, and trends (Conway & O'Connor, 2016; Ji, Chun, Cappellari, & Geller, 2017). Dai, Lee, and Hao (2017) used data from Twitter to analyze, and then predict, asthma prevalence in different geographical areas across the United States (American Community Survey) and in cross-referencing this data with Behavioral Risk Factor Surveillance System (BRFSS) survey data. Researchers developed an epidemiological model from these data sets to predict regional asthma prevalence (Dai et al., 2017). This information could be useful in distributing healthcare resources and planning asthma-related health interventions in clinics and community organizations in real time. In another study, researchers analyzed the use of different technologies (including social media) as ways to capture geographical and neighborhood data for public health measures (Schootman et al., 2016). Schootman et al. (2016) found that although social media was a powerful tool for gathering large amounts of user data in specific geographical locations, it can also be unrepresentative of different audiences depending on the use of specific platforms.

Health Behavior Interventions and Intervention Design

Intervention design has been impacted by the introduction of social media; for example, sample recruitment using social media platforms such as Facebook, Twitter, and quick response (QR) codes provided an additional option for Gu, Skierkowski, Florin, Friend, and Ye (2016). In this particular study, QR codes provided the highest return on investment compared with other social media platforms in recruiting adolescent populations (Gu et al., 2016). Providing a highly effective and cost-efficient recruitment tool is extremely helpful to adolescent health and behavioral researchers. Musiat et al. (2016) evaluated the use and cost-effectiveness of paid and unpaid online study recruitment among teens. This study found that unpaid online recruitment was more cost-effective, and that these two recruitment options can yield very different sample demographics depending on the study details, advertisement dissemination, exposure, message, visual esthetic, and social media platform used (Musiat et al., 2016). Broader health behavior interventions in different clinical settings use social media as a vehicle for chronic disease management (Kear, Harrington, & Bhattacharya, 2015; Patel et al., 2015), patient safety (Bell et al., 2014), support (Alvarez-Jimenez et al., 2014), prevention (Bull, Levine, Black, Schmiege, & Santelli, 2012), and education (Bell et al., 2014; Patel et al., 2015). Social media has also been used as a health behavior intervention delivery tool (Bull et al., 2012; Lelutiu-Weinberger et al., 2015). For example, Lelutiu-Weinberger et al. (2015) administered a sexual risk–reduction intervention to men having sex with men (MSM) using the live chat function on Facebook with significant reductions in drug and alcohol use, unprotected anal sex (sober or not) as well as increasing HIV knowledge among participants.

CONSIDERATIONS FOR SOCIAL MEDIA USE IN HEALTH INTERVENTIONS AND RESEARCH

The benefits of using social media to change health behavior or conduct clinical research should be contrasted with potential detriments. Researchers and health educators may have to compete with incorrect, misleading, and potentially dangerous independently generated content in many social media platforms (Fergie, Hilton, & Hunt, 2016). For instance, in one study of glaucoma patients' information uptake from social media, researchers found that many social media posts contained misleading or dangerous information about treatment and the disease (McGregor et al., 2014). The "net" can be cast too wide, and, therefore, the message can become diluted or conversely, social media data can be misleading when looking for specific audiences in inappropriate platforms (Schootman et al., 2016). One concern that many researchers face when designing interventions using social media is how to protect participant and patient privacy (Aase & Timimi, 2013). Although many social media platforms include their own privacy protections, it can be difficult for researchers to customize or ensure privacy is protected in highly sensitive research interventions (Lunnay, Borlagdan, McNaughton, & Ward, 2015). This concern should be acknowledged by researchers when recruiting and informing participants for a study. One way to alleviate this, for instance, is using Facebook ads that can redirect users to study websites with more confidential and privacy functions to protect participants when collecting data. Facebook ads can also target very specific gender, age, educational, and geographical areas, which help researchers ensure that they are reaching the appropriate audience (Kosinski, Matz, Gosling, Popov, & Stillwell, 2016). Using Facebook ad recruitment strategies for study protocol should include online privacy protection strategies including redirecting users to a website with a secure sockets layer (SSL) certificate (e.g., https vs. http) that encrypts user and organizational data such as IP address, health history, and other identifying information (Office for Human Research Protections, 2016). Identifying staff with social media knowledge and experience can significantly help researchers in implementing successful social media strategies in study design.

Social media can also be used by researchers to disseminate evidence-based research findings to scientific peers, the public, and practitioners. Promoting research can create networking opportunities for future collaboration, deliver critical research to communities and practitioners to implement evidence-informed practice and interventions, and accelerate research to practice (Kandeh, 2016). On average, it takes 17 years for research to be translated into evidence-based practice (Munro & Savel, 2016); therefore, technological communication methods such as social media may fast-track release of critical research findings to organizations and practitioners.

Key Points From This Chapter

- Social media is constantly changing in terms of user base, functionality, and popularity.
- Social media use in healthcare is multi-faceted; its use should be aligned with the mission or goals of the study or organization before implementation.
- The key uses for social media in healthcare are patient social support, health information dissemination and evaluation, data mining and surveillance, and health behavior and intervention design.

SUMMARY

Social media integration in healthcare must be adaptable, innovative, and strategic. Health communication, social marketing, and patient interaction are all avenues that would greatly benefit from using social media for messaging, cultural norming, and outreach. Data collection and mining provide health behavior and clinical researchers with large amounts of social, geographical, and various other types of data to analyze with other forms of traditional data sets. Although there is quite a deal of promise in using social media to deliver evidence-based health interventions, there must also be attention given to specific protocols developed to ensure patient privacy and safety, information accuracy, and account security.

REFERENCES

Aase, L., & Timimi, F. K. (2013). Health care social media: Engagement and health care in the digital era. *Clinical Obstetrics and Gynecology, 56*(3), 471–476. doi:10.1097/GRF.0b013e31829d6058

Alotaibi, N. M., Samuel, N., Wang, J., Ahuja, C. S., Guha, D., Ibrahim, G. M., ... Macdonald, R. L. (2017). The use of social media communications in brain aneurysms and subarachnoid hemorrhage: A mixed-method analysis. *World Neurosurgery, 98*, 456–462. doi:10.1016/j.wneu.2016.11.085

Alvarez-Jimenez, M., Alcazar-Corcoles, M. A., González-Blanch, C., Bendall, S., McGorry, P. D., & Gleeson, J. F. (2014). Online, social media and mobile technologies for psychosis treatment: A systematic review on novel user-led interventions. *Schizophrenia Research, 156*(1), 96–106. doi:10.1016/j.schres.2014.03.021

Arrington, M. (2006, July 15). Odeo releases Twttr. *TechCrunch.* Retrieved from https://techcrunch.com/2006/07/15/is-twttr-interesting

Bell, M., Douglas, J., & Cutts, C. (2014). How pharmacy's adoption of social media can enhance patient outcomes. *Integrated Pharmacy Research and Practice, 3*, 39–47. doi:10.2147/IPRP.S42774

Boyle, S. C., LaBrie, J. W., Froidevaux, N. M., & Witkovic, Y. D. (2016). Different digital paths to the keg? How exposure to peers' alcohol-related social media content influences drinking among male and female first-year college students. *Addictive Behaviors, 57*, 21–29. doi:10.1016/j.addbeh.2016.01.011

Bull, S. S., Levine, D. K., Black, S. R., Schmiege, S. J., & Santelli, J. (2012). Social media-delivered sexual health intervention: A cluster randomized controlled trial. *American Journal of Preventive Medicine, 43*(5), 467–474. doi:10.1016/j.amepre.2012.07.022

Conway, M., & O'Connor, D. (2016). Social media, big data, and mental health: Current advances and ethical implications. *Current Opinion in Psychology, 9*, 77–82. doi:10.1016/j.copsyc.2016.01.004

Dai, H., Lee, B. R., & Hao, J. (2017). Predicting asthma prevalence by linking social media data and traditional surveys. *Annals of the American Academy of Political and Social Science, 669*(1), 75–92. doi:10.1177/0002716216678399

Fergie, G., Hilton, S., & Hunt, K. (2016). Young adults' experiences of seeking online information about diabetes and mental health in the age of social media. *Health Expectations, 19*(6), 1324–1335. doi:10.1111/hex.12430

Gu, L. L., Skierkowski, D., Florin, P., Friend, K., & Ye, Y. (2016). Facebook, Twitter, & Qr codes: An exploratory trial examining the feasibility of social media mechanisms for sample recruitment. *Computers in Human Behavior, 60*, 86–96. doi:10.1016/j.chb.2016.02.006

Hales, S. B., Davidson, C., & Turner-McGrievy, G. M. (2014). Varying social media post types differentially impacts engagement in a behavioral weight loss intervention. *Translational Behavioral Medicine, 4*(4), 355–362. doi:10.1007/s13142-014-0274-z

Hamm, M. P., Chisholm, A., Shulhan, J., Milne, A., Scott, S. D., Given, L. M., & Hartling, L. (2013). Social media use among patients and caregivers: A scoping review. *BMJ Open, 3*(5), e002819. doi:10.1136/bmjopen-2013-002819

Instagram. (2018). Instagram: What is instagram? Retrieved from https://help.instagram.com/424737657584573.

Ji, X., Chun, S. A., Cappellari, P., & Geller, J. (2017). Linking and using social media data for enhancing public health analytics. *Journal of Information Science, 43*(2), 221–245. doi:10.1177/0165551515625029

Kandeh, D. (2016). Research dissemination: How social media can be a useful tool. Retrieved from http://blogs.springer.com/lst/research-dissemination-how-social-media-can-be-a-useful-tool

Kear, T., Harrington, M., & Bhattacharya, A. (2015). Partnering with patients using social media to develop a hypertension management instrument. *Journal of the American Society of Hypertension, 9*(9), 725–734. doi:10.1016/j.jash.2015.07.006

Kosinski, M., Matz, S. C., Gosling, S. D., Popov, V., & Stillwell, D. (2016). Facebook as a research tool. *Continuing Education Corner: Monitor on Psychology*, 70–75. Retrieved from https://www.apa.org/education/ce/facebook-research.pdf

Koskan, A., Klasko, L., Davis, S. N., Gwede, C. K., Wells, K. J., Kumar, A., … Meade, C. D. (2014). Use and taxonomy of social media in cancer-related research: A systematic review. *American Journal of Public Health, 104*(7), e20–e37. doi:10.2105/AJPH.2014.301980

Lelutiu-Weinberger, C., Pachankis, J. E., Gamarel, K. E., Surace, A., Golub, S. A., & Parsons, J. T. (2015). Feasibility, acceptability, and preliminary efficacy of a live-chat social media intervention to reduce HIV risk among young men who have sex with men. *AIDS and Behavior, 19*(7), 1214–1227. doi:10.1007/s10461-014-0911-z

Leonard, T. (2012, April 12). Instacash: The nerds who made a billion in 551 days from camera app. *Daily Mail.* Retrieved from http://www.dailymail.co.uk/sciencetech/article-2128518/Instagram-The-nerds-billion-551-days-camera-app.html

Lin, W.-Y., Zhang, X., Song, H., & Omori, K. (2016). Health information seeking in the Web 2.0 age: Trust in social media, uncertainty reduction, and self-disclosure. *Computers in Human Behavior, 56*, 289–294. doi:10.1016/j.chb.2015.11.055

LinkedIn. (2016a). About LinkedIn. Retrieved from https://press.linkedin.com/about-linkedin

LinkedIn. (2016b, June). How LinkedIn can help you. Retrieved from https://www.linkedin.com/help/linkedin/answer/45/how-linkedin-can-help-you?lang=en

Logsdon, M. C., Bennett, G., Crutzen, R., Martin, L., Eckert, D., Robertson, A., … Flamini, L. (2014). Preferred health resources and use of social media to obtain health and depression information by adolescent mothers. *Journal of Child and Adolescent Psychiatric Nursing, 27*(4), 163–168. doi:10.1111/jcap.12083

Lunnay, B., Borlagdan, J., McNaughton, D., & Ward, P. (2015). Ethical use of social media to facilitate qualitative research. *Qualitative Health Research, 25*(1), 99–109. doi:10.1177/1049732314549031

Madrigal, A. C. (2012, February 9). Know your internet: What is Pinterest and why should i care? *The Atlantic.* Retrieved from https://www.theatlantic.com/technology/archive/2012/02/know-your-internet-what-is-pinterest-and-why-should-i-care/252835/

McGregor, F., Somner, J. E., Bourne, R. R., Munn-Giddings, C., Shah, P., & Cross, V. (2014). Social media use by patients with glaucoma: What can we learn? *Journal of the College of Optometrists, 34*(1), 46–52. doi:10.1111/opo.12093

Munro, C. L., & Savel, R. H. (2016). Narrowing the 17-year research to practice gap. *American Journal of Critical Care, 25*(3), 194–196. doi:10.4037/ajcc2016449

Musiat, P., Winsall, M., Orlowski, S., Antezana, G., Schrader, G., Battersby, M., & Bidargaddi, N. (2016). Paid and unpaid online recruitment for health interventions in young adults. *Journal of Adolescent Health, 59*(6), 662–667. doi:10.1016/j.jadohealth.2016.07.020

Obar, J. A., & Wildman, S. (2015). Social media definition and the governance challenge: An introduction to the special issue. *Telecommunications Policy, 39*(9), 745–750. doi:10.1016/j.telpol.2015.07.014

Obar, J. A., Zube, P., & Lampe, C. (2012). Advocacy 2.0: An analysis of how advocacy groups in the United States perceive and use social media as tools for facilitating civic engagement and collective action. *Journal of Information Policy, 2*(2012), 1–25. doi:10.5325/jinfopoli.2.2012.0001

Office for Human Research Protections. (2016). *Use of electronic informed consent: Questions and answers.* Washington, DC: U.S. Department of Health & Human Services. Retrieved from https://www.hhs.gov/ohrp/regulations-and-policy/guidance/use-electronic-informed-consent-questions-and-answers/index.html#tocq10

Paige, S. R., Stellefson, M., Chaney, B. H., & Alber, J. M. (2015). Pinterest as a resource for health information on chronic obstructive pulmonary disease (COPD): A social media content analysis. *American Journal of Health Education, 46*(4), 241–251. doi:10.1080/19325037.2015.1044586

Patel, R., Chang, T., Greysen, S. R., & Chopra, V. (2015). Social media use in chronic disease: A systematic review and novel taxonomy. *American Journal of Medicine, 128*(12), 1335–1350. doi:10.1016/j.amjmed.2015.06.015

Pew Research Center. (2017, January 12). Social media fact sheet. Retrieved from http://www.pewinternet.org/fact-sheet/social-media

Pinterest. (2018). All about Pinterest. Retrieved from https://help.pinterest.com/en/guide/all-about-pinterest

Puljak, L. (2016). Using social media for knowledge translation, promotion of evidence-based medicine and high-quality information on health. *Journal of Evidence-Based Medicine, 9*(1), 4–7. doi:10.1111/jebm.12175

Robillard, J. M., Cabral, E., Hennessey, C., Kwon, B. K., & Illes, J. (2015). Fueling hope: Stem cells in social media. *Stem Cell Reviews and Reports, 11*(4), 540–546. doi:10.1007/s12015-015-9591-y

Schootman, M., Nelson, E. J., Werner, K., Shacham, E., Elliott, M., Ratnapradipa, K., … McVay, A. (2016). Emerging technologies to measure neighborhood conditions in public health: Implications for interventions and next steps. *International Journal of Health Geographics, 15*(1), 20. doi:10.1186/s12942-016-0050-z

Statista. (2018). Most famous social network sites worldwide as of April 2018, ranked by number of active users (in millions). Retrieved from https://www.statista.com/statistics/272014/global-social-networks-ranked-by-number-of-users

Twitter. (2017a). New user FAQs. Retrieved from https://help.twitter.com/en/new-user-faq

Twitter. (2017b). Using hashtags on Twitter. Retrieved from https://support.twitter.com/articles/49309

Weaver, B., Lindsay, B., & Gitelman, B. (2012). Communication technology and social media: Opportunities and implications for healthcare systems. *Online Journal of Issues in Nursing, 17*(3), 3. doi:10.3912/OJIN.Vol17No03Man03

Westgate, E. C., & Holliday, J. (2016). Identity, influence, and intervention: The roles of social media in alcohol use. *Current Opinion in Psychology, 9*, 27–32. doi:10.1016/j.copsyc.2015.10.014

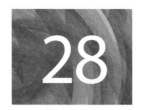

Speeding the Translation of Evidence-Based Interventions Into Real-World Practice Settings

Bernadette Mazurek Melnyk

> As long as we are persistent in our pursuit of our deepest destiny, we will continue to grow. We cannot choose the day or time when we will fully bloom. It happens in its own time. —*Denis Waitley*

At the outset of designing an intervention, investigators need to begin thinking about the translation of their intervention into real-world practice settings if findings from their research support positive intervention effects. Unfortunately, it typically takes several years to translate evidence-based interventions into clinical practice settings to improve care and outcomes. Therefore, this chapter reviews the common barriers that block the translation of evidence-based interventions into clinical practice and community settings as well as describes facilitators that enhance their uptake in the real world. Knowing these factors is important as new interventions are being designed. A case example of how a research-based intervention for parents of premature infants was adopted in neonatal intensive care units (NICUs) across the country and globe will be used to highlight important strategies for investigators whose dreams are to make a positive impact on outcomes in the real world with their interventions.

> Every day is a blessing and a chance to make a positive difference in the world. —*Jim Hamilton*

BARRIERS TO TRANSLATING RESEARCH-BASED INTERVENTIONS INTO REAL-WORLD SETTINGS

Although there is abundant evidence to support that the use of evidence-based interventions in clinical practice improves quality of care and patient outcomes as well as reduces healthcare costs and errors, **evidence-based practice** (EBP) is currently not the standard norm in numerous healthcare settings across the United States (McGinty & Anderson, 2008; Melnyk & Fineout-Overholt, 2015; Melnyk et al., 2016; Pravikoff, Pierce, & Tanner, 2005; PricewaterhouseCoopers' Health Research Institute, 2007). Although the goal set by the Institute of Medicine (IOM) is that 90% of healthcare decisions will be evidence based by 2020 (IOM, 2007), it has long been cited that it takes on an average of 17 years to translate research-based findings into clinical practice (Balas & Boren, 2000). Unfortunately, many evidence-based interventions never make it into real-world practice settings, even when high-quality intervention trials with excellent outcomes are achieved.

The translation of research-based interventions into clinical settings is a complex and challenging process because of multiple barriers that exist in both healthcare systems and individual clinicians. Barriers in healthcare systems include (a) lack of administrative/leadership/manager support, (b) cultures that do not support EBP, (c) lack of resources and tools necessary to implement EBP, (d) insufficient numbers of EBP mentors in healthcare systems to work with clinicians in implementing evidence-based interventions, (e) administrative leaders and managers who do not model EBP, and (f) inadequate insurance coverage (Beckett et al., 2011; Majid et al., 2011; Melnyk, 2007; Melnyk, Fineout-Overholt et al., 2004; Melnyk et al., 2016). Individual barriers within clinicians include (a) lack of adequate EBP knowledge and skills, (b) limited cognitive belief that EBP improves practice and patient outcomes, (c) perceived inadequate time for implementation, (d) inadequate authority to make practice changes, and (e) low self-efficacy (Atkins, Kupersmith, & Eisen, 2010; Klein et al., 2010; Melnyk, Fineout-Overholt et al., 2004). Research findings have shown that education of healthcare providers can increase self-efficacy but does not necessarily change practice behaviors (Klein et al., 2010). Therefore, it is currently unknown if increasing self-efficacy will improve the EBP behaviors of clinicians. Transferring efficacious interventions into real-world practice settings is a complicated process that requires dealing effectively with the multifaceted phases of program diffusion, including adoption, implementation, and sustainability as well as the culture and context within which the care is delivered (Melnyk, Fineout-Overholt, Giggleman, & Cruz, 2010).

FACTORS THAT FACILITATE THE ADOPTION OF RESEARCH-BASED INTERVENTIONS IN REAL-WORLD SETTINGS

There are multiple intervention characteristics that influence the degree to which clinicians adopt and sustain new evidence-based interventions, including the (a) strength and quality of the evidence, (b) complexity of the new intervention or its ease of administration, (c) adaptability of the intervention in clinical practice, (d) the significance of the intervention to the clinician's work (i.e., easy to use with existing task performance), and (e) relative advantage of the intervention to the user (McClellan, McGinnis, Nabel, & Olsen, 2007; McGinty & Anderson, 2008; Williams, 2004). If interventions are not adapted locally and tailored to real-world practice settings, they usually are a poor fit and resisted by the clinicians (McClellan et al., 2007).

Factors that facilitate the uptake of research-based interventions include (a) clinicians' beliefs that the research-based intervention has strong benefit, (b) resources and time to implement the intervention, (c) ease of administration, (d) reproducibility of the intervention, (e) skill-based training in the delivery of the intervention, and (f) the availability of mentors to assist in implementation (Cabana et al., 2006; Melnyk & Fineout-Overholt, 2015; Melnyk, Fineout-Overholt et al., 2010).

Dissemination of evidence or instruction in research-based interventions alone is not enough for the adoption or use of those interventions in the real world. One key facilitator of EBP, or the uptake of evidence-based interventions, is skill-based training of clinicians and access to tools that assist in implementation (Cabana et al., 2006; Lustig et al., 2001; Story et al., 2002). Moderate-to-intense skill-based training in the research-based intervention is necessary to stimulate behavioral change in clinicians to implement research-based interventions. Specifically, interactive skill-building sessions with clinicians and the use of mentors have been successful in facilitating implementation of research-based interventions in clinical practice settings (Iglehart, 2009; Melnyk, 2007; Schectman, Schroth, Verme, & Voss, 2003). Medical record systems that build in automatic reminders can also facilitate implementation of evidence-based interventions and guidelines (Atkins et al., 2010). However, if too many reminders are built into systems, clinicians could begin to ignore those messages.

The environment or practice setting also highly influences the ability of clinicians to implement evidence-based interventions (Melnyk, Fineout-Overholt et al., 2010; O'Connor, Creager, Mooney, Laizner, & Ritchie, 2006). Organizations with cultures that provide consistent support and resources for clinicians to implement evidence-based interventions are critical for the implementation and sustainability of EBP (Melnyk, Fineout-Overholt et al., 2010). Furthermore, EBP mentors (i.e., individuals with expertise in EBP as well as in individual behavioral change and organizational culture change) in clinical practice settings are also the key in increasing the translation of research-based findings into clinical practice (Melnyk, 2007; Melnyk, Fineout-Overholt, Giggleman & Choy, 2017). Finally, strategies for the implementation of research-based interventions "make the right thing the easy thing," as healthcare providers are overloaded (Atkins et al., 2010, p. 1911).

> Organizational and federal healthcare policies play an important role in enhancing the routine uptake of research-based interventions or evidence-based guidelines in clinical practice. For example, if it is written into healthcare policy that reimbursement will be provided only if certain evidence-based recommendations or guidelines are followed, clinicians will be more likely to adopt those practices. Similarly, if organizational policies and procedures include evidence-based interventions, clinicians are obligated to follow them. Therefore, investigators who develop research-based interventions should work with policy makers to formulate evidence-based recommendations for clinical practice that incorporate their findings.

THE COPE PROGRAM FOR PARENTS OF PREMATURE INFANTS: A CASE EXAMPLE

The Creating Opportunities for Parent Empowerment (COPE) program is an educational–behavioral skills-building intervention for parents of hospitalized/critically ill children and premature infants that began its development in the mid-1980s. Working as a nurse in the pediatric intensive care unit (PICU), I became troubled by the fact that we educated parents about the technology in the unit as well as their children's tubes and arterial/venous lines; however, very little of the teaching that we provided focused on the psychological needs and reactions of the children and parents to critical illness and painful distressing procedures. After a thorough search and synthesis of the literature on the needs and stressors of critically ill children and their parents, it was evident that the major stressors for parents that could be positively affected through an intervention are (a) uncertainty about their children's emotions and behaviors as they recovered from critical illness and (b) loss of parental role and not knowing how best to help their children cope during and following hospitalization. Therefore, based on the literature of the top stressors for parents of hospitalized/critically ill children, I developed a videotaped intervention entitled *Young Children's Reactions to Hospitalization* that prepared parents for (a) what to expect in their children's emotions and behaviors and (b) how they could best help their children adjust to hospitalization and their illness. Findings from my first small quasi-experimental pilot study with 40 mothers of young children experiencing an unplanned hospitalization indicated that mothers who received the videotaped intervention reported less state anxiety during their children's hospitalization than those who received the standard of care. Although small with multiple flaws, that pilot study launched a series of randomized controlled trials (RCT) funded by the National Institutes of Health (NIH)/National Institute of Nursing Research (NINR), testing my COPE program with parents of hospitalized/critically ill children and parents of low birth weight (LBW) premature infants.

The next study in my program of research was a 2 × 2 factorial experiment that tested the COPE Program with 108 mothers of unexpectedly hospitalized children. To that point in time, intervention studies focused on parents undergoing planned minor surgeries/procedures. As such, there was a huge gap in the literature regarding efficacious interventions for families whose children were experiencing unplanned hospitalizations. Findings from this study indicated that parents who received COPE, in comparison with those who received an attention-control program, reported less stress and anxiety as well as provided greater support to their children during hospitalization (Melnyk, 1994). In addition, COPE children had fewer negative behaviors than attention-control-group children following discharge. Along with studying the effects of COPE on child and parent outcomes, I studied the process through which COPE worked by empirically identifying maternal beliefs as the key mediator of the effects of the intervention on maternal state anxiety and participation in their children's care (Melnyk, 1995). Findings also supported that maternal anxiety and participation in their children's care mediated the effects of COPE on child outcomes. These findings filled a gap in the science of understanding the process through which a psychosocial intervention with parents of hospitalized children worked to positively impact their outcomes.

Because I was a pediatric critical care nurse earlier in my career, the next step in my research program was to adapt COPE for critically ill children and their parents. Following intensive pilot work refining the intervention for parents of children in the PICU, I received funding from NIH/NINR for a R01 grant to test the efficacy of COPE with 174 critically ill children and their mothers in a multisite RCT at two children's hospitals. In addition to short-term positive intervention effects, findings indicated that COPE mothers, in comparison with attention-control mothers, reported less adverse mental health outcomes up to a year following hospitalization (e.g., posttraumatic stress disorder), and their children had less negative behavioral mental health outcomes (e.g., fewer behavioral problems and less attention-deficit symptoms; Melnyk, Alpert-Gillis et al., 2004). This was the first intervention study with parents in the PICU that employed a manualized intervention and assessed the sustainability of the intervention following hospitalization. As part of this study, our team empirically supported and published a model to explain the process through which the intervention worked, which extended the science in the area (Melnyk, Crean, Feinstein, Fairbanks, & Alpert-Gillis, 2007).

Because COPE was efficacious for parents of critically ill children, the next step in my program of research was to adapt and test COPE with parents of LBW premature infants. With another R01 grant from NIH/NINR, I completed a multisite RCT testing the efficacy of COPE with 260 LBW premature infants and their mothers as well as their fathers. The original grant tested the short- and long-term efficacy of COPE, through the infants' 2 years of age. Because early findings were promising, I applied for and was awarded a supplemental grant to continue to study the impact of COPE through the children's third birthday. Findings from this study indicated that parents reported less stress, anxiety, depressive symptoms, and suicidal thoughts during and following hospitalization. Blind observers also rated COPE parents as more developmentally sensitive in their interactions with their infants than parents who received an attention-control program. In addition, COPE infants averaged a 4-day shorter length of stay in the NICU than the attention-control infants and 8 days shorter for preemies younger than 32 weeks, which resulted in a cost saving of nearly $5,000 per COPE infant (Melnyk et al., 2006; Melnyk & Feinstein, 2009).

Up until this point in my research career, not one hospital had adopted the COPE program for implementation with parents of hospitalized/critically ill children or premature infants. However, after my latest RCT was published that showed a decreased length of stay and substantial cost savings for infants whose parents received COPE, I began to receive calls from NICUs across the country who wanted to implement the COPE program. This is a classic example of how important it is to include the "so what" factor in research (i.e., measuring outcomes that the healthcare system deems important). Without measuring length of stay and conducting a cost analysis on my premature infant study, it is likely that no one would have begun to use the COPE intervention in real-world practice settings—a disheartening scenario for any researcher who dreams of making a positive difference in outcomes for the population he or she cares for deeply.

To determine the best strategy for rolling out the COPE program in NICUs, I then conducted an implementation study in which nurses were trained on providing COPE to parents of premature infants. From that study, our team learned that because of competing priorities in the care of preemies by NICU staff nurses, parents would often not receive the intervention. Therefore, we introduced a COPE mentor in the NICU (i.e., a clinician whose role was to track the implementation of COPE and work with the nurses to facilitate the delivery of the intervention to parents of preterm infants). After introduction of the COPE mentor, parents of preterms routinely received the intervention (Melnyk, Bullock et al., 2010). Without the mentor facilitating COPE, few parents would have received the intervention program. This is an excellent example of how important it is to consider factors that influence the translation of research-based interventions into real-world practice settings where local adaptations are often necessary to ensure consistent use.

COPE has been or is now being adopted for (a) burned children in the Shriner's Hospital system, (b) children with epilepsy at Boston Children's Hospital, (c) cardiac children at Barnes-Jewish Hospital, (d) cardiac infants at Children's Hospital of Philadelphia, and (e) children in rehabilitation at Emory Children's Hospital. In addition, COPE is being implemented in several other children's hospitals across the United States as well as in Switzerland, Sweden, Australia, the United Kingdom, China, the Netherlands, Canada, Iran, and Israel. Most recently, COPE has been translated into Spanish and German and is being tested with Spanish-speaking mothers. In addition, two insurers have integrated COPE for parents of preterms into their services.

To disseminate the COPE program into real-world practice settings, I, along with some of my wonderful colleagues who worked for years with me conducting research to evaluate the efficacy of COPE, launched a new corporation called COPE for HOPE, Inc. (www.copeforhope.com), which was a longtime dream for us. Because we did not have business degrees, we had to learn the process of how to start a corporation and seek legal assistance in forming it. Our team also did intense reading to learn about how to develop business and marketing plans and sought the consultation of others who had successfully launched corporations. Starting a corporation involves intense planning, time, and monetary investment. It also takes a common vision among the partners and a commitment of time as well as financial resources. The purpose of our corporation is to promote the health of children, teens, and families through stressful times. Through this corporation, training on COPE is provided to hospitals and COPE parent packs are distributed to those hospitals that choose to adopt it. The first hospital and NICU to adopt the COPE program was Nationwide Children's Hospital in Columbus, Ohio. After a year of implementation, this hospital realized an even shorter length of stay for the preemies whose parents received COPE than we found in our full-scale RCT—a researcher's dream. In addition, readmission rates for COPE preemies have decreased by over 10%.

On a side note, to encourage you, it took the maximum number of grant submissions allowed to obtain funding for all of my NIH grants. In fact, when I was in a tenure track position and writing my first NIH grant, I received a good first score. Our team responded to every comment/suggestion by the review panel and resubmitted the grant only to improve our score by two points. When we received the summary statement (i.e., the critique) from the grant review, my team was very discouraged. I shared that summary statement with five seasoned NIH-funded investigators for advice on next steps. Each of those senior researchers painted a bleak picture and discouraged me from resubmitting the application one last time. That is where the rubber met the road, and I had to decide on the next step in my research career. After much soul searching, I remained focused on my dream of improving outcomes for a highly vulnerable population and refused to give up. My thought was that if we did not swing the bat again, we stood no chance of funding and conducting this work. So, we worked tremendously hard on revising that grant and achieved a great fundable score on the final submission to NIH—exactly a month before my tenure materials were due to be submitted. There is no doubt that I would not have been tenured without that NIH grant, and there is also no doubt that the number of families now positively impacted by COPE would never have received the intervention. I share this story with you to give you hope, encourage you to follow your dreams, and persist in the face of adversity until those dreams become reality.

There are other excellent examples of research-based interventions that have been successfully adopted in real-world practice settings or influenced health policy after years of intensive work. After years of research and multiple trials, David Olds and Harriet Kitzman's research program on nurse home visitation influenced health policy to the extent that federal funding is now being provided to community agencies to implement nurse home-visitation interventions (Olds et al., 2010). In addition, Mary Naylor's research on transitioning older adults from hospital to home with advanced practice nurses is now being implemented in real-world practice settings and resulting in substantial savings for our healthcare system (Naylor, Aiken, Kurtzman, Olds, & Hirschman, 2011).

> Remember, with each rejection you receive, you are one step
> closer to getting funded and realizing your dream.
> —*Bernadette Mazurek Melnyk*

LESSONS LEARNED

There are many lessons to learn from my program of research. I wish someone had mentored me on the "so what" factor early in my career and encouraged me to incorporate cost and other key outcomes that the healthcare system deems important in my studies. If that were the case, it may not have taken 25 years to see my COPE program implemented in hospitals throughout the country and world to improve outcomes for vulnerable families. It was fortunate that from its inception, I intuitively knew to design the COPE program to be easily implemented in real-world practice settings because cumbersome or expensive interventions are less likely to be adopted. My "character-building experiences" from this long journey of translating my evidence-based COPE program for parents of preterm infants and critically ill children into practice prepared me well to design my next NIH/NINR-funded intervention study to include "so what" outcomes for high school teens (e.g., depression, academic performance) and to be easily adapted and taught by teachers in classroom settings. As a result of lessons learned, it took only a few years to translate my evidence-based COPE Healthy Lifestyle TEEN (Thinking, Emotions, Exercise, and Nutrition) Program, based on cognitive behavioral therapy, into real-world school settings and primary care practices. The National Cancer Institute now lists the COPE TEEN intervention program as an obesity control intervention for teens (see rtips.cancer.gov/rtips/programDetails.do?programId=22686590).

From the early seeds of an intervention idea, investigators need to think about the practicality and cost of the intervention that they are designing and create an intervention that is likely to be adopted by practicing clinicians and real-life communities if it is found to be efficacious. There are so many interventions that are cumbersome and costly, which reduces the probability that clinicians and communities will adopt them. However, there is always a fine line between designing a practical, easy to administer, reproducible intervention and one that is potent enough and possibly tailored to produce sustainable positive outcomes for a wide variety of individuals or communities. Finally, years ago, I wished that I had learned the strategy of cost-effective analysis along with how to create a sound business and marketing plan so that I would have been ready for a widespread dissemination initiative when hospitals started calling me to adopt COPE.

After 25 years of my research journey with the COPE intervention, the seeds from this program are blooming, and the intervention is being adopted in real-world practice settings to improve the outcomes and lives of high-risk children and families. It has been well worth the years of effort to see the realization of my dream—the uptake of the evidence-based COPE program to improve parent and child outcomes. So remember—your dreams of making a difference through your intervention work can come to fruition with belief, patience, and persistence through all of the "character builders" you are sure to encounter. Remember, success is going from one failure to the next with enthusiasm. So stay enthusiastic about your work, keep your dream bigger than your fears, and in the famous words of Winston Churchill, "Never, never, never, never, never, never, never quit!" until your dream comes to fruition.

Never, never, never, never, never, never, never
quit! —*Winston Churchill*

Key Points From This Chapter

- Right from the start of designing an intervention, it is critical to think about whether clinicians or communities will be able to easily adopt and implement it. Designing complex and costly interventions will decrease the probability of adoption in real-world settings.
- Make a strategic plan for how you will work to ensure that your intervention, if found to be efficacious through research, will be adopted and successfully implemented in real world-settings.
- Remember to include "so what" outcomes (i.e., those that the healthcare system deems important, e.g.: cost, adverse events) when studying the efficacy of your intervention.
- Persist through the "character builders" until your dream to make a difference in outcomes through your intervention work becomes a reality.

REFERENCES

Atkins, D., Kupersmith, J., & Eisen, S. (2010). The Veterans Affairs experience: Comparative effectiveness research in a large health system. *Health Affairs, 29*(10), 1906–1912. doi:10.1377/hlthaff.2010.0680

Balas, E. A., & Boren, S. A. (2000). Managing clinical knowledge for health care improvement. In J. Bemmel & A. T. McCray (Eds.), *Yearbook of medical informatics 2000: Patient-centered systems* (pp. 65–70). Stuttgart, Germany: Schattauer Verlagsgesellschaft.

Beckett, M., Quiter, E., Ryan, G., Berrebi, C., Taylor, S., Cho, M., … Kahn, K. (2011). Bridging the gap between basic science and clinical practice: The role of organizations in addressing clinician barriers. *Implementation Science, 6*, 35. doi:10.1186/1748-5908-6-35

Cabana, M. D., Slish, K. K., Evans, D., Mellins, R. B., Brown, R. W., Lin, X., … Clark, N. M. (2006). Impact of physician asthma care education on patient outcomes. *Pediatrics, 117*(6), 2149–2157. doi:10.1542/peds.2005-1055

Iglehart, J. K. (2009). Health insurers and medical-imaging policy: A work in progress. *New England Journal of Medicine, 360*(10), 1030–1037. doi:10.1056/NEJMhpr0808703

Institute of Medicine. (2007). *The learning healthcare system: Workshop summary*. Washington, DC: National Academies Press.

Klein, J. D., Sesselberg, T. S., Johnson, M. S., O'Connor, K. G., Cook, S., Coon, M., … Washington, R. (2010). Adoption of body mass index guidelines for screening and counseling in pediatric practice. *Pediatrics, 125*(2), 265–272. doi:10.1542/peds.2008-2985

Lustig, J. L., Ozer, E. M., Adams, S. H., Wibbelsman, C. J., Fuster, C. D., Bonar, R. W., & Irwin, C. E., Jr. (2001). Improving the delivery of adolescent clinical preventive services through skills-based training. *Pediatrics, 107*(5), 1100–1107. doi:10.1542/peds.107.5.1100

Majid, S., Foo, S., Luyt, B., Zhang, X., Theng, Y. L., Chang, Y. K., & Mokhtar, I. A. (2011). Adopting evidence-based practice in clinical decision making: Nurses' perceptions, knowledge, and barriers. *Journal of the Medical Library Association, 99*(3), 229–236. doi:10.3163/1536-5050.99.3.010

McClellan, M. B., McGinnis, M., Nabel, E. G., & Olsen, L. M. (2007). *Evidence-based medicine and the changing nature of health care*. Washington, DC: National Academies Press.

McGinty, J., & Anderson, G. (2008). Predictors of physician compliance with American Heart Association guidelines for acute myocardial infarction. *Critical Care Nursing Quarterly, 31*(2), 161–172. doi:10.1097/01.CNQ.0000314476.64377.12

Melnyk, B. M. (1994). Coping with unplanned childhood hospitalization: Effects of informational interventions on mothers and children. *Nursing Research, 43*(1), 50–55. doi:10.1097/00006199-199401000-00011

Melnyk, B. M. (1995). Coping with unplanned childhood hospitalization: The mediating functions of parental beliefs. *Journal of Pediatric Psychology, 20*(3), 299–312. doi:10.1093/jpepsy/20.3.299

Melnyk, B. M. (2007). The evidence-based practice mentor: A promising strategy for implementing and sustaining EBP in healthcare systems. *Worldviews on Evidence-Based Nursing, 4*(3), 123–125. doi:10.1111/j.1741-6787.2007.00094.x

Melnyk, B. M., Alpert-Gillis, L., Feinstein, N. F., Crean, H. F., Johnson, J., Fairbanks, E., … Corbo-Richert, B. (2004). Creating opportunities for parent empowerment: Program effects on the mental health/coping outcomes of critically ill young children and their mothers. *Pediatrics, 113*(6), e597–e607. doi:10.1542/peds.113.6.e597

Melnyk, B. M., Bullock, T., McGrath, J., Jacobson, D., Kelly, S., & Baba, L. (2010). Translating the evidence-based NICU COPE program for parents of premature infants into clinical practice: Impact on nurses' evidenced-based practice and lessons learned. *Journal of Perinatal & Neonatal Nursing, 24*(1), 74–80. doi:10.1097/JPN.0b013e3181ce314b

Melnyk, B. M., Crean, H. F., Feinstein, N. F., Fairbanks, E., & Alpert-Gillis, L. J. (2007). Testing the theoretical framework of the COPE program for mothers of critically ill children: An integrative model of young children's post-hospital adjustment behaviors. *Journal of Pediatric Psychology, 32*(4), 463–474. doi:10.1093/jpepsy/jsl033

Melnyk, B. M., & Feinstein, N. F. (2009). Reducing hospital expenditures with the COPE (Creating Opportunities for Parent Empowerment) program for parents and premature infants: An analysis of direct healthcare neonatal intensive care unit costs and savings. *Nursing Administration Quarterly, 33*(1), 32–37. doi:10.1097/01.NAQ.0000343346.47795.13

Melnyk, B. M., Feinstein, N. F., Alpert-Gillis, L., Fairbanks, E., Crean, H. F., Sinkin, R. A., … Gross, S. J. (2006). Reducing premature infants' length of stay and improving parents' mental health outcomes with the Creating Opportunities for Parent Empowerment (COPE) neonatal intensive care unit program: A randomized, controlled trial. *Pediatrics, 118*(5), e1414–e1427. doi:10.1542/peds.2005-2580

Melnyk, B. M., & Fineout-Overholt, E. (2015). *Evidence-based practice in nursing & healthcare: A guide to best practice* (3rd ed.). Philadelphia, PA: Wolters Kluwer.

Melnyk, B. M., Fineout-Overholt, E., Feinstein, N. F., Li, H., Small, L., Wilcox, L., & Kraus, R. (2004). Nurses' perceived knowledge, beliefs, skills, and needs regarding evidence-based practice: Implications for accelerating the paradigm shift. *Worldviews on Evidence-Based Nursing, 1*(3), 185–193. doi:10.1111/j.1524-475X.2004.04024.x

Melnyk, B. M., Fineout-Overholt, E., Giggleman, M., & Choy, K. (2017). A test of the ARCC Model improves implementation of evidence-based practice, healthcare culture, and patient outcomes. *Worldviews on Evidence-Based Nursing, 14*(1), 5–9. doi:10.1111/wvn.12188

Melnyk, B. M., Fineout-Overholt, E., Giggleman, M., & Cruz, R. (2010). Correlates among cognitive beliefs, EBP implementation, organizational culture, cohesion and job satisfaction in evidence-based practice mentors from a community hospital system. *Nursing Outlook, 58*(6), 301–308. doi:10.1016/j.outlook.2010.06.002

Melnyk, B. M., Gallagher-Ford, L., Thomas, B. K., Troseth, M., Wyngarden, K., & Szalacha, L. (2016). A study of chief nurse executives indicates low prioritization of evidence-based practice and shortcomings in hospital performance metrics across the United States. *Worldviews on Evidence-based Nursing, 13*(1), 6–14. doi:10.1111/wvn.12133

Naylor, M. D., Aiken, L. H., Kurtzman, E. T., Olds, D. M., & Hirschman, K. B. (2011). The care span: The importance of transitional care in achieving health reform. *Health Affairs, 30*(4), 746–754. doi:10.1377/hlthaff.2011.0041

O'Connor, P., Creager, J., Mooney, S., Laizner, A. M., & Ritchie, J. A. (2006). Taking aim at fall injury adverse events: Best practices and organizational change [Special issue]. *Healthcare Quarterly, 9*, 43–49. doi:10.12927hcq.2013.18458

Olds, D. L., Kitzman, H. J., Cole, R. E., Hanks, C. A., Arcoleo, K. J., Anson, E. A., … Stevenson, A. J. (2010). Enduring effects of prenatal and infancy home visiting by nurses on maternal life course and government spending: Follow-up of a randomized trial among children at age 12 years. *Archives of Pediatrics & Adolescent Medicine, 164*(5), 419–424. doi:10.1001/archpediatrics.2010.49

Pravikoff, D. S., Pierce, S. T., & Tanner, A. (2005). Evidence-based practice readiness study supported by academy nursing informatics expert panel. *Nursing Outlook, 53*(1), 49–50. doi:10.1016/j.outlook.2004.11.002

PricewaterhouseCoopers' Health Research Institute. (2007). What works: Healing the healthcare staffing shortage. Retrieved from https://council.brandeis.edu/pdfs/2007/PwC%20Shortage%20Report.pdf

Schectman, J. M., Schroth, W. S., Verme, D., & Voss, J. D. (2003). Randomized controlled trial of education and feedback for implementation of guidelines for acute low back pain. *Journal of General Internal Medicine, 18*(10), 773–780. https://doi.org/10.1046/j.1525-1497.2003.10205.x

Story, M. T., Neumark-Stzainer, D. R., Sherwood, N. E., Holt, K., Sofka, D., Trowbridge, F. L., & Barlow, S. E. (2002). Management of child and adolescent obesity: Attitudes, barriers, skills, and training needs among health care professionals. *Pediatrics, 110*(1), 210–214.

Williams, D. O. (2004). Treatment delayed is treatment denied. *Circulation, 109*(15), 1806–1808. doi:10.1161/01.CIR.0000126892.17646.83

Factors Influencing Successful Uptake of Evidence-Based Interventions in Clinical Practice

Sharon Tucker

> All is connected … no one thing can change by itself. —*Paul Hawken*
> *(Natural Capitalism, Yoga Journal, October 1994)*

As discussed throughout the preceding chapters, the ultimate goal of intervention research and evidence-based quality improvement (QI) projects is to improve healthcare practices that promote optimal health outcomes. An important expectation in improving outcomes is that the interventions discovered through research actually reach patients in routine clinical care and are adapted to meet patient needs. Unfortunately, research indicates that only about 55% to 57% of recommended evidence-based practices (EBPs) are implemented (McGlynn et al., 2003; Runciman et al., 2012) and about one-third of what the United States spends may be wasteful and even harmful (Lallemand, 2012). Such gaps noted in healthcare have been the impetus for the field of translation and implementation science. This final chapter specifically defines and elucidates this growing science associated with the study of methods to promote the use and integration of research evidence into policy and practice (Lobb & Colditz, 2013). A definition and characteristics of this area of research are provided, along with the complexities associated with implementing, and importantly adapting, interventions for unique patients and settings. The harnessing of implementation science to improve care is presented with examples of how implementation science has informed and improved intervention application. The chapter concludes with an overview of what is currently understood about promoting the uptake of evidence in real-world settings and where gaps exist for continued research.

IMPETUS FOR IMPLEMENTATION SCIENCE

Evidence-based interventions in nursing and the broader healthcare arena have grown exponentially in the past three decades. Many interventions have been identified as important for nursing and healthcare delivery such as bundles for preventing central-line associated bloodstream infections, ventilator-associated pneumonia, hospital-acquired pressure injuries, hospital falls with injuries, and catheter-associated urinary tract infections (Agency for Healthcare Research and Quality [AHRQ], 2014; Flodgren et al., 2013; Loveday et al., 2014). Many other interventions have been demonstrated to improve adult and pediatric pain management, patient self-management of chronic disease, physical activity levels in patients with cancer and other healthcare conditions, and coping with depression and anxiety, to name a few (AHRQ, 2017; Creating Opportunities for Parent Empowerment [COPE], 2017; Joanna Briggs Institute, 2017). Although such scientific advancements are improving care options and processes for patients and families, getting these interventions delivered routinely in real-world care settings has not kept up and has lagged behind (Metz & Bartley, 2012).

Redle (2013) stated "If the process of knowing what to do and actually doing it were perfect, there would be no need for knowledge translation or implementation research" (p. 1). A number of organizations beginning with the Institute of Medicine (IOM) have highlighted the gap between published reports of effective interventions and the care actually received by patients and vulnerable populations. In 2001, in their seminal report, *Crossing the Quality Chasm*, the IOM (2001) indicated it takes an average of 17 years for new knowledge that has been discovered through clinical trials to be applied in clinical practice, and even then, inconsistently. This gap has been repeatedly cited by many, and although some evidence, particularly nonpharmacological interventions, suggests a narrowing of the gap (Munro & Savel, 2016), there remains much concern about the lack of progress in identifying strategies to narrow the gap (Every-Palmer & Howick, 2014; Klein, Woods, Klein, & Perry, 2016).

Clinicians can play a major role in narrowing the gap by adopting new evidence into their routine practices. However, individual professionals usually work in complex systems and cannot simply decide to change their practices and decision making to be aligned with an innovation (Scott et al., 2012). Procedures exist in organizations to ensure practice changes are safe as well as for practical reasons such as electronic health records (EHRs) and the implications for documenting and communicating interventions. Clearly, there needs to be a balance between moving research into practice more quickly while not exposing patients to unnecessary harm (Munro & Savel, 2016), but how to do this needs a closer partnership between academics and clinicians (Rycroft-Malone, 2014), and more dedicated research (Redle, 2013).

DEFINING IMPLEMENTATION SCIENCE

A number of specific organizations (such as the AHRQ and the Patient-Centered Outcomes Research Institute) have grown out of the need for narrowing the research-to-practice gap. These groups have advocated for investigations dedicated to understanding and facilitating the cycle of scientific discovery to widespread adoption of healthcare innovations. Key stakeholders for these investigations are many and include recipients of healthcare, providers of healthcare, funders of healthcare, and those who set policy for healthcare. Investigators and clinicians are beginning to work together to promote EBP by discovering what factors and characteristics facilitate uptake of evidence by patients, clinicians, and organizations. This movement has created the implementation science field that continues to expand and grow. As the field has grown, concepts have been clarified and differentiated. Translation science has been forwarded by the National Institutes of Health (NIH), although implementation science has been supported by the AHRQ, the latter focusing more on human behavior and organizational issues such as limited resources, infrastructure challenges, and the basic messiness of real-world clinical settings with moving targets that make measurement difficult (Woolf, 2008).

Expanding a bit more on the history of translation science, in 2006, in recognition of the gap in translating research evidence into practice, the NIH made translational research a priority and launched the Clinical and Translational Science Award (CTSA) Program. This program converted existing specific NIH mechanisms, including the General Clinical Research Units and training programs (e.g., pre- and postdoc programs), to components of the CTSA Program. They describe the program as "...designed to develop innovative solutions that will improve the efficiency, quality and impact of the process for turning observations in the laboratory, clinic and community into interventions that improve the health of individuals and the public" (ncats.nih.gov/ctsa). To be funded as a CTSA Center, institutions are required to submit competitive applications and once funded, they are on continuing competitive renewal cycles with no guarantee of continued funding. Applications must demonstrate a number of outcomes in their programs including evidence of reaching patients with research findings and innovations, and involving families and communities in the implementation of clinical trials.

With the launch of translational science programs and funding, definitions have been forwarded that span a clinical research continuum with identified translational blocks of biomedical research, to human studies, to clinical science and knowledge, and ultimately to routine clinical practice. These blocks align with two major obstacles: (a) the transfer of new knowledge of disease mechanisms discovered in the laboratory into new clinical tools such as diagnostics, therapeutics, and prevention with first testing in humans (T1) and (b) the translation of knowledge from clinical studies into everyday health clinical decision making and practices (T2; Sung et al., 2003). For each of these major obstacles, research is needed; however, the goals, settings, study designs, and study teams differ (Woolf, 2008). For nursing science and practice, T2 studies are the primary focus. The settings and key stakeholders for T2 are hospitals, outpatient settings, practitioners, organizations, and patients/families. Initially, the T2 focus was endorsed by the AHRQ and given the title Translating Research Into Practice (TRIP). However, the T2 community has been inconsistent in endorsing this phrase as adequate and instead alternatives have emerged such as dissemination science, health services research, knowledge translation, implementation and even QI research (Woolf, 2008). Moreover, Westfall, Mold, and Fagnan (2007), introduced another T level (T3) and coined this level "practice-based research."

The term "implementation science" has been adopted by nursing to a large extent. Implementation science has been defined as "the methods to promote the systematic uptake of clinical research findings and other EBPs into routine practice and hence improve the quality and effectiveness of healthcare" (Eccles & Mittman, 2006).

IMPLEMENTATION SCIENCE: WHAT IS CURRENTLY KNOWN

EBP Uptake Facilitators

Multiple studies have been conducted on factors that facilitate uptake of healthcare evidence with consistent findings regarding important factors that organizations and providers can ensure are available to expedite the uptake of EBP. The most effective strategies include education that is interactive and continuous and include discussion of evidence, local consensus, feedback on performance (by peers), use of reminder and computerized decision support, multidisciplinary collaboration, mass media campaigns, educational outreach visits, and combined interventions. Table 29.1 includes a reprinted table published by Grol and Grimshaw (2003) that includes a summary of implementation strategies, the number of studies that examined the strategy, and conclusions about the strategy effectiveness in promoting uptake of EBP.

Scott et al. (2012) summarized eight general factors that facilitate EBP uptake:

- Adequate preparation for a practice change
- Human resource capacity with the appropriate expertise/skills to make the change
- Receptiveness to the practice change
- Type of tools for implementing the practice
- Overall human and fiscal resources for the implementation
- Support from organizational leaders to make the change and stick with the support before moving resources to a new initiative
- Support to sustain the practice once implemented
- Inclusion of several implementation strategies or features such as action planning, use of tools, communication, collaboration, teamwork, champions, monitoring, auditing with feedback, incentives, flexibility, standardizing, and adapting to populations and local context.

They also emphasized that use of a single factor or strategy to promote uptake is rarely sufficient to change behavior or practices and combining factors is highly recommended (Scott et al., 2012).

A common limitation of many EBP implementation initiatives is the heavy or sole reliance on education to make the practice change (Grol & Grimshaw, 2003; Novak & McIntyre, 2010; Scott et al., 2012). Novak and McIntyre (2010) in reviewing literature on the effects of continuing education (CE) for social workers stated, "In summary, CE appears to change what professionals know, but not what they do" (p. 387). Although education is needed for most providers, patients, and organizations, reliance on practice/behavioral change from education alone is highly unlikely to result in successful change (Scott et al., 2012).

Implementation Models and Phases

Implementation models have been presented that include phased approaches with multiple implementation strategies. For example, Braithwaite, Marks, and Taylor (2014) presented a phased approach that included preparing for change, ensuring the capacity for implementation, choosing the types of implementation, leveraging resources, and sustaining the change. Cullen and Adams (2012) similarly presented a four-phased approach to implementation along with recommended evidence-based implementation strategies categorized by system/organizational and provider/leader/key stakeholder perspectives for each phase. Their phases included creating awareness and interest, building knowledge and commitment, promoting action and adoption, and pursuing integration and sustained use. Within each phase are a number of suggested implementation strategies that can facilitate the goal of each phase related to a particular evidence-based intervention. For example, consider early mobility in critical care patients. The evidence strongly encourages mobility as important for healing and preventing further complications following any surgery or trauma. Using the Cullen and Adams framework, in phase one, "creating awareness and interest," strategies suggested for engaging clinicians and other key stakeholders could be highlighting the advantages or benefits of early mobility and highlighting the urgency along a number of dimensions for the patient (healing) and the unit (releasing ICU beds). From the organizational perspective, sharing announcements with key senior leaders is essential. Moving to phase two, "build knowledge and commitment," change agents could be created on each unit to provide education and local adoption (engaging clinician) about early mobility and strategies for implementing along with benchmarking and creating teamwork (organization

TABLE 29.1 Evidence for Implementation Strategies

STRATEGY	NUMBER OF REVIEWS[a]	NUMBER OF STUDIES	CONCLUSIONS
Educational materials	9	3–37	Mixed effects
Conferences, courses	4	3–17	Mixed effects
Interactive small group meetings	4	2–6	Mostly effective, but limited numbers of studies
Educational outreach visits	8	2–8	Especially effective for prescribing/prevention
Use of opinion leaders	3	3–6	Mixed effects
Education with different educational strategies	8	5–63	Mixed effects, dependent on combination of strategies
Feedback on performance	16	3–37	Mixed effects, most effective for test ordering
Reminders	14	4–68	Mostly effective, particularly for prevention
Computerized decision support	5	11–98	Mostly effective for drug dosing and prevention
Introduction of computers in practice	2	19–30	Mostly effective
Substitution of tasks	6	2–14	Pharmacist: effect on prescribing; nurse: mixed effects
Multiprofessional collaboration	5	2–22	Effective for a range of different chronic conditions
Mass media campaigns	1	22	Mostly effective
Total quality management/ continuous quality improvement	1	55	Limited effects, mostly single-site noncontrolled studies
Financial interventions	6	3–89	Fund holding and budgets effective, mainly on prescribing
Patient-mediated interventions	8	2–14	Mixed effects; reminding by patients is effective in prevention
Combined interventions	16	2–39	Most reviews: more effective than single interventions; not confirmed in recent reviews

[a]Number of reviews that included studies addressing the interventions. (Reprinted with permission).

and system level). In the third phase, "promote action and adoption," competencies could be created and assessed for nursing staff, reference or pocket guides could be created, and reminders on the unit could be placed (engaging clinicians) while auditing (system) key mobility indicators that could promote accountability. The final phase of "pursue integration and sustained use" may include celebrating the practice change, auditing patient records to ensure early mobility is occurring, and/or providing real-time feedback when there is a slip in the practice change.

In their study with social workers, Novak and McIntyre (2010) examined individual and workplace barriers that affect the uptake of EBP and evaluated the effects of a 1-day EBP workshop with workplace support on EBP knowledge and behavior among allied health professionals. As part of their overall EBP strategy, in addition to the 1-day workshop, they included a number of implementation strategies:

- Added to the strategic plan the outcome that all services were to be underpinned by best-available evidence
- Engaged managers and the senior leaders to embrace a culture of EBP implementation
- Provided computer and Internet resources to professionals
- Coached senior leaders to ensure they modeled EBP competently
- Provided frontline clinical staff mentoring.

Their findings suggested that the approach may lead to improvements in EBP knowledge and indirect implementation behavior as observed in health professionals' increased use of evidence to inform their peer-reviewed conference presentations and the number of critically appraised topics produced and loaded on the Intranet.

A very recent report demonstrated promise for accelerating uptake of evidence by adapting the Institute of Healthcare Improvement (IHI) QI campaign approach. Schneider et al. (2017) used the approach as an intervention to tackle surgical site infections (SSIs) prevention after joint replacement. This team conducted a cluster randomized trial including 10 states and 188 hospitals and evaluated adherence to three components of a bundle for SSI prevention. Compared with the control hospitals, they found in the intervention (campaign) states statistically significant improvements in adherence to the three EBP components. The researchers highlighted that campaigns can orchestrate multifaceted communication strategies that leverage professional and informal social networks within and across organizations; and they seem best for spreading relatively well-defined, reasonable clinical practices that can be easily messaged and implemented.

Patient Engagement, Values, and Preferences

Patient engagement has been lifted in the past 10 years as an essential component of EBP uptake. The National Academy of Medicine (Frampton et al., 2017) just released a framework for building and sustaining Patient and Family Engaged Care (PFEC). This framework essentially promotes the active engagement of patients and families/care partners in the planning, delivery, and evolving care for patients to ensure that patient values, preferences, and goals are integrated into the care. In a recent editorial about the framework, Allen, Sparling, and Montori (2017) praised Frampton and colleagues for correctly identifying that PFEC programs ultimately need to lead to better care. Allen et al. identified that through true engagement, not as a cost containment tactic, but rather as an "obligation to attend to a human situation of patients and family experiencing illness or the threat of illness," healthcare providers and organizations can "co-create careful and kind care for everyone" (p. 2).

A significant body of literature demonstrates that patients experience better health-care and health outcomes when they are actively involved in the decision making about their healthcare (James, 2013). Nowadays, many regulatory and quality organizations expect patient engagement as a quality metric of healthcare (Sherman & Hilton, 2014), and healthcare organizations are employing strategies to better engage patients (James, 2013). Nevertheless, much work is yet needed in the patient engagement process. For example, Jun et al. (2015) highlighted the lack of patient engagement even in the study of important intervention topics. Using a case study approach, they examined the extent to which recently completed and ongoing clinical research was consistent with research topics prioritized by patients, caregivers, and clinicians for patients on or nearing dialysis. They found that less than one quarter (21%) of published studies addressed topics consistent with the top 10 research priorities identified by patients, and four of the 10 (strategies to improve itching, increased access to kidney transplantation, assessing the psychosocial impact of kidney failure, and determining effects of dietary restrictions in kidney failure) received basically no attention.

Kunneman, Montori, Castaneda-Guarderas, and Hess (2016) discussed the need for shared decision making between patients and clinicians, emphasizing that in this model, clinicians and patients work together to understand the patient's situation and determine how to best address it. They also identified that for true shared decision making, key are clarifying the patient's situation and where the action is needed, understanding and exploring choices or options with the patient, discussing pros and cons of the available options, and being mindful of what the patient values that influence the best choice (Kunneman et al., 2016).

Looking more specifically at what patient engagement factors promote uptake of care that is most evidence supported includes two areas of focus: the active involvement of patients in choosing the intervention that fits best with their values and beliefs and resources and the behavioral change and patient activation processes (James, 2013). Patient activation involves characteristics of patient management of their own healthcare. Characteristics include knowledge, attitudes, skills, ability, willingness, and resources. Much research has been done in the areas of assisting patients with activation and behavioral change for illness and healthcare management (Bolen et al., 2014; Kinney, Lemon, Person, Pagoto, & Saczynski, 2015).

One highly promising patient engagement approach that has grown substantially in the patient engagement field is motivational interviewing (MI). MI grew out of the problem-drinking literature as an alternative counseling approach to the confrontation method of helping patients examine and change their drinking patterns (Miller & Rollnick, 2008). Building on Carl Rogers's work, MI was identified as a humanistic approach to assist people to think about their behaviors in new ways and move them toward resolving ambivalence about their unhealthy behaviors and choose to make healthier (evidence-based) choices that make sense to them and are consistent with their values, beliefs, and ability.

The role of the counselor is to serve as a helper in the change process and to express acceptance of the patient. The counselor is directive, with a goal of eliciting self-motivational statements that reflect the patient's intrinsic motivations and values. There are five basic principles in the MI to help facilitate change: expressing empathy through reflective listening, developing discrepancies between the patient's current behaviors and his or her goals and values, avoiding argument and confrontation, rolling with resistance rather than opposing it, and supporting self-efficacy and optimism (Miller & Rollnick, 2008). The MI approach has been adapted for many health issues beyond substance use/abuse problems. A number of systematic reviews have been published about MI effectiveness for various health behaviors with overall support for even brief interventions across healthcare settings (Lee, Choi, Yum, Yu, & Chair, 2016; Lundahl et al., 2013; Rubak, Sandbaek, Lauritzen, & Christensen, 2005).

Clinician Expertise and Perspective

Clinician expertise, attitudes, and perspectives also significantly influence the uptake of EBP. Foy et al. (2002) aimed to identify which attributes of clinical practice recommendations influenced changes in practice following audit and feedback provided to clinicians. Adherence to the practice recommendation was their primary outcome and they found that clinician values and not requiring changes to fixed routines were independently associated with greater compliance at baseline and follow-up. They also found that recommendations that were incompatible with clinician values were independently associated with greater change in practice following audit and feedback, suggesting that the auditing process can facilitate change.

Katz et al. (2016) examined perceptions of inpatient nurses with regard to evidence-based tobacco treatment. They surveyed 164 Veterans Administration (VA) nurses and conducted semistructured interviews with a purposeful sample of 33 nurses with different attitudes toward cessation counseling. Findings included the following barrier themes: a perceived lack of skills, skepticism about the effectiveness of cessation guidelines in hospitalized veterans, behavioral and organizational barriers to guideline adherence, resistance from patients, insufficient time and resources, smoking allowed on the VA campus, and lack of coordination with primary care. The findings highlighted the issues among clinicians in implementing evidence-based smoking cessation, and the authors encouraged hospitals to train nurses in behavioral change techniques, integrate tobacco cessation into nurses' workflow, develop referral mechanisms for after discharge, and adopt hospital policies to promote patient abstinence, such as not permitting smoking on the hospital grounds.

Another example of an evidence-based intervention adherence challenge for hospitals is clinician hand hygiene (HH) practices. HH is recognized as an important strategy for preventing hospital-acquired infections (HAIs) and is estimated to prevent 15% to 30% of HAIs (Lautenbach, 2001). Yet, consistent studies outline HH adherence rates as being below desired rates and without intervention likely to be about 50% (Larson, 1988; Larson, 1995; Randle, Arthur, Vaughan, Wharrad, & Windle, 2014; Teare, Cookson, & French, 1999). A systematic review of HH adherence conducted by Huis et al. (2012) mirrored previous implementation studies and identified that focusing on one single target for behavioral change is unlikely to be successful. The median effect size of strategies to increase HH compliance increased from 17.6% (relative difference) when addressing only one determinant to 49.5% for the studies that addressed five determinants. They concluded that more creative strategies are needed in the application of alternative improvement activities, emphasizing that the focus only on knowledge, awareness, action control, or facilitation is insufficient and strategies need to also address determinants such as social influence, attitude, self-efficacy, or intention. Similarly, Luangasanatip et al. (2015) conducted a systematic review to evaluate the relative efficacy of the World Health Organization campaign (WHO-5) and other interventions to promote HH among hospital healthcare workers. Their review allowed for different methods, and 41 studies met inclusion criteria. Findings indicated improvements in HH compliance rates from WHO-5 occurred especially when additional interventions such as goal setting, rewarding incentives, and holding clinicians accountable were included.

There are numerous other examples of how adherence by nurses to practice changes influences EBP uptake and sustainability. For example, sustaining fall prevention among hospitalized patients is consistently cited as a challenge and a problem that can be very costly for patients, family members, healthcare teams, and organizations (Wong et al., 2011). Hempel et al. (2013) completed a systematic review to document the implementation, components, comparators, adherence, and effectiveness of published fall prevention approaches in U.S. acute care hospitals. Of 59 studies that met inclusion criteria, only about one-third documented their comprehensive implementation strategies, 49% reported primarily education as their implementation strategy, and 17% reported no implementation documentation. A vast majority (81%) included multiple components in their programs, 54% did not report on comparison group measures, and about 40% did not report fidelity or adherence data. As summarized by Healey (2011), the key challenge in fall prevention is consistently applying the available evidence in practice. The assessment process itself does not often translate into application of interventions, and this includes even the basics such as keeping call lights in patient reach and promptly responding to them (Healey, 2011).

There are also clinician deviations from the EBP based on their own beliefs. Returning to fall prevention, I led a study with colleagues on implementing evidence-based structured nursing rounds as a fall reduction strategy (Meade, Bursell, & Ketelsen, 2006) in an orthopedic unit of a large Midwestern academic medical center (AMC; Tucker, Bieber, Attlesey-Pries, Olson, & Dierkhising, 2012). We found that fall rates declined during the implementation of the 6-month structured nursing rounds; however, by the end of the first year, postintervention rates drifted back toward baseline. Nursing staff expressed in focus groups that the structured rounds felt like an imposition and unnecessary mandate and many resisted documenting according to the study protocol. They stressed the need for a balance between standardizing the intervention and providing individualized patient care. Building on these findings, I led a study at another AMC that aimed to understand factors that influence sustainable uptake of evidence-based intervention related to fall prevention, after observing fall rates moving up over time following a 5-year period of low fall rates from a robust fall prevention program (Farrington, Tucker, & Cullen, 2014). In this study, we collected data from multiple sources about perspectives of fall prevention strategies including from patients, staff, and medical records of patients who experienced a fall while hospitalized on one of the study units over a 4-year period. Key findings indicated that patients do not necessarily see themselves at risk even when they have had a previous fall, interdisciplinary ownership and communication for fall prevention was lacking, and reinfusion of education about effective strategies including leaving patients unobserved while toileting was needed.

Grol and Grimshaw (2003) studied strategies for improving adherence to best evidence and clinical guidelines. They found that for clinical guideline adherence, better compliance occurs with (a) select health problems (acute better than chronic), (b) stronger quality evidence for the recommendation, (c) compatibility of the evidence with existing values, (d) less complexity to the decision-making process, and (e) fewer new skills and organizational change expectations needed to implement the practice guideline. Klein et al. (2016) more recently framed the importance of similar issues, which they described as "cognitive challenges" in EBP implementation. These challenges included managing the "wicked problems" of today's hospitalized patients; giving providers adequate time to gain confidence in the evidence and its application; managing the discrepancies between provider expertise and best evidence recommendations; applying simple solutions to complex and messy clinical situations; the reality of evolving clinical problems and need for changing treatment plans when they are not working; and considering remedies that lack evidence but clinicians believe in. They encouraged use of cognitive engineering science and principles to strengthen best practices. These include:

1. Develop and sustain expertise of clinicians
2. Support adaptations to meet local needs
3. Support combining evidence with clinical experience
4. Balance generic evidence with clinician experience and evidence
5. Represent data for clinicians to be able to use
6. Appraise the evidence for adaptability for populations
7. Share evidence using creative information exchange mechanisms
8. Support collaborative decision making among healthcare teams including the patient

FUTURE DIRECTIONS

There are reasons to be positive about the uptake of EBP with examples of where it has occurred relatively expeditiously. Munro and Savel (2016) recently discussed examples where the research to practice gap is narrowing. For example, they point out that early mobility of critically ill patients has become a major initiative with mobility protocols implemented widely in many intensive/critical care units across the country, despite that early mobility has been the subject of research for less than a decade. Additional examples include oral care and support of family involvement in the intensive care unit (ICU). These authors recommend conducting larger, multisite studies rather than small single-site studies to continue to narrow the gap; promoting new experimental designs such as adaptive trials, stepped wedge, or comparative effectiveness trials; and presenting research findings in formats that include actionable information for clinicians. Ultimately, the goal is "a delicate balance of incorporating new findings quickly enough to maximally benefit patients, but not so quickly that we expose patients to unnecessary harm" (p. 196).

Advancing EBP uptake will require consideration of the implementation strategies discussed in this chapter. In addition, adapting concepts and processes from the QI framework has merit. The QI field has paralleled implementation science in terms of goals to improve healthcare uptake of evidence and patient outcomes by enhancing overall systems and processes. Adapted from other industries such as the auto industry, QI methods are designed to ultimately improve healthcare practice and outcomes, and efficiencies and costs. Dixon-Woods, McNicol, and Martin (2012) from the United Kingdom wrote about the gaps that remain in quality and safety despite the decades of continuous improvement efforts in healthcare. They conducted a review of findings of several reports created in the United Kingdom about the effectiveness of improvement efforts and focused on 10 challenges to implementation with recommended solutions (Exhibit 29.1). These quality methods and tools are critical to integration and sustainability of EBP changes.

Merging concepts from implementation science and QI is a reasonable approach to narrow the research to practice gap and improve the uptake of evidence into practice. As implied in the definitions of EBP, the scientific evidence is insufficient to change practice. The scientific evidence needs to be adapted and integrated within a local context, tailored to patient situation, values and preferences, and blended with the clinical expertise of those providing care. In addition, the organizational resources, data information systems, healthcare models, and leadership support are powerful factors that will influence the uptake, integration, and sustainability of EBP. A final discussion for this chapter encourages merging concepts and shifting EBP from a "project" focus to embrace integration of EBP into daily thinking and practicing using the full components of EBP along with QI methods and tools to guide improving patient care and outcomes while containing costs.

Taylor, Priefer, and Alt-White (2016) presented an expanded view of EBP to move beyond interpreting EBP as process-driven projects to a "way of practicing," where the ownership of EBP is assumed and embraced by nurses. Their work emerges after several years of efforts to create an EBP culture and observing consistent themes that (a) EBP was observed by some staff as projects completed by select nurses and (b) a number of projects completed reflected leadership commitment and support of EBP. They asked the question as to why EBP in their institutions and in the literature was still being viewed as a project rather than a process that was used daily and that integrated scientific evidence, patient preferences and values, and clinician expertise. Moreover, how to merge these concepts is essentially not well defined in the literature.

Taylor and colleagues differentiated the word "practice," highlighting that it can narrowly refer to repeated actions or it can more broadly reflect the exercise of one's discipline. They proposed that viewing EBP as a way of practicing rather than an action with a beginning

EXHIBIT 29.1 How to Address 10 Challenges in Improvement

DESIGN AND PLANNING OF IMPROVEMENT INTERVENTIONS

Challenge 1: Convincing people that there is a problem

Use hard data and secure emotional engagement by using patient stories and voices.

Challenge 2: If you do it, will it work? Convincing people of the solution

Come prepared with clear facts and figures; have convincing measures of impact; and be able to demonstrate the advantages of your solution.

Challenge 3: Data collection and monitoring systems

This always takes much more time and energy than anyone anticipates. It is worth investing heavily in data from the outset. Assess local systems, train people, and have quality assurance.

Challenge 4: "Projectness" and ambitions

Over-ambitious goals and too much talk of "transformation" can alienate staff if they feel the change is impossible. Instead match goals and ambitions to what is realistically achievable and focus on bringing everyone along with you. Avoid giving the impression that the improvement activity is unlikely to survive the time span of the project.

ORGANIZATIONAL AND INSTITUTIONAL CONTEXTS, PROFESSIONS, AND LEADERSHIP

Challenge 5: Organizational context, culture, and capacities

Staff may not understand the full demands of improvement when they sign up, and team instability can be very disruptive. Explain requirements to people and then provide ongoing support. Make sure improvement goals are aligned with the wider goals of the organization, so people do not feel pulled in too many directions.

Challenge 6: Tribalism and lack of staff engagement

Overcoming a perceived lack of ownership and professional or disciplinary boundaries can be very difficult. Clarify who owns the problem and solution, agree on roles and responsibilities at the outset, work to common goals, and use shared language.

Challenge 7: Leadership

Getting leadership for quality improvement right requires a delicate combination of setting out a vision and sensitivity to the views of others. "Quieter" leadership, oriented toward inclusion, explanation, and gentle persuasion, may be more effective.

Challenge 8: Incentivizing participation and "hard edges"

Relying on the intrinsic motivations of staff for quality improvement can take you a long way, especially if "carrots" in the form of incentives are provided—but they may not always be enough. It is important to have "harder edges"—sticks—to encourage change, but these must be used judiciously.

BEYOND THE INTERVENTION: SUSTAINABILITY, SPREAD, AND UNINTENDED CONSEQUENCES

Challenge 9: Securing sustainability

Sustainability can be vulnerable when efforts are seen as "projects" or when they rely on particular individuals.

Challenge 10: Side effects of change

It is not uncommon to successfully target one issue while also causing new problems elsewhere. This can cause people to lose faith in the project. Be vigilant about detecting unwanted consequences and be willing to learn and adapt.

Source: Dixon-Woods, M., McNicol, S., & Martin, G. (2012). Ten challenges in improving quality in healthcare: Lessons from the Health Foundations' programme evaluations and relevant literature. *British Medical Journal Quality & Safety, 21,* 876–884. doi: 10.1136/bmjqs-2011-000760. Reprinted with permission from BMJ Publishing Group Ltd.

and end (such as an EBP project) allows thinking to expand beyond projects and process to a more fluid and dynamic practice that successfully considers and integrates evidence, patient preferences, and clinician expertise. This then moves away from EBP being isolated to select projects led by select people and proposes an ownership for all within the discipline and as part of their daily work with patients. And, in turn, embracing EBP in daily practice can help illuminate how to actually adapt evidence to patient needs, values and preferences, and clinician perspectives. For example, by talking with patients and truly engaging with what matters to them, it is possible to learn why they are not achieving recommended daily physical activity levels. Other responsibilities, pain, or fear may be limiting the patient and thus a caring conversation (perhaps using evidence-based MI) with the patient may help identify alterative solutions that will work for the patient to meet physical activity goals. The clinician may also better appreciate the situation and help problem solve through his or her knowledge of community resources or past experiences with other patients that have been successful. Much more work in this area is needed to build cultures and systems that consider the evidence with each patient encounter. Toolkits of implementation strategies along with effective use of information systems can further augment the uptake of EBP by patients and clinicians, as well as organizations.

Information systems with decision support have been recognized as a system strategy for aiding clinicians in the uptake of EBP. Bates et al. (2003) identified that with the electronic health record (EHR) as the platform, clinical decision makers can be provided with tools making it possible to improve clinical performance, narrow the gap between knowledge and practice, and improve safety. In their study at a 720-bed tertiary care hospital, they evaluated their EHR and its effects on improvement on care. Through their project, they presented 10 lessons important for effective clinical decision support:

- Users value speed as a top priority
- Applications must anticipate clinician needs and bring information to clinicians just in time
- Alerts, guidelines, algorithms, and so fortht must integrate into clinician practice and workflow
- Changes, even minor ones, can have a major impact on provider workflow and actions
- Providers are creatures of habit and will resist change including stopping a routine practice even when not useful
- Computer support can be powerful in getting providers to change directions
- Users want simplicity and will resist using any complex guidelines
- Users want to access information when they need it
- It is important to monitor decision support tools, obtain feedback from users, and modify accordingly
- It is essential to monitor, maintain, and upgrade knowledge-based systems routinely

In examining effects of EHRs and specifically of computerized decision support systems (CDSS), Moja et al. (2014) systematically reviewed 28 randomized controlled trials assessing the effectiveness of CDSS featuring rule- or algorithm-based software integrated with EHR and evidence-based knowledge. Their findings indicated that across clinical settings, new generation CDSS integrated with EHRs did not affect mortality and might moderately improve morbidity outcomes. They acknowledged the method limitations including underpowered studies that were not long enough to observe or exclude an effect on mortality and overall studies were limited by diverse morbidity outcomes. They also pointed out that their review differed from many others that have favored effects of CDSS and postulated this might be because of the strict methodological parameters they used. They recommended that further research is needed and that CDSS not be currently observed as a confident approach to improving morbidity and mortality.

From a nursing perspective, O'Brien, Weaver, Settergren, Hook, and Ivory (2015) identified how EHRs have increased the burden of documentation for nursing while providing limited support to identify needs of patients and deliver evidence-based care. They encouraged nurse leaders and informatics partners to be engaged at all levels to ensure redesign is interdisciplinary and integrates best evidence into seamless workflows that do not further burden staff but instead capture coded nursing data and provide decision support that improves quality and patient safety as well as optimal outcomes.

SUMMARY

This chapter reviews the growing field of implementation science, why it emerged, what it is, what is known about factors that facilitate and impede the implementation and uptake of EBP, and directions for future research. As reflected in the chapter, there is neither a single obstruction nor resistance to the desire of bringing best evidence to clinical practice to improve patient outcomes. However, there is also not a one-size-fits-all or simple approach to implement EBP in most settings because of the enormous complexity of the clinical profile of today's patients, multiple and complicated systems and processes that make overnight change unlikely, and patient engagement needs to fully assist patients in their healthcare journeys and recovery or adjustment to illness and disease. As it is well established that scientific discovery improves clinical outcomes and trajectories for patients, continued efforts to bring the latest and best science to the point of care are needed. Research that illuminates how to address complexity, embrace EBP as a daily practice in each patient encounter, and engage patients and clinicians in the change process is gradually unfolding and necessary.

REFERENCES

Agency for Healthcare Research and Quality. (2014). *Advances in the prevention and control of HAIs* (AHRQ Publication No. 14-0003). Rockville, MD: Author.

Agency for Healthcare Research and Quality. (2017). Clinical guidelines and recommendations. Retrieved https://www.ahrq.gov/professionals/clinicians-providers/guidelines-recommendations/index.html

Allen, S. V., Sparling, K., & Montori, V. (2017). Patient and family engaged care: Going beyond tactical buzzwords. *British Medical Journal, 356*, 1–2. doi:10.1136/bmj.j1155

Bates, D. W., Kuperman, G. J., Wang, S., Gandhi, T., Kittler, A., Volk, L., … Middleton, B. (2003). Ten commandments for effective clinical decision support: Making the practice of evidence-based medicine a reality. *Journal of the American Medical Informatics Association, 10*(6), 523–530. doi:10.1197/jamia.M1370

Bolen, S. D., Chandar, A., Falck-Ytter, C., Tyler, C., Perzynski, A. T., Gertz, A. M., … Windish, D. M. (2014). Effectiveness and safety of patient activation interventions for adults with type 2 diabetes: Systematic review, meta-analysis, and meta-regression. *Journal of General Internal Medicine, 29*(8), 1166–1176. doi:10.1007/s11606-014-2855-4

Braithwaite, J., Marks, D., & Taylor, N. (2014). Harnessing implementation science to improve care quality and patient safety: A systematic review of targeted literature. *International Journal for Quality in Healthcare, 26*(3), 321–329. doi:10.1093/intqhc/mzu047

Creating Opportunities for Personal Empowerment. (2017). Intervention studies supporting positive effects of the program. Retrieved from http://www.cope2thrive.com/published-papers

Cullen, L., & Adams, S. L. (2012). Planning for implementation of evidence-based practice. *Journal of Nursing Administration, 42*(4), 222–230. doi:10.1097/NNA.0b013e31824ccd0a

Dixon-Woods, M., McNicol, S., & Martin, G. (2012). Ten challenges in improving quality in healthcare: Lessons from the Health Foundation's programme evaluations and relevant literature. *British Medical Journal Quality & Safety, 10*, 876–884. doi:10.1136/bmjqs-2011-000760

Eccles, M. P., & Mittman, B. S. (2006). Welcome to Implementation Science. *Implementation Science, 1*, 1. doi:10.1186/1748-5908-1-1

Every-Palmer, S., & Howick, J. (2014). How evidence-based medicine is failing due to biased trials and selective publication. *Journal of Evaluation in Clinical Practice, 20*(6), 908–914. doi:10.1111/jep.12147

Farrington, M., Tucker, S., & Cullen, L. (2014). *Sustaining evidence-based nursing practices for fall prevention in hospitalized oncology patients.* Poster presented at the Midwest Nursing Research Society Annual Conference, St. Louis, MO.

Flodgren, G., Conterno, L. O., Mayhew, A., Omar, O., Pereira, C., R., & Shepperd, S. (2013). Interventions to improve professional adherence to guidelines for prevention of device-related infections. *Cochrane Database of Systematic Reviews. 2013*(3), CD006559. doi:10.1002/14651858.CD006559.pub2

Foy, R., Maclennan, G., Grimshaw, J., Penney, G., Campbell, M., & Grol, R. (2002). Attributes of clinical recommendations that influence change in practice following audit and feedback. *Journal of Clinical Epidemiology, 55*(7), 717–722. doi:10.1016/S0895-4356(02)00403-1

Frampton, S. B., Guastello, S., Hoy, L., Naylor, M., Sheridan, S., & Johnston-Fleece, M. (2017, January 31). Harnessing evidence and experience to change culture: A guiding framework for patient and family-engaged care. *National Academy of Medicine Perspectives.* Retrieved from https://nam.edu/harnessing-evidence-and-experience-to-change-culture-a-guiding-framework-for-patient-and-family-engaged-care/

Grol, R., & Grimshaw, J. (2003). From best evidence to best practice: Effective implementation of change in patients' care. *Lancet, 362*, 1225–1230. doi:10.1016/S0140-6736(03)14546-1

Healey, F. (2011). Implementing a fall prevention program. *AHRQ Patient Safety Network.* Retrieved from https://psnet.ahrq.gov/perspectives/perspective/114/implementing-a-fall-prevention-program

Hempel, S., Newberry, S., Wang, Z., Booth, M., Shanman, R., Johnsen, B., ... Ganz, D. A. (2013). Hospital fall prevention: A systematic review of implementation, components, adherence, and effectiveness. *Journal of the American Geriatrics Society, 61*(4), 483–494. doi:10.1111/jgs.12169

Huis, A., van Achterberg, T., de Bruin, M., Grol, R., Schoonhoven, L., & Hulscher, M. (2012). A systematic review of hand hygiene improvement strategies: A behavioural approach. *Implementation Science, 7*(92), 1–14. doi:10.1186/1748-5908-7-92

Institute of Medicine. (2001). *Crossing the quality chasm: A new health system for the 21st century.* Washington, DC: National Academies Press.

James, J. (2013, February). Health policy brief: Patient engagement. *Health Affairs*, 1–6.

Joanna Briggs Institute. Retrieved from http://joannabriggs.org

Jun, M., Manns, B., Laupacis, A., Manns, L., Rehal, B., Crowe, S., & Hemmelgarn, B. R. (2015). Assessing the extent to which current clinical research is consistent with patient priorities: A scoping review using a case study in patients on or nearing dialysis. *Canadian Journal of Kidney Health and Disease, 2*(35), 1–10. doi:10.1186/s40697-015-0070-9

Katz, D. A., Stewart, K., Paez, M., Holman, J., Adams, S. L., Vander Weg, M. W., ... Ono, S. (2016). "Let me get you a nicotine patch": Nurses' perceptions of implementation smoking cessation guidelines for hospitalized Veterans. *Military Medicine, 181*(4), 373–382. doi:10.7205/MILMED-D-15-00101

Kinney, R. L., Lemon, S. C., Person, S. D., Pagoto, S. L., & Saczynski, J. S. (2015). The association between patient activation and medication adherence, hospitalization, and emergency room utilization in patients with chronic illness: A systematic review. *Patient Education and Counseling, 98*(5), 545–552. doi:10.1016/j.pec.2015.02.005

Klein, D. E., Woods, D. D., Klein, G., & Perry, S. J. (2016). Can we trust best practices? Six cognitive challenges of evidence-based approaches. *Journal of Cognitive Engineering and Decision Making, 10*(3), 244–254. doi:10.1177/1555343416637520

Kunneman, M., Montori, V. M., Castaneda-Guarderas, A., & Hess, E. P. (2016). What is shared decision making? (and what is it not). *Academic Emergency Medicine, 23*(12), 1320–1324. doi:10.1111/acem.13065

Lallemand, N. C. (2012, December 13). Health policy brief: Reducing waste in health care. *Health Affairs.* Retrieved from https://www.healthaffairs.org/do/10.1377/hpb20121213.959735/full/

Larson, E. (1988). A causal link between handwashing and risk of infection? Examination of the evidence. *Infection Control and Hospital Epidemiology, 9*, 28–36. doi:10.1086/645729

Larson, E. L.. (1995). APIC guideline for handwashing and hand antisepsis in healthcare settings. *American Journal of Infection Control, 23*, 251–269. doi:10.1016/0196-6553(95)90070-5

Lautenbach, E. (2001). Practices to improve handwashing compliance. In K. Shojania, B. Duncan, K. McDonald., & R. M. Wachter (Eds.), *Making healthcare safer: A critical analysis of patient safety practices* (pp. 119–126). Rockville, MD: Agency for Healthcare Research and Quality.

Lee, W. W., Choi, K. C., Yum, R. W., Yu, D. S., & Chair, S. Y. (2016). Effectiveness of motivational interviewing on lifestyle modification and health outcomes of clients at risk or diagnosed with cardiovascular diseases: A systematic review. *International Journal of Nursing Studies, 53,* 331–341. doi:10.1016/j.ijnurstu.2015.09.010

Lobb, R., & Colditz, G. A. (2013). Implementation science and its application to population health. *Annual Review of Public Health, 34,* 235–251. doi:10.1146/annurev-publhealth-031912-114444

Loveday, H. P., Wilson, J. A., Pratt, R. J., Golsorkhi, M., Tingle, A., Bak, A., … Wilcox, M. (2014). Epic3: National evidence-based guidelines for preventing healthcare-associated infections in NHS hospitals in England. *Journal of Hospital Infection, 86*(Suppl. 1), S1–S70. doi:10.1016/S0195-6701(13)60012-2

Luangasanatip, N., Hongsuwan, M., Limmathurotsakul, D., Lubell, Y., Lee, A. S., Harbarth, S., … Cooper, B. S. (2015). Comparative efficacy of interventions to promote hand hygiene in hospital: Systematic review and network meta-analysis. *British Medical Journal, 351,* h3728. doi:10.1136/bmj.h3728

Lundahl, B., Moleni, T., Burke, B. L., Butters, R., Tollefson, D., Butler, C., & Rollnick, S. (2013). Motivational interviewing in medical care settings: A systematic review and meta-analysis of randomized controlled trials. *Patient Education and Counseling, 93,* 157–168. doi:10.1016/j.pec.2013.07.012

McGlynn, E. A., Asch, S. M., Adams, J., Keesey, J., Hicks, J., DeCristofaro, A., & Kerr, E. A. (2003). The quality of health care delivered to adults in the United States. *New England Journal of Medicine, 348*(26), 2635–2645. doi:10.1056/NEJMsa022615

Meade, C. M., Bursell, A. L., & Ketelsen, L. (2006). Effects of nursing rounds: On patients' call light use, satisfaction, and safety. *American Journal of Nursing, 106*(9), 58–70.

Metz, A., & Bartley, L. (2012). Active implementation frameworks for program success: How to use implementation science to improve outcomes for children. *Zero to Three, 32*(4), 11–18.

Miller, W. R., & Rollnick, S. (2008). *Motivational interviewing in health care: Helping patients change behavior.* New York, NY: Guilford Press.

Moja, L., Kwag, K. H., Lytras, T., Bertizzolo, L., Brandt, L., Pecoraro, V., … Bonovas, S. (2014). Effectiveness of computerized decision support systems linked to electronic health records: A systematic review and meta-analysis. *American Journal of Public Health, 104*(12), e12–e22. doi:10.2105/AJPH.2014.302164

Munro, C. L., & Savel, R. H. (2016). Narrowing the 17-year research to practice gap. *American Journal of Critical Care, 25*(3), 194–196. doi:10.4037/ajcc2016449

Novak, I., & McIntyre, S. (2010). The effect of education with workplace supports on practitioners' evidence-based practice knowledge and implementation behaviours. *Australian Occupational Therapy Journal, 57*(6), 386–393. doi:10.1111/j.1440-1630.2010.00861.x

O'Brien, A., Weaver, C., Settergren, T. T., Hook, M. L., & Ivory, C. H. (2015). EHR Documentation: The hype and the hope for improving nursing satisfaction and quality outcomes. *Nursing Administration Quarterly, 39*(4), 333–339. doi:10.1097/NAQ.0000000000000132

Randle, J., Arthur, A., Vaughan, N., Wharrad, H., & Windle, R. (2014). An observational study of hand hygiene adherence following the introduction of an educational intervention. *Journal of Infection Prevention, 15*(4), 142–147. doi:10.1177/1757177414531057

Redle, E. E. (2013, November). Improving practice through implementation science and knowledge translation. Retrieved from http://www.asha.org/Articles/Improving-Practice-Through-Implementation-Science-and-Knowledge-Translation

Rubak, S., Sandbaek, A., Lauritzen, T., & Christensen, B. (2005). Motivational interviewing: A systematic review and meta-analysis. *British Journal of General Practice, 55,* 305–312.

Runciman, W. B., Hunt, T. D., Hannaford, N. A., Hibbert, P. D., Westbrook, J. I., Coiera, E. W., … Braithwaite, J. (2012). CareTrack: Assessing the appropriateness of healthcare delivery in Australia. *Medical Journal of Australia, 197,* 100–105. doi:10.5694/mja12.10510

Rycroft-Malone, J. (2014). From knowing to doing—from the academy to practice. Comment on "The many meanings of evidence: implications for the translational science agenda in healthcare". *International Journal of Health Policy and Management, 2*(1), 45–46. doi:10.15171/ijhpm.2014.08

Schneider, E. C., Sorbero, M. E., Haas, A., Ridgely, M. S., Khodyakov, D., Setodji, C. M., … Goldmann, D. (2017). Does a quality improvement campaign accelerate take-up of new evidence? A ten-state cluster-randomized controlled trial of the IHI's Project JOINTS. *Implementation Science, 12*(1), 1–10. doi:10.1186/s13012-017-0579-7

Scott, S. D., Albrecht, L., O'Leary, K., Ball, G. D., Hartling, L., Hofmeyer, A., … Dryden, D. M. (2012). Systematic review of knowledge translation strategies in the allied health professions. *Implementation Science, 7,* 1–17. doi:10.1186/1748-5908-7-70

Sherman, R. O., & Hilton, N. (2014). The patient engagement imperative. *American Nurse Today, 9*(2), 1–4.

Sim, I. (2016). Two ways of knowing: Big data and evidence-based medicine. *Annals of Internal Medicine, 164*(8), 562–563. doi:10.7326/M15-2970

Sung, N. S., Crowley, W. F., Jr, Genel, M., Salber, P., Sandy, L., Sherwood, L. M., … Rimoin, D. (2003). Central challenges facing the national clinical research enterprise. *Journal of the American Medical Association, 289*(10), 1278–1287. doi:10.1001/jama.289.10.1278

Taylor, M. V., Priefer, B. A., & Alt-White, A. C. (2016). Evidence-based practice: Embracing integration. *Nursing Outlook, 64*(6), 575–582. doi:10.1016/j.outlook.2016.04.004

Teare E., Cookson, B., & French, G. (1999). Hand washing: A modest measure with big effects. *British Medical Journal, 318,* 686–710. doi:10.1136/bmj.318.7185.686

Tucker, S. J., Bieber, P. L., Attlesey-Pries, J. M., Olson, M. E., & Dierkhising, R. A. (2012). Outcomes and challenges in implementing hourly rounds to reduce falls in orthopedic units. *Worldviews on Evidence-Based Nursing, 9*(1), 18–29. doi:10.1111/j.1741-6787.2011.00227.x

Westfall, J. M., Mold, J., & Fagnan, L. (2007). Practice-based research: "Blue Highways" on the NIH roadmap. *Journal of the American Medical Association, 297*(4), 403–406. doi:10.1001/jama.297.4.403

Wong, C. A., Recktenwald, A. J., Jones, M. L., Waterman, B. M., Bollini, M. L., & Dunagan, W. C. (2011). The cost of serious fall-related injuries at three Midwestern hospitals. *Joint Commission Journal on Quality and Patient Safety, 37*(2), 81–87. doi:10.1016/S1553-7250(11)37010-9

Woolf, S. H. (2008). The meaning of translational research and why it matters. *Journal of the American Medical Association, 299*(2), 211–213. doi:10.1001/jama.2007.26

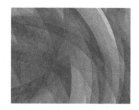

Glossary

2 × 2 Factorial Experiment: A true experiment that allows an investigator to study the separate and combined effects of the interventions (i.e., two or more interventions or treatments).

Absolute risk reduction (ARR): Measures the absolute difference in outcome rates between the intervention and control group.

Adaptive intervention: An intervention in which participant-specific modifications to the intervention are built into the intervention protocol based on process, mediator, or outcome measures taken on participants over the course of the study.

Alpha (α): Level of statistical significance that is the probability of making a Type I error (rejection of a null hypothesis when it is actually true).

Alternative hypothesis: A hypothesis that is different from the statistical null hypothesis; predicts that there is an association between the intervention and outcome variables.

Alzheimer's disease: The most common form of dementia; a neurologic disease characterized by loss of mental ability severe enough to interfere with normal activities of daily living, lasting at least 6 months, and not present from birth. Alzheimer's disease usually occurs in old age, and is marked by a decline in cognitive functions such as remembering, reasoning, and planning.

Assent: The affirmative agreement of a vulnerable subject to participate in research, especially a child older than 7 years who is not cognitively capable of giving informed consent.

Assurance: A document that institutions must have in place for clinical research with Common Rule agency funding. The document explains how the institution will comply with U.S. federal regulations. State of assurance is issued by Federal Wide Assurance (FWA) under the Department of Health and Human Services (DHHS) to protect human subjects in research.

Attention-control group: A group which receives an intervention that is different from that which is received by the intervention group, but similar in amount of time and attention received by the intervention group; used as a comparison to assess the effectiveness of the tested intervention.

Attrition: In the context of an intervention study, this refers to the loss of participants from the control or intervention group.

Authorship agreement: A written document that establishes a clear set of guidelines concerning who is eligible to be a lead or coauthor on papers, how eligible individuals earn authorship for a given paper, and how authorship order will be established.

Baseline equivalence: The result of intervention data analysis used to demonstrate that the intervention and control groups were not statistically different on key demographic variables at baseline.

Belmont Report: A report issued in 1979 that shaped human subjects research and identified ethical requirements in research protocols to include respect for persons, beneficence, and justice.

Beta (β): The probability of making a Type II error (accepting the null hypothesis when it is false).

Bias: Influence leading to a divergence of results from the true values.

Big data: Sets of data too large and complex for traditional data-processing software to deal with. Machine-learning algorithms are used to search the data for patterns, trends, and associations, especially relating to human behavior.

Biomarkers: Measurable and quantifiable biological parameters (e.g., specific enzyme concentration, specific hormone concentration, specific gene phenotype distribution in a population, presence of biological substances), which serve as indices for health- and physiology-related assessments, such as disease risk, psychiatric disorders, environmental exposure and its effects, disease diagnosis, metabolic processes, substance abuse, pregnancy, cell line development, epidemiologic studies, and so forth.

Blind study: A study during which details identifying participants who are receiving the intervention and participants who are receiving the control or comparison condition are concealed from the investigator, data collectors, or participants to reduce the risk of bias.

Blinding: Occurs when details regarding which participants are receiving the experimental intervention versus those receiving the control or comparison condition are concealed from the investigator, data collectors, or participants (or some combination of these entities).

Carryover request: A request, made at the end of a grant's budget year, to carry over unspent funds to the next budget year.

Case report form (CRF): Data collection document or tool used in a clinical study that contains all data to be analyzed.

Categorical variable: A variable in which values can be placed into groups (e.g., gender, race, profession) rather than values measured along a continuum (e.g., weight). They are measured as unordered categories.

Cause and effect relationship: A relationship between variables in which a change in one variable results in a change in another variable.

Causal mechanisms: The processes through which changes in behavioral or health outcomes occur as a result of an intervention.

Causality: The reason certain treatments or intervention strategies (the independent variable) create changes in selected outcomes (the dependent variable).

Center for Epidemiologic Studies Depression Scale (CES-D): A short self-report scale designed to measure depressive symptomatology in the general population.

Centers for Medicare & Medicaid Services (CMS): The operating division of the Department of Health and Human Services whose mission is to promote the timely delivery of quality health care to Medicare and Medicaid beneficiaries and to ensure that the Medicare and Medicaid programs are administered in an efficient manner.

Clinical measures: Data collected as part of the clinical care of a patient.

Clinical research: A branch of healthcare science that determines the safety and effectiveness of medications, devices, diagnostic products, and treatment regimens intended for human use.

Clinical trial: A research study in which one or more human subjects are arbitrarily assigned to one or more interventions to evaluate the effects of those interventions on health-related biomedical or behavioral outcomes.

Coefficient: A number in front of a variable used as a multiplicative factor.

Cohen's *d*: Used with *t*-tests, this measures the standardized effect size of the difference between two means and is used with *t*-tests. It is calculated by subtracting the mean of the control group from the mean of the experimental group and dividing the resultant by the pooled standard deviation. Small, medium, and large effects are designated as 0.2, 0.5, and 0.8, respectively.

Common Rule (45 CFR 46): The ethical ruling resulting from the Belmont Report that refined and enhanced human research subjects' protections and rights.

Community Advisory Board (CAB): Typically serves in an advisory capacity to provide assistance and counsel concerning project goals, to inform about local issues ensuring the program is attentive to community concerns, needs, and priorities, to suggest how to improve recruitment and retention efforts, and to assist with the dissemination of information to the community.

Community-based participatory research (CBPR): A collaborative approach to research that involves researchers and community members in the process. The process usually involves a topic of importance to the community and seeks to combine knowledge with action to improve health outcomes.

Comparative effectiveness research: The comparison of effective interventions among patients in typical patient care settings, with decisions that are tailored to meet individual patients' needs (i.e., which interventions are most effective for which patients).

Compensatory intervention: Control group receives an intervention that might affect outcome; a threat to internal validity.

Compensatory rivalry: Control group "tries harder" to affect outcome; a threat to internal validity.

Computer-assisted personal interviewing (CAPI): In-person interviewing in which interviewers read questions from, and enter responses into, a computer.

Computer-assisted self-interviewing (CASI): Interviewing in which the respondent reads questions from, and enters responses into, a computer.

Computer-assisted telephone interviewing (CATI): Interviewing completed over the telephone in which interviewers read questions from, and enter responses into, a computer.

Concurrent validity: A type of criterion-related validity that demonstrates that a measure correlates with a previously validated "gold standard" measure. In contrast to predictive validity, data are collected at one time using both the predictor measure and "gold standard" criterion measure.

Confidentiality: Assurance made to study participants that identifying information about them acquired through the study will not be released to anyone outside of the study.

Confirmatory factor analysis: A theory testing form of factor analysis used to test whether measures of a construct are consistent with the researcher's understanding of the nature of the factors.

Confounding variables: Extraneous variables that are statistically related to (correlated with) the independent variable and may influence the study's results.

Construct validity: The degree to which an instrument measures the theoretical construct it claims to measure. In social research, the degree to which inferences legitimately can be made from the operationalizations in the study to the theoretical constructs on which those operationalizations are made.

Contamination: Control group receives actual, or imitation of the, intervention.

Content validity: The degree to which items on an instrument adequately represent the scope and range of the concept being measured.

Continuous variable: A variable that is ranked with quantifiable intervals and can take on an infinite range of values along a specified continuum (e.g., weight, pulse rate).

Control group: Equivalent group of subjects against whom a treated group outcome is compared.

Convergent validity: A type of construct validity; the degree to which scores on a test correlate positively with scores on other tests that are designed to assess the same construct.

Cost–benefit analysis (CBA): Values all consequences in monetary units, and thus, multiple effects that may not be common to both alternatives can be investigated.

Cost-consequence analysis (CCA): Costs and consequences are not aggregated, and the decision maker must make the value judgment trade-offs to integrate all costs and consequences in rendering a final decision.

Cost-effectiveness analysis (CEA): A form of economic analysis used to compare the relative cost and value of various clinical strategies used in creating better health. The outcome is expressed as cost per unit of health outcome.

Cost-minimization analysis (CMA): The outcomes of interest are basically equivalent and there is interest only in examining costs.

Cost-utility analysis (CUA): CUA is a special type of CEA that includes a quality-of-life measure in the analysis.

Covariate: A variable that correlates with the outcome variable and whose relationship to the outcome variable must be controlled for in the analysis so it does not interfere with the relationship between the independent and dependent variables of interest.

Cramer's phi (ϕ_c) or V: Measures the standardized effect size of association for the chi-square test.

Criterion variable: See dependent variable.

Criterion-related validity: The validation of a measure based on its relationship to the "gold standard" measure for assessing the construct of interest.

Cronbach's coefficient alpha: A coefficient of reliability; it is generally used to determine the reliability of a measure with multiple items.

Cross-contamination: When some part of the experimental intervention diffuses to subjects in the control group.

Cultural targeting: The identification of a particular cultural group for the purposes of ensuring exposure of an intervention to that group.

Data coordinating site: The place where data are shipped, processed, and analyzed.

Data integrity: The completeness and accuracy of all data elements.

Data mining and surveillance: From the enormous amount of information provided by social media, researchers, communities, and for-profit industries can collect data to analyze and to use for their purposes. In healthcare, providers can use data for better understanding public health indicators, information, and trends.

Dementia: A loss of mental ability severe enough to interfere with normal activities of daily living, lasting more than 6 months, not present at birth, and not associated with a loss or alteration of consciousness.

Dependent variable: The variable that changes as the independent variable is manipulated by the researcher. It is the variable of most interest in intervention studies and is measured to assess impact of the treatment.

Derived variables: Those that are constructed from a number of different items.

Descriptive research: Nonexperimental research design used to accurately describe the characteristics of persons, situations, or groups, and/or the frequency with which certain phenomena occur using systematic methods.

Divergent validity: A type of construct validity; the degree to which scores on a measure have a low or no correlation with scores from other tests that are not designed to assess the same construct.

Dose: The amount of the intervention that the participants received—whether it be hours, sessions, videos watched, phone calls made, pills taken, meals eaten, miles swum—and needed to change the dependent variable/outcome.

Dropout: Subject failure to complete a research study.

Effect size: An estimation of the strength of impact that the intervention will have on the primary outcome variable; usually best gathered from a pilot study or literature of similar interventions.

Effectiveness: The degree of beneficial effect that an intervention achieves under actual practice, "real world" conditions.

Effectiveness trial: Pragmatic trials; conducted in real-world practice settings to determine if the outcomes that were achieved in an efficacy randomized controlled trial (RCT) can be reproduced in real-world settings.

Efficacy: The extent to which an intervention produces the expected result under ideal circumstances, such as a clinical trial or in a laboratory setting.

Equipoise: An important ethical requirement in randomized intervention studies; means that one study arm has the potential to be as beneficial as any other study arm.

Eta-squared (η^2): Measure of effect size in analysis of variance (ANOVA). It is typically calculated as a ratio of variance terms and is the standardized effect size of the shared variance between a continuous outcome and categorical predictor(s).

Ethical approval: The affirmative result, by a designated committee, of a review of a research study involving human subjects. Approval indicates the study meets guidelines to protect the rights and welfare of the participating subjects.

Evidence-based clinical practice guidelines: Specific practice recommendations that are systematically developed by rigorous review of the best evidence available and used to assist practitioner and patient decisions about health care.

Evidence-based information: Information derived from research that provides evidence of the effectiveness, benefits, and harms of different treatment options to assist consumers, clinicians, and payers in making better informed clinical and health policy decisions.

Evidence-based intervention: An intervention that is based on the best available evidence, with an emphasis on evidence from disciplined research.

Evidence-based practice (EBP): A problem-solving approach to the delivery of care that integrates the best evidence from well-designed research studies with a clinician's expertise, which includes assessment of a patient's history and condition as well as availability of healthcare resources and a patient's preferences and values.

Evidence-based quality improvement (EBQI): Happens when improvements are based on a thorough search for and critical appraisal and synthesis of the literature and the best evidence is implemented along with the monitoring of outcomes.

Experimental design: Research used when an investigator would like to establish causality between certain treatments or intervention strategies and changes in selected outcomes.

Experimental research (also known as intervention studies): The only type of research that allows conclusions to be drawn about cause and effect relationships between an intervention or treatment and an outcome.

Exploratory factor analysis: A theory-generating statistical method in which the data can be analyzed without any preconceived ideas about the underlying constructs. It can be used to reduce and refine a group of items within a new measure.

External validity: The degree to which study results can be generalized from a study to the larger population from which the sample was drawn.

Extraneous/confounding findings: Factors that interfere with the relationship between the independent and dependent variables and could influence study results. Extraneous variables should be controlled for in the study design or statistical procedures to lessen or eliminate their influence on study results.

Face validity: The approach of obtaining subjective feedback from individuals who "possess" the construct of interest on whether the items on the measure reasonably assess or cover components of their experience.

Facilities and Administration (F&A) costs: Indirect costs that are general expenses that cannot be directly attributed to a specific research project but are collectively used by many research projects at an academic institution. These costs may include allocations for capital improvement, maintenance, and operation of facilities used for research. They may also support expenses for administration costs including financial management, institutional review board (IRB), and environmental health and safety management.

Factor analysis: A statistical method that can be used to assess whether the items in a measure cluster into predetermined variable groupings. It also can be used to confirm how multiple items conceptually "hang together"; that is, it can provide evidence for the items serving as a cohesive representation of the construct.

Feasibility: The likelihood that an intervention or a component of a study can be carried out.

Fidelity: Adherence and conformity to the intervention's protocols, including monitoring strategies.

Generalizability: Evidence that an intervention approach is effective and shows promise across multiple settings and in different regions of the country.

Gerontology: The branch of science that deals with aging and the problems of aged persons; the study in aging including the biological, psychological, and social aspects.

Group equivalence: Research groups are the same on dimensions likely to impact the outcome.

Health Insurance Portability and Accountability Act (HIPAA): Enacted in 1996; it provides federal protection of the privacy and security of health information yet permits sharing of information for patient care or other important purposes.

Health literacy: The ability to understand health information and use it to make decisions about health and health care.

History: Those events that transpire during the course of a study, which may impact the outcome variable; a threat to internal validity.

Hospice: An interdisciplinary team focusing on palliative care (symptom management).

Human subjects: Participants consenting to be in a specified research study, having rights to protection of their welfare from unnecessary risks or harm and oversight maintained by the IRB to ensure compliance. Keywords include respect for persons, beneficence, and justice.

Hypothesis: A supposition or tentative explanation for (a group of) phenomena; a statement of the predicted relationship between two variables under study.

Impact: The effect of a program or intervention on outcomes of interest.

Implementation: Taking the study from the preparation and planning stage to beginning the intervention stage.

Implementation science: A term favored by nursing describing how clinical research findings and other evidence-based practices make their way into routine practice to improve the quality and effectiveness of healthcare. Alternative terms are dissemination science, health services research, knowledge translation, implementation, quality improvement research, and practice-based research.

Inclusion enrollment report: A report summarizing the number of subjects enrolled in a study to date by race and ethnicity.

Incremental cost-effectiveness ratio (ICER): This ratio is calculated by dividing the net cost of a health care intervention by the total number of incremental health outcomes prevented by the intervention.

Independent variable: Those that precede or are antecedents to the dependent variable; the variable that is manipulated and believed to influence the dependent variable.

Indices: An index is composed of the sum of a group of items, most often binary, to measure a single construct.

Informed consent: A subject's voluntary decision about participating in a research study based on the understanding of what is involved in the study, including the potential risks and benefits and subject's rights and responsibilities. The informed consent process is based on ethics drawn from the Belmont Report and is regulated by federal code (45 CFR 46).

Innovation: In research, how a study extends the science in the related area of investigation.

Institutional review board (IRB): A committee of clinical providers (including physicians), statisticians, researchers, community advocates, and others that ensures that a clinical trial is ethical and that the rights of study participants are protected. Federal code (45 CFR 46) provides regulations regarding IRBs and requires that biomedical or behavioral research involving human participants must, by federal regulation, initially be approved and periodically reviewed by an IRB.

Instrumentation threat: Decay or change in measures or subject response to measures over the course of a research study; a threat to internal validity.

Intention-to-treat (ITT) analysis: Analyses of all subjects randomized into a study at the outcome of the study, including dropouts.

Interaction effect: The effect of one independent variable on the dependent variable depends on the level of another independent variable.

Interobserver reliability: Estimates comparability of scores on a measure between different observers. Statistical results indicating 90% agreement or higher between observers provide evidence of the measure's reliability.

Internal validity: The ability to say that it was the intervention or treatment that caused a change in the dependent variable or outcome, not other confounding variables.

Intervention: The experimental treatment in a research study.

Intervention fidelity: The extent to which every intervention is carried out in exactly the same way every time for every subject.

Intervention manual: Includes all study materials used in implementation of the intervention and the control-group activities.

Intervention research: A systematic process to find treatments or strategies that work best to improve outcomes.

Intervention studies (also known as "experimental research"): The only type of research that allows conclusions to be drawn about cause and effect relationships between an intervention or treatment and an outcome.

Intra-rater reliability: Assesses, in a similar manner, comparability or consistency of scores on a measure between the same rater across multiple time points. Statistical results indicating 90% agreement or higher within raters provide evidence of the measure's reliability.

Level: A subdivision of a variable into components or features. For example, if participants received 5 mL or 10 mL doses of a study medication, there would be two levels.

Level I evidence: Evidence generated from systematic reviews or meta-analysis of all relevant RCTs or evidence-based clinical practice guidelines based on systematic reviews of randomized controlled trials; the strongest level of evidence to guide clinical practice.

Level II evidence: Evidence generated from at least one well-designed RCT (i.e., a true experiment).

Level III evidence: Evidence obtained from well-designed controlled trials without randomization.

Level IV evidence: Evidence obtained from well-designed case-control and cohort studies.

Level V evidence: Evidence from systematic reviews of descriptive and qualitative studies.

Level VI evidence: Evidence from a single descriptive or qualitative study.

Level VII evidence: Evidence from the opinion of authorities and/or expert committees.

Likert-type scale: A method of scaling in which the items are assigned interval level scale values, and the responses are gathered using an interval level response format. Often assesses the respondent's agreement or belief in an item's statement.

Local health department (LHD): A government-funded agency that provides a broad range of health services to diverse populations.

Manipulation checks: Strategies for assuring that participants in a study actually processed the intervention content and/or are adhering to prescribed activities. For example, if educational content comprised the intervention, a multiple choice test might be administered to subjects after they received the educational content to determine whether they received and processed the information.

Manual of operations (MOPs): Describes methods and instruments used to complete each task, including a recruitment manual that records all procedures used and contacts made while recruiting and retaining the participants.

Maturation: Changes in the subject over time in the study; a threat to internal validity.

Maximum likelihood (ML) estimates: The value of the parameter that is most likely to have resulted in the observed data.

Maximum likelihood (ML) estimation: A method used to address missing data in which each participant's available data is analyzed to compute maximum likelihood estimates.

Measurement: The process of observing and recording observations collected as part of a research study and assignment of numbers according to specified rules.

Measurement error: The difference between the true value of a variable and the value obtained during data collection, whether classified as random, caused by chance, systematic, or a component of measurement itself.

Mediating variable: When a third variable is intermediate in the causal path from an independent variable to a dependent variable.

Mediators: Variables that identify the essential processes that must occur for a predictor to have an effect on an outcome.

Mock review: A process that many colleges have established where a grant is reviewed by seasoned investigators before it is actually submitted to the funding agency in order to give helpful feedback to the investigator for improvement. Often, the same criteria and process that is used by the National Institutes of Health is used for the mock review process.

Moderated mediation: When the process of mediation for producing the effect of the intervention on outcome depends on the level of a moderator variable.

Moderating variable: A quantitative or qualitative variable that affects the direction and/or strength of the relationship between the independent and dependent variables.

Moderator: An independent variable that affects the strength and/or direction of the association between a predictor and an outcome. Moderators identify for whom and under which circumstances treatments have different effects.

Moderators: See moderating variable.

Mortality: Attrition or dropout of subjects during a research trial and may include failure to follow the treatment protocol (lack of adherence); a threat to internal validity.

Multiple imputation (MI): This is the process of replacing missing data by estimating a distribution of probable values to allow statistical analysis that includes all participants.

Multisite intervention trial: A study that involves at least two intervention sites that employ separate research staff, a common data collection protocol that is shared across sites, and a separate data coordinating site, where data are shipped, processed, and analyzed.

Multisite trial: Trials that recruit study participants from two or more geographically distinct sites. Participants are randomized and study protocols are followed at each site.

National Institute of Mental Health (NIMH): A federally funded agency whose mission is to transform the understanding and treatment of mental illnesses through basic and clinical research, paving the way for prevention, recovery, and cure.

National Institute of Nursing Research (NINR): A federally funded agency whose mission is to promote and improve the health of individuals, families, communities, and populations.

National Institutes of Health (NIH): Federal governing agency of the Department of Health and Human Services. Its mission is to seek fundamental knowledge about the nature and behavior of living systems and the application of that knowledge to enhance health, lengthen life, and reduce the burdens of illness and disability. There are 27 different institutes and centers, each with its own research agenda.

Nonexperimental design: Research that can be qualitative, descriptive, or predictive and is best suited when constructs need to be described or there is a desire to determine relationships among variables.

Notice of award (NOA) or notice of grant award (NGA): Legal documents issued to notify the grantee that an award has been made and that funds may be requested from the funding agency.

Null hypothesis: A prediction that there is no association between the treatment and outcome variables. In statistical testing, it is the hypothesis to be rejected.

Number needed to treat (NNT): The average number of patients who would need to be treated to prevent one additional bad outcome.

Operationalization: The translation of an idea or construct into something real, concrete, and measurable.

Optical character recognition (OCR): Translation of scanned images of handwritten, typed, or printed text into machine-encoded text so it may be manipulated for desired use.

Ordinal variables: Variables that can be categorized and placed in order but cannot be quantified; intervals are not clearly equal. For example, mild, moderate, or severe anxiety.

Outcome: The result of a healthcare intervention, practice, or treatment that can be quantified, or can be assessed by objective measures or self-report.

Outcome management (OM): Quality improvement programs or committees that are responsible for monitoring quality of care and patient outcomes and making practice changes to improve them.

Outcome variable: See dependent variable.

Palliative care: Management of symptoms at the end of someone's life, usually the final 6 months of life.

Parallel forms: Alternative versions of the same instrument that have means and standard deviations that are approximately the same.

Partial eta-squared (η_p^2): Measure of effect size in ANOVA. It is typically calculated as a ratio of variance terms and is the standardized effect size of the shared variance between a continuous outcome and categorical predictor(s).

Passive consent: Parents are notified of research and given an opportunity to refuse consent. If they do not remove their child from participation then consent is implied.

Patient engagement: Recently seen as an essential component of evidence-based practice, it promotes patients and families/caregivers being involved in the planning and delivery of care.

Per-protocol (PP) analysis: Analysis focusing only on the fully compliant subjects that can be used to determine the maximal efficacy of a treatment; also called "efficacy analysis."

Phi (ɸ): See Cramer's phi.

PICO(T): A mnemonic for questions to be asked that stands for patient population; intervention or area of interest; comparison intervention or group; outcomes; and time, if indicated. It is commonly used in the planning phase of the PDSA model.

Pilot study: A small study carried out in preparation for a larger study allowing a researcher to assess the preliminary effects of a new intervention as well as provide opportunity to assess study burden and the best times for collecting measures.

Plan, Do, Study, Act (PDSA) model: One of the quality improvement models used by healthcare institutions to improve care and outcomes.

Portable Document Format (PDF): A file format created in 1993. It fixes the layout of the document including text, font, and graphics, making the file easier to share with others.

Power: The probability that a research study will successfully detect a statistically significant difference between study groups, assuming that a difference truly exists, typically set at .80 or .90.

Predictive research: Research that is undertaken when an investigator is interested in determining whether one variable predicts another variable.

Predictive validity: A type of criterion-related validity that demonstrates a measure correlates with a previously validated "gold standard" measure. In contrast to concurrent validity, data is collected at two different time points where the criterion measure is administered some time after the predictor measure.

Pretesting: Gathering of assessments from subjects on the study measures prior to the start of the intervention; collection of baseline data.

Principal investigator (PI): The lead person who is responsible and accountable for the scientific integrity of a study as well as the oversight of that study.

Process measures: Different from outcomes, they are those factors or variables that influence outcomes.

Project director (PD): The role of the PD is to flesh out all aspects of the study implementation, including a recruitment plan, human subjects' approvals from the organization's IRB, detailing activities for subcontracts, development of all study procedure manuals, including protocol manual and intervention manuals, making all data collection instruments suitable and orderly for collection and transfer to the database, recruiting and training both data collectors and interventionists, conducting fidelity and manipulation checks, and coordinating team meetings.

Protected health information (PHI): Any health information, in any form or medium including written or oral, that may individually identify an individual. There are 18 identifiers that should be protected under HIPAA.

Protocol: A study plan on which all clinical trials are based. The plan is carefully designed to safeguard the health of the participants as well as answer specific research questions. A protocol describes what types of people may participate in the trial; the schedule of tests, procedures, medications, and dosages; and the length of the study.

Quality-adjusted life year (QALY): A common measure that combines life years gained as a result of health interventions/health care programs and adjusted for quality of life.

Quality assurance/quality control manual: A manual that describes training procedures to assure accurate data collection

Quality improvement (QI): A systematic process used by healthcare systems to analyze existing data and improve its processes and/or outcomes for a specific patient population.

Qualitative research: A method in which data is collected in nonnumeric form, such as personal interviews and observations, with the intention to identify aspects of the phenomenon under study from the participant's point of view and to describe the phenomenon.

Quasi-experiments: Studies in which the independent variable is manipulated (an intervention or treatment delivered), but there is a lack of at least one of the other two properties of true experiments (i.e., random assignment or comparison/control group).

Quorum: When a research-related decision is made by a majority of IRB members.

Random assignment: A procedure used to arbitrarily place participants in either an experimental group or a comparison/control group.

Random error: Variability in measurement because of chance.

Randomization: The random assignment of subjects to treatment conditions. See also random assignment.

Randomized controlled trial (RCT): The strongest type of intervention study for testing cause and effect relationships. Participants are randomly assigned to experimental and control groups.

Ratio level variables: Variables measured with a level of measurement that has quantified intervals on an infinite scale in which there are equal distances between points and a "true" zero point (e.g., temperature, ounces of water, height).

Regression to the mean: The tendency of extreme scores to move closer to the population mean upon repeat testing; a threat to internal validity.

Relative risk reduction (RRR): Measures how much the risk is reduced in the intervention group compared to a control group.

Reliability: The ability of an instrument to consistently measure what it claims to measure; the degree to which it would give the same result over and over again.

Research: A systematic process used to generate new knowledge or evidence.

Research coordinator (RC): A member of the research team who is responsible for the organization, coordination, and overall integrity of the study. The RC works under the overall direction of the PI but plays a significant role in carrying out study activities.

Research design: The overall plan for answering the study question(s) or testing the hypotheses.

Research Electronic Data Capture (REDCap): A web-based application designed to support data capture for research studies.

Research hypothesis: Predicts the researcher's actual expectations about the study outcome, including the direction of the relationship between the intervention and outcome.

Research question: The statement of the specific question that the researcher wants to answer in the study.

Response shift: Change in internal standard for personal assessment of personal qualities, particularly quality of life.

Scales: Measures composed of a number of items measuring the same construct. The purpose of a scale is to obtain a more reliable and valid measure of the construct than is possible from any single item.

Scaling: The process of measuring quantitative traits.

Self-administered questionnaires (SAQ): Surveys used to gather information from participants and can include those presented in paper/pencil format; administered through handheld or laptop computer devices or by cell phone.

Significance: The probability that an observed relationship could be caused by chance (i.e., as a result of a sampling error).

Site principal investigator (PI): The person charged with supervising the site project coordinator, other staff, and for ensuring that the trial is carried out as planned within a given site, maintaining all correspondence with local institutional review boards, and serving as a liaison for the project within a given community.

"So what" factor: In research, an investigator must ask the "So what?" question before entering into a new research venture to ensure that the intended research project addresses a "big picture" issue that will be of interest and benefit to many individuals and will be a wise use of money and resources.

Social marketing: Recruitment strategy by researchers that has been shown to assist researchers in developing interventions that are well received in the community.

Social media: A term difficult to define because of its ever-changing nature. Since its inception, the Internet provides a wealth of information and connects people around the globe. In healthcare, various venues include support groups for patients, dissemination and evaluation of health information, data mining and surveillance, and health behavior and intervention design.

Split-half reliability: A measure of internal consistency reliability where a test is split in half, and scores from each half are correlated with one another.

Split-half technique: A method used for assessing homogeneity within a measure by taking one-half of the items in a measure and correlating the scores between the two halves.

Statistical Analysis System (SAS): Analytic software package.

Statistical assumptions: Those characteristics of the data and the design that should be present for accurate use and valid interpretation of a statistical test.

Statistical conclusion validity: An integrated approach to analysis accounting for power, statistical assumption, measurement variability, and effect sizes in forming inferences.

Statistical Package for the Social Sciences (SPSS): Statistical software package.

Steering committee: Provides scientific oversight of a study and usually include the PI, site PI, statisticians, and key research team members who also have responsibilities that include voting and dissemination of study information.

Streamlined Noncompeting Award Process (SNAP): A process implemented by the NIH to simplify requirements of the noncompeting application and financial reporting processes. One of its main benefits is that it eliminated the need for annual financial status reporting and requires it only at the end of the competitive segment.

Structural equation modeling (SEM): A set of statistical techniques for testing and estimating causal relationships. SEM allows confirmatory and exploratory modeling useful in theory testing and development.

Structurally equivalent attention control intervention: An intervention that is different from that which is received by the intervention group, but similar in amount of time and attention received by the intervention group.

Structured Query Language (SQL): A programming language designed to manage data in a database system.

Sunshine laws: Allow the public to make formal requests for information and allow public access to certain government meetings and records.

Surrogate decision maker: An individual who acts on behalf of a subject to provide consent for participation in research when the subject is unable to provide consent for self. U.S. state laws vary in identification of who may act as a surrogate decision maker for research.

Systematic reviews: A summary of evidence on a particular topic of interest. Reviews are typically conducted by an expert or expert panel and use a rigorous process (to minimize bias) for identifying, appraising, and synthesizing studies to answer a specific clinical question and draw conclusions about the data gathered.

Tailored interventions: The adaptation or redesign of an intervention to best fit the specific needs of an individual or group to improve health or change behavior.

Targeted health messages: Health messages that are tailored for a homogenous group based on factors such as age, gender, ethnicity, and so forth.

Testing: Practice effect or reactivity due to pretesting. A threat to internal validity.

Test–retest reliability: Assesses the stability or consistency of a measure from one time to another. In this approach, one would ask the same participants to respond to the same measure at a specified time interval.

Theoretical models: Represent an integrated set of concepts, existence statements, and relational statements that link a problem to be addressed with relevant intervention strategies and expected changes in outcomes.

Theory: Reflects a body of knowledge that organizes, describes, predicts, and explains a phenomenon.

Theory of the problem: Models the processes that produce the problem addressed by an intervention.

True experiment: The strongest type of experimental design for testing cause and effect relationship; true experiments possess three characteristics: (a) treatment or intervention, (b) a control or comparison group, and (c) random assignment.

U.S. Centers for Disease Control and Prevention: The federal agency authority charged with tracking and investigating public health trends in disease, injury, and disability; may provide funding resources if appropriate.

Validity: In a data analytic context, this is the degree to which the results of measurement correspond to the true state of the phenomenon being measured.

Variable: Any entity that can take on different values; characteristics or attributes that differ among persons being studied (e.g., age, gender).

Visual analog scale (VAS): Measurement using a horizontal line with anchors at each end. The study participant places a hatch mark on the line closest to the preferred choice in the range.

Vulnerable populations: A group of people with higher-than-average risk for adverse effects who require special protection of their rights in research studies. Examples include children, pregnant women, and the mentally retarded.

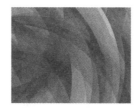

Index